CLINICAL ANATOMY EXPLAINED!

NETTER'S INTEGRATED MUSCULOSKELETAL SYSTEM

CLINICAL ANATOMY EXPLAINED!

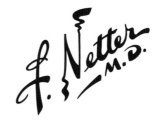

NETTER'S
INTEGRATED MUSCULOSKELETAL SYSTEM

Peter J. Ward, PhD
Professor of Anatomy
West Virginia School of Osteopathic Medicine
Lewisburg, West Virginia

Illustrations by
Frank H. Netter, MD

Contributing Illustrators
Carlos A. G. Machado, MD
DragonFly Media Group
Kristen Wienandt Marzejon, MS, MFA
James A. Perkins, MS, MFA
John A. Craig, MD

ELSEVIER

ELSEVIER

1600 John F. Kennedy Blvd.
Ste 1600
Philadelphia, PA 19103-2899

NETTER'S INTEGRATED MUSCULOSKELETAL SYSTEM:
CLINICAL ANATOMY EXPLAINED!

ISBN: 978-0-323-69661-6

Notice

Practitioners and researchers must always rely on their own experience and knowledge in evaluating and using any information, methods, compounds or experiments described herein. Because of rapid advances in the medical sciences, in particular, independent verification of diagnoses and drug dosages should be made. To the fullest extent of the law, no responsibility is assumed by Elsevier, authors, editors or contributors for any injury and/or damage to persons or property as a matter of products liability, negligence or otherwise, or from any use or operation of any methods, products, instructions, or ideas contained in the material herein.

ISBN: 978-0-323-69661-6

Publisher: Elyse O'Grady
Senior Content Strategist: Marybeth Thiel
Publishing Services Manager: Catherine Jackson
Senior Project Manager: Kate Mannix
Design Direction: Patrick Ferguson

Printed in India

Last digit is the print number: 9 8 7 6 5 4 3 2 1

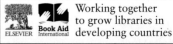

Sarah, Archer, and Dashiell, this book would have been impossible without your love and enthusiasm. You are my whole world. I'd also like to express my gratitude to the rest of my family, Lucinda, Robert, and Christopher Ward, whose lifelong encouragement has meant so much. Many thanks to Rene Koressel for cheerfully giving time and assistance; and also to Robert and Janette Koressel for their unflagging support.

ABOUT THE AUTHOR

Peter J. Ward, PhD grew up in Casper, Wyoming, graduating from Kelly Walsh High School and then attending Carnegie Mellon University in Pittsburgh, graduating with a BS in biology in 1996. He began graduate school at Purdue University, where he first encountered gross anatomy, histology, embryology, and neuroanatomy. Having found a course of study that engrossed him, he attended and helped to teach those courses in the veterinary and medical programs at Purdue. Dr. Ward completed a MS in molecular biology and then began a PhD program in anatomy education. In 2005, he completed his thesis and joined the faculty at the West Virginia School of Osteopathic Medicine (WVSOM) in Lewisburg, West Virginia. There he has taught gross anatomy, embryology, neuroscience, histology, and the history of medicine. Dr. Ward has received numerous teaching awards, including the WVSOM Golden Key Award, the Basmajian Award from the American Association of Anatomists, and has been a two-time finalist in the West Virginia Merit Foundation's Professor of the Year selection. Dr. Ward has also been director of the WVSOM plastination facility, coordinator of the anatomy graduate teaching assistants, chair of the curriculum committee, chair of the faculty council, creator and director of a clinical anatomy elective course, and host of several anatomy-centered events between WVSOM and two Japanese Colleges of Osteopathy. Dr. Ward has also served as council member and association secretary for the American Association of Clinical Anatomists. His research program explores how medical students learn effectively, differences in medical school curricula, and he also investigates anatomical variations and the importance of little-studied structures. In conjunction with Bone Clones, Inc., Dr. Ward has produced tactile models that mimic the feel of anatomical structures encountered in the physical examination in their intact or ruptured state. He created the YouTube channel, *Clinical Anatomy Explained!* and continues to pursue interesting ways to present the anatomical sciences to the public. Dr. Ward was the Senior Associate Editor for the three-part volume of *The Netter Collection: The Digestive System,* 2nd Edition, a contributor to *Gray's Anatomy,* 42nd Edition, and is one of the editors of *Netter's Atlas of Human Anatomy,* 8th Edition. In his spare time, he enjoys reading and teaches martial arts at the Yatagarasu Dojo in Lewisburg, WV. He is exceedingly lucky to be the husband of Sarah Koressel, DVM, and father to Dashiell and Archer Ward, who make him proud every day.

Frank H. Netter, MD

Frank H. Netter was born in 1906 in New York City. He studied art at the Art Student's League and the National Academy of Design before entering medical school at New York University, where he received his MD degree in 1931. During his student years, Dr. Netter's notebook sketches attracted the attention of the medical faculty and other physicians, allowing him to augment his income by illustrating articles and textbooks. He continued illustrating as a sideline after establishing a surgical practice in 1933, but he ultimately opted to give up his practice in favor of a full-time commitment to art. After service in the United States Army during World War II, Dr. Netter began his long collaboration with the CIBA Pharmaceutical Company (now Novartis Pharmaceuticals). This 45-year partnership resulted in the production of the extraordinary collection of medical art so familiar to physicians and other medical professionals worldwide.

In 2005, Elsevier, Inc. purchased the Netter Collection and all publications from Icon Learning Systems. There are now more than 50 publications featuring the art of Dr. Netter available through Elsevier, Inc.

Dr. Netter's works are among the finest examples of the use of illustration in the teaching of medical concepts. The 13-book *Netter Collection of Medical Illustrations*, which includes the greater part of the more than 4,000 paintings created by Dr. Netter, became and remains one of the most famous medical works ever published. *Netter's Atlas of Human Anatomy*, first published in 1989, presents the anatomical paintings from the Netter Collection. Now translated into 16 languages, it is the anatomy atlas of choice among medical and health professions students the world over.

The Netter illustrations are appreciated not only for their aesthetic qualities, but, more important, for their intellectual content. As Dr. Netter wrote in 1949, "…clarification of a subject is the aim and goal of illustration. No matter how beautifully painted, how delicately and subtly rendered a subject may be, it is of little value as a medical illustration if it does not serve to make clear some medical point." Dr. Netter's planning, conception, point of view, and approach are what inform his paintings and what makes them so intellectually valuable.

Frank H. Netter, MD, physician and artist, died in 1991.

Learn more about the physician-artist whose work has inspired the Netter Reference collection:

https://netterimages.com/artist-frank-h-netter.html.

Carlos A.G. Machado, MD

Carlos Machado was chosen by Novartis to be Dr. Netter's successor. He continues to be the main artist who contributes to the Netter collection of medical illustrations.

Self-taught in medical illustration, cardiologist Carlos Machado has contributed meticulous updates to some of Dr. Netter's original plates and has created many paintings of his own in the style of Netter as an extension of the Netter collection. Dr. Machado's photorealistic expertise and his keen insight into the physician/patient relationship inform his vivid and unforgettable visual style. His dedication to researching each topic and subject he paints places him among the premier medical illustrators at work today.

Learn more about his background and see more of his art at: https://netterimages.com/artist-carlos-a-g-machado.html.

ACKNOWLEDGMENTS

This textbook is the product of many people who assisted in different aspects of its production and helped me develop a love for the topic. I must thank my "anatomy dads," James Walker and Kevin Hannon, who taught me that high academic standards can co-exist with humor and earnest concern for the learning of their students; also my "academic sister," Rebecca Pratt, for always providing inspiration and a good laugh when challenges arose. I especially wish to thank my colleagues in the American Association of Clinical Anatomists for their insightful and ceaseless research into the human body. It has been a pleasure to be amongst such people and learn from their efforts. This textbook is also inspired by Nels Hennum, Joseph Urich, and David White, dedicated teachers who gave me a new appreciation for the musculoskeletal system and how to apply that knowledge to a variety of situations.

There are far too many colleagues, both past and present, at the West Virginia School of Osteopathic Medicine to list here, but it would have been impossible to complete this book without the personal and institutional support I've received from them; I am extraordinarily fortunate to work with such dedicated professionals. Particular thanks are due to Joyce Morris-Wiman for her insights into the nervous system and for tracking down resources that seemed impossible to find.

Special thanks are due to the hardworking team at Elsevier, especially Marybeth Thiel and Elyse O'Grady, who were kind enough to take my rough outline seriously and kept this project moving forward (and me on-track), as well as Kate Mannix for seeing it past the finish line to publication. Being permitted to make use of the incomparable illustrations of Frank Netter and Carlos Machado was an unexpected, but very welcome, boon. These illustrations are as vibrant as ever and several questions that arose during the preparation of the text were resolved by referring to the images and giving them a voice. Revisiting the Netter illustrations allowed me to renew the fascination I experienced during my first gross anatomy course. I hope that this textbook helps bring these works of medical art to a new generation of students as they begin investigating the awesome enigma of the human body.

This textbook is meant to fill a need for resources for integrated health science curricula. The medical school at which I work went through the process of curricular reform in 2012. We moved from teaching the standard medical courses of gross anatomy, physiology, microbiology, etc. into an integrated curriculum that consisted of courses with titles like "Urogenital," "Blood, Lymph, Immunology, and Bone," "Rheumatology," and "Musculoskeletal." One of the difficulties we encountered in this process was that nearly all the available materials were centered around the traditional course topics. This is difficult for students since readings for an integrated course tend to be scattered across several texts and their attention is continually disrupted as they shift from one resource to another. The process is also onerous for the teaching faculty and course directors, who were probably trained in one of the traditional biomedical fields but are unlikely to have a comprehensive understanding of an entire body system from the macroscopic to the microscopic level.

To fill this void in teaching resources, I decided (in equal parts ambition and hubris) to create a textbook that would bring together most of the content that would be needed to teach an integrated course. I made the choice to begin with the musculoskeletal system for several reasons. It is a major focus of osteopathic medical education at my home institution. The musculoskeletal system is of vital importance not only to surgeons and physicians, but also to physician assistants, physical therapists, occupational therapists, athletic trainers, masseuses, chiropractors, and many others; it has a significant presence in many health professions. Also, musculoskeletal complaints include not only disorders of the muscle and bone, but the nerves that allow the muscles to contract, and the connective tissue structures that convey muscle contraction and stabilize the skeleton. In addition, dysfunctions of the molecules within the muscle and bone will often manifest clinically and a variety of movement disorders are distinguished from each other based on their effect on the musculoskeletal system.

This book is meant as a starting place for both teaching faculty and health science students to investigate the musculoskeletal system without the dissonance from switching between sources. It presents the gross anatomy, histology, physiology, biochemistry, neuroanatomy, and embryology of the musculoskeletal system in a fluid and sequential manner. Since this is a lot of ground to cover, it has been done as efficiently as possible and if a topic has not received the attention that some readers believe it deserves, I look forward to their feedback. Sadly, a line had to be drawn somewhere to keep the text from expanding indefinitely, so it excludes pharmacology, microbiology, and detailed histopathology.

Another facet of this textbook is that it is intended for a beginning student with no background in the topic. The text is organized in a novel, spiral manner, with early introductory chapters that form a solid foundation of human structures by working through the bones, muscle groups, major nerves, and major vessels of the back and limbs. At that point, the book shifts focus to investigate the histology, physiology, biochemistry, embryology, and neuroscience related to the musculoskeletal system. Finally, we finish the spiral with four detailed chapters cataloging the structures and functions of the back, upper limb, lower limb, and torso. Throughout the text I have done my utmost to highlight the clinical relevance of the topics. While we all fall short of our ideals, I believe that every line in this text should be able to stand the "so what?" test. If I cannot give a reason why any point of data (a "datum" for you language purists) is important to a health professional, it should not be present. The relevance of the detailed points in the later chapters may be of interest to specialists, but relevancy remains the focus of the text.

It would be hard to overstate the importance of the accompanying illustrations in learning the musculoskeletal system. In fact, there are many places in this text where the actual verbiage over which I have agonized is ancillary to a detailed inspection of the images. I hope that together the art program and text will make the mastery of this topic not just more interesting, but actively pleasant. I have tried to make the text as conversational as possible without getting too jokey or going off on tangents. If you are able to envision me sitting next to you at a table, avidly discussing the mysteries of how the body moves and why it breaks down in complicated but understandable ways, then my efforts will have been successful. I truly hope you enjoy reading this book.

Peter Ward, PhD

CONTENTS

Introduction

INTRODUCTION AND BASIC TERMINOLOGY

This book is laid out in a very specific manner to help you learn this content in a lasting and engaging way. We will introduce topics, use them as a foundation to introduce new topics, and revisit them later in more detail. If the content seems basic and unsophisticated initially, rest assured that it will become more and more rigorous as we move along. We will begin with a quick introduction to the skeleton and joints, then investigate the muscle compartments as well as their innervation and blood supply. Along the way, embryonic development, histology (microscopic anatomy), physiology, biochemistry, and neuroscience will be presented as they relate to the musculoskeletal system. Finally, we will revisit the back, upper limbs, lower limbs, and torso in greater detail.

If you have already taken a human anatomy course, you may be able to scan the early sections. If you are new to the topic, these will provide a solid foundation that will be revisited and heavily elaborated upon in subsequent chapters. This book highlights the form and the function of the musculoskeletal system, what happens when structures "go bad" in various clinical conditions, and how these maladies can be diagnosed. Although I might find anatomy interesting for its own sake (which I absolutely do), this book is for medical and health science students who will need to apply this information practically. When we are done, a clinically grounded understanding of the musculoskeletal system will have become a powerful tool for your career.

THE REGIONS OF THE BODY

The human body is a conundrum. To function properly, every system and region must interact as part of a whole. However, it can be subdivided into organ systems and regions that each have distinctive actions and characteristics. To begin a proper study of anatomy, we will divide the entire body into 8 regions (Fig. 1.1) and then into 11 organ systems. The focus of this book is on the musculoskeletal system, particularly in the back and limbs, but other systems will be discussed as they influence and impact it.

The **head** consists of the face, bones of the skull, and mandible. It is attached to the back and neck through the cervical vertebrae, large vessels, muscles, nerves, and the pharynx (throat). The cranium surrounds the brain and brainstem along with the other tissues and fluid that supports them. The brainstem extends into the back as the spinal cord.

The **back** contains the vertebrae, or spinal column. The muscles and nerves of the back stabilize the vertebrae but also allow them some mobility. The vertebrae surround the spinal cord and its associated spinal nerves. It is segmented into the cervical, thoracic, lumbar, sacral, and coccygeal vertebral regions.

The **upper limbs** are subdivided into the shoulder, arm (brachium), forearm (antebrachium), wrist (carpus), and hand (manus). The hand has a palmar and dorsal aspect. The bones, muscles, ligaments, and nerves of the upper limb link it to the lower cervical vertebrae and the upper thorax at the **axilla** or armpit. The muscles of the upper limb attach to the bones and move them using the joints in the shoulder, elbow, wrist, and digits.

The **lower limbs** are subdivided into the gluteal region, thigh, leg (crus), ankle (tarsus), and foot (pes), which has a plantar and dorsal aspect. The bones, muscles, ligaments, and nerves of the lower limb link it to the pelvis, lumbar vertebrae, and sacrum. Muscles that attach to the bones of the lower limb allow strong and stable movements to occur at the joints of the hip, knee, ankle, and digits.

The **neck** extends inferiorly from the head and connects it to the thorax, allowing the head a degree of both movement and stability. It contains the cervical vertebrae of the back (they are shared by both regions) and the carotid arteries and jugular veins. The neck conveys air between the head and lungs via the larynx and trachea; it also conveys food and beverages from the head to the stomach via the esophagus. The neck also contains the hyoid bone, thyroid gland, and a variety of muscles and ligaments.

The **thorax** or **chest** consists of the thoracic vertebrae, ribs, and sternum along with their associated muscles, which form a cage around the heart, lungs, large blood vessels, esophagus, and other organs in this region. Several muscles connect the

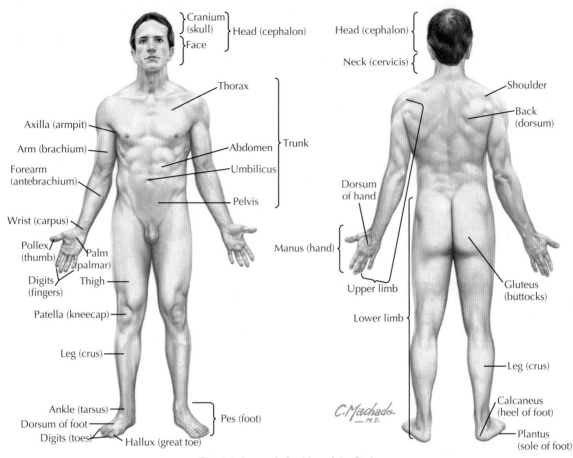

Fig. 1.1 Anatomic Position of the Body.

thorax to the neck, back, upper limb, and abdomen. It is separated from the abdomen by the diaphragm.

The **abdomen** is inferior to (below) the diaphragm and consists of lumbar vertebrae and muscles of the abdominal wall, which surround the stomach, small intestines, large intestines, liver, gall bladder, pancreas, spleen, kidneys, ureters, and adrenal glands. The umbilicus is located on its central, anterior aspect. The abdomen is continuous with the pelvis.

The **pelvis** consists of the sacrum and pelvic bones that form a protective bowl around the internal reproductive organs, urinary bladder, and rectum. Several muscles connect it to the abdomen and lower limb. The external aspect of the pelvis, which includes the external genitalia, anus, and urinary openings is referred to as the **perineum**.

THE SYSTEMS OF THE BODY

The **cardiovascular (circulatory) system** is primarily associated with the heart and blood vessels. The heart pumps blood to the lungs and then throughout the body in a (mostly) closed system of vessels, with arteries leading to capillaries and then to veins, then back to the heart. This system exchanges nutrients and oxygen for metabolic wastes and carbon dioxide in the tissues of the body and transports them where they can be removed or recycled.

The **lymphatic system** is a subset of the cardiovascular system. Cellular debris and "junk" proteins that are too large to be carried away by veins enter open-ended lymphatic vessels and travel into progressively larger lymphatic vessels until they empty into a large vein. As lymphatic fluid travels through lymphatic vessels, it is filtered through immune organs called lymph nodes, which are part of the immune system.

The **immune system** allows the body to defend itself from foreign pathogens by producing specific and nonspecific defenses against invaders. The widely distributed cells and organs of the immune system produce substances that actively fight infection and screen for invasive organisms.

The **integumentary system** consists of the skin and its associated structures such as hair, fingernails, toenails, and sweat glands. These form and maintain a protective barrier while preventing the loss of water and heat.

The **musculoskeletal system** protects the other systems while allowing for controlled movement. **Skeletal muscles** attach to bones by means of tendons. When muscles contract, they pull their attachment points closer to each other, allowing deliberate motions. **Bones** of the skeleton both support the body against gravity and form a protective cage around some organs. Bone is a metabolically active tissue that serves as a reservoir for calcium and phosphorus. Bones meet other bones at a variety of **articulations** or **joints**. Frequently this involves a layer of cartilage lining bony surfaces, contained within a fibrous capsule full of synovial fluid, which minimizes friction between bones.

The **nervous system** is composed of specialized cells, called **neurons**, and their support structures. The central nervous system is the brain, brainstem, and spinal cord. The peripheral nervous system is composed of nerves that travel to and from the central nervous system as well as clusters of nerve cell bodies, called ganglia. In general, efferent (motor) neurons travel to peripheral tissues (e.g., muscle, glands) and cause a change to that tissue, such as muscle contraction. Afferent (sensory) neurons carry information from the periphery back to the central nervous system, alerting the brain to changes in the environment.

The **respiratory (pulmonary) system** conveys air to and from the lungs and allows gas exchange (oxygen is inhaled, carbon dioxide is exhaled) while simultaneously preventing particulate matter and pathogens from reaching deep into the lungs. Vibrations caused by the flow of air through one portion of the respiratory system, the larynx, is what allows us to speak.

The organs of the **digestive (gastrointestinal) system** mechanically and chemically digest solid and liquid nutrients that enter the body through the mouth before releasing the remnants at the anus. The **alimentary tract** extracts nutrients and transports them to nearby blood vessels while simultaneously protecting the body from foreign pathogens. Associated **gastrointestinal glands** release exocrine and endocrine products that help to break down and store nutrients.

The cells and organs of the **endocrine system** release signaling molecules, hormones, that modulate the activity of neighboring target cells or enter the circulation to reach target cells further away. The endocrine and nervous systems are responsible for modulating the body's responses to external stimuli, coordinating bodily cycles, and maintaining homeostasis.

The **urogenital system** is sometimes used to denote two separate but interconnected body systems: the reproductive and urinary systems.

In the **reproductive (sexual) system**, germ cells are produced or maintained by specialized organs called the gonads (testes/ovaries). The other organs and cells of the reproductive system transport and sustain these germ cells to allow the process of sexual reproduction. The organs and supporting structures of this system differ between males and females.

The **urinary system** removes metabolic wastes that the blood picks up from the tissues of the body. Kidneys filter the blood to produce urine, which is transported through the ureters to be stored in the urinary bladder. It is released from the urinary bladder via the urethra.

ANATOMIC TERMINOLOGY AND THE "ANATOMIC POSITION"

Because terms such as "up," "down," "behind," and "over" can mean different things depending on the position of the speakers and the person about whom they are speaking, anatomists use a precise set of terms to describe the position of the human body. Becoming fluent in these terms helps prevent mistakes in surgery or when interpreting imaging studies.

Structures are described as though the body is always in an "anatomic position" (Fig. 1.2). In this position we assume that the body is standing, facing forward with the head looking straight ahead. The legs are parallel and the toes directed straight ahead. The arms are described as hanging at the side of the body with the palms directed straight ahead. The following terms are used to describe the body in the **anatomic position.**

- **Superior/Inferior**: Structures that are *superior* to others are located closer to the topmost part of the head. Things that are located *inferior* to others are positioned closer to the soles of the feet. For example, the mouth is superior to the heart and inferior to the eyes. The terms *cranial/caudal* are largely synonymous with *superior/inferior,* with the caveat that "caudal" is more commonly used in comparative anatomy and refers to something closer to the tail. Similarly, the term "rostral" refers to structures close to the tip of the nose.
- **Anterior/Posterior**: Structures that are *anterior* to others are located closer to the front of the body. *Posterior* things are located closer to the back of the body. For example, the heart is posterior to the sternum but anterior to the thoracic vertebrae. The terms *ventral/dorsal* are largely synonymous with *anterior/posterior* and are used more commonly in comparative anatomy.
  - The superior-most aspect of structures that extend from the body (tongue, nose, penis) are also often referred to as having dorsal and ventral sides.
  - The anterior aspect of the hand is frequently referred to as the *palmar* side, and the posterior side as the *dorsum* of the hand.
  - The inferior aspect of the foot is frequently referred to as the *plantar* side, and the superior side as the *dorsum* of the foot.
- **Proximal/Distal**: Structures that are *proximal* are located closer to the center of the body than other things, such as the scapula or hip. *Distal* structures, such as the fingernails and toenails, are located further away from the center of the body. For example, the elbow is distal to the shoulder but proximal to the fingers.
- **Deep/Superficial**: *Deep* structures are located closer to the core of the body. *Superficial* things are located closer to the outside surface of the body. For example, the abdominal muscles are deep to the overlying skin but they are superficial to the abdominal organs.
- **Median/Medial/Lateral**: Unlike many of the other terms in this section, *median* is not a relative term. Instead, *median* refers to being located on the exact midline of the body or one of the limbs. In contrast, *medial* and *lateral* are relative terms. Structures that are medial are closer to the body or limb's midline (the median plane), whereas lateral structures are located further away from the midline. For example, in the upper limb the middle finger (third digit) is a median structure, the thumb (first digit) is lateral, and the little finger (fifth digit) is medial. Don't forget that in anatomic position, the palms are directed anteriorly!
- **Unilateral/Bilateral**: Something that is *unilateral* exists only on one side of the body, such as the spleen on the left. *Bilateral* structures, such as the kidneys, are present on both the left and right sides.
- **Ipsilateral/Contralateral**: This one is a bit conceptually difficult. Something that is *ipsilateral* is located on the same side of the body relative to something else. For example, an injury

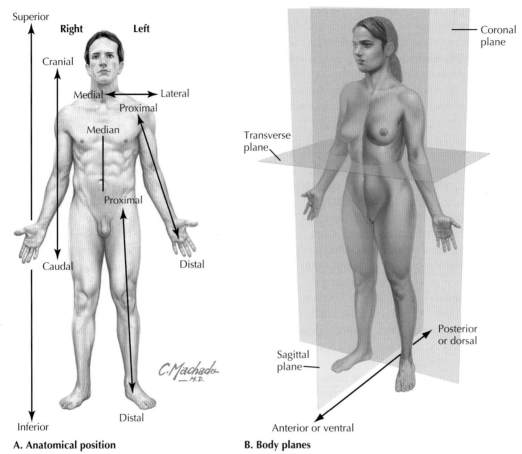

A. Anatomical position   **B. Body planes**

Fig. 1.2 Terms of Relationship and Body Planes.

to the right side of the spinal cord will often cause motor problems on the ipsilateral (right) side. *Contralateral* refers to something located on the opposite side of the body relative to something else. An injury to the right frontal lobe of the brain will often cause motor problems on the contralateral (left) side.

PLANES OF THE BODY

One common way in which anatomists and medical professionals conceptualize the body is by creating "planes" that section the body into two or more parts (see Fig. 1.2B). This is particularly true when viewing computed tomography (CT) or magnetic resonance imaging (MRI) cross-sections.

- The **sagittal plane** divides the body into a right and left side. The "slice" occurs along a vertical plane that passes along the anterior/posterior axis.
  - Midsagittal/median—a sagittal plane that is on the exact midline.
  - Parasagittal—a sagittal plane that is to one side (right or left) of the midline.
- The **coronal plane** divides the body into an anterior and a posterior part. This slice occurs along a vertical plane that passes along the left/right axis.
- The **axial/horizontal/transverse plane** divides the body into superior and inferior parts. This slice occurs along a horizontal plane.

- An **oblique plane** is neither vertical nor horizontal. It can exist along any combination of axes. Oblique views are used clinically to view structures in a specific way.

TERMS DESCRIBING MOTION

Muscles contract and move the bones around their articulations in a variety of ways (Fig. 1.3). Although each joint is unique (and we will talk about them in later chapters), there are some common ways to describe these movements. Motions that are unique to specific regions of the body will be discussed in the relevant sections.

Flexion/Extension

- Primarily occurs in the sagittal plane.
- *Flexion* occurs when contraction causes a decrease in the angle between two bones or regions of the body (see Fig. 1.3A–E, H, N, and O). For example, curling your wrist up toward your shoulder occurs due to flexion of the elbow joint (see Fig. 1.3C); likewise, if you were to curl up into the fetal position, your trunk would be in flexion (see Fig. 1.3B).
- *Extension* occurs when contraction causes an increase in the angle between two bones or regions of the body (see Fig. 1.3A–E, I, and O). For example, if you are doing a push-up, you extend the elbow as you move away from the ground (see Fig. 1.3C); likewise, if you look up into the sky while standing, you are extending the neck (see Fig. 1.3B).

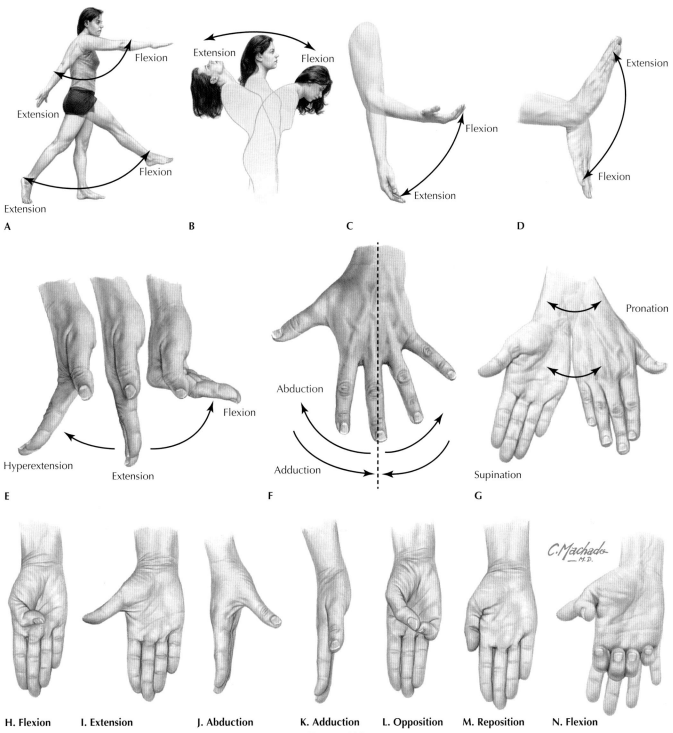

Fig. 1.3 Terms of Movement.

Continued

- *Plantarflexion* and *dorsiflexion* (see Fig. 1.3Q) are motions that occur at the ankle. Plantarflexion is "straightening" the ankle, as when you stand on tiptoes. Dorsiflexion refers to "bending" the ankle, such as when initially trying to get a sock over your toes.

Abduction/Adduction/Lateral Flexion
- Primarily occurs in the coronal plane.
- *Abduction* occurs when a limb, or a portion of a limb, is moved away from the midline (see Fig. 1.3F, J, and S). For

example, if you kick your right lower limb out to the right, it is being abducted (see Fig. 1.3S).
- *Adduction* occurs when a limb, or portion of a limb, is moved closer to the midline (see Fig. 1.3F, K, and S). For example, if you clamp your upper limb strongly against the side of your body, it has been adducted (see Fig. 1.3S).
- *Lateral flexion (side-bending)* refers to leaning the body to the right or to the left. This occurs due to movement of the vertebrae, with one side becoming concave (curved inward),

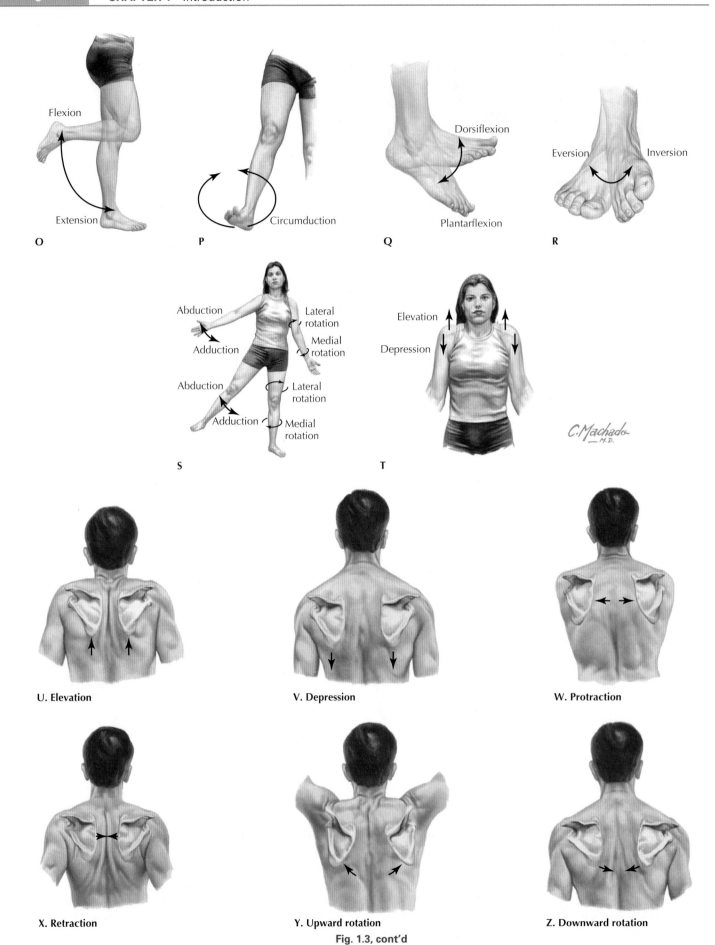

O

Flexion

Extension

P

Circumduction

Q

Dorsiflexion

Plantarflexion

R

Eversion   Inversion

S

Abduction

Adduction

Lateral rotation

Medial rotation

Abduction

Adduction

Lateral rotation

Medial rotation

T

Elevation

Depression

C. Machado
— M.D.

U. Elevation

V. Depression

W. Protraction

X. Retraction

Y. Upward rotation

Z. Downward rotation

Fig. 1.3, cont'd

and the other side becoming convex (curved outward). Side-bending is frequently coupled with rotation of the vertebrae.

Rotation

- Primarily occurs in the horizontal plane.
- *Left* and *right rotation* of the body occurs when the vertebrae rotate around their vertical axis, allowing us to twist from side to side and turn our head right and left.
- *Medial* and *lateral rotation* occur at the arm of the upper limb and thigh of the lower limb (see Fig. 1.3S). As medial rotation occurs, the arm twists to move the elbow laterally, and lateral rotation works in the opposite direction to move the elbow medially. In the lower limb, medial rotation of the thigh would move the patella (kneecap) to face medially, and lateral rotation would result in the patella pointing laterally.
- *Supination* and *pronation* are special rotary motions of the forearm (see Fig. 1.3G) that can be seen if you alternate between a palms-up and palms-down position. Even though the hand moves dramatically, the motion originates in the forearm. Rotating the palm superiorly is supination, rotating the palm inferiorly is pronation.
- *Eversion* and *inversion* are special motions of the ankle (see Fig. 1.3R). Eversion occurs when the sole of the foot is rotated laterally. Inversion occurs when the sole of the foot is rotated medially.

Elevation/Depression, Protraction/Retraction, Upward/Downward Rotation

- These motions are primarily seen in the shoulders.
- *Elevation* occurs when the scapula is moved superiorly, "lifting" the shoulders (see Fig. 1.3T and U).

- *Depression* occurs when the scapula is pulled inferiorly along the thorax (see Fig. 1.3T and V).
- *Protraction* occurs when the shoulder blade moves anteriorly along the thoracic wall. This motion "fixes" the scapula in place, stabilizing the base of the upper limb (see Fig. 1.3W).
- *Retraction* occurs when the shoulder blade is moved posteriorly and medially. This often happens bilaterally, bringing the two scapulae close together medially (see Fig. 1.3X).
- *Upward (superior) rotation* of the scapula directs the lateral point of the shoulder superiorly, as when elevating the arms (see Fig. 1.3Y).
- *Downward (inferior) rotation* of the scapula directs the lateral point of the shoulder inferiorly, as when reaching down (see Fig. 1.3Z).

Circumduction

- This motion occurs at the shoulder and hip.
- *Circumduction* results in the entire upper or lower limb moving in a rotary motion (see Fig. 1.3P). As such, it is a coordinated combination of flexion, abduction, extension, and adduction.

Opposition/Reposition

- A motion of the thumb.
- *Opposition* is a motion that brings the entire first digit (thumb) of the hand medially, toward the fifth digit (see Fig. 1.3L).
- *Reposition* is the opposite motion, moving the first digit laterally, back into the anatomic position (see Fig. 1.3M).

Overview of Skeletal Anatomy

SKELETON GENERAL

To understand the musculoskeletal system, we must pick a place to begin. Although this choice is somewhat arbitrary, the skeletal system serves as an excellent starting place. It supports and protects the other organ systems and serves as the scaffolding onto which our muscles attach. This chapter will introduce the major bones and joints of the body so that in Chapter 3 we can understand how large muscle groups move the bones. In subsequent chapters we will revisit these topics in more detail.

We can generally group the features of the skeleton into processes, depressions, and holes.

Processes are projections extending off of a bone:
- *Rami* are large, angled extensions of a bone
- *Trochanters* are very large processes extending exclusively from the proximal femur
- *Tuberosities* are broad and rounded (sometimes plateau-like) processes
- *Tubercles* are medium-sized, distinct bony elevations
- *Protuberances* are very small but distinct elevations (sometimes tent-shaped) that come to a blunted tip
- *Crests* are large elongated processes that are noticeably elevated from the nearby bone
- *Ridges/Lines* are similar to crests but are less pronounced and elevated from nearby bone. Ridges tend to be rougher than lines.
- *Spines* can be as large as tuberosities or as small as protuberances, but they come to an elongated, sharp point. A major exception is the spine of the scapula, which is a very broad wall of bone along the scapula's posterior side.

Depressions are areas of bone that are at a lower elevation compared with surrounding bone.
- *Fossae* (singular, fossa) are depressions that are generally wider than deep

- *Foveae* (singular, fovea) are very shallow, round depressions
- *Grooves/Sulci* (singular, sulcus) are elongated depressions. Sulci tend to be particularly broad and deep (sometimes canyon-like) grooves, but there is not always a clear distinction between the terms.
- *Notches* are particularly large grooves

Holes are perforations or hollow spaces within bones
- *Foramens* are holes in bones
- *Fissures* are elongated clefts through bones
- *Canals/Meati* (singular, meatus) are tunnels through bone.
- *Cavities* are hollow spaces within bones
- Bony *sinuses* are hollow spaces inside bone that are lined by a mucous membrane and connect to another space in the body

BONES OF THE HEAD AND ANTERIOR NECK

The skull (Figs. 2.1 and 2.2) is a complex skeletal structure that is made of many fused bones and one true articulated joint, the temporomandibular joint. It also articulates with the top-most vertebral bone, the atlas. The skull can be divided into two regions that reflect functional and developmental differences, the neurocranium and viscerocranium. The **neurocranium** (braincase) is the portion of the skull that surrounds the brain, and the **viscerocranium** (facial skeleton) consists of the facial bones inferior to the neurocranium. The bones of the skull base contribute to both the neurocranium and viscerocranium. The upper part of the neurocranium, the **calvarium**, is sometimes called the "skull cap."

The left and right **frontal bones** make up the forehead and brow line. They contribute to the anterior portion of the neurocranium and the superior part of the facial skeleton. The inferior portion of the facial bones contain an air space, the **frontal sinus**. These paired bones generally fuse during fetal development to create a single frontal bone.

A. Anterior view

Frontal bone

Nasal bone

Lacrimal bone

Orbit

Zygomatic bone

Maxilla

Piriform aperture

Parietal bone

Sphenoid bone

Temporal bone

Ethmoid bone

Nasal septum

Inferior nasal concha

Vomer

Ramus

Mandible

B. Lateral view

Parietal bone

Coronal suture

Frontal bone

Pterion

Sphenoid bone

Lacrimal bone

Nasal bone

Zygomatic bone

Maxilla

Mandible

Coronoid process

Head of mandible

Ramus

Body

Angle of mandible

Occipital bone

Temporal bone

Lambdoid suture

Squamous part

External acoustic meatus

Mastoid process

Styloid process

C. Sagittal section

Grooves for branches of
middle meningeal vessels

Coronal suture

Parietal bone

Sphenoid bone

Sella turcica

Sphenoidal sinus

Frontal bone

Frontal sinus

Ethmoid bone

Nasal bone

Inferior
nasal concha

Maxilla

Vomer

Palatine bone

Temporal bone

Squamous part

Petrous part

Lambdoid suture

Occipital bone

Foramen magnum

Occipital condyle

D. Sagittal section

Nasal bone

Ethmoid bone

Superior nasal concha

Middle nasal concha

Lacrimal bone

Inferior nasal concha

Maxilla

Frontal bone

Opening of
sphenoidal sinus

Sphenoid bone

Body

Palatine bone

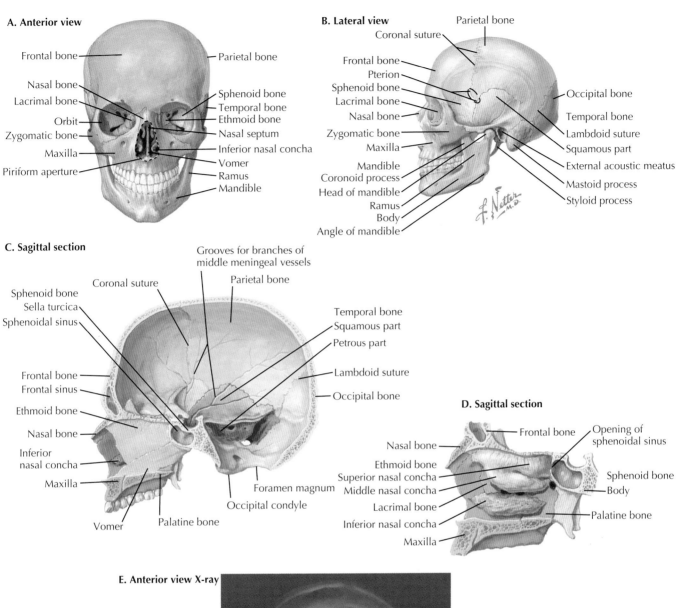

E. Anterior view X-ray

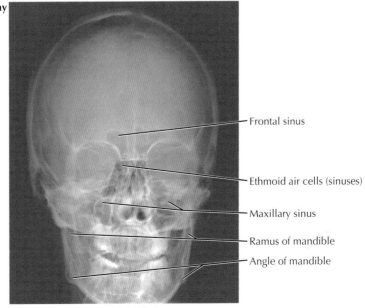

Frontal sinus

Ethmoid air cells (sinuses)

Maxillary sinus

Ramus of mandible

Angle of mandible

Fig. 2.1 Skull.

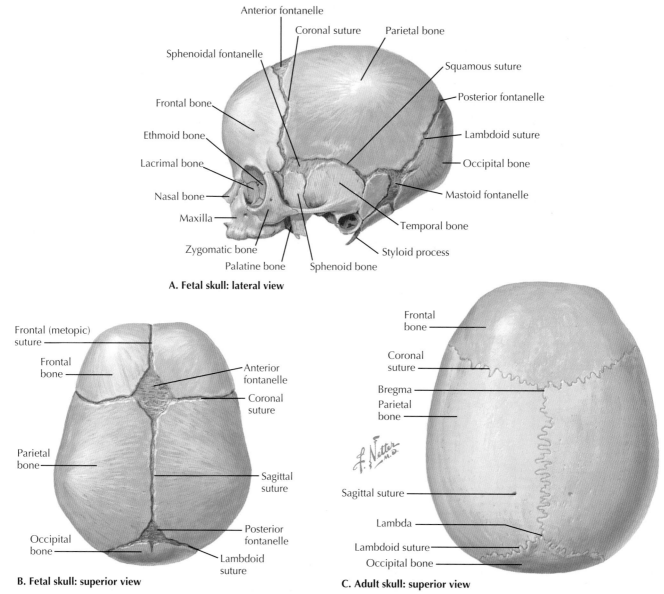

A. Fetal skull: lateral view

B. Fetal skull: superior view

C. Adult skull: superior view

Fig. 2.2 Bones of the Skull.

The left and right **parietal bones** are very flat and contribute to the superior and lateral portion of the neurocranium.

The single **occipital bone** forms the posterior and inferior neurocranium. The base of this bone also contributes to the facial skeleton. Inferiorly, it has a large opening, the **foramen magnum**, flanked by two **occipital condyles** that articulate with the first cervical vertebra, the atlas.

The (somewhat) bat-shaped **sphenoid bone** contributes to the anterolateral neurocranium as well as the skull base and facial skeleton. Its central area contains an air-filled cavity, the **sphenoid sinus**. It also supports the pituitary gland in a small depression, the **sella turcica**, which is connected to the inferior aspect of the brain.

The single **ethmoid bone** is located just anterior to the body of the sphenoid bone. It contains many small air-filled **ethmoid air cells**. The ethmoid bone contributes to the skull base and facial skeleton, particularly the upper portion of the nasal cavity and nasal septum. The small **vomer bone** forms

the rest of the nasal septum. The ethmoid bone also forms part of the medial orbits of the eyes, along with the paired **lacrimal bones**.

The left and right **temporal bones** contribute to the lateral aspect of the neurocranium and the skull base, including part of the facial skeleton. The flat **squamous part** of the temporal bone interacts with the parietal and sphenoid bones. On the lateral aspect of the temporal bone is the **external acoustic opening** that leads into the hard, **petrous part** of the temporal bone. Within the petrous part of the temporal bone is the middle ear, which contains the three tiny bones that allow us to hear: the **incus, malleus,** and **stapes**. Immediately posterior to the external acoustic opening is the large and broad **mastoid process**, and inferior to the opening is the spike-shaped **styloid process**. Both are important sites for muscle attachment. Anterior to the opening is the **mandibular fossa**, where the condylar process of the mandible articulates with the rest of the skull.

The left and right **zygomatic bones** are frequently called the cheekbones and connect the temporal bone to the maxilla and facial bones on each side.

The left and right **maxillae** (singular: maxilla) are part of the facial skeleton. They contain the upper arcade of teeth, contain a large **maxillary sinus**, and contribute to the nasal cavity, oral cavity, and hard palate. Two smaller **palatine bones** form the rest of the hard palate. The maxillae also form the opening of the nasal cavity along with the paired **nasal bones**.

The single **mandible** or jaw bone has a **body** that contains the lower arcade of teeth. At the **angle of the mandible**, the mandibular **ramus** turns superiorly, dividing into a **coronoid process** and **condylar process**, separated by a **mandibular notch**. The condylar process narrows before expanding to form the **head of the mandible**, which articulates with the right and left temporal bones of the skull. It is connected to the skull and moved by the muscles that allow us to chew, the **muscles of mastication**.

The single **hyoid bone** is unique. It is a bone of the anterior neck that is not connected directly with any other bone; instead, it is connected to the mandible, sternum, larynx, and scapula by muscles.

Sutures of the Skull

During development, the bones of the skull enlarge and grow closer together. If the bones fused as soon as they met, the skull would be too small for the human brain to enlarge. To accommodate this, the cartilage of the facial skeleton grows with the rest of the head and ossifies after puberty (see Figs. 2.1 and 2.2). The flat bones of the neurocranium meet at sutures and do not completely fuse until very late in life, if at all.

The two frontal bones meet at the **metopic suture**, which is present in the sagittal plane. This suture typically disappears as the right and left frontal bones fuse to form a single bone. It remains distinct in approximately 14% of people.

The two parietal bones meet at the midline **sagittal suture**, which (no surprise here) runs through the sagittal plane.

The frontal bone meets the two parietal bones at the **coronal suture**, which is present in the coronal plane.

The occipital bone meets each parietal bone at the **lambdoidal sutures**, it is not present in any one plane but runs inferiorly and laterally from the terminus of the sagittal suture.

The superior edge of the temporal bone meets the occipital, parietal, and sphenoid bones at the curved **squamous suture**.

There are several important points where various sutures intersect. The coronal and sagittal sutures meet at the **anterior fontanelle**. In newborns, this area is the "soft spot" because the nearby parietal and frontal bones have not yet completely fused. In adults it is termed the **bregma**.

The sagittal suture meets the lambdoidal suture at the **posterior fontanelle**, which also forms a soft spot in newborns, but is much smaller than the anterior fontanelle. In adults it is termed the **lambda**.

The lambdoidal and squamous sutures meet at the **mastoid fontanelle**, which does not form an appreciable soft spot. It is called the **asterion** in the adult. The frontal, sphenoid, parietal, and temporal bones meet at the **sphenoidal fontanelle**. It also does not form an appreciable soft spot but in adults is a weak area that is prone to fracture when trauma occurs near the temple. It is known as the **pterion**.

Major Foramina of the Skull

There are many foramina, fissures, and other features of the skull. To begin, there are six major openings in the skull that we need to know. Note that the mouth is not among them because it is formed primarily by soft tissues (skin, muscle, connective tissues) around the articulation of the mandible and maxilla.

The **piriform aperture** (see Fig. 2.1A) marks the opening of the nasal cavities and is a single, pear-shaped opening in the front of the skull. Its opening is bounded by the maxilla and nasal bones. Within the piriform recess you should be able to see the (mostly) midline **nasal septum** and the **superior, middle, and inferior nasal conchae** (see Fig. 2.1A, C, and D), which are spiral bony structures that extend from the lateral nasal wall.

Superior and lateral to the piriform recess are the right and left **orbits** (see Fig. 2.1A). In life, these contain the eyes and the muscles that move them. The frontal, sphenoid, ethmoid, lacrimal, maxillary, and zygomatic bones all contribute to the bony orbit.

The left and right **external acoustic meati** (see Fig. 2.1B) are the openings of each ear canal into the middle ear. The opening is completely surrounded by the petrous portion of the temporal bone, along with all the other structures of the middle and internal ear.

The easily identified **foramen magnum** (literally "large hole") is a feature of the occipital bone (see Fig. 2.1C). The spinal cord exits the skull through this opening and descends into the vertebral canal.

BONES OF THE BACK—THE VERTEBRAE

The **vertebral** (spinal) **column** is made from a series of individual **vertebrae** (Fig. 2.3). These bones surround and protect the spinal cord and its associated structures. It also mechanically supports and maneuvers the head, transmits forces from the limbs, and resists compression. There are five distinct regions of the vertebral column. From superior to inferior, they are the **cervical** (7 vertebrae), **thoracic** (12), **lumbar** (5), **sacral** (5), and **coccygeal** (3 to 5) regions. When the whole group is viewed from the side, the different regions have distinctive curves. The cervical and lumbar regions appear concave (scooped out) posteriorly and convex (bulging) anteriorly. This sort of curvature is called a **lordosis.** Conversely, the thoracic and sacral regions appear concave anteriorly and convex posteriorly. This sort of curvature is called a **kyphosis.**

The "Generic" Vertebra

Before delving into the specifics of each region, let's review the features that are common to almost all vertebrae (Fig. 2.4). The anterior-most part of each vertebrae is the **vertebral body**. It is the largest part of each vertebra and is cylindrical in shape. Each vertebral body supports the weight of the vertebrae superior to it and transmits forces from the vertebrae inferior to it. Neighboring vertebrae are connected by **intervertebral discs**.

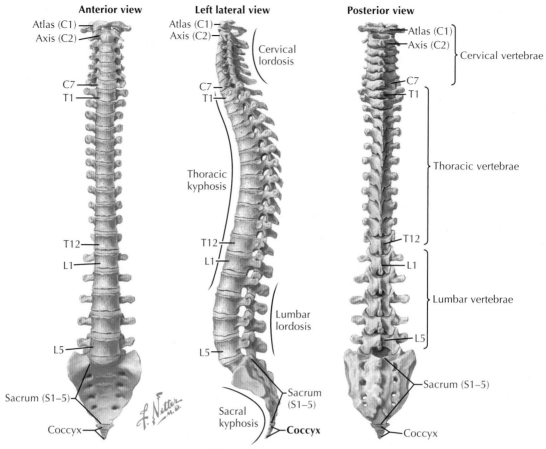

Anterior view

- Atlas (C1)
- Axis (C2)
- C7
- T1
- T12
- L1
- L5
- Sacrum (S1–5)
- Coccyx

Left lateral view

- Atlas (C1)
- Axis (C2)
- Cervical lordosis
- C7
- T1
- Thoracic kyphosis
- T12
- L1
- Lumbar lordosis
- L5
- Sacrum (S1–5)
- Sacral kyphosis
- **Coccyx**

Posterior view

- Atlas (C1)
- Axis (C2)
- Cervical vertebrae
- C7
- T1
- Thoracic vertebrae
- T12
- L1
- Lumbar vertebrae
- L5
- Sacrum (S1–5)
- Coccyx

Fig. 2.3 Vertebral Column.

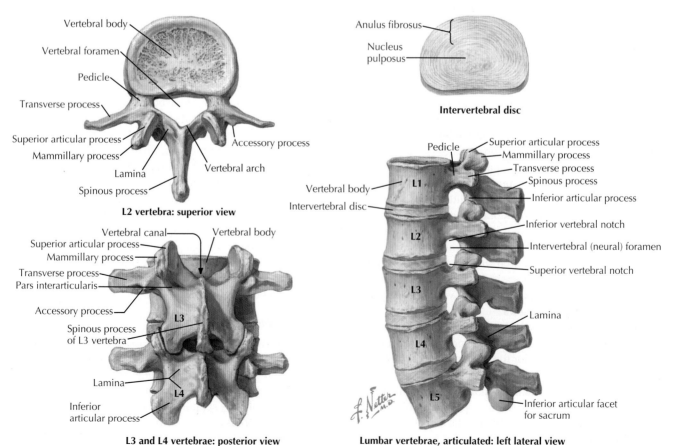

L2 vertebra: superior view

- Vertebral body
- Vertebral foramen
- Pedicle
- Transverse process
- Superior articular process
- Mammillary process
- Lamina
- Spinous process
- Accessory process
- Vertebral arch

Intervertebral disc

- Anulus fibrosus
- Nucleus pulposus

L3 and L4 vertebrae: posterior view

- Vertebral canal
- Superior articular process
- Mammillary process
- Transverse process
- Pars interarticularis
- Accessory process
- Spinous process of L3 vertebra
- Vertebral body
- Lamina
- Inferior articular process

Lumbar vertebrae, articulated: left lateral view

- Pedicle
- Superior articular process
- Mammillary process
- Transverse process
- Spinous process
- Inferior articular process
- Vertebral body
- Intervertebral disc
- Inferior vertebral notch
- Intervertebral (neural) foramen
- Superior vertebral notch
- Lamina
- Inferior articular facet for sacrum
- L1
- L2
- L3
- L4
- L5

Fig. 2.4 Lumbar Vertebrae and Intervertebral Disc Spine: Osteology.

These serve as "shock absorbers" for the forces that are transmitted along the vertebral column. They have a gelatinous core, the **nucleus pulposus**, which is surrounded by concentric rings of connective tissue, the **anulus fibrosis**. This allows the disc to rebound when it experiences compressive forces.

The **vertebral arch** is the portion of the vertebra that projects off the vertebral body to surround and protect the spinal cord. The space that is surrounded by the arch is the **vertebral foramen**. The sections of the vertebral arch that connect directly to the vertebral body on each side are the right and left **pedicles**; they form the "walls" around the cord. The right and left **laminae** (singular: lamina) continue from the pedicles and meet each other on the midline to form the "roof" over the cord.

There are several bony processes extending from the vertebral arch for muscle and ligament attachment. A single **spinous process** extends posteriorly off of the vertebral arch at the point where the right and left laminae meet. The right and left **transverse processes** extend laterally off of the arch at the points where the pedicles meet the laminae on each side. Near the transverse processes are two additional processes that connect to neighboring vertebrae. The **superior articular process**, as its name suggests, extends superiorly and articulates with the next-most superior vertebra through a **superior articular facet**. The **inferior articular process** extends inferiorly and articulates with the next-most inferior vertebra through an **inferior articular facet**.

Superior and inferior to each pedicle are the superior vertebral notch and inferior vertebral notch. Adjacent inferior and superior vertebral notches create a space, the **intervertebral foramen**, shared by two neighboring vertebrae that allows the spinal nerves to leave the spinal cord and extend to the body.

Cervical Vertebrae

There are seven cervical vertebrae connecting the head to the thoracic vertebrae. The lower cervical vertebrae (3rd to 7th) have many features in common, but the upper cervical vertebrae (1st and 2nd) are unlike the other five cervical vertebrae, so they will be discussed separately.

Lower Cervical Vertebrae

Each of the 3rd to 7th cervical vertebrae (C3–C7) have all the features of a "generic" vertebra (vertebral body, vertebral arch, pedicles, laminae, transverse processes, spinous process, superior and inferior articular processes and facets, intervertebral disc) as well as few distinctive features (Fig. 2.5). Vertebrae C1–C6 typically have a **transverse foramen** in their transverse processes that surrounds vessels that ascend toward the head and central nervous system. The transverse foramen splits the transverse processes into an **anterior and posterior tubercle**. The superior aspect of the bodies of the lower cervical vertebrae have raised lateral edges that cradle the intervertebral disc. These **uncinate processes** extend superiorly and may form tiny

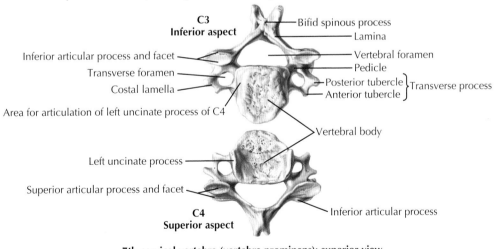

Inferior aspect of C3 and superior aspect of C4 showing the sites of the facet and uncovertebral articulations

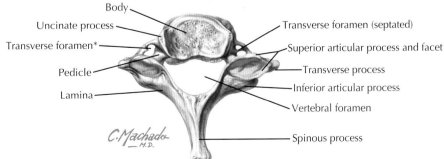

7th cervical vertebra (vertebra prominens): superior view

The Transverse foramen of C7 transmit vertebral veins, but usually not the vertebral artery, and are asymmetrical in this specimen.

Fig. 2.5 Cervical Vertebrae.

articulations with the disc or vertebral body above it. The spinous processes of C3–C6 are typically **bifid**, meaning that they split posteriorly into two processes, resembling a snake's forked tongue. This allows a cervical vertebra's spinous processes to straddle the spinous process of its inferior neighbor during full extension of the neck.

Upper Cervical Vertebrae

The axis (C2) and atlas (C1) are unique vertebrae (Fig. 2.6). The **axis** (C2) appears to be a regular cervical vertebra as described earlier, including a bifid spinous process and transverse foramen, but is distinguished by a large, thumb-shaped process extending superiorly from its vertebral body. This is the **dens** or **odontoid process**, which is actually the C1 vertebral body that was taken by the axis during development. The dens has **anterior and posterior articular facets** that allow it to interact with the atlas and an associated ligament. C2 interacts with C1 via its superior articular facet and the dens; there is no intervertebral disc between C2 and C1.

The **atlas** (C1) is a hoop-shaped bone that lacks most of the generic features of a vertebra. It has no vertebral body but instead has large **lateral masses** that host the transverse processes, transverse foramina, and articular facets, which articulate with the occipital bone of the skull and C2, respectively. The lateral masses are connected anteriorly by a short **anterior arch**, which has a distinct **anterior protuberance** at its midpoint. The inner surface of the anterior arch has a smooth **articular facet for the dens**. A larger **posterior arch** extends from each lateral mass to surround the spinal cord and enclose the vertebral foramen. It has a **posterior protuberance** on its posterior midline, as well as a notable **groove for the vertebral artery** running along its superior aspect.

Thoracic Vertebrae

There are 12 thoracic vertebrae between the cervical and lumbar regions (Fig. 2.7). They have all the features of a "generic" vertebra as well as a few distinctive features, most of which are related to their interaction with the ribs. Each thoracic vertebra articulates with one or two **ribs** via a costal facet or demifacets.

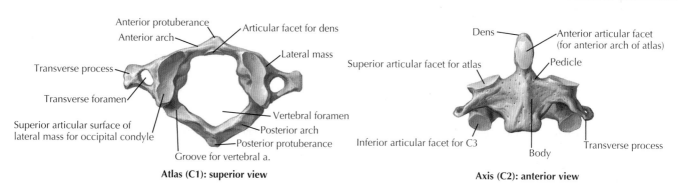

Atlas (C1): superior view

Axis (C2): anterior view

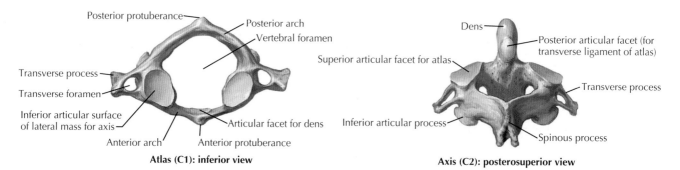

Atlas (C1): inferior view

Axis (C2): posterosuperior view

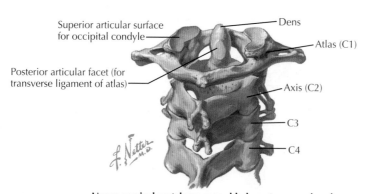

Upper cervical vertebrae, assembled: posterosuperior view

Fig. 2.6 Cervical Vertebrae: Atlas and Axis Spine: Osteology.

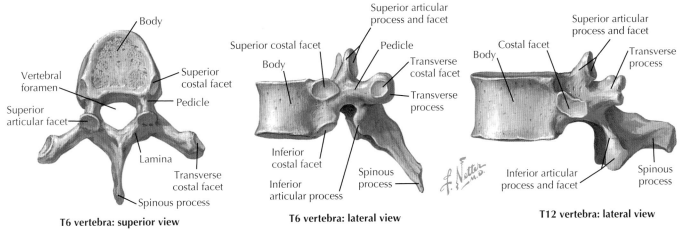

Fig. 2.7 Thoracic Vertebrae.

Costal facets (T1, T11, T12) are seen when the entire head of a rib articulates with a single vertebral body, whereas **superior and inferior demifacets** (T1–T10) are seen when the head of a rib straddles two adjacent vertebral bodies and their intervertebral disc. The ribs also articulate with the transverse processes at a point called the **transverse costal facet**. The transverse costal facets become less distinct in the lower thoracic vertebrae. From a lateral viewpoint, the upper and middle spinous processes are long and angled inferiorly, especially the middle (T4–T9) thoracic spinous processes. The lower thoracic spinous processes are smaller and square-shaped.

Lumbar Vertebrae

There are five lumbar vertebrae, and they have all the features of a "generic" vertebra (see Fig. 2.4). Their vertebral bodies are very large because they have to support the upper half of the body's weight. The transverse processes of the lumbar vertebrae are very elongated and flat. The spinous processes of the lumbar vertebrae are very large and square-shaped. Because there are many muscles and ligaments attaching to the lumbar vertebrae, they carry some additional processes that are distinctive. The small bumps that project posteriorly from the superior articular processes are called **mammillary processes**. Just inferior to them and located on the base of the transverse processes are **accessory processes**.

Sacral Vertebrae

The **sacrum** is a unique bone that consists of five vertebrae (Fig. 2.8) that fuse during early development. The sites of fusion, marking where intervertebral discs would have been, are the **transverse ridges** on the anterior surface of the sacrum. At the lateral limits of each transverse line are large openings for the nerves leaving the sacrum and traveling to the pelvic organs and lower limbs, the **anterior sacral foramina**. The large superior portion of the sacrum is the **sacral base**, and it terminates anteriorly as the **sacral promontory**. The inferior tip of the sacrum is called the **apex of the sacrum**. The large bony wings, **alae** (singular ala), that extend laterally from the sacral vertebral bodies articulate with the ilium, one of the bones of the pelvis. This surface is large and ear-shaped; hence it is called the **auricular surface**.

Because the sacral vertebrae are fused, the vertebral foramina create a completely enclosed **sacral canal** that surrounds nerves extending from the spinal cord. Its inferior opening is the **sacral hiatus**; it is surrounded by two or more bony processes, the **sacral horns** or **cornua**. The posterior aspect of the sacrum has a large ridge of bone running along its median aspect. This is the **median sacral crest** and is formed by the fused (sometimes incompletely) spinous processes of the sacral vertebrae. On either side of the median sacral crest are smaller right and left **intermediate sacral crests**, which are formed by fused sacral articular processes. The intermediate sacral crests terminate superiorly as **superior articular processes** and facet, which articulate with the inferior articular facets of L5. Further lateral are the right and left **lateral sacral crests**, formed by fusion of the sacral transverse processes. Between the intermediate and lateral sacral crests are the **posterior sacral foramina**, which transmit nerves from the sacrum to the lower back.

Coccygeal Vertebrae

The **coccyx** (tailbone) is a series of three to five fused and vestigial vertebrae (see Fig. 2.8). They are like tiny, conjoined vertebral bodies with none of the other characteristics of a vertebra. The first coccygeal vertebra may have a stunted transverse process on each side. The posterosuperior aspect of the first coccygeal vertebra may also have left and right **coccygeal horns**, or **cornua**, extending superiorly.

BONES OF THE THORAX

The thoracic vertebrae, ribs, and sternum are the bony components of the thorax. They protect the thoracic organs, serve as sites for muscle attachment, and help to anchor the upper limbs.

Ribs

The **ribs** (Fig. 2.9) extend from the thoracic vertebrae and wrap around the lungs and heart. However, the ribs themselves do not complete the journey. Instead, **costal cartilages** continue from the bony ribs to meet the **sternum**. In truth, only the costal

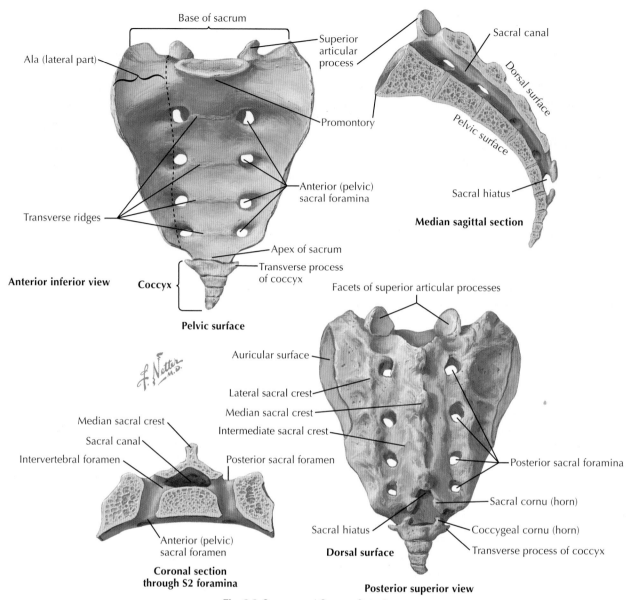

Fig. 2.8 Sacrum and Coccyx Osteology.

cartilages of ribs 1 to 7 (**true ribs**) actually reach the sternum directly. The costal cartilages of ribs 8 to 12 (**false ribs**) fuse to the costal cartilages of their superior neighbors, creating the **costal arch**. Ribs 11 and 12 (**floating ribs**) do not complete the journey to the sternum at all.

The "generic" rib has a **costal head** that articulates with its associated thoracic vertebral bodies via a costal facet or demifacet. Just lateral to the head is the narrower costal **neck**. Thereafter is the pronounced costal **tubercle** and its articular facet joint, which articulates with the transverse costal facets of the associated thoracic vertebrae. Then is an elongated costal **body**, which initially projects laterally and posteriorly but makes an anterior turn, creating a U-bend that is convex posteriorly, the **costal angle**. Along the inferomedial aspect of the entire costal body is a shallow **costal groove** that protects the intercostal vessels and nerves that travel alongside each rib. Compared with the others, ribs 1 and 2 are broad and flat. On

rib 1 there are visible grooves made by the large subclavian vessels as they pass across its superior surface toward the upper limbs. Ribs 11 and 12 do not have pronounced necks, tubercles, angles, or grooves.

Sternum

The sternum is actually three fused bones, the **manubrium, sternal body**, and **xiphoid process** (see Fig. 2.9). The superior aspect of the manubrium has a midline depression, the **jugular notch**. On either side of the jugular notch are the left and right **clavicular notches** that articulate with the left and right clavicles. Continuing inferiorly along the manubrium and sternum's lateral sides are costal notches for ribs 1 to 7. The manubrium meets the sternal body at the **sternal angle**. From a superior view, the first ribs, first thoracic vertebra, and manubrium surround the **superior thoracic aperture**. Likewise, the inferior ribs, costal arch, and xiphoid process surround the much larger **inferior thoracic aperture**.

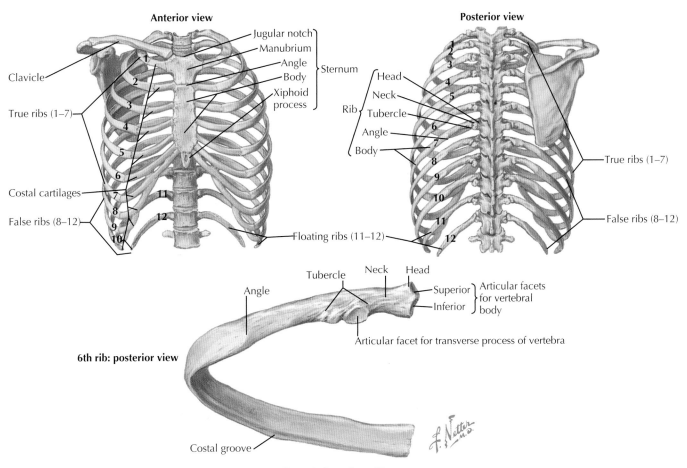

Fig. 2.9 Osteology: Thorax.

BONES OF THE UPPER LIMB

The five segments of the upper limb extend from the back and thorax with a core of bone surrounded by the muscles, vessels, nerves, and skin of the limb itself. The segments and their associated bones are the shoulder girdle (clavicle and scapula), arm (humerus), forearm (radius and ulna), wrist (carpal bones), and hand (metacarpal bones and phalanges).

Clavicle

Despite its slender and elongated appearance, the clavicle is the only direct bony attachment of the upper limb to the rest of the body (Figs. 2.9 and 2.10). It has a **sternal end** and **facet** that articulate with the clavicular notch of the manubrium. Its **body** or **shaft** extends laterally, terminating in its **acromial end** and **facet** to articulate with the scapula.

Scapula

The scapula, or shoulder blade, has an unusual shape (see Fig. 2.10). Seen from an anterior view, it appears to be triangular. It has a distinct **medial border**, **lateral border**, and **superior border**. The lateral and medial borders meet at the **inferior angle**, and the medial and superior borders meet at the **superior angle**. Traveling laterally along the superior border, there is a notable depression, the **suprascapular notch**, followed by a prominent thumb-shaped extension of bone, the **coracoid**

process. The superior and lateral borders meet laterally at a narrowed area, the **neck of the scapula**, which expands to form a broad depression that faces laterally, the **glenoid cavity**. This is where the scapula articulates with the head of the humerus. Superior and inferior to it are two sites for muscle attachment, the **supraglenoid tubercle** and **infraglenoid tubercle**. The flat, anterior aspect of the scapula is the **subscapular fossa**.

The posterior aspect has a similar overall outline but with a long strut of bone crossing laterally from the medial border of the scapula; this is the **scapular spine**. The spine divides the posterior aspect of the scapula into a **supraspinous fossa** and an **infraspinous fossa**. It extends laterally and superiorly, swooping over the glenoid fossa, terminating in the broad **acromion** that articulates with the acromial end of the clavicle.

Humerus

The bone at the core of the arm is the humerus (see Fig. 2.10). The most prominent aspect of the proximal humerus is its smooth and rounded **head** that articulates with the glenoid cavity of the scapula. More laterally are two sites for muscle attachment, the **lesser tubercle** and **greater tubercle**, which continue inferiorly as the **crest of the lesser tubercle** and **crest of the greater tubercle**. Between the two tubercles is the deep **intertubercular sulcus**, also known as the bicipital groove. The head and tubercles are separated from each other by the **anatomic**

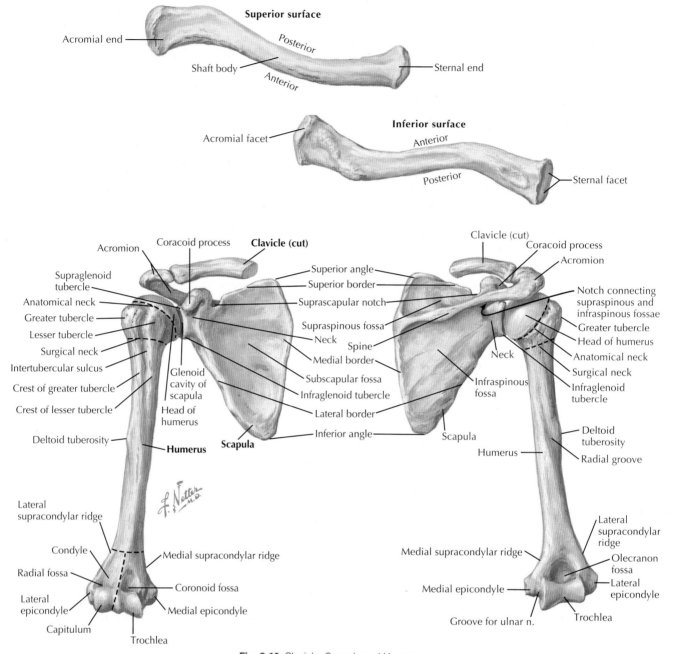

Fig. 2.10 Clavicle, Scapula and Humerus.

neck of the humerus, marking where bony growth centers fused to create a continuous bone. The tubercles and their crests narrow as they extend inferiorly into the **shaft** of the humerus. This narrowing marks the **surgical neck** of the humerus, a common site for fractures and orthopedic operations. On the lateral aspect of the shaft is a moderate elevation, the **deltoid tuberosity**. The distal end of the humerus, the **humeral condyle**, articulates with the radius and the ulna. Specifically, the **capitulum** is the portion that interacts with the radius and the **trochlea** with the ulna. Just proximal to the condyles are two pronounced ridges of bone that connect to the shaft, the **medial epicondyle** and **lateral epicondyle**. These are connected to the shaft by the **medial supracondylar ridge** and **lateral supracondylar ridge**, respectively. Between the two epicondyles, there are two

anterior depressions, the **radial fossa** and **coronoid fossa,** as well as a posterior depression, the single **olecranon fossa.**

Ulna

The most prominent part of the proximal ulna (Fig. 2.11) is the massive **olecranon process**. During full extension of the elbow, it comes to rest in the olecranon fossa of the humerus. On its anterior, proximal side is a C-shaped **trochlear notch** that fits into the trochlea of the humerus. The distal trochlear notch ends with a bony process, the sharp **coronoid process**. Just distal to the coronoid process is the **ulnar tuberosity**. On the lateral, proximal side of the ulna is the **radial notch**, which (not surprisingly) articulates with the head of the radius. The **shaft/body** of the ulna extends distally and becomes narrower as it approaches

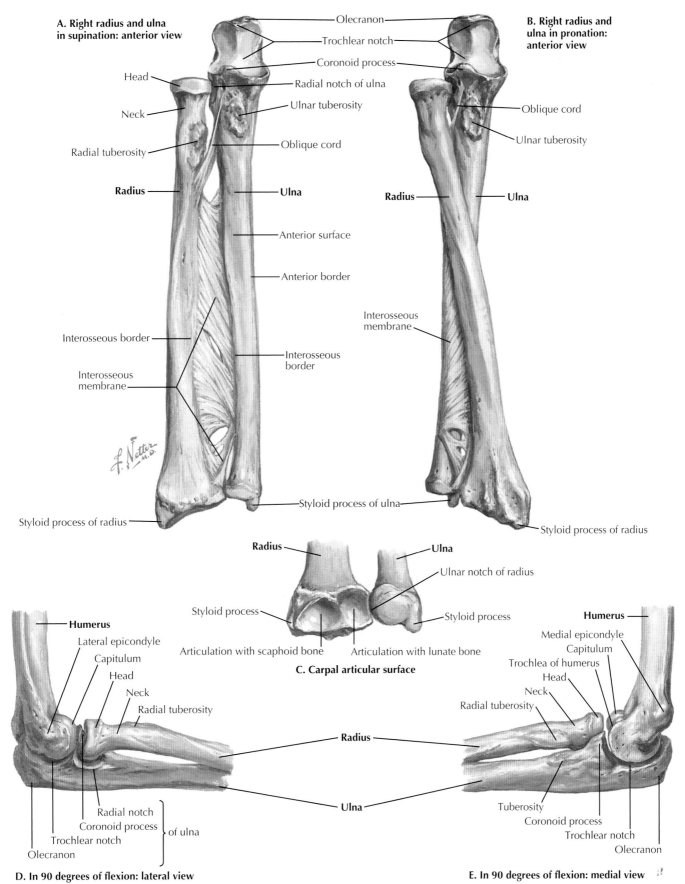

A. Right radius and ulna in supination: anterior view

Olecranon

Trochlear notch

Coronoid process

Head

Neck

Radial notch of ulna

Ulnar tuberosity

Radial tuberosity

Oblique cord

Radius

Ulna

Anterior surface

Anterior border

Interosseous border

Interosseous border

Interosseous membrane

Interosseous membrane

Styloid process of ulna

Styloid process of radius

B. Right radius and ulna in pronation: anterior view

Oblique cord

Ulnar tuberosity

Radius

Ulna

Interosseous membrane

Styloid process of radius

Radius

Ulna

Ulnar notch of radius

Styloid process

Styloid process

Articulation with scaphoid bone

Articulation with lunate bone

C. Carpal articular surface

Humerus

Lateral epicondyle

Capitulum

Head

Neck

Radial tuberosity

Radius

Ulna

Radial notch

Coronoid process

} of ulna

Trochlear notch

Olecranon

D. In 90 degrees of flexion: lateral view

Humerus

Medial epicondyle

Capitulum

Trochlea of humerus

Head

Neck

Radial tuberosity

Radius

Ulna

Tuberosity

Coronoid process

Trochlear notch

Olecranon

E. In 90 degrees of flexion: medial view

Fig. 2.11 Bones of the Forearm and Elbow Joint.

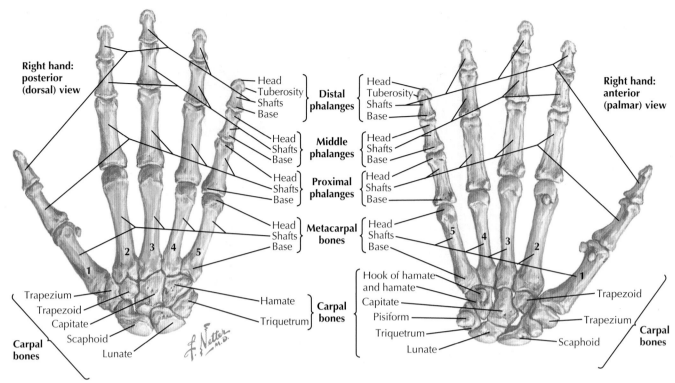

Right hand: posterior (dorsal) view

Right hand: anterior (palmar) view

Head / Tuberosity / Shafts / Base } **Distal phalanges**

Head / Shafts / Base } **Middle phalanges**

Head / Shafts / Base } **Proximal phalanges**

Head / Shafts / Base } **Metacarpal bones**

Trapezium
Trapezoid
Capitate
Scaphoid
Lunate

Carpal bones

Hamate / Triquetrum } **Carpal bones**

Hook of hamate and hamate
Capitate
Pisiform
Triquetrum
Lunate

Trapezoid
Trapezium
Scaphoid

Carpal bones

Fig. 2.12 Bones of the Wrist and Hand.

the smaller **head** of the ulna at its distal end. The medial side of the head ends with a small but distinct **ulnar styloid process**.

Radius

The proximal part of the radius (see Fig. 2.11) is the **head** that articulates with the capitulum of the humerus. It narrows considerably at the **neck** before expanding again as the **shaft** of the radius. The proximal shaft has a notable process, the **radial tuberosity**. The distal end of the radius flares outward, enlarging as it goes. On the medial, distal end is the **ulnar notch** of the radius, which articulates with the head of the ulna. On the opposite, lateral side is a bony process, the **radial styloid process**. The concave, distal extremity of the radius is its **carpal articular surface** that articulates with the proximal row of carpal bones. The shafts of the radius and ulna are connected along their **interosseous borders** by an interosseous membrane.

Carpal Bones

The carpal, or wrist, bones are a collection of eight bones that fit together very tightly and connect the forearm to the hand (Fig. 2.12). Their proximal row is formed by (from lateral to medial) the **scaphoid, lunate, triquetrum,** and **pisiform** bones. The pisiform "breaks rank" with the other bones of the proximal row and sits anteriorly on the triquetrum. The distal row (again, from lateral to medial) is formed by the **trapezium, trapezoid, capitate,** and **hamate** bones. The hamate bone has a very elongated process that extends anteriorly, the **hook of the hamate**.

BONES OF THE HAND AND DIGITS

The hand itself (see Fig. 2.12) contains five long **metacarpal bones** that form the core of the palm. The **base** of each

metacarpal bone associates with one or more distal carpal bones. Each metacarpal has a long **body/shaft** and a **head**, which enlarges as it comes to associate with the bones of the fingers, the **phalanges**. The thumb or **pollux** (first digit) has two segments, formed by a **proximal phalanx** (singular of phalanges) and **distal phalanx**. The fingers (second to fifth digits) have three segments, a **proximal phalanx, middle phalanx,** and **distal phalanx**. Each phalanx appears like a shrunken metacarpal, with a proximal **base, shaft/body,** and distal **head**. The distal phalanges have a flared-out region just proximal to their heads, the **tuberosity of the distal phalanges**.

BONES OF THE PELVIS AND LOWER LIMB

The five segments of the lower limb extend from the vertebrae with a core of bone surrounded by the muscles, vessels, nerves, and skin of the limb itself. The pelvic girdle (sacrum and os coxae) contributes to both the pelvis and the lower limb. The sacrum has already been described in the section on the vertebrae. The segments and their associated bones are the hip (pelvic bones: ilium, ischium, pubis), thigh (femur), leg (tibia and fibula), ankle (tarsal bones), and foot (metatarsal bones and phalanges).

Os Coxae/Hip Bones

The os coxae are complex bones formed by the fusion of three distinct bones, the ilium, ischium, and pubis, that connect to the sacrum, surround the pelvic organs, and meet anteriorly, forming a complete bony ring in the pelvis (Fig. 2.13).

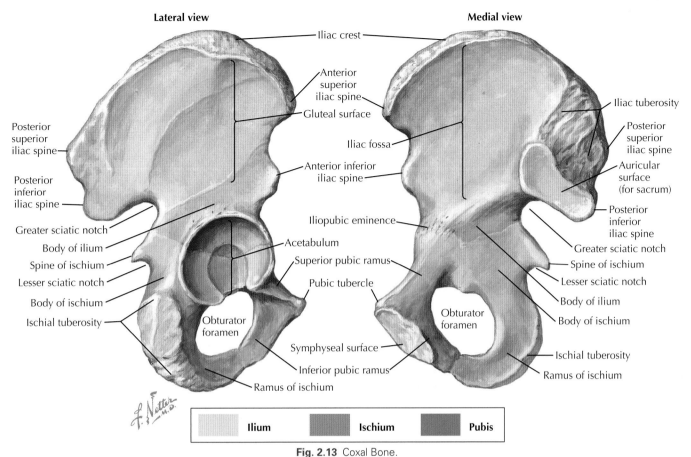

Lateral view

Medial view

Iliac crest

Anterior superior iliac spine

Gluteal surface

Iliac fossa

Anterior inferior iliac spine

Iliopubic eminence

Acetabulum

Superior pubic ramus

Pubic tubercle

Obturator foramen

Symphyseal surface

Inferior pubic ramus

Ramus of ischium

Posterior superior iliac spine

Posterior inferior iliac spine

Greater sciatic notch

Body of ilium

Spine of ischium

Lesser sciatic notch

Body of ischium

Ischial tuberosity

Obturator foramen

Iliac tuberosity

Posterior superior iliac spine

Auricular surface (for sacrum)

Posterior inferior iliac spine

Greater sciatic notch

Spine of ischium

Lesser sciatic notch

Body of ilium

Body of ischium

Ischial tuberosity

Ramus of ischium

Ilium   Ischium   Pubis

Fig. 2.13 Coxal Bone.

Ilium

The ilium is the largest of the three os coxae, and it meets the auricular (ear-shaped) surface of the sacrum at its own **auricular surface** to form a synovial joint between the two. Immediately posterior to it is the **iliac tuberosity**, which gives off a great mass of fibrous connective tissue that anchors the ilium to the sacrum. The **ala/wing** of the ilium extends laterally with smooth inner and outer surfaces that give rise to very large proximal limb muscles. The inner surface of the ala is the **iliac fossa** and the outer surface is the **gluteal surface**. Separating the two fossae is a massive, rough line of bone, the **iliac crest**—extending from posterior to anterior—that anchors many of the abdominal muscles. The iliac crest terminates anteriorly as the **anterior superior iliac spine** and a slightly lower **anterior inferior iliac spine**. Similarly, the iliac crest terminates posteriorly as the **posterior superior iliac spine** with a smaller **posterior inferior iliac spine** just inferior to it. Inferior to the posterior inferior iliac spine is a large indentation, the **greater sciatic notch**. In this area, the ilium transitions into the ischium.

Ischium

At the inferior end of the greater sciatic notch is a very sharp bony extension, the **ischial spine**. The portion of bone just inferior to the ischial spine is another indentation, the **lesser sciatic notch**. At the end of this notch is the most inferior part of the os coxae, the massive **ischial tuberosity**, which is a site of muscle attachment as well as the part of the skeleton that supports our weight when seated. It is often called the "sits" bones by trainers, dancers, and others. Continuing anteriorly from the ischial tuberosity is a strut of bone that connects the ischium and pubis, the **ischial ramus**.

Pubis

The pubis is a V-shaped bone with one leg of the V formed by the **inferior pubic ramus** and the other leg formed by the **superior pubic ramus**. Between the two rami and the ischium is the huge and round **obturator foramen**. The body of the pubis is located where the two rami converge. The left and right pubic bodies meet each other at their **symphyseal surfaces**. On the superior aspect of the pubic body is a bump, the **pubic tubercle**. The superior pubic ramus meets the ilium at the **iliopubic eminence**, just superior to the acetabulum.

Acetabulum

The acetabulum is not a separate bone but is a massive depression in the lateral os coxae at the point where all three bones converge. The depression itself is properly called the **acetabular fossa** and has a surrounding rim of bone that allows it to form a massive ball-in-socket joint with the femoral head.

Femur

The femur is the largest bone in the body (Fig. 2.14). The almost-spherical **head of the femur** articulates with the acetabulum.

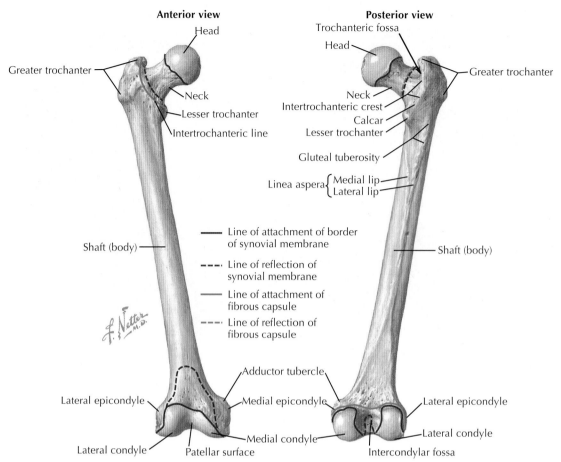

Fig. 2.14 Osteology of the Femur.

An extended **neck** connects the head of the femur to a large knot of bone at the its superior end that is dominated by two large processes: the **greater trochanter** extends superiorly while the **lesser trochanter** projects medially and a bit posteriorly. The medial side of the greater trochanter has a depression, the **trochanteric fossa**. Anteriorly, the two trochanters are connected by a roughened **intertrochanteric line**. Posteriorly the trochanters are connected by a large **intertrochanteric crest**. Inferior to the intertrochanteric crest is the **gluteal tuberosity** that extends inferiorly down the posterior **shaft** of the femur as a line for bony attachment, the **linea aspera**, which has a medial and lateral lip.

The distal end of the femur terminates in two large, smooth articular surfaces, the **medial condyle** and **lateral condyle**. Both femoral condyles extend posteriorly and are separated by the **intercondylar fossa**. Anteriorly the two condyles come together at the smooth **patellar surface**. Extending from each femoral condyle is a ridge of bone that extends superiorly along the shaft, the **lateral epicondyle** and **medial epicondyle**, the latter of which has a prominent **adductor tubercle** projecting superiorly.

Patella

The patella (kneecap) (Fig. 2.15) has a posterior **articular surface** that glides along the patellar surface of the femur. The **anterior surface** is considerably rougher than its posterior articular

surface with a rounded **base** along its superior aspect and an **apex** pointing inferiorly.

Tibia

The tibia (Fig. 2.16) has broad, flat **superior articular surfaces** superior to a **medial condyle** and **lateral condyle** that articulate with the medial and lateral femoral condyles. The tibial condyles are separated from each other by an **intercondylar eminence**. On the proximal tibia, the **anterolateral tubercle** is located inferior to the lateral tibial condyle and the **fibular articular facet** is located just inferior to it. The large **tibial tuberosity** is seen on the proximal, anterior midline of the tibia. A pronounced **soleal line** is present on the upper, posterior shaft and marks one attachment site of the large soleus muscle. The **shaft** continues inferiorly, ending with a lateral **fibular notch**, an **inferior articular surface** for the talus, and a prominent bony process on the medial side, the **medial malleolus**, with its own **articular facet**.

Fibula

The fibula (see Fig. 2.16) is the slender, lateral companion to the tibia. Its **head** has an **articular facet** that meets the fibular articular facet of the tibia. A slight **neck** connects the head to the **body/shaft** of the fibula, which continues inferiorly to end as the **lateral malleolus**, with its own **articular facet**. The shafts of the fibula and tibia are connected along their **interosseous borders** by an interosseous membrane. The lateral malleolus is tethered to the lateral fibular notch of the tibia by connective tissue. The lateral malleolus joins the tibia's inferior articular surface and the medial malleolus to surround and articulate with the first tarsal bone, the talus.

Tarsal Bones

The tarsal, or ankle, bones are a collection of seven bones (talus, calcaneus, navicular, cuboid, medial cuneiform, intermediate cuneiform, and lateral cuneiform) that connect the leg to the rest of the foot (Fig. 2.17). The **talus** has several prominent articular surfaces. On its superior aspect is the large **trochlea of the talus**

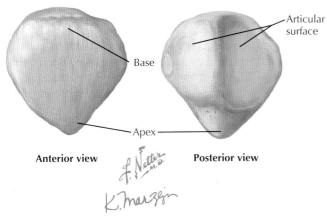

Fig. 2.15 Osteology of the Leg and Knee.

that articulates with the inferior articular surface of the tibia and is wedged in on either side by the medial and lateral malleoli. Anteriorly it articulates with the navicular bone and inferiorly with the calcaneus. The **calcaneus** (heel bone) is the largest tarsal bone. Its posterior side is dominated by the **calcaneal tuberosity**. Anteriorly it articulates with the talus and cuboid bones. Medially it has a shelf of bone, the **sustentaculum tali**, that supports and stabilizes the talus. The **navicular** bone has a broad and concave articular surface where it interacts with the talus. On its opposite, anterior side, it has a convex articular surface for the **medial cuneiform**, **intermediate cuneiform**, and **lateral cuneiform** bones. The anterior aspects of the cuneiform bones have articular surfaces for the first to third metatarsal bones. The **cuboid bone** is located lateral to the navicular and lateral cuneiform bones and has a saddle-shaped **articular surface for the calcaneus** on its posterior aspect. The cuboid bone's anterior surface has articular surfaces for the fourth and fifth metatarsal bones.

BONES OF THE FOOT AND DIGITS

The bones of the foot (see Fig. 2.17) are laid out similarly to the bones of the hand, with five long **metatarsal bones** forming its core. The **base** of each metatarsal bone associates with the cuboid or cuneiform bones. There is a prominent **tuberosity of the fifth metatarsal bone** on its lateral base. Each metatarsal has a long **body/shaft** and a **head** that enlarges as it comes to

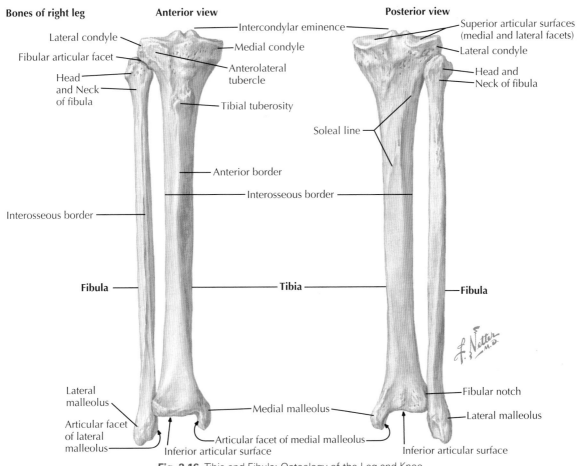

Fig. 2.16 Tibia and Fibula: Osteology of the Leg and Knee.

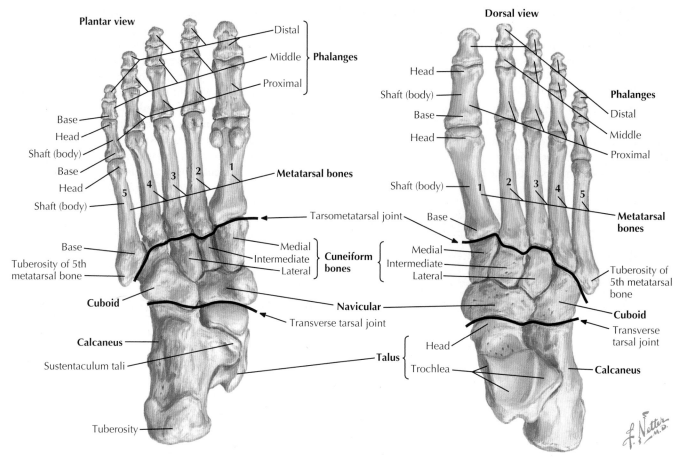

Fig. 2.17 Bones of the Foot.

associate with the bones of the toes, the **phalanges**. The big toe or **hallux** (first digit) has two segments, formed by a **proximal phalanx** and **distal phalanx**. The toes (second to fifth digits) have three segments, a **proximal phalanx**, **middle phalanx**, and **distal phalanx**. Each phalanx has a proximal **base**, **shaft/body**, and distal **head**.

MAJOR JOINTS AND STABILIZING LIGAMENTS

We will discuss how the bones interact, the movements that are allowed by their articulations, and the major connective tissue structures that protect them. Synovial joints (Fig. 2.18) allow smooth movements between adjacent bones. They are surrounded by an outer **fibrous layer** and an inner **synovial layer** that secretes the lubricating **synovial fluid**. The surfaces of bones within the capsule are typically covered by smooth **articular cartilage**. We will revisit the joints and ligaments in more detail in the chapters on the back, upper limbs, lower limbs, and torso.

JOINTS AND LIGAMENTS OF THE HEAD AND UPPER CERVICAL VERTEBRAE

There are many bones in the skull that are connected by connective tissue within the sutures. The only true synovial joint of the skull is the **temporomandibular joint**, which allows the condylar process of the mandible to articulate with the mandibular

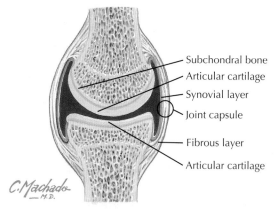

Fig 2.18 Synovial Joint.

fossa of the temporal bone (Fig. 2.19). In life the two bones are separated by an **articular disc** made of tough fibrocartilage and surrounded by the **temporomandibular joint capsule**. The capsule and disc allow the jaw to open and close in a hinge-like motion, but when the mouth is opened wide, the condylar process of the mandible glides anteriorly out of the fossa across the **articular tubercle** of the temporal bone. When the mouth is closed, the condyle returns to a posterior position.

The inferior aspect of the occipital bone has two occipital condyles that flank the foramen magnum. These condyles are biconvex and sit primarily in an anteroposterior orientation. Each occipital condyle meets the biconcave superior articular facets

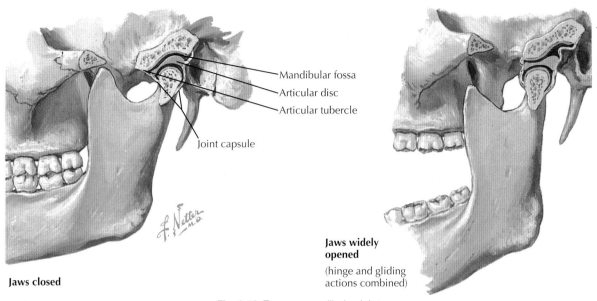

Jaws closed

Mandibular fossa
Articular disc
Articular tubercle
Joint capsule

Jaws widely opened

(hinge and gliding actions combined)

Fig. 2.19 Temporomandibular Joint.

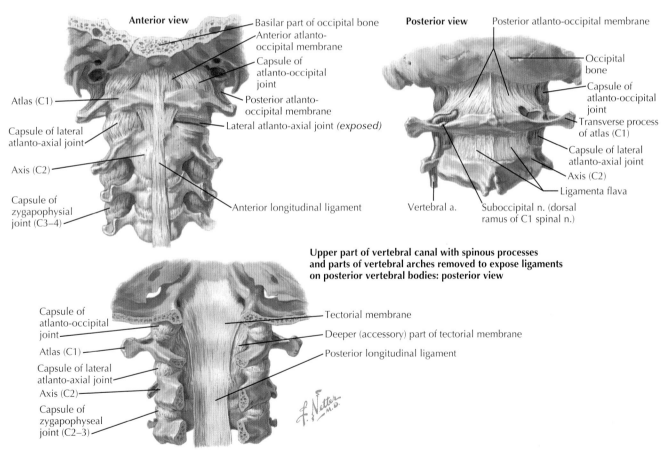

Anterior view

Basilar part of occipital bone
Anterior atlanto-occipital membrane
Capsule of atlanto-occipital joint
Posterior atlanto-occipital membrane
Lateral atlanto-axial joint (exposed)

Atlas (C1)
Capsule of lateral atlanto-axial joint
Axis (C2)
Capsule of zygapophysial joint (C3–4)

Anterior longitudinal ligament

Posterior view

Posterior atlanto-occipital membrane
Occipital bone
Capsule of atlanto-occipital joint
Transverse process of atlas (C1)
Capsule of lateral atlanto-axial joint
Axis (C2)
Ligamenta flava

Vertebral a.
Suboccipital n. (dorsal ramus of C1 spinal n.)

Upper part of vertebral canal with spinous processes and parts of vertebral arches removed to expose ligaments on posterior vertebral bodies: posterior view

Capsule of atlanto-occipital joint
Atlas (C1)
Capsule of lateral atlanto-axial joint
Axis (C2)
Capsule of zygapophyseal joint (C2–3)

Tectorial membrane
Deeper (accessory) part of tectorial membrane
Posterior longitudinal ligament

Fig. 2.20 External Craniocervical Ligaments.

of the atlas (C1) to form the **atlantooccipital joint and capsule**. These joints primarily allow flexion and extension of the head. To test this motion, nod "yes" to signify your understanding. There is a **posterior atlantooccipital membrane** connecting the posterior arch of the atlas to the occipital bone, just posterior to the foramen magnum. A smaller **anterior atlantooccipital membrane** connects the anterior arch of the atlas to the occipital bone.

The **atlantoaxial joint** is composed of three separate articulations (Fig. 2.20). The left and right lateral atlantoaxial joints are formed by the superior facets of the axis (C2) as they meet the inferior facets of the atlas (C1). The dens of the axis extends superiorly from its vertebral body and forms a **median altantoaxial joint** with the **facet for the dens** on the posterior aspect of the anterior arch of the atlas. This allows a great deal of rotation, using the dens as a pivot point,

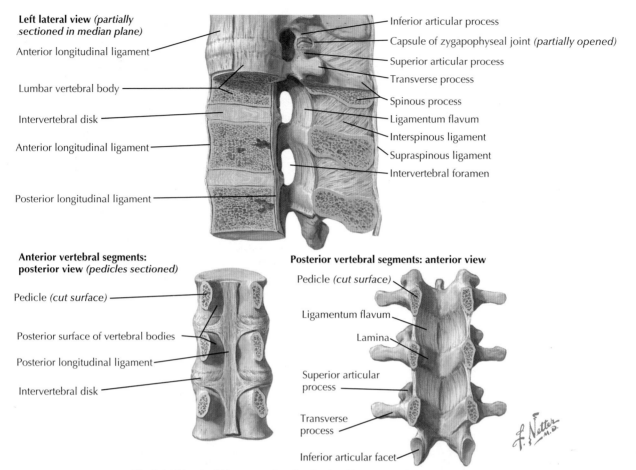

Left lateral view *(partially sectioned in median plane)*

Anterior longitudinal ligament

Lumbar vertebral body

Intervertebral disk

Anterior longitudinal ligament

Posterior longitudinal ligament

Inferior articular process

Capsule of zygapophyseal joint *(partially opened)*

Superior articular process

Transverse process

Spinous process

Ligamentum flavum

Interspinous ligament

Supraspinous ligament

Intervertebral foramen

Anterior vertebral segments: posterior view *(pedicles sectioned)*

Pedicle *(cut surface)*

Posterior surface of vertebral bodies

Posterior longitudinal ligament

Intervertebral disk

Posterior vertebral segments: anterior view

Pedicle *(cut surface)*

Ligamentum flavum

Lamina

Superior articular process

Transverse process

Inferior articular facet

Fig. 2.21 Vertebral Ligaments: Lumbar Region Ligaments of the Spinal Column.

such as when you shake your head "no." The dens is tethered to the atlas and occipital bone by several ligaments that allow movement of the upper cervical vertebra but prevent posterior displacement of the dens. These will be discussed in detail in Chapter 9.

JOINTS AND LIGAMENTS OF THE BACK

The facet joints of the vertebrae from C1 to S1 share several features in common. The articular facet on the inferior articular process of a vertebra meets the articular facet on the superior articular process of the vertebra that is immediately inferior to it. Repeat that tongue twister until it becomes clear. The interaction of an inferior and superior facet is called a vertebral **facet joint** (a.k.a. zygapophyseal joint) and is surrounded by a fibrous joint capsule.

The anterior aspects of the vertebral bodies from the axis (C2) to the sacrum, including their **intervertebral discs**, are connected by a very strong **anterior longitudinal ligament**. It limits extension of the vertebrae. There is a corresponding **posterior longitudinal ligament** on the posterior side of the vertebral bodies that extends from the axis to the sacrum, also including the intervertebral discs (Figs. 2.20 and 2.21). The **tectorial membrane** continues superiorly from the posterior longitudinal ligament and covers the ligaments of the dens before it inserts on the inside of the occipital bone, anterior to the foramen magnum.

Each vertebral arch is connected to its neighboring vertebra by an elastic **ligamentum flavum** that allows flexion to occur

while keeping the vertebral arches connected. Adjacent transverse processes are connected by **intertransverse ligaments** that limit side-bending/lateral flexion. Similarly, adjacent spinous processes are connected by **interspinous ligaments** that limit flexion. Most posteriorly is a long **supraspinous ligament** that connects the tip of each spinous process and significantly limits flexion. In the cervical region it forms a broad, fan-shaped **nuchal ligament** (see Fig. 2.20) that connects the spinous processes of the cervical vertebrae and serves as a site of muscle attachment for the muscles of the posterior neck. The fibers of the nuchal ligament are elastic, allowing a greater degree of flexion than is typically present in the thoracic and lumbar regions.

The lower cervical vertebrae are able to flex and extend, although extension is limited by contact of adjacent spinous processes. Flexion is significant but eventually limited by tension in the nuchal ligament and cervical muscles. Although the majority of head rotation occurs at the atlantoaxial joint, some rotation and lateral flexion (side-bending) does occur in the lower cervical region. In the thoracic region, flexion is permitted but limited by tension of the supraspinous ligament, while extension is severely limited by the inferiorly directed spinous processes of the thoracic vertebrae. The ribs constrain movements of the thoracic vertebrae, allowing only a small degree of lateral flexion and rotation. The lumbar vertebrae are able to flex and extend easily but are more limited in lateral flexion and rotation.

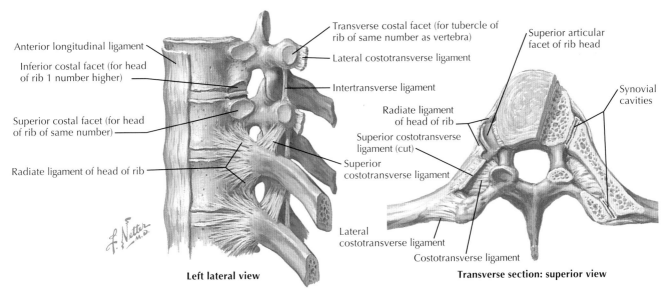

Left lateral view

Transverse section: superior view

Fig. 2.22 Joints of the Thoracic Spine.

JOINTS AND LIGAMENTS OF THE THORAX

Each thoracic vertebra articulates with one or two ribs (Fig. 2.22) at the **joint of the head of the rib**. The head of each rib is covered by a **radiate ligament of the head of the rib** that extends from the costal neck to the vertebral bodies at the costal facet or demifacet joints. It keeps the head of the rib in place and allows a bit of superior and inferior "rocking." The ribs also articulate with the anterior side of each thoracic vertebra's transverse processes at a point called the **transverse costal facet**. Several **costotransverse ligaments** connect the neck and tubercle of the rib to the transverse processes of nearby thoracic vertebrae. These ligaments stabilize the ribs and prevent gross movements but allow the ribs to pivot into an elevated and depressed position during inspiration and expiration, respectively. Because the body of the rib extends so far anteriorly, a small amount of movement posteriorly at the costal head can translate to large movements anteriorly.

Anteriorly, the body of each rib gives off a cartilaginous continuation, the **costal cartilages** (Fig. 2.23). The left and right first costal cartilages attach to the lateral side of the manubrium. The second costal cartilages attach at the point where the manubrium and sternal body articulate. The costal cartilages of the "true" ribs 3 to 7 attach along the sternal body and are anchored in place by the **radiate sternocostal ligaments**. The costal cartilages of the remaining "false" ribs 8 to 10 insert on the costal cartilage of their superior neighbor. Costal cartilages of the "floating" ribs 11 and 12 do not meet the sternum or other costal cartilages.

JOINTS AND LIGAMENTS OF THE UPPER LIMB

Sternoclavicular Joint

The **sternoclavicular joint** is the only direct bone-to-bone link that the upper limb has to the torso (see Fig. 2.23). The clavicular notch of the manubrium forms a depression in which the sternal end of the clavicle sits. Because the surfaces

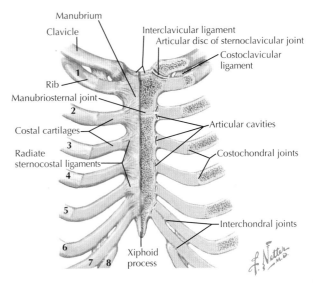

Note: On left side of the rib cage, the sternum and proximal ribs have been shaved down and the ligaments removed to show the bone marrow and articular cavities.

Fig. 2.23 Ribs and Sternocostal Joints: Anterior View.

of these bones do not fit together, there is an **articular disc** present between the two bones that allows them to interact. The articular disc is connected to the articular capsule of the joint, which is reinforced by capsular ligaments on its anterior, posterior, and superior side. Just lateral to the sternoclavicular joint is a stout **costoclavicular ligament** connecting the inferior side of the clavicle to the first rib. The presence of the articular disc proximally allows the distal clavicle to move anteriorly, posteriorly, superiorly, or inferiorly along with a little bit of rotation (Biomechanics Box 2.1).

Acromioclavicular Joint

The **acromioclavicular joint** (Fig. 2.24) is formed by the distal, acromial end of the clavicle and the acromion of the scapula. It is enclosed by a very strong and tight acromioclavicular

---

BIOMECHANICS 2.1   **Clavicular Movement and the Shoulder**

Place the thumb of one hand on the sternal end of the clavicle on the opposite side of your body. Leaving it there, place another finger on the acromion. Now move your shoulder in a superior, inferior, anterior, and posterior direction while palpating and noting the motions occurring at the sternal end of the clavicle. Wave your arm up and down to feel the rotation that occurs with small movements at the sternal end becoming more expansive at the acromial end.

capsule, reinforced by a strong acromioclavicular ligament. It is nearly immobile and serves to keep the two bones tightly connected. There is often fibrocartilage between the bones but not always a complete disc. The inferior side of the distal clavicle is tethered to the superior aspect of the scapula's coracoid process by two **coracoclavicular ligaments** (Clinical Correlation 2.1). Although these two ligaments, the trapezoid and conoid ligaments, are distinct, they are very close together, have similar functions, and tend to be damaged simultaneously. A broad and surprisingly strong **coracoacromial ligament** connects the acromion to the lateral aspect of the coracoid process. Because both the acromion and coracoid process are part of the scapula, damage to this ligament is infrequent. Just medial to the coracoid process is the suprascapular notch, which is covered by a small but strong **superior transverse scapular ligament**.

Scapulothoracic Joint

The **scapulothoracic joint** is a very unusual articulation. It is not a synovial joint and has no capsule. Rather, it denotes the interaction between the anterior aspect of the scapula (which in life is covered by muscles and fascia) and the lateral ribcage. This interaction allows the motions of the scapula (elevation, depression, protraction, retraction, superior rotation, inferior rotation) as it glides.

Glenohumeral Joint

As we have seen, there are several articulations around the shoulder, but when people talk casually about the "shoulder joint" they are typically referring to the **glenohumeral joint** (see Fig. 2.24), where the head of the humerus articulates with the glenoid cavity. Because this fossa is so shallow, this joint is tremendously mobile. It can flex and extend, abduct and adduct, and internally and externally rotate. It can also circumduct, moving through several motions simultaneously. As it approaches limits in abduction, flexion, and extension, the scapula itself moves to shift the angle of the glenohumeral joint. This mobility comes at the cost of stability (Clinical Correlation 2.2). To deepen the articulation and provide a bit more surface area, there is a fibrocartilage ring around the outside of the glenoid fossa named the **glenoid labrum** (Clinical Correlation 2.3). The glenohumeral joint capsule surrounds the joint and has strong intracapsular ligaments that are not visible from the outside but are more distinct from within the joint. The capsule and overlying muscles keep the head of the humerus settled in the glenoid fossa to prevent dislocation. Nearby, the **transverse humeral ligament** forms a bridge across the greater tubercle and lesser tubercle on the proximal humerus.

Elbow Joint

The **elbow joint** is often treated as a single joint that primarily allows flexion and extension. However, it is more properly treated as a combination of three distinct articulations: the humeroulnar, humeroradial, and proximal radioulnar joints (Fig. 2.25).

The **humeroulnar joint** occurs between the trochlea of the humerus and trochlear notch of the ulna. This joint allows a great deal of flexion and extension. Flexion is limited by the coronoid process reaching the coronoid fossa of the distal humerus. Likewise, extension is limited by the olecranon process reaching the olecranon fossa of the humerus. The medial side of the ulna is connected to the medial, distal side of the humerus by a strong, fan-shaped ligament, the **ulnar collateral ligament** (also known as the medial collateral ligament of the elbow).

The **humeroradial joint** occurs between the capitulum of the humerus and the articular facet of the head of the radius. The radial head rotates around the capitulum, causing the forearm and hand to supinate (palm facing superiorly) or to pronate (palm facing inferiorly). A **radial collateral ligament** (a.k.a. lateral collateral ligament of the elbow) connects the annular

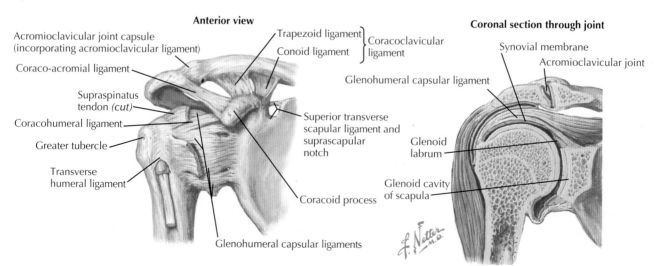

Fig. 2.24 Joints and Ligaments of the Shoulder.

CLINICAL CORRELATION 2.1   Shoulder Separation

Damage to the **acromioclavicular joint** and ligament, potentially also involving the **coracoclavicular ligaments**, is called a **shoulder separation**. This occurs when downward pressure is placed on the lateral shoulder, depressing the acromion. In a grade I shoulder separation, the acromioclavicular capsule is damaged but not ruptured. A grade II separation occurs when the acromioclavicular capsule is completely disrupted; the coracoclavicular ligaments may be stretched but keep the clavicle attached to the scapula. Additional downward force can cause a grade III separation, which causes complete rupture of the acromioclavicular and the coracoclavicular ligaments. The shoulder, now detached from the clavicle, will drop while the trapezius and sternocleidomastoid muscles will elevate the distal clavicle, creating a bump in the lateral neck.

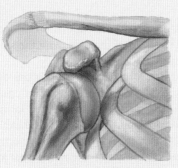

Injury to acromioclavicular joint. Usually caused by fall on tip of shoulder, depressing acromion (shoulder separation)

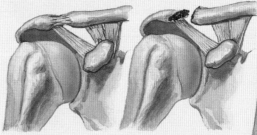

Grade I. Acromioclavicular ligaments stretched but not torn; coracoclavicular ligaments intact

Grade II. Acromioclavicular ligaments ruptured and joint separated; coracoclavicular ligaments intact

Grade III. Coracoclavicular and acromioclavicular ligaments rupture with wide separation of joint

Fig. CC2.1 Acromioclavicular Joint Injuries.

CLINICAL CORRELATION 2.2   Shoulder Dislocation

When the **head of the humerus** is displaced from the **glenoid fossa**, a **shoulder dislocation** has occurred. Depending on the nature of the dislocation, the humeral head may rest posteriorly, inferiorly, or anteriorly. Anteriorly, it may come to rest inferior to the coracoid process, glenoid cavity, or the clavicle.

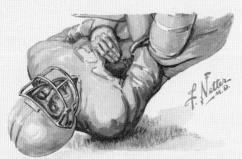

Subcoracoid dislocation

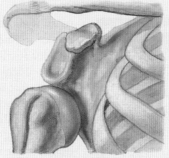

Subglenoid dislocation

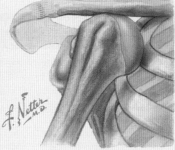

Subclavicular dislocation

Fig. CC2.2 Anterior Dislocation of Glenohumeral Joint.

CLINICAL CORRELATION 2.3   Labral Tears

The **glenoid labrum** can become damaged by excessive movement of the humeral head, arthritis, or trauma. **Fibrocartilage** heals slowly, and damage to the labrum often results in pain, clicking, and "catching" of the joint as the arm moves.

ligament to the distal, lateral aspect of the humerus (Clinical Correlation 2.4).

A circular **annular ligament** wraps around the head and neck of the radius. This keeps the radial head in place during pronation and supination. Medially the annular ligament attaches to either side of the ulna's radial notch, and on the lateral side it is connected to the radial collateral ligament. This keeps the head of the radius in close contact with the radial notch of the ulna, forming the **proximal radioulnar joint**, which also allows for pronation and supination.

The **interosseous membrane** is not a joint per se but is a collection of connective tissue fibers that tether the shaft of the ulna to the shaft of the radius. It allows pronation and supination but keeps the two bones connected even when one or both are fractured.

Wrist Joint

Like the elbow, the wrist is a complex joint that is formed from a number of smaller articulations (Fig. 2.26). The distal radius and ulna interact with the proximal row of carpal bones, and each carpal bone articulates with its neighbors. There are many small ligaments connecting these bones (Clinical Correlation 2.5). To

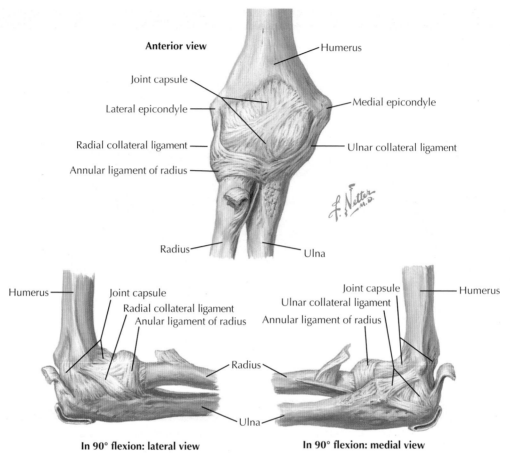

Anterior view

Humerus

Joint capsule

Lateral epicondyle

Medial epicondyle

Radial collateral ligament

Ulnar collateral ligament

Annular ligament of radius

Radius

Ulna

Humerus

Joint capsule

Radial collateral ligament

Anular ligament of radius

Joint capsule

Ulnar collateral ligament

Annular ligament of radius

Humerus

Radius

Ulna

In 90° flexion: lateral view

In 90° flexion: medial view

Fig. 2.25 Ligaments of the Elbow.

CLINICAL CORRELATION 2.4   Nursemaid's Elbow

The **radial head** of children is scarcely any larger than the **radial neck**. Because of this, sudden traction on the hand or forearm can **displace the radial head from the annular ligament**. This causes immediate pain and guarding of the affected elbow.

Fig. CC2.4 Dislocation of Radius at Elbow (Nursemaid's Elbow).

simplify this situation, we will divide the wrist into the following joints: the distal radioulnar, radiocarpal, midcarpal, and carpometacarpal articulations, and examine only a few ligaments.

The **distal radioulnar joint** is formed by the head of the ulna, the ulnar notch of the radius, and the **articular disc** of the wrist; it allows pronation and supination to occur. The radius rotates around the head of the ulna, with the styloid process of the ulna serving as the axis of rotation.

The articular disc forms a fibrocartilage cap over the head of the ulna that is continuous with the carpal articular surface of the radius; this articular surface is concave and forms the proximal side of the **radiocarpal joint**. The scaphoid, lunate, and triquetrum form the joint's distal, convex surface. The pisiform does not contribute to the radiocarpal joint. The radiocarpal joint has a great degree of freedom because the bones that form it are concave/convex in two planes. This allows the wrist to flex and extend (better at flexion) as well as to abduct and adduct, which is referred to as radial deviation and ulnar deviation (better at ulnar deviation).

The **midcarpal joint** is the collection of articulations of the proximal row of carpal bones with the distal row. Its complex articular surface does not allow as much movement as the radiocarpal joint, but it does allow some flexion/extension (better at extension) and ulnar/radial deviation (better at radial deviation).

For both the radiocarpal and intercarpal joint, flexion/extension is limited by muscle tension as well as some ligaments on both sides of the wrist, the **dorsal radiocarpal**, **dorsal ulnocarpal**, **palmar radiocarpal**, and **palmar ulnocarpal ligaments**. Many other ligaments connect the carpal and metacarpal bones to each other but will not be discussed here. Radial/ulnar deviation is significantly limited by collateral ligaments on each side. The **radial collateral ligament** of the wrist connects the radial styloid process to the scaphoid, trapezium, and first metacarpal, while the **ulnar collateral ligament** connects the ulnar styloid process to the triquetrum and pisiform.

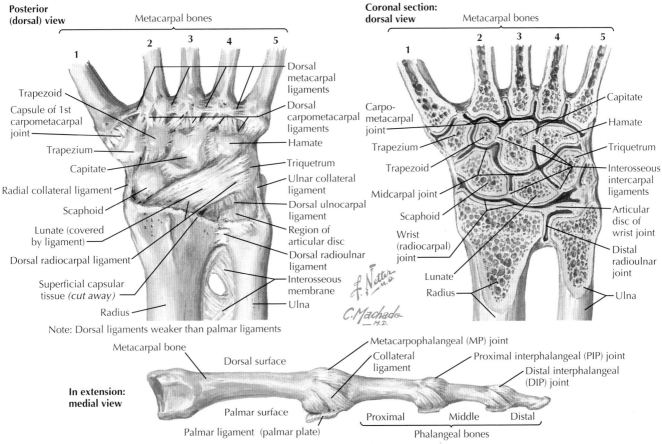

Fig. 2.26 Joints and Ligaments of the Wrist and Hand.

Labels (left, Posterior (dorsal) view — Metacarpal bones): Trapezoid; Capsule of 1st carpometacarpal joint; Trapezium; Capitate; Radial collateral ligament; Scaphoid; Lunate (covered by ligament); Dorsal radiocarpal ligament; Superficial capsular tissue (cut away); Radius; Dorsal metacarpal ligaments; Dorsal carpometacarpal ligaments; Hamate; Triquetrum; Ulnar collateral ligament; Dorsal ulnocarpal ligament; Region of articular disc; Dorsal radioulnar ligament; Interosseous membrane; Ulna. Note: Dorsal ligaments weaker than palmar ligaments

Labels (right, Coronal section: dorsal view — Metacarpal bones): Carpometacarpal joint; Trapezium; Trapezoid; Midcarpal joint; Scaphoid; Wrist (radiocarpal) joint; Lunate; Radius; Capitate; Hamate; Triquetrum; Interosseous intercarpal ligaments; Articular disc of wrist joint; Distal radioulnar joint; Ulna.

Labels (bottom, In extension: medial view): Metacarpal bone; Dorsal surface; Palmar surface; Palmar ligament (palmar plate); Metacarpophalangeal (MP) joint; Collateral ligament; Proximal interphalangeal (PIP) joint; Distal interphalangeal (DIP) joint; Proximal; Middle; Distal; Phalangeal bones.

CLINICAL CORRELATION 2.5 Carpal Tunnel Syndrome

Despite its narrow bore, there are nine tendons and one nerve that travel through the **carpal tunnel** to reach the hand. Because the **flexor retinaculum** is so strong, the carpal tunnel cannot expand when there is inflammation in the space. Therefore inflammation associated with the tendons will put pressure on the nerve, causing motor and sensory losses in the lateral palm.

Flexor retinaculum (transverse carpal ligament)
Median n.*
Flexor tendons*
Hamate
Capitate
Trapezoid
Trapezium
*Contents of carpal tunnel

Fig. CC2.5 Cross Section of Wrist: Carpal Tunnel.

The **carpometacarpal joints** are the articulations that exist between the distal row of carpal bones and the bases of metacarpals 1 to 5. The articulation involving the first metacarpal and thumb is often treated separately because it has several unique features. The first metacarpal articulates only with the trapezium via a saddle-shaped surface that allows flexion/extension and adduction/abduction. A combination of thumb abduction, flexion, and adduction creates a movement that brings the thumb in contact with the other digits, called opposition.

The bases of metacarpals 2 to 5 each articulate with the distal row of carpal bones and their neighboring metacarpals. The carpometacarpal joints allow a small degree of flexion/extension (biased toward flexion) so that objects can be "cupped" in the palm. Abduction of metacarpals 2 to 5 is prevented by the **deep transverse metacarpal ligament**, which connects their heads. Palmar and dorsal metacarpal ligaments and carpometacarpal ligaments stabilize these joints. As a whole, the carpal and metacarpal bones are concave on the palmar side. This is reinforced by the **flexor retinaculum**, a very strong band of connective tissue that connects the trapezium to the pisiform and hamate bones more medially. This forms a "roof" over the space, the **carpal tunnel**.

Joints of the Digits

Digits 2 to 5 each have metacarpophalangeal (MCP), proximal interphalangeal (PIP), and distal interphalangeal (DIP) joints that allow the fingers to move (see Fig. 2.26). Digit 1, the thumb or pollux, has an MCP joint but only one interphalangeal joint because it has no middle phalanx.

At the MCP joints, the head of each metacarpal is rounded and fits into a shallow depression at the base of each proximal phalanx. There are stout **medial collateral** and **lateral collateral ligaments** on each side of the MCP. These ligaments allow for significant flexion and extension. The collateral ligaments of the MCP joint are tense in flexion and loose in extension. This makes adduction/abduction of the digits possible when the MCP is extended but not when flexed. Lastly, there are **palmar ligaments** (palmar plates) that stabilize the palmar side of the MCP. They limit extension of the MCP and also connect to the deep transverse metacarpal ligament.

CLINICAL CORRELATION 2.6   Damage to the Palmar Ligaments

Hyperextension of the metacarpophalangeal, proximal interphalangeal, or distal interphalangeal can tear the fibers of the palmar ligaments. If the digit is not kept in an extended position shortly thereafter, these ligaments may heal in a contracted state, leaving the affected joint permanently flexed to some degree.

The PIP and DIP **joints** are very similar to the MCP, with **medial collateral**, **lateral collateral**, and **palmar ligaments** limiting abduction, adduction, and extension. One difference is that the collateral ligaments of the PIP and DIP are tight in both flexion and extension, so no abduction or adduction is possible at those joints unless the result of trauma (Clinical Correlation 2.6).

JOINTS AND LIGAMENTS OF THE PELVIS AND LOWER LIMB

Sacroiliac Joint

The articulation of the auricular (ear-shaped) surface of the sacrum with the auricular surface of the ilium forms the synovial **sacroiliac joint**. Because this joint has to accommodate the forces transferred between each lower limb to the rest of the body, it needs to be very stable. The synovial joint is reinforced by strong ligaments (Fig. 2.27). The **posterior**

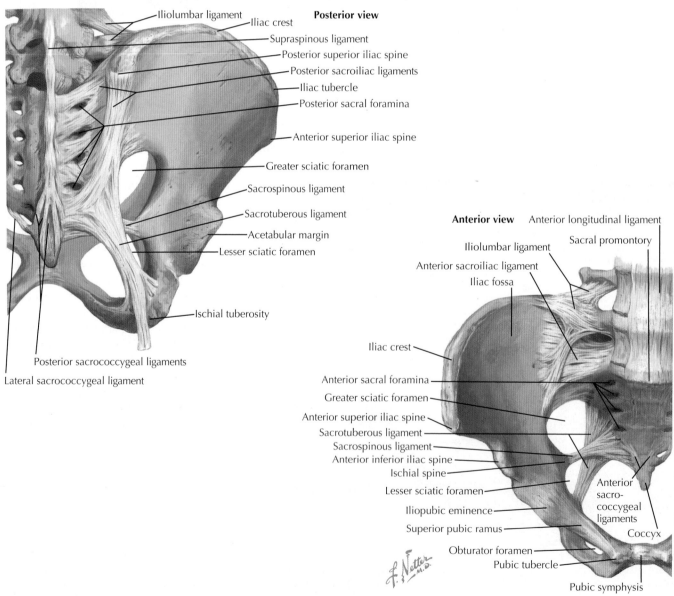

Fig. 2.27 Bones and Ligaments of the Pelvis.

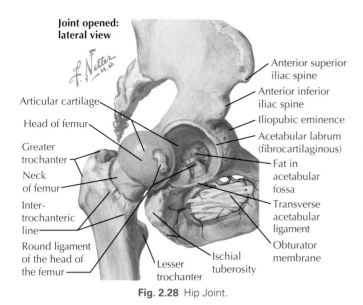

Joint opened: lateral view

Articular cartilage
Head of femur
Greater trochanter
Neck of femur
Intertrochanteric line
Round ligament of the head of the femur
Lesser trochanter
Ischial tuberosity
Anterior superior iliac spine
Anterior inferior iliac spine
Iliopubic eminence
Acetabular labrum (fibrocartilaginous)
Fat in acetabular fossa
Transverse acetabular ligament
Obturator membrane

Fig. 2.28 Hip Joint.

sacroiliac ligaments fill in the deep space between the ilium and the posterior aspect of the sacrum. The **anterior sacroiliac ligament** connects the iliac crest to the ala of the sacrum and forms the anterior border of the synovial sacroiliac joint. It is supplemented by ligaments extending from the transverse processes of L4 and L5 to the iliac crest, the **iliolumbar ligaments**.

The sacrum is further stabilized by two strong ligaments that pass between it and the ischium. The **sacrotuberous ligament** continues inferiorly from the posterior sacroiliac ligament and tethers the lateral sacrum to the ischial tuberosity. The nearby **sacrospinous ligament** connects the anterolateral sacrum to the ischial spine. In addition to stabilization, these ligaments form two foramina that are not visible when examining dry bones. They enclose the greater and lesser sciatic notches to create the **greater sciatic foramen** and **lesser sciatic foramen**, which allow muscles, nerves, and vessels to leave the pelvis and reach the lower limb. Lastly, **anterior, lateral,** and **posterior sacrococcygeal ligaments** keep the coccyx attached to the apex of the sacrum.

Hip Joint

The **coxofemoral joint** (Fig. 2.28) is commonly known as the hip joint but can be confused with the nearby sacroiliac joint when people are describing pain in the region. It is formed by the articulation of the head of the femur with the acetabulum. A stout **acetabular labrum** made of fibrocartilage deepens the cavity in which the head of the femur sits, allowing this ball-and-socket joint to flex/extend, abduct/adduct, and internally/externally rotate without dislocating. The acetabular labrum is discontinuous along its inferior border but is bridged by the **transverse acetabular ligament**. Along with the labrum, the capsule surrounding the joint is one of the major factors in limiting its motion. It has strong intracapsular ligaments that are not visible from the outside but are more distinct from within the joint. A small **round ligament of femur** connects a shallow fovea on the head of the femur to the acetabular notch.

Nearby is the ligamentous **obturator membrane** covering the obturator foramen.

Knee Joint

The knee joint (Fig. 2.29) consists of the **patellofemoral** and **tibiofemoral** articulations. The articular surface of the patella sits within the aptly named patellar surface of the femur. The two femoral condyles on either side keep the patella "on track" as it glides during flexion and extension of the knee. The patella is linked directly to the tibial tuberosity by the **patellar ligament**.

The **tibiofemoral articulation** allows a tremendous degree of flexion and extension. This occurs as the medial and lateral femoral condyles glide across the medial and lateral articular surfaces of the tibial condyles. Because the tibial articular surfaces are flat, this joint tends to be unstable and requires considerable support from connective tissue structures. The **medial meniscus** and **lateral meniscus** are fibrocartilage discs that slightly deepen the articulations between the femur and the tibia.

In between the medial and lateral menisci and on either side of the intercondylar eminence of the tibia are two ligaments that connect the tibial and femur. The **anterior cruciate ligament** originates anteriorly on the tibia and inserts more posteriorly on the intercondylar fossa of the femur. Likewise, the **posterior cruciate ligament** originates just posterior to the tibia's intercondylar eminence and inserts more anteriorly on intercondylar fossa of the femur. These ligaments prevent the tibia from sliding anteriorly or posteriorly relative to the femur.

A very strong thickening of the capsule of the knee forms an intracapsular ligament on its medial side that connects the medial tibia and femur. This is the **tibial (medial) collateral ligament** of the knee, and it also connects to the medial meniscus. A **fibular (lateral) collateral ligament** of the knee connects the fibular head to the lateral, distal femur. It is not part of the knee joint capsule and does not connect to the lateral meniscus (Clinical Correlation 2.7).

Tibiofibular Joints

The tibia and fibula have three distinct articulations (Fig. 2.30). The **proximal tibiofibular joint** is a synovial joint that is connected by two intracapsular ligaments, the **anterior ligament of the fibular head** and the **posterior ligament of the fibular head**. It allows a small degree of shifting superiorly and inferiorly as the ankle moves through the full range of dorsiflexion and plantarflexion. The **interosseous membrane**, like its counterpart in the upper limb, is a sheet of connective tissue that tethers the medial aspect of the fibular shaft to the lateral tibia. It keeps the two bones connected even when fractured.

Inferiorly, the **distal tibiofibular joint** keeps the lateral malleolus in contact with the fibular notch of the distal tibia. This is not a synovial joint but a synchondrosis, an articulation created entirely by connective tissue that tethers the two bones together. Two strong ligaments, the **anterior tibiofibular ligament** and **posterior tibiofibular ligament** are part of this joint.

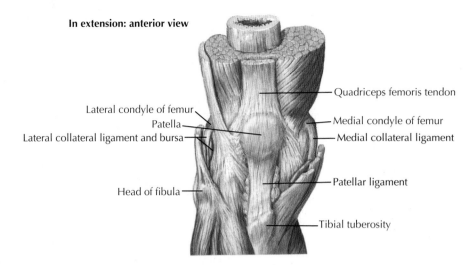

In extension: anterior view

Lateral condyle of femur
Patella
Lateral collateral ligament and bursa

Head of fibula

Quadriceps femoris tendon
Medial condyle of femur
Medial collateral ligament

Patellar ligament

Tibial tuberosity

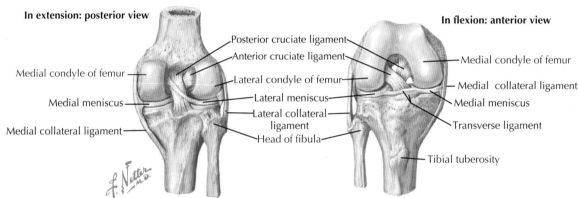

In extension: posterior view

Posterior cruciate ligament
Anterior cruciate ligament
Medial condyle of femur
Lateral condyle of femur
Medial meniscus
Lateral meniscus
Lateral collateral ligament
Medial collateral ligament
Head of fibula

In flexion: anterior view

Medial condyle of femur
Medial collateral ligament
Medial meniscus
Transverse ligament
Tibial tuberosity

Fig. 2.29 Leg: Knee Joint and Ligaments.

CLINICAL CORRELATION 2.7   Damage to the Connective Tissue Structures of the Knee

Ligaments are relatively inelastic. Because of the powerful forces that the knee encounters and its high degree of mobility, damage to the menisci or nearby ligaments is common. If the leg is deflected laterally, the **tibial (medial) collateral ligament** will be stretched and possibly ruptured. Likewise, medial deflection will stress the **fibular (lateral) collateral ligament**. Continued lateral or medial deflection and rotation may cause the femur and tibia to pinch and damage the menisci. Rotation, deflection, or anterior/posterior translation of the tibia can also damage the **anterior cruciate ligament** or **posterior cruciate ligament**.

Posterior cruciate ligament
Anterior cruciate ligament (ruptured)

Fig. CC2.7 Rupture of the Anterior Cruciate Ligament.

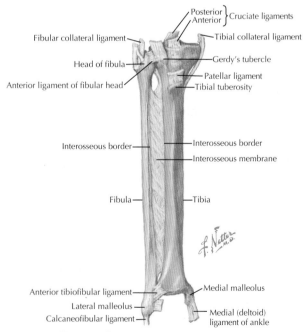

Posterior
Anterior } Cruciate ligaments
Fibular collateral ligament
Tibial collateral ligament
Head of fibula
Gerdy's tubercle
Patellar ligament
Anterior ligament of fibular head
Tibial tuberosity
Interosseous border
Interosseous border
Interosseous membrane
Fibula
Tibia
Anterior tibiofibular ligament
Medial malleolus
Lateral malleolus
Medial (deltoid) ligament of ankle
Calcaneofibular ligament

Fig. 2.30 Tibia and Fibula: Anterior View.

Ankle Joints

The ankle (Fig. 2.31) or **tibiotarsal joint** occurs between the inferior articular surface of the tibia and the trochlea of the talus. The trochlea of the talus is confined by the medial and lateral malleoli but is able to plantarflex and dorsiflex the foot. Because the trochlea is narrow posteriorly, the foot can be moved from side-to-side when plantarflexed. However, because the trochlea is wider anteriorly, when the foot is dorsiflexed it is difficult to move the foot medially or laterally.

Because the movements of the ankle are sophisticated, the ligaments that stabilize the area are complex. On the lateral side is a set of three ligaments. The **anterior talofibular ligament (ATFL)** connects the lateral malleolus to the anterior body of the talus. Just posterior to it is the **calcaneofibular ligament (CFL)**, which connects the lateral aspect of the calcaneus to the inferior tip of the lateral malleolus. Most posteriorly is the very deep **posterior talofibular ligament (PTFL)**, connecting the posterior aspect of the lateral malleolus to the posterior body of the talus (Clinical Correlation 2.8).

On the medial side of the ankle is a complex of four ligaments that connect the medial malleolus of the tibia to the talus, calcaneus, and navicular bones. Because these ligaments are fused and shaped (approximately) like a triangle, they are given the group name, the **deltoid ligament**.

Joints of the Foot

A staggering number of joints and ligaments connect the tarsal bones (see Fig. 2.31). We will discuss only a few of the more clinically important ones. The **subtalar joint** is most commonly defined as the articulations between the talus and calcaneus bones, and it is where most inversion/eversion of

the foot occurs. On the plantar aspect of the foot are several ligaments that keep the tarsal bones together and maintain the longitudinal arch of the foot. Of these, the **long plantar ligament** passes from the calcaneus to the cuboid and third and fourth metatarsal bases. Deep to it is the **short plantar ligament**, which also passes between the calcaneus and cuboid. More medially is the **plantar calcaneonavicular (spring) ligament** that prevents the calcaneus and navicular bones from separating from each other despite the significant weight the talus places on them with each step.

Joints of the Digits

Digits 2 to 5 each have metatarsophalangeal, PIP, and DIP joints that allow the toes to move (Fig. 2.32). Digit 1, the big toe or hallux, has a metatarsophalangeal joint but only one interphalangeal joint because it has no middle phalanx.

At the **metatarsophalangeal** joints, the head of each metatarsal is rounded and fit into a shallow depression at the base of each proximal phalanx. There is a stout **medial collateral ligament** and **lateral collateral ligament** on each side. These ligaments allow for a significant amount of flexion and extension. Lastly, there are **plantar ligaments (plates)** that stabilize the palmar side of the metatarsophalangeal joint and limit extension. The **PIP** and **DIP joints** are very similar to the metatarsophalangeal joint, with **medial collateral**, **lateral collateral**, and **plantar ligaments** limiting abduction, adduction, and extension.

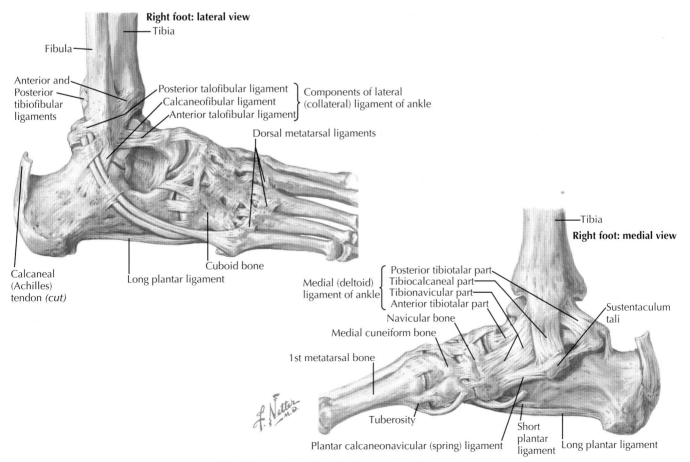

Fig 2.31 Ankle and Foot: Ankle Joints and Ligaments.

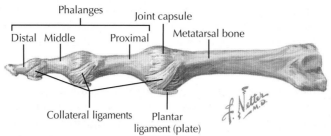

Fig. 2.32 Capsules and Ligaments of the Metatarsophalangeal and Interphalangeal Joints.

CLINICAL CORRELATION 2.8   Damage to Ligaments of the Ankle

When the foot and ankle are forced into **inversion/adduction**, the ligaments on the lateral aspect of the ankle rupture from anterior to posterior: first the **anterior talofibular ligament**, then the **calcaneofibular**, and finally the **posterior talofibular ligament**. The ankle becomes more unstable as more ligaments are ruptured. When the foot and ankle are forced into **eversion/abduction**, the **deltoid ligament** on the medial aspect of the ankle is stressed. Because this ligament is so strong, it is very common for the ligament to rip the medial malleolus from the tibia. A fracture of this type, where a ligament or tendon pulls and fractures a bone, is an **avulsion fracture**. A different injury occurs when the distal fibula and tibia are pulled apart, rupturing the distal tibiofibular ligaments. This is called a "**high ankle sprain.**"

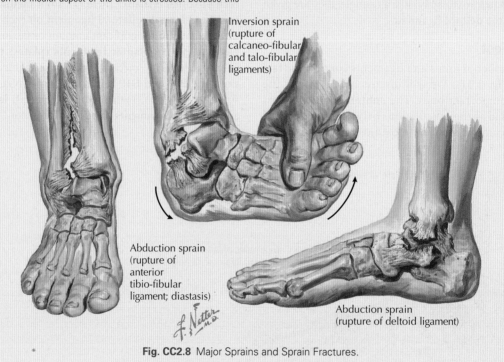

Fig. CC2.8 Major Sprains and Sprain Fractures.

Overview of Muscle Groups and Their Functions

INTRODUCTION

There are many individual muscles in the body, and each has distinctive sites of attachment. When muscles are active, they contract and pull those attachment sites together. They are unable to actively lengthen and are typically stretched passively as their attachment sites move away from each other. Muscles attach to bones through tendons, which are dense bundles of connective tissue that are continuous with the connective tissue within the muscle itself. These are different from ligaments, which attach from bone to bone without an intervening muscle.

The specifics of each muscle will be explored in detail in later chapters. In this chapter we will investigate the large muscles and muscle groups in each region of the body to get a big-picture view of their function. Muscle compartments are separated from each other by sheets of connective tissue that surround them and attach to the underlying bones. These sheets of connective tissue are called **deep fascia**. The individual muscles within a compartment are separated by thinner layers of connective tissue called **epimysium**. An important sheet of deep fascia, the **thoracolumbar fascia**, surrounds and supports many muscles in the back. Once the locations and functions of these muscle groups are understood, we will move on to the nerves that innervate each compartment.

MUSCLE GROUPS OF THE BACK

Extrinsic Back Muscles

The most superficial muscles of the back are the **extrinsic back muscles: latissimus dorsi, trapezius, rhomboid major and minor, and levator scapulae** (Fig. 3.1). They are called extrinsic because they did not originate in the back but migrated there and primarily act to move the upper limb rather than the back itself.

Latissimus Dorsi

- *Attachments*: The latissimus dorsi is a broad, flat muscle that originates from the iliac crest and the superficial layer of the thoracolumbar fascia, which itself is anchored to the lumbar and lower thoracic spinous processes. The muscle narrows to insert on the intertubercular sulcus of the proximal humerus.

- *Functions*: From the anatomic position, the latissimus dorsi cannot accomplish much because its fibers are already shortened. However, it is a very strong extensor of the shoulder from a flexed position, and it is a very strong adductor of the upper limb when it is in an abducted position. It is very active when rowing or performing a pull-up/chin-up.
- *Innervation*: Thoracodorsal nerve

Trapezius

- *Attachments*: The trapezius originates from the posterior aspect of the occipital bone and stretches down the nuchal ligament to the spinous processes of the lower thoracic vertebrae. Muscle fibers from this broad origin converge onto the distal clavicle, acromion, and spine of the scapula.
- *Functions*: Because it has such a broad origin focusing onto a smaller insertion area, the trapezius has multiple functions. The upper fibers travel in an inferolateral direction and elevate the scapula, the middle fibers are oriented horizontally and retract the scapula, and the inferior fibers travel in a superolateral direction and will depress the scapula when contracted.
- *Innervation*: Cranial nerve XI, the spinal accessory nerve.

Rhomboid Major and Minor

- *Attachments*: The rhomboid muscles originate from the lower cervical and upper thoracic spinous processes. They travel in a slightly inferolateral direction to insert on the medial border of the scapula near the scapular spine (minor) and medial to the infraspinatus fossa (major).
- *Functions*: Contraction of the rhomboid muscles will strongly retract the scapula and (slightly) tilt the glenoid fossa of the scapula inferiorly.
- *Innervation*: Dorsal scapular nerve

Levator Scapulae

- *Attachments*: The levator scapulae muscle originates from the lateral aspect and transverse processes of C1–C4 as four separate muscle bellies. These bellies fuse and insert on the superior angle and upper medial border of the scapula.

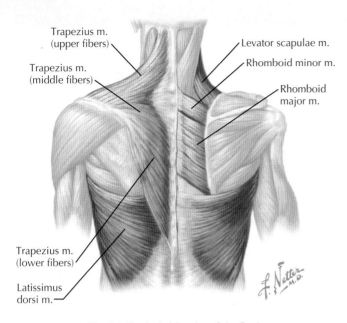

Fig. 3.1 Extrinsic Muscles of the Back.

- *Functions*: As its name suggests, it elevates the scapula and (slightly) tilts the glenoid fossa inferiorly.
- *Innervation*: Dorsal scapular nerve

Intrinsic Back Muscles

The **intrinsic back muscles** develop in the back and are located deep to the extrinsic muscles. These are the erector spinae, transversospinalis, splenius, and suboccipital muscle groups (Fig. 3.2). These muscles attach to the vertebrae and ribs and will move the back when they contract.

Erector Spinae Muscle Group

- *Attachments*: The three muscles of the **erector spinae group (iliocostalis, longissimus, spinalis)** are composed of many small muscle fibers that originate from the sacrum, iliac crest, thoracolumbar fascia, transverse processes, spinous processes, and ribs. These fibers join the muscles and ascend in a superolateral direction and insert on more lateral and superior structures such as transverse processes, spinous processes, and ribs. The iliocostalis group is most lateral,

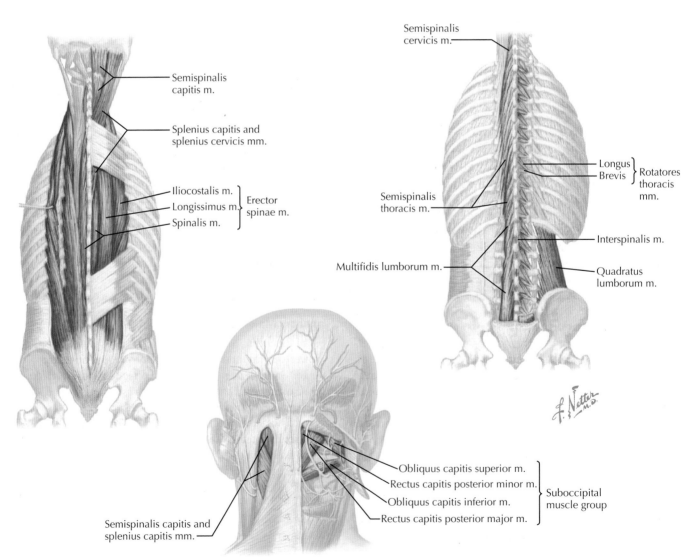

Fig. 3.2 Intrinsic Muscles of the Back.

followed by the longissimus group, and finally the spinalis group is the most medial, as it originates from spinous processes and inserts on more superior spinous processes.

- *Functions*: If these muscles are contracted unilaterally, they will laterally flex (side-bend) the torso to the ipsilateral side. If these muscles are contracted bilaterally, they strongly extend the back (Biomechanics Box 3.1).
- *Innervation*: Posterior rami

Splenius Muscle Group

- *Attachments*: The splenius cervicis and capitis muscles ascend superolaterally from their origin on the spinous processes of the midthoracic and lower cervical spinous processes and insert onto the transverse processes of C1–C4 (splenius cervicis) as well as the occipital bone and mastoid process of the temporal bone (splenius capitis).
- *Functions*: If these muscles contract unilaterally, they laterally flex (side-bend) and rotate the head and neck to the ipsilateral side. Contracted bilaterally, they extend the head and neck (see Biomechanics Box 3.1).
- *Innervation*: Posterior rami

Transversospinalis Muscle Group

- *Attachments*: The muscles in this group are composed of many small muscle fibers that originate from the sacrum as well as transverse processes along the entire length of the vertebral column. They ascend in a superomedial direction to insert on a superior spinous process. The deeper muscles in this group, **rotatores**, ascend only one to two vertebral levels and appear almost horizontal sometimes. Members that ascend two to four levels are called **multifidi**. The most superficial muscles, **semispinalis**, are nearly vertical in appearance, ascending four or six vertebral levels before inserting on a spinous process. One unique member of the transversospinalis group is the large **semispinalis capitis** muscle, which is located deep to the trapezius and splenius muscles. It originates from the transverse processes of the upper thoracic and cervical vertebrae, and instead of inserting on a spinous process, it inserts onto the occipital bone. When contracted bilaterally, this muscle is a very strong extensor of the head and neck.
- *Functions*: If the shorter transversospinalis muscles contract unilaterally, they may rotate the spine contralaterally. The longer muscles will laterally flex the spine to the ipsilateral side. Muscle fibers of intermediate length will do a bit of both. Transversospinalis muscles extend the back when they are contracted bilaterally (see Biomechanics Box 3.1). The smallest members of the group are not capable of moving the spine appreciably but act in a proprioceptive manner, updating the central nervous system regarding the position of the vertebrae as the muscles are stretched by movements of the spine.
- *Innervation*: Posterior rami

Suboccipital Muscle Group

- *Attachments*: The **suboccipital muscles** are a group of four small and deep muscles that connect the atlas and axis to the occipital bone. As a group they originate from the spinous processes of C1 and C2 and insert on the posterior occipital bone. Some individual members of the group take a more indirect pathway, which will be covered in Chapter 9.
- *Functions*: If these muscles are contracted unilaterally, they will laterally flex (side-bend) and rotate the head to the ipsilateral side. If these muscles are contracted bilaterally, they will extend the head. These muscles are too small to move the head in a wide range of motion and act largely as proprioceptive muscles. They are often involved in muscle tension headaches.
- *Innervation*: Posterior ramus of C1—the suboccipital nerve

MUSCLE GROUPS OF THE ANTERIOR NECK

In addition to the muscles of the cervical region of the back, there are several important muscles in the anterior neck (Fig. 3.3). While these also maneuver the head and neck, several attach to the hyoid bone, which lacks bony articulations and is entirely suspended by muscles and connective tissue.

Sternocleidomastoid Muscle

- *Attachments*: The sternocleidomastoid is a large and palpable muscle of the anterior neck. It originates from the sternum and proximal clavicle, ascends in a superolateral-posterior direction, and inserts onto the mastoid process of the temporal bone.
- *Functions*: Because it ascends in multiple directions, the sternocleidomastoid has several functions. Unilateral contraction will laterally flex the head and neck ipsilaterally but rotate the head contralaterally. Normally, bilateral contraction will flex the head and neck; however, if the head and neck are already extended, bilateral contraction will strongly extend them even further.
- *Innervation*: Cranial nerve XI, the spinal accessory nerve

Suprahyoid Muscles

- *Attachments*: These muscles originate from the mandible (**anterior belly of digastric** and **mylohyoid**) and temporal bone (**posterior belly of digastric** and **stylohyoid**) and insert directly or indirectly onto the body of the hyoid bone.
- *Functions*: Bilateral contraction of these muscles will elevate the hyoid bone and underlying laryngeal cartilages. This helps to close the laryngeal opening during swallowing.

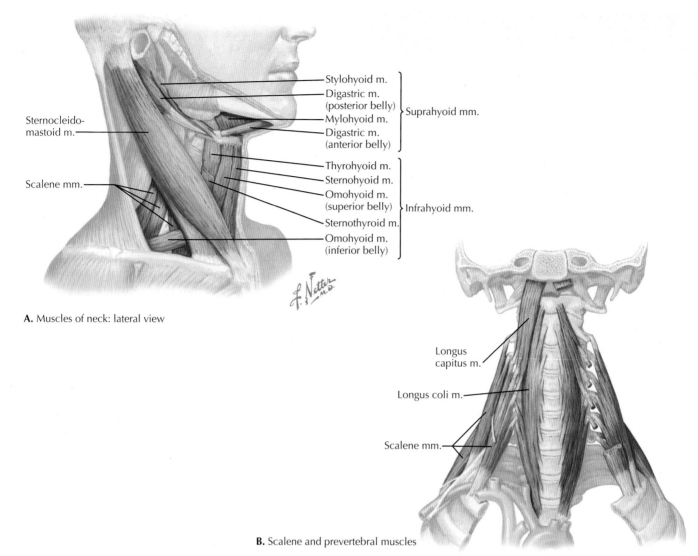

A. Muscles of neck: lateral view

B. Scalene and prevertebral muscles

Fig. 3.3 Muscle Groups of the Anterior Neck.

- *Innervation*: Several. Cranial nerve V, cranial nerve VII, C1 anterior rami.

Infrahyoid Muscles

- *Attachments*: As a group, these muscles originate from the superior sternum (**sternohyoid** and **sternothyroid**), laryngeal cartilage (**thyrohyoid**) and superior border of the scapula (**inferior and superior bellies of omohyoid**) and insert on the body of the hyoid bone.
- *Functions*: Bilateral contraction of these muscles will depress the hyoid bone and underlying laryngeal cartilages.
- *Innervation*: C1–C3 anterior rami

Longus Capitis and Coli Muscles

- *Attachments*: These muscles originate as slips of muscles from the transverse processes and vertebral bodies of upper thoracic and cervical vertebrae and insert on more superior transverse processes, vertebral bodies, and the base of the occipital bone.
- *Functions*: These muscles are primarily oriented vertically. Unilateral contraction will laterally flex the head and neck ipsilaterally; bilateral contraction will flex head and neck.

- *Innervation*: Anterior rami of C1–C6

Scalene Muscles

- *Attachments*: These muscles are located posterior to the sternocleidomastoid muscle. They originate from the transverse processes of the lower cervical vertebrae and insert on ribs 1 and 2.
- *Functions*: These muscles elevate the upper ribs during inspiration and side-bend the neck to the ipsilateral side.
- *Innervation*: Anterior rami of C3–C8
  See Clinical Correlation 3.1

MUSCLE GROUPS OF THE UPPER LIMB
Muscles of the Shoulder

These muscles connect the torso and scapula to the proximal humerus (Figs. 3.4 and 3.5). The latissimus dorsi and trapezius might also have been included here but were discussed in the extrinsic back muscle section. Flexion of the shoulder occurs when the arm is directed anteriorly and extension occurs when the arm is directed posteriorly. Abduction of the shoulder

CLINICAL CORRELATION 3.1   Respiration and Accessory Muscles of Respiration

Respiration consists of cycles of inhalation, wherein the pleural spaces of the thorax expand, followed by exhalation, when the thoracic spaces and lungs contract. Under normal circumstances, the lungs expand and contract along with the thorax. The diaphragm is the major muscle of inhalation because it flattens as it contracts, increasing the pleural spaces of the thorax tremendously and compressing the abdominal organs. The exact role of each group of intercostal muscles in this process is unclear; however, the current understanding is that the external intercostal, parasternal region of the internal intercostal, scalene, and sternocleidomastoid muscles help to elevate the ribs, which also increases the thoracic spaces. During labored breathing, such as intense exercise, these muscles contract faster and more forcefully with each inhalation. Quiet exhalation is mostly passive because the elastic tissues in the lungs pull them and the ribcage inward once the muscles of inhalation have stopped contracting. During labored breathing, the lateral aspect of the internal intercostal, innermost intercostal,

and transversus thoracis muscles contract to quickly pull the ribs and sternum inward. At the same time, the abdominal oblique and rectus abdominis muscles contract to compress the abdominal organs. This pressure causes the diaphragm to shoot upward as it relaxes with each exhalation and forces air from the lungs.

In obstructive conditions of the lungs, patients will have difficulty inhaling sufficient air due to expansion of lung air spaces and lack of lung recoil. They will compensate by inhaling as fully as possible with each breath. This will cause enlargement (hypertrophy) of muscles that insert on the ribs and sternum, such as the sternocleidomastoid and scalene muscles. In addition, they may use upper limb muscles to act as accessory muscles of respiration. To do this, the patient will fix the upper limb against a stationary object such as a desk so that the origin-insertion relationship of those muscles is reversed. Thereafter, contraction of the pectoralis major, pectoralis minor, and serratus anterior muscles will elevate the ribs during inspiration rather than moving the upper limb.

Muscles of inspiration

Accessory

Sternocleidomastoid (elevates sternum and medial clavicle) Scalene mm.
  Anterior
  Middle
  Posterior (elevate and fix upper ribs)

Principal

External intercostals, most superficial (elevate ribs, thus increasing width of thoracic cavity and aiding deep inspiration)

Interchondral parts of internal intercostals are deep to external intercostals (also elevate ribs and aid external intercostals with deep inspiration)

Respiratory diaphragm (domes descend, thus increasing vertical dimension of thoracic cavity; also elevates lower ribs)

Muscles of expiration

Quiet breathing

Expiration results from passive recoil of lungs and rib cage

Active breathing

Internal intercostal mm., except interchondral part (aid forced expiration)

Abdominals (depress lower ribs, compress abdominal contents, thus pushing up respiratory diaphragm, aiding forced expiration)

Rectus abdominis
External abdominal oblique m.
Internal abdominal oblique m.
Transversus abdominis m.

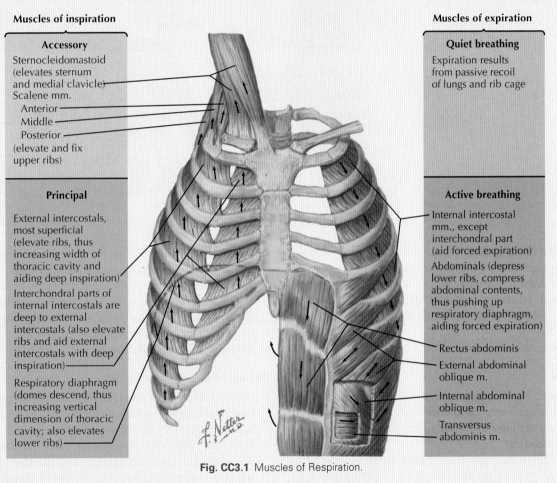

Fig. CC3.1 Muscles of Respiration.

occurs when the arm is directed laterally away from the body, and adduction occurs when it is pulled closer to the body.

Rotator Cuff Muscles

- *Attachments*: All members of this group (**subscapularis, supraspinatus, infraspinatus, and teres minor**) are functionally and clinically important and will be discussed in detail in Chapter 10. They originate from the subscapular, supraspinous, and infraspinous fossae of the scapula and insert on the greater and lesser tubercles of the humerus.

- *Function*: The subscapularis internally rotates, the supraspinatus abducts (Biomechanics Box 3.2), and the infraspinatus and teres minor externally rotate the humerus. As a group they hold the head of the humerus tight in the glenoid fossa to prevent dislocation.

- *Innervation*: Axillary, suprascapular, and subscapular nerves

Deltoid

- *Attachments*: The **deltoid muscle** has three bellies that originate from the distal clavicle, acromion, and lateral spine of

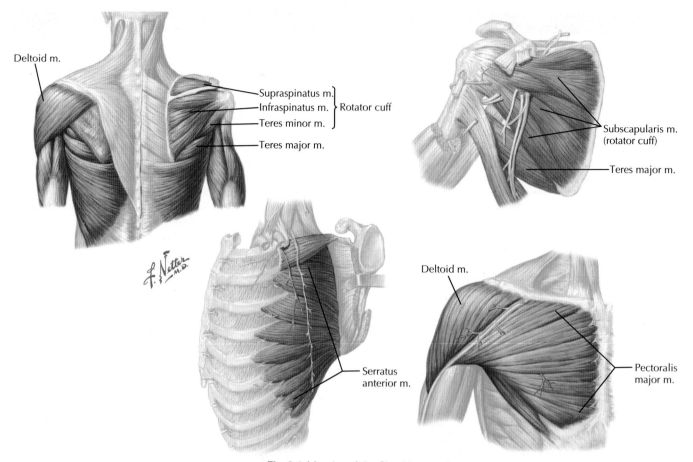

Fig. 3.4 Muscles of the Shoulder.

the scapula. All three bellies fuse and insert onto the deltoid tuberosity on the lateral midshaft of the humerus.

- *Function*: Because the three bellies lie across the anterior, lateral, and posterior aspect of the glenohumeral joint, they flex, abduct (see Biomechanics Box 3.2), and extend it, respectively.
- *Innervation*: Axillary nerve

Teres Major

- *Attachments*: The **teres major** originates from the lateral border of the scapula near its inferior angle. It extends laterally to insert on the intertubercular sulcus alongside the latissimus dorsi tendon.
- *Function*: The teres major has similar functions as the latissimus dorsi, moving the shoulder from a flexed position to an extended one, as well as moving it from abduction into adduction.
- *Innervation*: Lower subscapular nerve

Pectoralis Major and Minor

- *Attachments*: The **pectoralis major** is a broad and powerful muscle that originates from the anterior ribs, sternum, and clavicle. Its fibers insert on the humerus along the medial aspect of the crest of the greater tubercle. The **pectoralis minor** (see Fig 3.7A) is deep to the pectoralis major. It originates from the anterior aspect of ribs 3 to 5 and inserts on the coracoid process of the scapula.

- *Functions*: The pectoralis major primarily acts to flex the shoulder, as when doing a push-up. Like the latissimus dorsi, it also returns the humerus to an adducted position from abduction. It also assists members of the rotator cuff in medially rotating the humerus. The pectoralis minor brings the scapula close to the upper thoracic wall and rotates the glenoid fossa inferiorly.
- *Innervation*: Lateral and medial pectoral nerves

Serratus Anterior (See Fig. 3.4)

- *Attachments*: The **serratus anterior** originates from the anterior aspect of the scapula's medial border. From there it fans out to insert on the lateral aspect of ribs 1 to 8.
- *Functions*: When the serratus anterior contracts, it causes the scapula to glide anteriorly across the thorax. If it contracts in conjunction with the rhomboid muscles, it "fixes" the scapula to the posterior thorax. If the most inferior region of the muscle contracts in isolation, it will rotate the glenoid fossa superiorly, abducting (see Biomechanics Box 3.2) the arm.
- *Innervation*: Long thoracic nerve

Muscle Compartments of the Arm and Forearm

The muscles of the anterior compartments of the arm and forearm are flexors, while the muscles of the posterior compartments are extensors (see Fig. 3.5). The compartments of the arm and forearm are surrounded by very tough deep fascia that tethers them to the underlying bones.

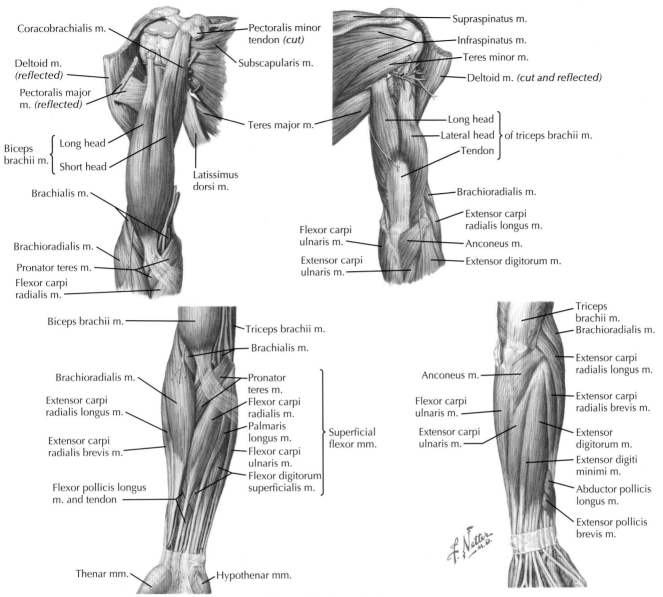

Fig. 3.5 Muscles of the Arm.

Anterior Compartment of the Arm

- *Attachments*: There are three muscles in the anterior compartment of the arm. The **coracobrachialis** stretches between the coracoid process and the medial shaft of the humerus. The **biceps brachii** has a short head originating from the coracoid process and a long head that originates from the supraglenoid tubercle of the scapula and descends in the intertubercular sulcus. The two heads fuse, and the strong bicipital tendon inserts on the radial tuberosity while a broad bicipital aponeurosis connects to the deep fascia of the forearm. The **brachialis** originates from the anterior, distal humerus and inserts on the ulnar tuberosity. Despite its significant size, it is almost entirely covered by the biceps brachii.
- *Functions*: Although each muscle has distinctive functions, the major function of the component as a whole is flexion of the forearm at the elbow.
- *Innervation*: Musculocutaneous nerve

Posterior Compartment of the Arm

- *Attachments*: The **triceps brachii** is the major muscle in the posterior arm. Its long head originates from the infraglenoid tubercle, and the lateral and medial heads originate from the posterior humerus. The three heads fuse and insert onto the olecranon. The small **anconeus** muscle is also present in this compartment very close to the elbow.

- *Functions*: The major function of the posterior arm muscles is extension of the forearm at the elbow.
- *Innervation*: Radial nerve

Posterior Compartment of the Forearm

- *Attachments*: There are many muscles in the posterior compartment of the forearm. They originate from the lateral epicondyle of the humerus and the posterior aspect of the radius, ulna, and interosseous membrane. The **extensor carpi radialis longus, extensor carpi radialis brevis**, and **extensor carpi ulnaris** insert on the posterior carpal bones. The **extensor digitorum, extensor digiti minimi, extensor pollicis longus** and **brevis**, and **abductor pollicis longus** insert on the dorsal aspect of the digits. The **supinator** attaches to the proximal radius.
- *Functions*: Although each muscle has distinctive functions, the major functions of the compartment are extension of the wrist, extension of all digits, abduction of the thumb, and forearm supination.
- *Innervation*: Radial nerve and its branches

One unique muscle of the posterior arm and forearm is the **brachioradialis muscle**. It originates from the lateral supracondylar ridge of the humerus and inserts on the distal radius. Although it is in the posterior compartment of the forearm with the extensor muscles and is innervated by the radial nerve, it actually acts to flex the elbow.

Anterior Compartment of the Forearm

- *Attachments*: There are also many muscles in the anterior compartment of the forearm. They originate from the medial epicondyle of the humerus and anterior aspect of the radius, ulna, and/or interosseous membrane. The **flexor carpi radialis** and **flexor carpi ulnaris** insert on the anterior carpal bones, while the **palmaris longus** blends into the fascia of the palm. The **superficial and deep digital flexors** and the **flexor pollicis longus** insert onto the palmar aspect of the middle and distal phalanges. The **pronator teres** inserts onto the proximal radius.
- *Functions*: While each muscle has distinctive functions, the major functions of the muscles in this compartment are flexion of the wrist, flexion of all digits, and pronation of the forearm.
- *Innervation*: Median and ulnar nerves

Muscle Compartments of the Hand

We will categorize the muscles of the hand as the **thenar muscles, hypothenar muscles**, and **intrinsic muscles of the hand** (Fig. 3.6). The palm itself is protected by a tough sheet of connective tissue, the **palmar aponeurosis**.

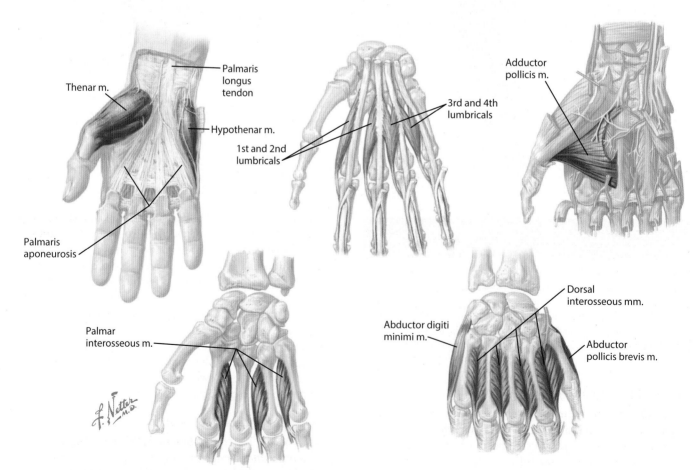

Fig. 3.6 Muscles of the Hand.

Thenar Muscles

- *Attachments:* These muscles form the "pad" of the thumb, called the **thenar eminence**, and originate from the palmar aspect of the lateral carpal bones and the first and second metacarpals. They insert onto the first metacarpal and proximal phalanx of the thumb.
- *Functions:* The **abductor pollicis brevis** and **flexor pollicis brevis** muscles abduct and flex the proximal phalanx of the thumb, respectively. The **opponens pollicis** brings about opposition of the first metacarpal, all of which allow fine motions of the thumb to occur.
- *Innervation:* Recurrent branch of the median nerve

Hypothenar Muscles

- *Attachments:* The muscles of the **hypothenar eminence** originate from the palmar aspect of the medial carpal bones and fifth metacarpal. They insert onto the fifth metacarpal and proximal phalanx of the fifth digit.
- *Functions:* The **abductor digiti minimi** and **flexor digiti minimi** muscles will abduct and flex the phalanges of the fifth digit. The **opponens digiti minimi** brings about opposition of the fifth metacarpal.
- *Innervation:* Ulnar nerve

Intrinsic Muscles of the Hand

- *Attachments:* The unusual **lumbrical muscles** originate from the tendons of the deep digital flexor muscle and insert onto the extensor tendons covering the posterior side of digits 2 to 5. The other intrinsic muscles of the hand originate from the bones of the hand itself and insert on the metacarpals and the proximal phalanges of all five digits. The **adductor pollicis** originates from the palmar side of metacarpals 2 and 3 and inserts on the ulnar side of the proximal phalanx of the pollicis. The **palmar and dorsal interosseous muscles** originate between the metacarpals and insert onto the proximal phalanges of digits 2 to 5.
- *Functions:* Due to their odd pathway, the lumbrical muscles flex the metacarpophalangeal joints but also extend the proximal and distal interphalangeal joints. The adductor pollicis does exactly what its name implies, bringing the pollicis closer to the second digit. The palmar interossei adduct digits 2, 4, and 5 toward the midline of the hand, digit 3. The dorsal interossei abduct digits 2 to 4 away from the midline of the hand.
- *Innervation:* Ulnar nerve, except for the first and second lumbrical muscles, which are innervated by the median nerve.

MAJOR MUSCLE GROUPS OF THE TORSO

Intercostal Muscles (Fig. 3.7A and B)

- *Attachments:* As their name suggests, these muscles are located between adjacent ribs. The **external intercostal muscles** are angled in an inferoanterior direction and project anteriorly from the vertebrae to the border of the costal cartilages. The **internal intercostal muscles** are angled in an inferoposterior direction and project posteriorly from the sternum to within 5 to 6 cm of the vertebrae. The **innermost intercostal muscles** are also directed inferoposteriorly but are seen only along the lateral aspect of the intercostal space.
- *Functions:* Different parts of the intercostal muscles will elevate the ribs during inspiration and depress them in expiration.
- *Innervation:* Intercostal nerves

Thoracic Diaphragm (See Fig. 3.7B and D)

- *Attachments:* This dome-shaped muscle separates the thoracic and abdominal cavities but allows the esophagus, aorta, and inferior vena cava to pass between the two cavities. It attaches around the periphery of the ribcage starting at the xiphoid process, along the inferior margin of the ribs, passing across the quadratus lumborum and psoas major muscles, and finally onto the T12 and upper lumbar vertebral bodies via two strong muscular slips that surround the aorta, the **right crus** and **left crus of the diaphragm.** It has a central tendon that is sandwiched between the heart and the liver.
- *Function:* When the diaphragm contracts during inspiration, it flattens to expand the thoracic cavity and compress the abdominal organs. When it relaxes during expiration, the abdominal organs push the dome superiorly.
- *Innervation:* Phrenic nerve
  See Clinical Correlation 3.1 Muscles of Respiration

Abdominal Oblique Muscles (See Fig. 3.7C and D)

- *Attachments:* These muscles form the lateral and anterior body wall around the abdomen. The **external abdominal oblique** muscle is directed in an inferoanterior direction, the **internal abdominal oblique** muscle is directed in an inferoposterior direction, and the **transversus abdominis** is primarily horizontal in orientation. They extend around the abdomen from the lumbar vertebrae, iliac crest, and thoracolumbar fascia. Their broad flat tendons, aponeuroses, surround the rectus abdominis muscles on each side before fusing along a line that extends from the xiphoid process to the pubic bones, the **linea alba.**
- *Functions:* As a group, these muscles compress and support the abdominal organs. Contracting in various combinations they are able to flex, side-bend (laterally flex), and rotate the torso (Biomechanics Box 3.3).
- *Innervation:* Intercostal (T6 to T11), subcostal (T12) nerves, and L1 anterior ramus

Rectus Abdominis Muscle (See Fig. 3.7A and C)

- *Attachments:* This segmented muscle extends from the anterior aspect of the lower ribs and costal cartilages along the anterior abdominal wall to the left and right pubic bones. The aponeuroses of the abdominal oblique muscles surround the anterior and posterior aspects of the rectus abdominis to form the **rectus sheath** before they converge to form the linea alba, which separates the left and right rectus abdominis muscles.
- *Functions:* The rectus abdominis muscles flex the torso bringing the thorax closer to the pelvis (see Biomechanics Box 3.3).
- *Innervation:* Intercostal (T6 to T11), subcostal (T12) nerves

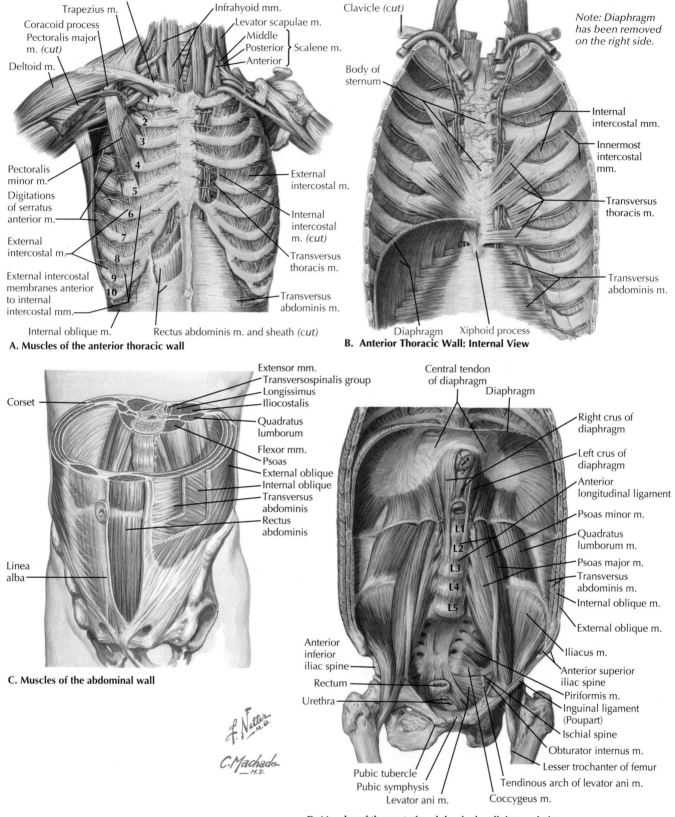

A. Muscles of the anterior thoracic wall

Clavicle
Trapezius m.
Coracoid process
Pectoralis major m. *(cut)*
Deltoid m.
Infrahyoid mm.
Levator scapulae m.
Middle
Posterior } Scalene m.
Anterior
Pectoralis minor m.
Digitations of serratus anterior m.
External intercostal m.
External intercostal membranes anterior to internal intercostal mm.
Internal oblique m.
External intercostal m.
Internal intercostal m. *(cut)*
Transversus thoracis m.
Transversus abdominis m.
Rectus abdominis m. and sheath *(cut)*

B. Anterior Thoracic Wall: Internal View

Clavicle *(cut)*
Note: Diaphragm has been removed on the right side.
Body of sternum
Internal intercostal mm.
Innermost intercostal mm.
Transversus thoracis m.
Transversus abdominis m.
Diaphragm   Xiphoid process

C. Muscles of the abdominal wall

Corset
Linea alba
Extensor mm.
Transversospinalis group
Longissimus
Iliocostalis
Quadratus lumborum
Flexor mm.
Psoas
External oblique
Internal oblique
Transversus abdominis
Rectus abdominis

D. Muscles of the posterior abdominal wall: internal view

Central tendon of diaphragm
Diaphragm
Right crus of diaphragm
Left crus of diaphragm
Anterior longitudinal ligament
Psoas minor m.
Quadratus lumborum m.
Psoas major m.
Transversus abdominis m.
Internal oblique m.
External oblique m.
Iliacus m.
Anterior superior iliac spine
Piriformis m.
Inguinal ligament (Poupart)
Ischial spine
Obturator internus m.
Lesser trochanter of femur
Tendinous arch of levator ani m.
Coccygeus m.
Anterior inferior iliac spine
Rectum
Urethra
Pubic tubercle
Pubic symphysis
Levator ani m.
L1
L2
L3
L4
L5

Fig. 3.7 Muscles of the Torso.

BIOMECHANICS BOX 3.3   Abdominal Muscles and Sit Ups

Although sit-ups are a basic exercise that many people learn at an early age, the combination of muscles involved can be very complex. The rectus abdominis muscles (the "six pack") are engaged when the thorax and pelvis are brought closer together during flexion of the torso. The abdominal oblique muscles assist in flexion but are more active when a rotation to one side is added to the flexion. When twisting to the right, the left external abdominal oblique and right internal abdominal oblique will be activated. The opposite combination occurs when twisting to the left. The rectus femoris and iliopsoas muscles (the hip flexors) are also frequently active during sit-ups, particularly when the feet are anchored by a bar or another object.

Quadratus Lumborum (See Fig. 3.7C and D)

- *Attachments*: This muscle extends superiorly from the posterior iliac crest to insert on the inferior aspect of the 12th rib.
- *Function*: Side-bends the lumbar vertebrae.
- *Innervation*: Anterior rami from T12 to L4

Psoas Major and Iliacus Muscles (See Fig. 3.7C and D)

- *Attachments:* The stout psoas major muscle originates from the bodies and transverse processes of the T12–L5 vertebrae and descends along the medial aspect of the ilium. The iliacus muscle originates from the iliac fossa of the ilium and fuses with the psoas major as it descends. The fused muscle, often called the **iliopsoas** passes across the anterior aspect of the pubic bone to insert on the lesser trochanter of the femur.
- *Function:* The iliopsoas muscle flexes the thigh at the hip (see Biomechanics Box 3.3).
- *Innervation:* Anterior rami from L1 to L3

Pelvic Diaphragm (Fig. 3.8A and B)

- *Attachments:* The pelvic diaphragm is a collection of muscles, the **levator ani** and **coccygeus muscles**, that form the floor of the abdominopelvic cavity, support the pelvic organs, but still allow the anus, vagina, and urethra to transit through it. This diaphragm is "domed" inferiorly, somewhat like a funnel with the anal opening at its inferior limit. It originates from the pubis anteriorly and then passes along the lateral wall of the pelvis before finally reaching the coccyx.
- *Function:* Normally, the pelvic diaphragm supports the pelvic organs and prevents organ prolapse. When the pelvic diaphragm contracts, it flattens and elevates the anal area. Some slips of muscle from the pelvic diaphragm also surround the urethra and vagina.
- *Innervation:* Pudendal nerve and other sacral branches

Muscles of the Urogenital and Anal Triangles (See Fig. 3.8C and D)

- *Attachments:* This collection of muscles is found on the inferior side of the pelvis, called the perineum. The urogenital triangle is formed by the left and right inferior pubic rami, ischial rami, and a line connecting the left and right ischial tuberosities. It contains a **deep transverse perineal muscle** that surrounds the opening of the vagina and ureter, which it surrounds to create the urethral sphincter. There are also muscles that cover the bases of the external genitalia, the **bulbospongiosus** and **ischiocavernosus muscles.** Posterior to the urogenital triangle is the anal triangle. It contains a great deal of adipose tissue but also the **external and internal anal sphincter muscles.**
- *Function:* The sphincter muscles tend to keep the urethral and anal openings closed until they are relaxed during willful urination and defecation. The other muscles compress the vaginal opening and erectile tissues of the external genitalia.
- *Innervation*: Pudendal nerve and other sacral branches

MUSCLE GROUPS OF THE LOWER LIMB

Gluteal Region (Fig. 3.9)

These muscles connect the posterior pelvis to the lower limb. This area contains several small muscles that will be examined in detail in Chapter 11. Similar to the shoulder, flexion of the thigh at the hip will move it anteriorly, whereas extension of the hip will direct the thigh posteriorly. Abduction of the thigh will raise it laterally while adduction returns it to the midline.

Gluteus Maximus

- *Attachments*: The massive gluteus maximus originates from the posterior ilium, posterior sacrum, and sacrotuberous ligament. It travels inferolaterally to insert on the gluteal tuberosity and the tough fascia on the lateral side of the thigh, called the **iliotibial band**. The iliotibial band eventually inserts on the anterolateral tubercle of the tibia.
- *Function:* From a flexed position, the gluteus maximus strongly extends the thigh at the hip (Biomechanics Box 3.4).
- *Innervation:* Inferior gluteal nerve

Gluteus Medius and Minimus

- *Attachments*: These muscles are located deep to the gluteus maximus. They both originate from the gluteal fossa on the lateral aspect of the ilium and insert onto the greater trochanter of the femur.
- *Function:* These muscles will abduct an unweighted lower limb. When standing on one leg, these muscles are very active on the support limb to prevent the pelvis from dropping toward the unsupported side (see Biomechanics Box 3.4).
- *Innervation:* Superior gluteal nerve

Lateral Rotators of the Thigh

- *Attachments:* Deep to the gluteus maximus and inferior to the gluteus medius and minimus are several smaller muscles that originate from the area of the lateral sacrum, obturator foramen, ischial spine, and ischial tuberosity. These are the **piriformis, obturator internus, obturator externus, superior gemellus, inferior gemellus**, and **quadratus femoris muscles**, and they all insert on the medial aspect of the greater trochanter and intertrochanteric crest.

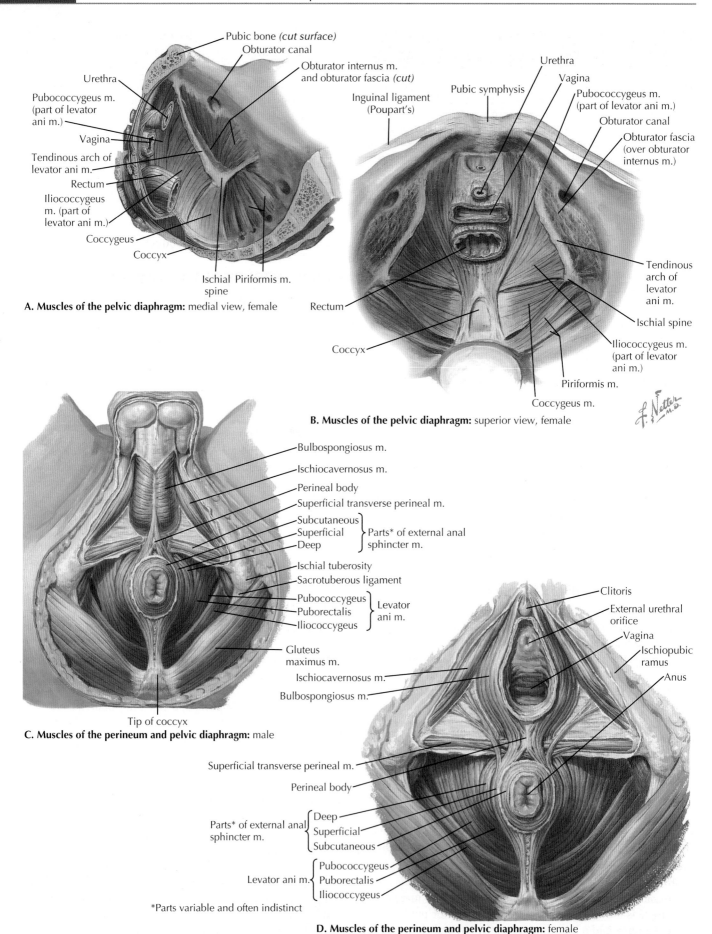

Pubic bone *(cut surface)*
Obturator canal
Urethra
Pubococcygeus m.
(part of levator
ani m.)
Vagina
Tendinous arch of
levator ani m.
Rectum
Iliococcygeus
m. (part of
levator ani m.)
Coccygeus
Coccyx
Obturator internus m.
and obturator fascia *(cut)*
Ischial Piriformis m.
spine

A. Muscles of the pelvic diaphragm: medial view, female

Inguinal ligament
(Poupart's)
Rectum
Coccyx
Pubic symphysis
Urethra
Vagina
Pubococcygeus m.
(part of levator ani m.)
Obturator canal
Obturator fascia
(over obturator
internus m.)
Tendinous
arch of
levator
ani m.
Ischial spine
Iliococcygeus m.
(part of levator
ani m.)
Piriformis m.
Coccygeus m.

B. Muscles of the pelvic diaphragm: superior view, female

Bulbospongiosus m.
Ischiocavernosus m.
Perineal body
Superficial transverse perineal m.
Subcutaneous
Superficial   Parts* of external anal
Deep   sphincter m.
Ischial tuberosity
Sacrotuberous ligament
Pubococcygeus
Puborectalis   Levator
Iliococcygeus   ani m.
Gluteus
maximus m.
Ischiocavernosus m.
Bulbospongiosus m.
Tip of coccyx

C. Muscles of the perineum and pelvic diaphragm: male

Clitoris
External urethral
orifice
Vagina
Ischiopubic
ramus
Anus
Superficial transverse perineal m.
Perineal body
Deep
Parts* of external anal   Superficial
sphincter m.   Subcutaneous
Pubococcygeus
Levator ani m.   Puborectalis
Iliococcygeus

*Parts variable and often indistinct

D. Muscles of the perineum and pelvic diaphragm: female

Fig. 3.8 Muscles of the Torso (Continued).

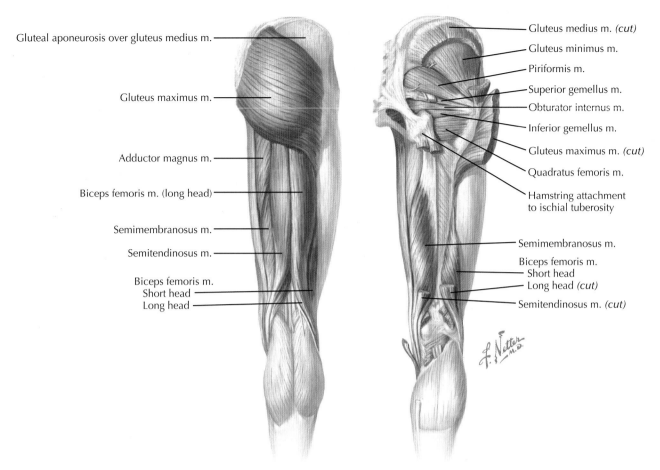

Gluteal aponeurosis over gluteus medius m.

Gluteus maximus m.

Adductor magnus m.

Biceps femoris m. (long head)

Semimembranosus m.

Semitendinosus m.

Biceps femoris m.
Short head
Long head

Gluteus medius m. *(cut)*

Gluteus minimus m.

Piriformis m.

Superior gemellus m.

Obturator internus m.

Inferior gemellus m.

Gluteus maximus m. *(cut)*

Quadratus femoris m.

Hamstring attachment
to ischial tuberosity

Semimembranosus m.

Biceps femoris m.
Short head
Long head *(cut)*

Semitendinosus m. *(cut)*

Fig. 3.9 Gluteal and Posterior Thigh Muscles.

- *Function:* These muscles rotate the thigh, and therefore the entire lower limb, laterally (see Biomechanics Box 3.4).
- *Innervation:* Anterior rami of L5–S1

Muscle Groups of the Thigh (See Figs. 3.9 and 3.10A and B)

The thigh contains three muscle groups divided into distinct compartments by the deep fascia that surrounds each.

Posterior Compartment of the Thigh

- *Attachments:* The most prominent muscles of the posterior thigh are the three hamstring muscles. The **semimembranosus, semitendinosus**, and the **long head of biceps femoris** originate from the ischial tuberosity and the **short head of biceps femoris** from the posterior shaft of the femur. The semitendinosus descends, fuses with two other muscles (the sartorius and gracilis, which will be discussed later), and inserts on the medial aspect of the superior tibia. The semimembranosus inserts nearby on the posteromedial tibia. The long and short heads of the biceps femoris insert on the head of the fibula. The deep **popliteus muscle** stretches from the lateral femoral epicondyle across the proximal posterior tibia.
- *Functions:* When the lower limb is bearing weight, the hamstring muscles extend the hip. When it is not bearing weight, the hamstrings flex the leg at the knee. The popliteus muscle

> ### BIOMECHANICS BOX 3.4 **Gluteal Muscles**
>
> Despite its massive size, weakness of the gluteus maximus can be somewhat subtle. It is most active when extending the hip from a flexed position, such as ascending the stairs and standing from a seated position. Patients may compensate (often unknowingly) by consistently stepping up with their strong side when ascending the stairs and bringing the weaker leg thereafter. When rising from a seat, they may use their upper limbs for assistance.
>
> If the limb is unweighted, the gluteus medius and minimus muscles abduct the thigh at the hip. However, when standing on one leg and supporting the body's weight, the stance side's gluteus medius and minimus are very active in keeping the hip level by pulling the ilium toward the greater trochanter. If those muscles are weak, the hip and body will fall away from the affected side anytime an afflicted person attempts to stand on the weak limb. This is called the Trendelenburg sign.

internally rotates the tibia relative to the femur and resists external rotation of the tibia.
- *Innervation:* Sciatic nerve and its branches

Anterior Compartment of the Thigh

- *Attachments:* The muscles of the anterior thigh are the sartorius and quadriceps. The **quadriceps** is further subdivided into four muscles: **rectus femoris, vastus lateralis, vastus medialis, and vastus intermedius**, which originate from the anterior

inferior iliac spine and anterior femur. The **sartorius** originates from the anterior superior iliac spine and travels inferomedially, fusing with the semitendinosus and gracilis muscles as they insert on the medial aspect of the superior tibia. The quadriceps muscles fuse into a **quadriceps tendon** that surrounds the superior base of the patella. The **patellar ligament** extends inferiorly from the patellar apex to the tibial tuberosity.
- *Functions*: The sartorius and rectus femoris flex the hip. The quadriceps muscles act as a group to strongly extend the leg at the knee.
- *Innervation*: Femoral nerve

Medial Compartment of the Thigh
- *Attachments:* The most prominent muscles of the medial thigh are the **gracilis, pectineus**, and **adductor group** (**adductor longus, adductor brevis**, and **adductor magnus muscles**). They originate from the pubis and iliopubic ramus. The gracilis travels inferiorly and joins the sartorius

and semitendinosus muscles to insert on the medial aspect of the superior tibia. The fused tendon of these three muscles is called the **pes anserinus.** The pectineus and adductor muscles insert along the medial aspect of the femur, the medial epicondyle, and adductor tubercle.
- *Functions:* The muscles of the medial compartment of the thigh adduct the thigh at the hip and help maintain pelvic stability while walking.
- *Innervation:* Obturator nerve

Muscle Groups of the Leg (See Figs. 3.10C and D and 3.11)
The leg also contains three muscle groups divided into distinct compartments by the deep fascia that surrounds each.

Posterior Compartments of the Leg
- *Attachments:* There are actually two compartments in the posterior leg.

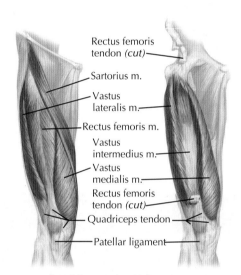

A. Muscles of the anterior thigh

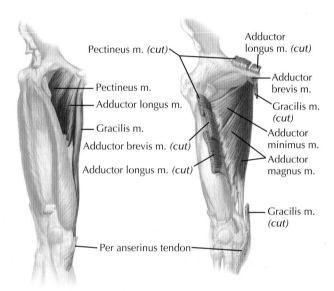

B. Muscles of the medial thigh

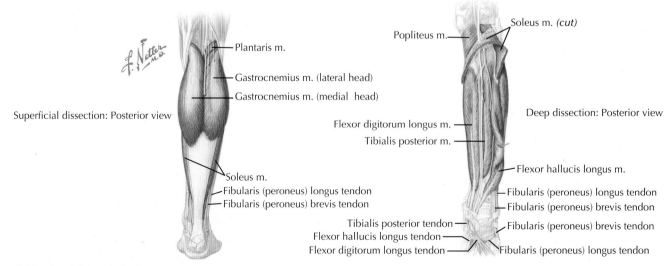

C. Muscles of the posterior leg

Fig. 3.10 Muscles of the Thigh.

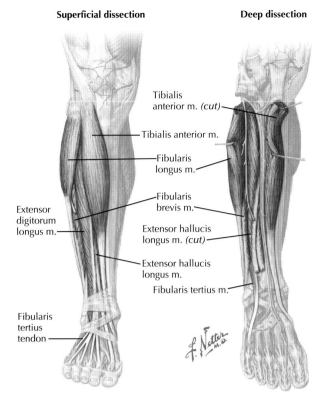

Superficial dissection   **Deep dissection**

Tibialis anterior m. *(cut)*

Tibialis anterior m.

Fibularis longus m.

Fibularis brevis m.

Extensor hallucis longus m. *(cut)*

Extensor hallucis longus m.

Fibularis tertius m.

Extensor digitorum longus m.

Fibularis tertius tendon

Fig. 3.11 Muscles of the Anterior and Lateral Compartments of the Leg.

- The superficial posterior compartment contains the **gastrocnemius, soleus**, and **plantaris muscles.** These originate from the medial and lateral femoral epicondyles as well as the posterior tibia, fibula, and interosseous membrane. All of these muscles converge to form the massive **calcaneal (Achilles) tendon** that inserts onto the superior aspect of the calcaneal tuberosity.
- The deep posterior compartment contains the **flexor hallucis longus, flexor digitorum longus**, and **tibialis posterior muscles.** They originate from the posterior tibia, fibula, and interosseous membrane. They insert, respectively, on the plantar aspect of the distal phalanx of the hallucis (big toe), distal phalanges of digits 2 to 5, and the medial tarsal bones and base of the first metatarsal.
- *Functions*: Muscles of the superficial posterior compartment of the leg are strong plantarflexors. The muscles of the deep posterior compartment flex all the digits of the foot and help to invert the foot. The entire compartment assists in toeing off while walking or running.
- *Innervation*: Tibial nerve

Anterior Compartment of the Leg

- *Attachments*: The muscles of the anterior compartment are the **extensor hallucis longus, extensor digitorum longus**, and **tibialis anterior.** They originate from the anterolateral tibia, fibula, and interosseous membrane. They insert, respectively, on the dorsal side of the distal phalanx of the hallucis (big toe), distal phalanges of digits 2 to 5, and the medial tarsal bones and first metatarsal.

- *Functions*: Muscles of the anterior compartment strongly dorsiflex the foot, extend all the digits of the foot, and help to invert the foot.
- *Innervation*: Deep fibular nerve

Lateral Compartment of the Leg

- *Attachments*: The muscles of the lateral compartment are the **fibularis longus** and **fibularis brevis**, which originate from the lateral shaft of the fibula. The fibularis brevis inserts onto the tuberosity of the base of the fifth metatarsal. The fibularis longus tendon passes inferior to the lateral malleolus and crosses along the deep plantar surface of the foot to insert on the medial cuneiform and first metatarsal.
- *Functions*: Muscles of the lateral compartment strongly evert the foot and resist inversion.
- *Innervation*: Superficial fibular nerve

Compartments of the Foot

The foot contains several compartments. For the moment we will group the muscles of the foot into two broad groups, those on the dorsum of the foot and those on the plantar side.

Muscles of the Dorsum of the Foot (Fig. 3.12)

- *Attachments*: The dorsal aspect of the foot has two muscles, the **extensor hallucis brevis** and **extensor digitorum brevis**, which originate from the superior aspect of the calcaneus. They insert on the extensor hood of the hallucis and digits 2 to 5, respectively.
- *Functions*: These muscles assist in extending the digits of the foot.
- *Innervation*: Deep fibular nerve

Muscles of the Plantar Foot (See Figs. 3.12 and 3.13)

- *Attachments*: There are many muscles on the plantar side of the foot. They originate from tarsal and metatarsal bones and insert more distally along the metatarsals and digits. Each has a distinctive origin and insertion and will be discussed in detail in Chapter 11. Note that the plantar muscles are protected by a strong **plantar aponeurosis** that is just deep to the skin and subcutaneous tissue of the plantar foot.
- *Function*: The muscles on the plantar side of the foot are named for the motion each would produce if they contracted in isolation. The **flexor digitorum brevis, flexor hallucis brevis,** and **flexor digiti minimi brevis** all flex the digits. The **abductor hallucis** and **abductor digiti minimi** pull their respective digits away from the midline of the foot while the **adductor hallucis** will pull the great toe toward the midline. Other muscles have the same functions as their counterparts in the hand. The **lumbricals** flex the metatarsophalangeal joints and extend the proximal and distal interphalangeal joints. **Plantar interossei** adduct digits 3 to 5, and the **dorsal interossei** abduct digits 2 to 4. Although each of these muscles can operate individually, they act strongly as a group to tether the tarsal and metatarsal bones together, to flex the digits, and to assist in toe-off during walking or running.
- *Innervation*: Medial and lateral plantar nerves, which are branches of the tibial nerve

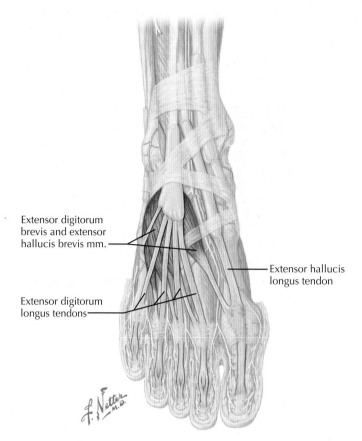

Extensor digitorum
brevis and extensor
hallucis brevis mm.

Extensor hallucis
longus tendon

Extensor digitorum
longus tendons

Fig. 3.12 Muscles of the Dorsum of the Foot.

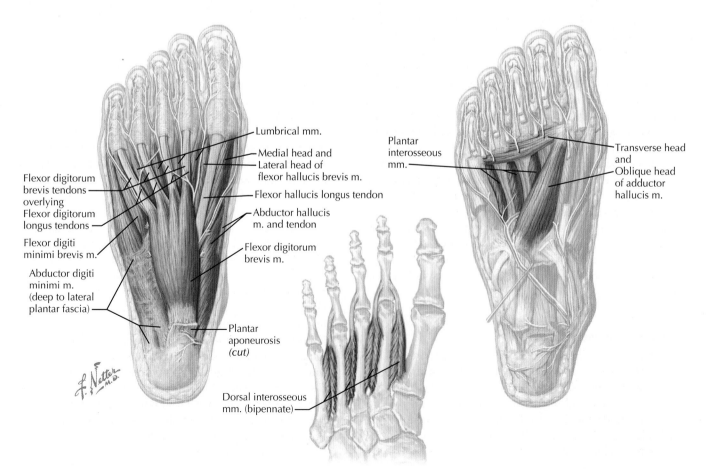

Lumbrical mm.

Medial head and
Lateral head of
flexor hallucis brevis m.

Flexor hallucis longus tendon

Flexor digitorum
brevis tendons
overlying
Flexor digitorum
longus tendons

Abductor hallucis
m. and tendon

Flexor digiti
minimi brevis m.

Flexor digitorum
brevis m.

Abductor digiti
minimi m.
(deep to lateral
plantar fascia)

Plantar
aponeurosis
(cut)

Dorsal interosseous
mm. (bipennate)

Plantar
interosseous
mm.

Transverse head
and
Oblique head
of adductor
hallucis m.

Fig. 3.13 Muscles of the Plantar Foot.

Innervation of the Muscle Compartments

INTRODUCTION

There are several ways to divide the nervous system and how it relates to the musculoskeletal system. The **central nervous system** (CNS) is the brain/cortex, brainstem, and spinal cord. The **peripheral nervous system** (PNS) is composed of nerves that travel to and from the CNS, as well as clusters of nerve cell bodies located throughout the body. Afferent (sensory) neurons carry information from the skin and muscles (somatic sensory), while others bring information from the organs (visceral sensory) back to the CNS. Likewise, efferent (motor) neurons can innervate skeletal muscles (somatic motor) or organs (visceral motor, also known as the autonomic nervous system). The autonomic nervous system is subdivided into parasympathetic and sympathetic divisions (Fig. 4.1).

The typical nerve cell, or neuron, has a large cell body with multiple dendrites and a single axon extending from it. The dendrites tend to receive inputs, depolarizations, from other neurons, which they convey to the nerve cell body. If the neuron depolarizes, this is propagated down the axon, which will then interact with another neuron or target tissue. The details of this process will be presented in Chapter 6. Compression or damage to a nerve will cause altered sensation and motor loss distal to the lesion. In this book we will focus almost exclusively on somatic motor and sensory activity.

SOMATOSENSORY ACTIVITY

The cell bodies of somatosensory nerves are located in the posterior root ganglia, a collection of nerve cell bodies at every vertebral level. Their axons split and project laterally to their target tissues and also medially to the spinal cord. This allows them to sense fine touch, vibration, pressure, pain, and temperature from the skin and proprioceptive inputs from the muscles and tendons, and to convey that information from the PNS to the CNS. They eventually reach the cerebral cortex, where sensation is consciously perceived. The details of this process will be explained in Chapter 8.

SOMATOMOTOR ACTIVITY

Upper motor neurons largely originate in the cerebral cortex and project through descending motor tracts to reach the spinal cord. Lower motor neurons in the brainstem and spinal cord send their axons through peripheral nerves, often branching and recombining, to reach their muscular targets.

CRANIAL NERVES

The cranial nerves (Fig. 4.2) exit the skull and tend to innervate structures of the head and neck. They will not be discussed in detail in this volume. In brief,

- **Cranial nerve I**, the **olfactory nerve** and its **olfactory tract**, conveys the sense of smell from the nasal cavity.
- **Cranial nerve II**, the **optic nerve**, conveys visual information from the retina. Some axons in each optic nerve cross at the **optic chiasm** to reach the contralateral **optic tract**, while the others will continue in the ipsilateral optic tract.
- **Cranial nerve III**, the **oculomotor nerve**, innervates five of the seven extraocular muscles that surround the eye.
- **Cranial nerve IV**, the **trochlear nerve**, innervates one of the seven extraocular muscles.
- **Cranial nerve V**, the **trigeminal nerve**, splits into three large branches that convey sensation from the face and internal structures of the head. It also innervates the muscles of mastication, which allow us to chew.
- **Cranial nerve VI**, the **abducens nerve**, innervates one of the seven extraocular muscles.
- **Cranial nerve VII**, the **facial nerve**, innervates the muscles of the face, the lacrimal gland, and two salivary glands. It also mediates the sense of taste from the anterior tongue.
- **Cranial nerve VIII**, the **vestibulocochlear nerve**, conveys hearing and balance sensations from the inner ear.
- **Cranial nerve IX**, the **glossopharyngeal nerve**, conveys sensation from the pharynx, middle ear, and posterior tongue, including taste. It also innervates one of the salivary glands.

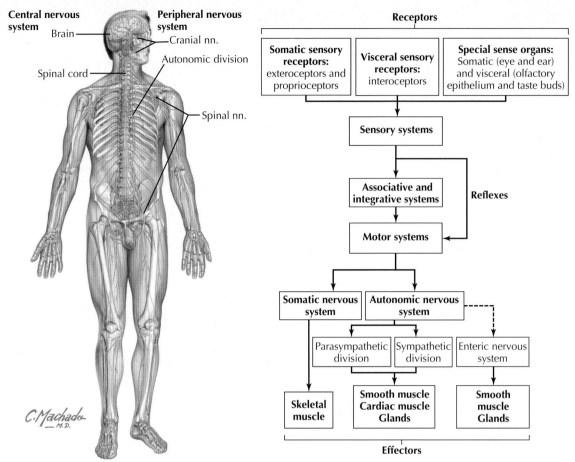

Fig. 4.1 Nervous System: Organization.

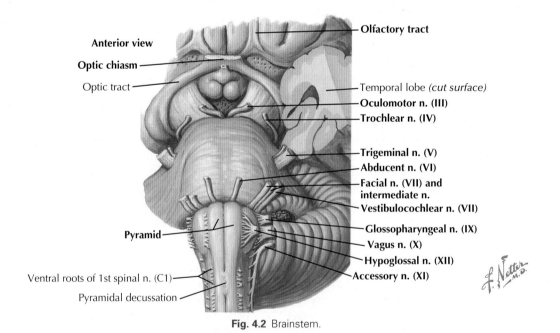

Fig. 4.2 Brainstem.

- **Cranial nerve X**, the **vagus nerve**, innervates muscles of the palate, pharynx, and larynx. It also provides visceral motor innervation to the organs of the thorax and several organs of the abdomen.
- **Cranial nerve XII**, the **hypoglossal nerve**, innervates the muscles of the tongue.

- **Cranial nerve XI**, the **accessory nerve** (Fig. 4.3), has been purposefully shuffled to the end of this list because it directly affects two of the muscles we have previously discussed and will be described in more detail. The accessory nerve originates from nerve cell bodies in the gray matter of the C1–C5 spinal cord. Axons from these nerve cells exit the lateral

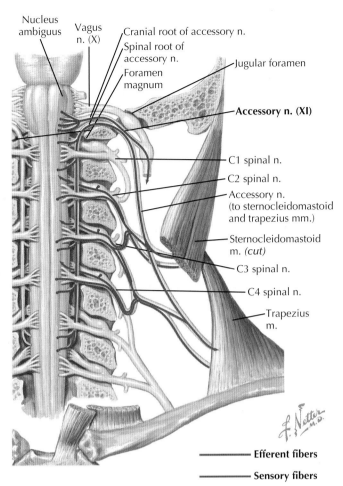

Fig. 4.3 Accessory Nerve (XI) Schema.

aspect of the spinal cord. Instead of exiting between the vertebrae, which is the normal route, these axons instead ascend within the vertebral canal and fuse with each other to form the **spinal root of the accessory nerve.** This nerve enters the foramen magnum of the skull from below and then turns to exit through the jugular foramen alongside cranial nerves IX and X. It receives some fibers from the brainstem, the **cranial root of the accessory nerve,** but these join the vagus nerve shortly after leaving the jugular foramen. It then descends and sends axons that innervate the **trapezius** and **sternocleidomastoid muscles.** If the spinal accessory nerve is damaged, either muscle or both muscles can be paralyzed, depending on the exact site of the injury (Clinical Correlation 4.1).

SPINAL CORD

Gray Matter, White Matter, and Posterior Root Ganglia

The spinal cord extends inferiorly from the brainstem, out the foramen magnum, and down within the vertebral canal. The nerve cell bodies, or gray matter, of the spinal cord are found inside the cord. They form a (roughly) butterfly-shaped structure with posterior horns and anterior horns on each side. Superficial to the gray matter are tracts that ascend and descend along the entire length of the cord. This is the white matter of the spinal cord and is made of axons and their supporting cells.

Alongside the vertebral column at each spinal level are collections of sensory cell bodies in the **posterior root ganglia.** Their axons project in two directions. The lateral side of each

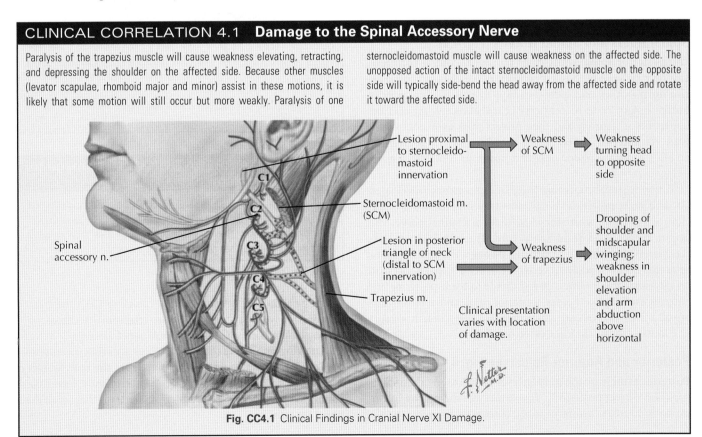

CLINICAL CORRELATION 4.1 Damage to the Spinal Accessory Nerve

Paralysis of the trapezius muscle will cause weakness elevating, retracting, and depressing the shoulder on the affected side. Because other muscles (levator scapulae, rhomboid major and minor) assist in these motions, it is likely that some motion will still occur but more weakly. Paralysis of one sternocleidomastoid muscle will cause weakness on the affected side. The unopposed action of the intact sternocleidomastoid muscle on the opposite side will typically side-bend the head away from the affected side and rotate it toward the affected side.

Fig. CC4.1 Clinical Findings in Cranial Nerve XI Damage.

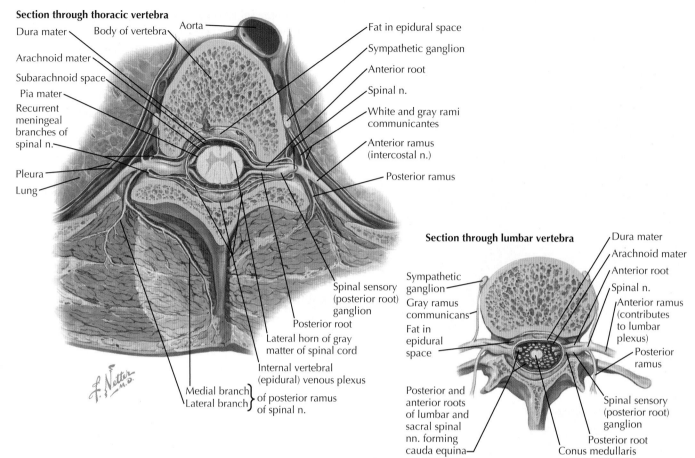

Fig. 4.4 Spinal Nerve Origin: Cross Sections Exit of Spinal Nerves.

axon projects to the skin and muscles, while the medial side projects to the spinal cord as posterior nerve roots.

Spinal Roots and Spinal Nerves (Fig. 4.4)

The **posterior spinal roots** enter the spinal cord at each level and may synapse with other sensory nerve cells in the **posterior horn**, or they may ascend without synapsing. The **anterior horns** contain lower motor nerve cells that receive inputs from upper motor neurons and then project their axons out of the cord via **anterior roots**. Spinal roots are strictly segregated: anterior roots are motor only and posterior roots are sensory only.

Anterior spinal roots that leave the spinal cord travel laterally and meet posterior spinal roots traveling toward a posterior root ganglion where they fuse to form a **spinal nerve**. This occurs at each level of the spinal cord. The spinal nerves leave the vertebral column by traveling through the intervertebral foramina between adjacent vertebrae. After a spinal nerve exits an intervertebral foramen, it will divide to form posterior and anterior rami. Spinal nerves, posterior rami, and anterior rami are all mixed nervous structures because they contain sensory and motor axons (Clinical Correlation 4.2).

Posterior and Anterior Rami (see Fig. 4.4)

Posterior rami leave the spinal nerves at each level of the spinal cord and project posteriorly. They innervate the nearby intrinsic back muscles before sending cutaneous branches to the

> ### CLINICAL CORRELATION 4.2 **Spinal Nerve Compression**
>
> Compression of the spinal nerves will affect the skin and muscles innervated by the affected spinal level. This commonly manifests as sensory changes along a dermatome as the ability of the nerve to reach the central nervous system is compromised immediately. Motor losses due to spinal nerve compression will also occur eventually, but muscle atrophy takes more time to visibly develop.

> ### CLINICAL CORRELATION 4.3 **Damage to the Posterior Rami**
>
> Paralysis of the intrinsic back muscles would result in weakness extending, rotating, and side-bending the back at the affected levels. Because the posterior rami innervate muscles in a segmental manner, loss of one posterior ramus might not entirely deinnervate the larger muscles.

overlying skin. Damage to posterior rami can affect the erector spinae, transversospinalis, splenius, semispinalis capitis, and suboccipital muscles (Clinical Correlation 4.3).

Anterior rami leave the spinal nerves at each level and project anteriorly. They innervate the muscles of the body wall and limbs. Unlike the posterior rami, they frequently form interconnected plexi before forming terminal nerves that reach their target muscles.

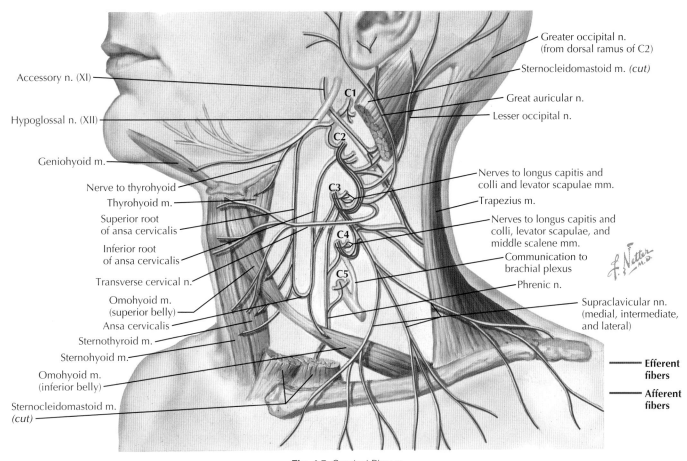

Accessory n. (XI)

Hypoglossal n. (XII)

Geniohyoid m.

Nerve to thyrohyoid

Thyrohyoid m.

Superior root
of ansa cervicalis

Inferior root
of ansa cervicalis

Transverse cervical n.

Omohyoid m.
(superior belly)

Ansa cervicalis

Sternothyroid m.

Sternohyoid m.

Omohyoid m.
(inferior belly)

Sternocleidomastoid m.
(cut)

Greater occipital n.
(from dorsal ramus of C2)

Sternocleidomastoid m. *(cut)*

Great auricular n.

Lesser occipital n.

Nerves to longus capitis and
colli and levator scapulae mm.

Trapezius m.

Nerves to longus capitis and
colli, levator scapulae, and
middle scalene mm.

Communication to
brachial plexus

Phrenic n.

Supraclavicular nn.
(medial, intermediate,
and lateral)

C1
C2
C3
C4
C5

Efferent
fibers

Afferent
fibers

Fig. 4.5 Cervical Plexus.

CERVICAL PLEXUS AND PHRENIC NERVE

The **cervical plexus** (Fig. 4.5) arises from the C1–C4 anterior rami. They combine to create several nerves that are only cutaneous (innervate the skin). These convey sensations from a variety of regions.

The **lesser occipital nerve** conveys sensation from the area of the scalp immediately behind the ear; the **great auricular nerve** covers most of the external ear, the **transverse cervical nerve** is sensory to the skin of the anterior neck, and the **supraclavicular nerves** convey sensations from the skin on the neck in the region of the clavicles. The cervical plexus also supplies some sensory nerves to the sternocleidomastoid, although its motor fibers come exclusively from the spinal accessory nerve.

The motor axons of the cervical plexus arise from C1 to C3 and form a loop, the **ansa cervicalis** (see Fig. 4.5), that sits just anterior to the large vessels of the neck, the external jugular vein and common carotid artery. The contribution from C1 travels along the hypoglossal nerve (cranial nerve XII) and peels away to form the superior limb of the ansa cervicalis. Other cervical plexus axons travel along the hypoglossal nerve a bit further to innervate the **geniohyoid** (suprahyoid muscle group) and **thyrohyoid** (infrahyoid muscle group). The inferior limb of the ansa cervicalis is formed by axons from C2 to C3. The ansa innervates the remaining infrahyoid muscles, the sternohyoid, **sternothyroid**, and the **superior and inferior bellies of the omohyoid muscle**. Small motor branches also leave the cervical

CLINICAL CORRELATION 4.4 Damage to the Cervical Plexus

The cutaneous branches of the cervical plexus travel just posterior to the midpoint of the sternocleidomastoid muscle. Damage at that point could affect any or all of the nerves, resulting in sensory loss distal to the lesion. Damage to the ansa cervicalis can occur in trauma to the anterior neck or during surgery to the large vessels that are deep to it. This would result in weakness in adjusting the hyoid bone during swallowing and tilting of the hyoid bone.

CLINICAL CORRELATION 4.5 Damage to the Phrenic Nerve

Dysfunction of the phrenic nerve can occur if it is impinged or damaged anywhere along its length between the cervical vertebrae and diaphragm. This will cause difficulty breathing due to paralysis of the diaphragm on the affected side. The paralysis will cause the muscles of the diaphragm to relax and dome upward into the thorax, pushed by the underlying abdominal organs.

plexus to innervate the longus coli, longus capitis, and scalene muscles (Clinical Correlation 4.4).

The **phrenic nerve** (see Fig. 4.5) arises from branches of the C3 to C5 anterior rami. These branches converge and fuse to form the nerve. It descends along the anterior surface of the anterior scalene muscle and enters the thorax. It travels through the central thorax, along the outer lining of the heart, and reaches the **thoracic diaphragm**, which it innervates (Clinical Correlation 4.5).

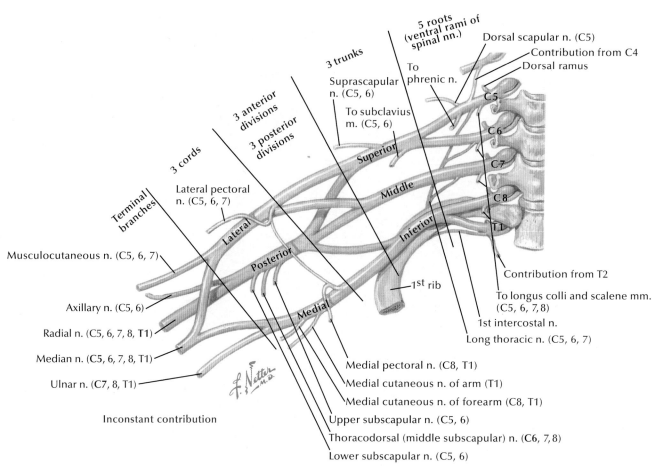

Fig. 4.6 Brachial Plexus: Schema.

BRACHIAL PLEXUS

The anterior rami of C5–T1 provide the majority of the axons that create the **brachial plexus** (Fig. 4.6), the collection of nerves that innervate the skin and muscles of the upper limb. The brachial plexus can be divided into five distinct regions: **roots, trunks, divisions, cords,** and **terminal nerves.** These "roots" are not to be mixed up with "spinal roots" but are instead a collection of anterior rami that create the "roots of the brachial plexus." I apologize for the confusing terminology; I do not care for it either.

C5 and C6 roots fuse to create the **superior trunk** of the brachial plexus. The superior trunk contains axons that tend to innervate proximal and lateral limb structures. The C7 root continues laterally and becomes the **middle trunk.** C8 and T1 roots fuse to create the **inferior trunk.** The inferior trunk contains axons that tend to innervate distal and medial limb structures.

Branches From the Roots of the Brachial Plexus

The C5–C7 roots give off branches that consolidate to form the **long thoracic nerve** (Figs. 4.6 and 4.7) which descends along the thoracic wall to innervate the **serratus anterior muscle.** The **dorsal scapular nerve** (see Figs. 4.6 and 4.8) arises as a branch from the C5 root and weaves along the **levator scapulae, rhomboid minor,** and **rhomboid major muscles,** which it innervates.

Branches From the Trunks of the Brachial Plexus

The superior trunk gives off the **suprascapular nerve** (see Figs. 4.6–4.8), which innervates the **supraspinatus** and **infraspinatus muscles.** This nerve travels posteriorly and passes through the scapular notch, inferior to the superior transverse scapular ligament, to reach the supraspinatus muscle and then passes lateral to the scapular spine to reach the infraspinatus. A nerve to the small subclavius muscle on the inferior aspect of the clavicle also arises from the superior trunk. No other important nerves leave the middle or inferior trunks.

Each trunk now divides into a posterior division and an anterior division (see Fig. 4.6). The **posterior cord** is formed by the fusion of all three of the posterior divisions and innervates the extensor muscles of the upper limb. The anterior divisions of the superior and middle trunks fuse to form the **lateral cord** while the anterior division of the inferior cord continues as the **medial cord.** The nerves derived from the anterior divisions, and thereafter the lateral and medial cords, innervate flexor muscles.

Branches From the Cords and Terminal Nerves of the Brachial Plexus

The posterior cord gives off three small but important nerves before terminating (see Figs. 4.6 and 4.7). The **upper subscapular** and **lower subscapular nerves** innervate the nearby subscapularis and teres major muscles. In between the subscapular

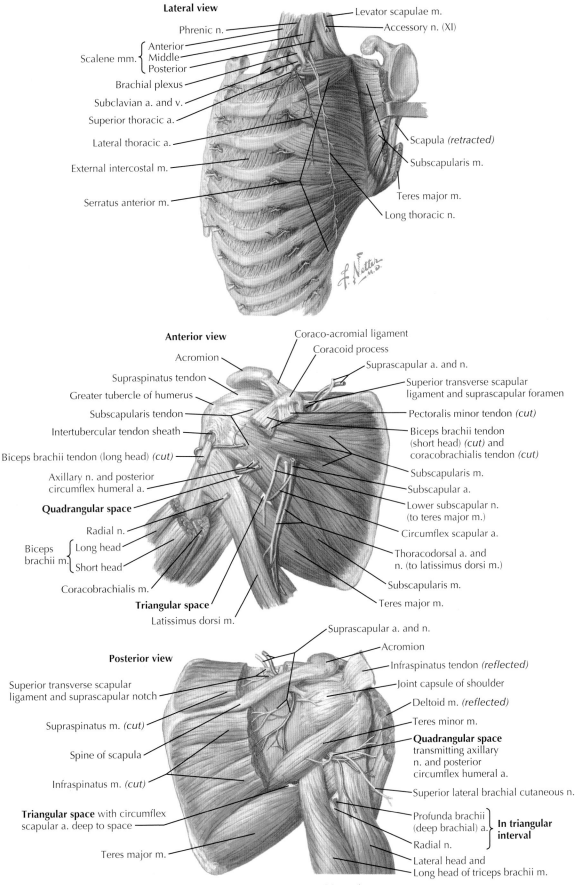

Lateral view

Levator scapulae m.

Phrenic n.

Accessory n. (XI)

Scalene mm. { Anterior — Middle — Posterior

Brachial plexus

Subclavian a. and v.

Superior thoracic a.

Lateral thoracic a.

Scapula *(retracted)*

Subscapularis m.

External intercostal m.

Serratus anterior m.

Teres major m.

Long thoracic n.

Anterior view

Coraco-acromial ligament

Coracoid process

Acromion

Suprascapular a. and n.

Suprasinatus tendon

Superior transverse scapular ligament and suprascapular foramen

Greater tubercle of humerus

Subscapularis tendon

Pectoralis minor tendon *(cut)*

Intertubercular tendon sheath

Biceps brachii tendon (short head) *(cut)* and coracobrachialis tendon *(cut)*

Biceps brachii tendon (long head) *(cut)*

Axillary n. and posterior circumflex humeral a.

Subscapularis m.

Subscapular a.

Quadrangular space

Lower subscapular n. (to teres major m.)

Radial n.

Circumflex scapular a.

Biceps brachii m. { Long head — Short head

Thoracodorsal a. and n. (to latissimus dorsi m.)

Coracobrachialis m.

Subscapularis m.

Triangular space

Teres major m.

Latissimus dorsi m.

Suprascapular a. and n.

Acromion

Posterior view

Infraspinatus tendon *(reflected)*

Joint capsule of shoulder

Superior transverse scapular ligament and suprascapular notch

Deltoid m. *(reflected)*

Teres minor m.

Suprasinatus m. *(cut)*

Quadrangular space transmitting axillary n. and posterior circumflex humeral a.

Spine of scapula

Infraspinatus m. *(cut)*

Superior lateral brachial cutaneous n.

Triangular space with circumflex scapular a. deep to space

Profunda brachii (deep brachial) a. } **In triangular interval**

Radial n.

Teres major m.

Lateral head and Long head of triceps brachii m.

Fig. 4.7 Scapulohumeral Dissection.

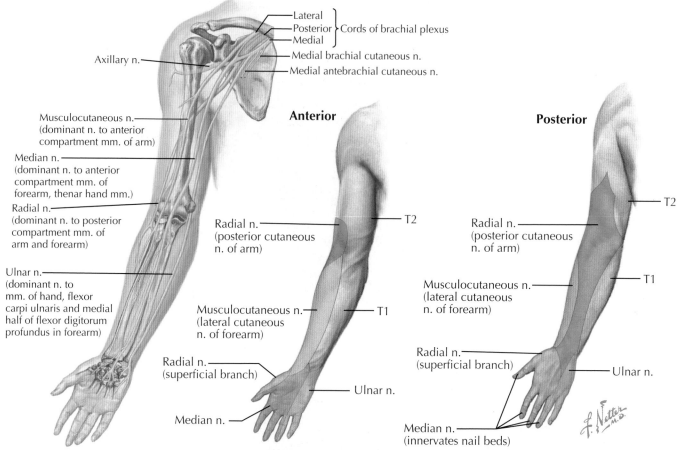

Fig. 4.8 Nerves of the Upper Limb.

nerves is the **thoracodorsal nerve**, which innervates the **latissimus dorsi muscle**. The posterior cord ends when it bifurcates to form its two terminal branches, the axillary and radial nerves.

The **axillary nerve** (see Figs. 4.6 and 4.8) wraps around the posterior aspect of the surgical neck of the humerus to innervate the **teres minor** and **deltoid muscles**. It also has cutaneous branches that convey sensation from the lateral shoulder. The massive **radial nerve** (Figs. 4.6 and 4.8) descends along the posterior aspect of the humeral shaft, innervating the muscles of the posterior compartment of the arm, such as the **triceps brachii muscle**. It continues across the lateral epicondyle of the humerus and splits into a superficial and deep branch. The radial nerve and its two motor branches, the **deep branch of the radial nerve** and **posterior interosseous nerve**, innervate the brachioradialis, extensor muscles of the wrist and digits, and the supinator muscle. The **superficial branch of the radial nerve** is cutaneous only and conveys sensations from the dorsum of the hand (excluding the fifth and the medial half of the fourth digits), posterior forearm, and posterolateral arm (Clinical Correlation 4.6).

The lateral cord gives off a **lateral pectoral nerve** (see Fig. 4.6) that innervates the part of the **pectoralis major muscle** that originates from the clavicle. The lateral cord then bifurcates as the musculocutaneous nerve and a lateral contribution to the median nerve. The **musculocutaneous nerve** (see Figs. 4.6 and 4.8) dives into the anterior compartment of the arm and

innervates the muscles of that compartment, the **coracobrachialis, biceps brachii,** and **brachialis muscles**. Its cutaneous branch, the **lateral cutaneous nerve of the forearm** continues inferiorly on the lateral forearm (Clinical Correlation 4.7).

The medial cord gives off a **medial pectoral nerve** (see Fig. 4.6), which innervates the **pectoralis minor** and the sternocostal portion of the **pectoralis major muscle**. Two cutaneous nerves, the **medial cutaneous nerve of the arm** and the **medial cutaneous nerve of the forearm**, arise from the medial cord just distal to the medial pectoral nerve. The cord terminates as the ulnar nerve and a medial contribution to the median nerve.

The **ulnar nerve** (see Figs. 4.6 and 4.8) continues inferiorly on the medial side of the arm, passing posterior to the medial epicondyle of the humerus and then into the anterior compartment of the forearm, where it innervates two muscles, **flexor carpi ulnaris** and the ulnar side of the **deep digital flexor**, before crossing the wrist. As it crosses the wrist, it gives off a deep branch and superficial branch. The **deep branch of the ulnar nerve** innervates all the **hypothenar muscles**, and nearly all **intrinsic muscles of the hand**, including the **adductor pollicis**. The **superficial branch of the ulnar nerve** innervates the skin of the fifth digit and medial half of the fourth digit, on both the palmar and dorsal sides (Clinical Correlation 4.8).

Branches from the lateral and medial cords combine to create the **median** nerve (see Fig. 4.6 and 4.8). This nerve travels inferiorly along the medial aspect of the humerus and then along the anterior midline of the forearm. As it descends, it gives off a small motor branch, the **anterior interosseous nerve**. Aside from the two forearm muscles innervated by the ulnar nerve, the median nerve innervates all the muscles of the forearm, the **pronators, carpal flexors, superficial digital flexor, flexor pollicis longus**, and radial half of the **deep digital flexor muscles**. The median nerve then travels through the carpal tunnel alongside the tendons of the digital flexors and flexor pollicis longus. In the hand, it gives off a **recurrent branch** that innervates the **thenar muscles**. Cutaneous branches of the median nerve innervate the palmar aspect of digits 1 to 3 and the lateral half of the fourth digit (Clinical Correlation 4.9).

INTERCOSTAL NERVES

The **intercostal nerves** (Fig. 4.9) are the anterior rami of T1–T11, and they travel along the inferior edge of their corresponding rib as they project anteriorly. They are not exclusively associated with the rib cage but continue inferomedially through the abdominal oblique muscles to reach the rectus abdominis muscles. In the thorax, these nerves innervate the **external, internal, innermost intercostal muscles**, as well as other muscles inside the thorax. In the abdomen they innervate the **external abdominal oblique, internal abdominal oblique, transversus abdominis**, and **rectus abdominis muscles**. They also give off **lateral cutaneous** and **anterior cutaneous branches** that convey sensations from the lateral and anterior body wall (Clinical Correlation 4.10).

LUMBAR PLEXUS

The anterior rami immediately inferior to the intercostal nerves form the lumbar plexus (Figs. 4.10 and 4.11); they are the **subcostal, ilioinguinal, iliohypogastric, genitofemoral**, and **lateral cutaneous nerve of the thigh**. Like the intercostal muscles, the first four of those nerves innervate the muscles and skin of the anterior body wall. Damage to these nerves would result in muscle weakness and sensory loss along the length of the nerve. The lateral cutaneous nerve of the thigh does exactly what its name implies. The genitofemoral nerve also innervates the skin of the anterior pelvic region and proximal, medial thigh.

Lumbar anterior rami from L1 to L3 innervate the **psoas major** and **iliacus muscles**. The large **femoral nerve** (see Figs. 4.10 and 4.11) passes through that abdominal wall into the thigh. It innervates muscles of the anterior compartment of the thigh, the **sartorius** and **quadriceps muscles**. Damage to this nerve would result in difficulty flexing the thigh at the hip as well as profound weakness extending the leg at the knee. It has sensory branches that cover the anterior thigh as well as a long sensory branch, the **saphenous nerve**, which extends inferiorly along the lateral thigh, leg, and onto the medial ankle and heel (Clinical Correlation 4.11).

The **obturator nerve** (Figs. 4.10 and 4.12) exits the pelvis through the obturator foramen to enter the medial compartment of the thigh. It innervates the **pectineus, gracilis, adductor longus, adductor brevis**, and **adductor magnus muscles**. It also carries sensory input from a patch of skin along the medial thigh (Clinical Correlation 4.12).

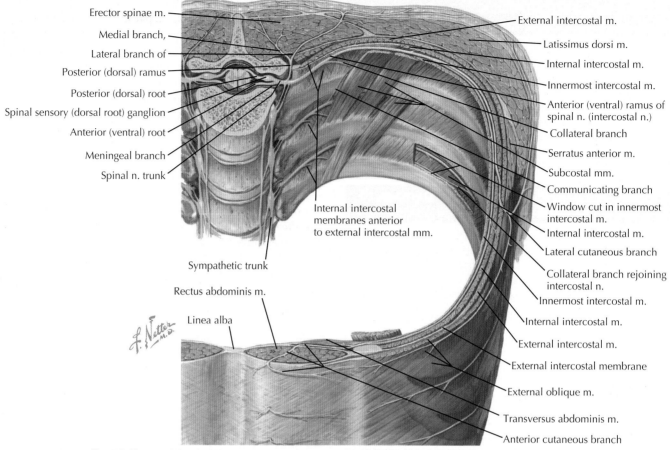

Erector spinae m.
Medial branch,
Lateral branch of
Posterior (dorsal) ramus
Posterior (dorsal) root
Spinal sensory (dorsal root) ganglion
Anterior (ventral) root
Meningeal branch
Spinal n. trunk

Internal intercostal
membranes anterior
to external intercostal mm.

Sympathetic trunk
Rectus abdominis m.
Linea alba

External intercostal m.
Latissimus dorsi m.
Internal intercostal m.
Innermost intercostal m.
Anterior (ventral) ramus of
spinal n. (intercostal n.)
Collateral branch
Serratus anterior m.
Subcostal mm.
Communicating branch
Window cut in innermost
intercostal m.
Internal intercostal m.
Lateral cutaneous branch
Collateral branch rejoining
intercostal n.
Innermost intercostal m.
Internal intercostal m.
External intercostal m.
External intercostal membrane
External oblique m.
Transversus abdominis m.
Anterior cutaneous branch

Fig. 4.9 Thoracoabdominal Nerves: Course of Typical Thoracic Nerve Innervation of Abdomen and Perineum.

LUMBOSACRAL PLEXUS

The anterior rami of L4 and L5 fuse and descend into the pelvis. Here they fuse with the sacral anterior rami to create the lumbosacral plexus. It provides motor and sensory innervation to the pelvis and posterior thigh, as well as the entire leg and foot.

The **superior gluteal nerve** (Fig. 4.13) exits the pelvis immediately superior to the piriformis muscle and innervates the **piriformis** and **gluteus medius and minimus muscles**. Correspondingly, the **inferior gluteal nerve** (see Fig. 4.13) exits inferior to the piriformis and innervates the **gluteus maximus muscle** (Clinical Correlation 4.13). Small **cluneal nerves** innervate the skin of the gluteal region.

The **posterior cutaneous nerve of the thigh** (see Figs. 4.13 and 4.14) descends parallel but superficial to the sciatic nerve.

The massive **sciatic nerve** (see Figs. 4.13 and 4.14) typically exits the pelvis just inferior to the piriformis muscle and descends deep to the gluteus maximus before entering the posterior thigh. It innervates the hamstring muscles in the posterior thigh, the **semimembranous, semitendinosus,** and **biceps femoris**

muscles. Although the sciatic nerve appears to be a single nerve, it is actually two nerves bundled together, the tibial and common fibular nerves, that split near the popliteal fossa of the posterior knee. Just after they split, they each send a cutaneous branch to the skin overlying the posterior leg. These branches often combine to form a single **sural nerve** (see Fig. 4.14) but may also remain separate.

The **tibial nerve** (Figs. 4.14 and 4.15) travels down the midline of the posterior leg and innervates all muscles of the posterior leg: **gastrocnemius, soleus, plantaris, tibialis posterior, flexor digitorum longus,** and **flexor hallucis longus**. It crosses inferior to the medial malleolus to reach the plantar foot, where it divides to become the **medial and lateral plantar nerves**. These nerves innervate **all muscles of the plantar foot** along with the overlying skin.

From the division of the sciatic nerve, the **common fibular nerve** (Figs. 4.14 and 4.15) travels laterally and crosses the superior aspect of the fibular head. It then splits into a superficial and deep fibular nerve. The **superficial fibular nerve** (see Fig. 4.15) innervates the muscles of the lateral leg, the **fibularis longus and brevis**, and the skin of the anterolateral leg and dorsum of the foot. The **deep fibular nerve** (Fig. 4.15) passes into the anterior leg and innervates, the **tibialis anterior, extensor hallucis longus,** and **extensor digitorum longus muscles**. It also innervates the small **extensor hallucis brevis** and **extensor digitorum brevis muscles** on the dorsum of the foot and conveys sensations from a tiny patch of skin between the first and second digits (Clinical Correlation 4.14).

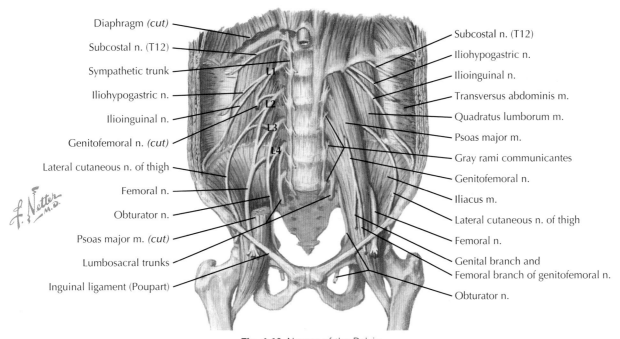

Diaphragm *(cut)*
Subcostal n. (T12)
Sympathetic trunk
Iliohypogastric n.
Ilioinguinal n.
Genitofemoral n. *(cut)*
Lateral cutaneous n. of thigh
Femoral n.
Obturator n.
Psoas major m. *(cut)*
Lumbosacral trunks
Inguinal ligament (Poupart)

L1
L2
L3
L4

Subcostal n. (T12)
Iliohypogastric n.
Ilioinguinal n.
Transversus abdominis m.
Quadratus lumborum m.
Psoas major m.
Gray rami communicantes
Genitofemoral n.
Iliacus m.
Lateral cutaneous n. of thigh
Femoral n.
Genital branch and
Femoral branch of genitofemoral n.
Obturator n.

Fig. 4.10 Nerves of the Pelvis.

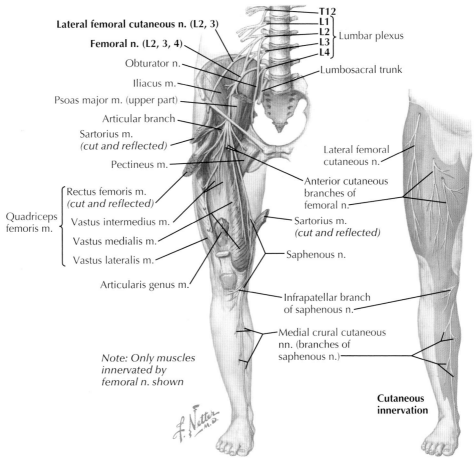

Lateral femoral cutaneous n. (L2, 3)
Femoral n. (L2, 3, 4)
Obturator n.
Iliacus m.
Psoas major m. (upper part)
Articular branch
Sartorius m. *(cut and reflected)*
Pectineus m.

Rectus femoris m. *(cut and reflected)*
Quadriceps femoris m. {
Vastus intermedius m.
Vastus medialis m.
Vastus lateralis m.

Articularis genus m.

T12
L1
L2
L3
L4
} Lumbar plexus

Lumbosacral trunk

Lateral femoral cutaneous n.
Anterior cutaneous branches of femoral n.
Sartorius m. *(cut and reflected)*
Saphenous n.
Infrapatellar branch of saphenous n.
Medial crural cutaneous nn. (branches of saphenous n.)

Note: Only muscles innervated by femoral n. shown

Cutaneous innervation

Fig. 4.11 Femoral and Lateral Femoral Cutaneous Nerves.

CLINICAL CORRELATION 4.11 Damage to the Femoral Nerve

Damage to the femoral nerve in the proximal thigh would result in profound weakness extending the knee due to loss of the quadriceps motor innervation. Some weakness in hip flexion may also be present. Sensory losses would include the anterior and medial thigh, medial leg, ankle, and heel. Because the branches to the sartorius and quadriceps muscles leave the femoral nerve very proximally in the thigh, distal damage would likely not affect knee extension but would result in sensory loss distal to the injury.

The **pudendal nerve** (Figs. 4.13 and 4.16) exits the pelvis through the greater sciatic foramen but immediately returns via the lesser sciatic foramen to innervate the skin and muscles around the **external anal sphincter** through the **inferior rectal (anal) nerve**. The pudendal nerve and some of its other branches such as the **perineal nerve** and **dorsal nerve of the clitoris/penis** will innervate parts of the **pelvic diaphragm (coccygeus and levator ani muscles)** and **the urogenital triangle**. This region will be described in detail in Chapter 12. Damage to the pudendal nerve and its branches can result in urinary and rectal incontinence and loss of sensation in the perineal region and most of the external genitalia.

CLINICAL CORRELATION 4.12 Damage to the Obturator Nerve

Damage to the obturator nerve in the pelvis or near the obturator foramen would result in profound weakness adducting the thigh and instability in supporting one's weight. Sensory losses may be noted along the medial thigh.

CLINICAL CORRELATION 4.13 Damage to the Gluteal Nerves

Damage to the superior gluteal nerve and weakness of the gluteus medius and minimus would result in an inability to abduct the thigh. That would result in difficulty keeping the pelvis level when standing on one leg, something we do with every step. Damage to the inferior gluteal nerve and gluteus maximus would prevent strong extension of the hip from a flexed position. This may not be obvious when walking but makes ascending stairs and standing from a seated position very difficult.

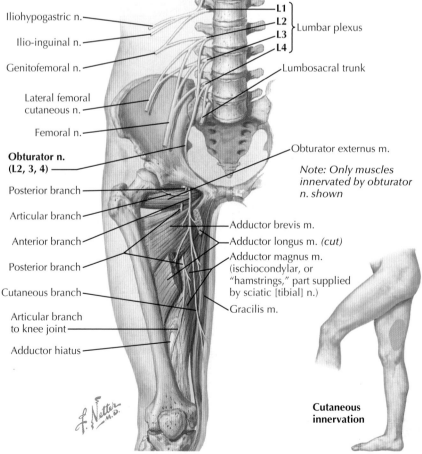

Iliohypogastric n.

Ilio-inguinal n.

Genitofemoral n.

Lateral femoral cutaneous n.

Femoral n.

Obturator n. (L2, 3, 4)

Posterior branch

Articular branch

Anterior branch

Posterior branch

Cutaneous branch

Articular branch to knee joint

Adductor hiatus

L1
L2
L3
L4

} Lumbar plexus

Lumbosacral trunk

Obturator externus m.

Note: Only muscles innervated by obturator n. shown

Adductor brevis m.

Adductor longus m. *(cut)*

Adductor magnus m. (ischiocondylar, or "hamstrings," part supplied by sciatic [tibial] n.)

Gracilis m.

Cutaneous innervation

Fig. 4.12 Obturator Nerve.

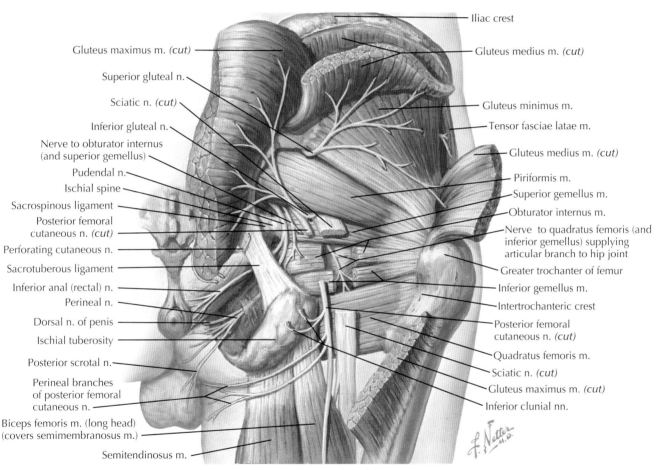

Iliac crest

Gluteus maximus m. *(cut)*

Gluteus medius m. *(cut)*

Superior gluteal n.

Sciatic n. *(cut)*

Gluteus minimus m.

Inferior gluteal n.

Tensor fasciae latae m.

Nerve to obturator internus
(and superior gemellus)

Gluteus medius m. *(cut)*

Pudendal n.

Piriformis m.

Ischial spine

Superior gemellus m.

Sacrospinous ligament

Obturator internus m.

Posterior femoral
cutaneous n. *(cut)*

Nerve to quadratus femoris (and
inferior gemellus) supplying
articular branch to hip joint

Perforating cutaneous n.

Greater trochanter of femur

Sacrotuberous ligament

Inferior gemellus m.

Inferior anal (rectal) n.

Intertrochanteric crest

Perineal n.

Posterior femoral
cutaneous n. *(cut)*

Dorsal n. of penis

Quadratus femoris m.

Ischial tuberosity

Sciatic n. *(cut)*

Posterior scrotal n.

Gluteus maximus m. *(cut)*

Perineal branches
of posterior femoral
cutaneous n.

Inferior clunial nn.

Biceps femoris m. (long head)
(covers semimembranosus m.)

Semitendinosus m.

Fig. 4.13 Nerves of the Buttock.

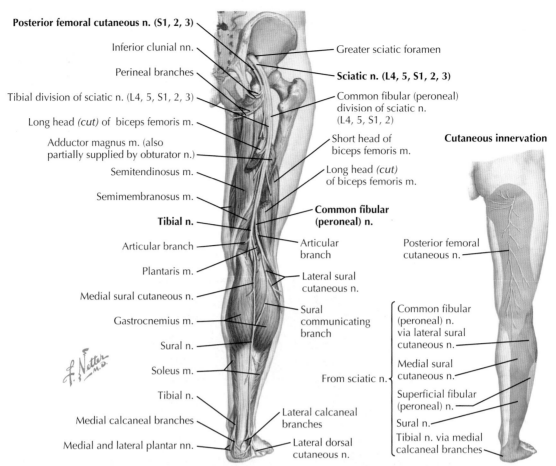

Posterior femoral cutaneous n. (S1, 2, 3)

Inferior clunial nn.

Perineal branches

Tibial division of sciatic n. (L4, 5, S1, 2, 3)

Long head *(cut)* of biceps femoris m.

Adductor magnus m. (also partially supplied by obturator n.)

Semitendinosus m.

Semimembranosus m.

Tibial n.

Articular branch

Plantaris m.

Medial sural cutaneous n.

Gastrocnemius m.

Sural n.

Soleus m.

Tibial n.

Medial calcaneal branches

Medial and lateral plantar nn.

Greater sciatic foramen

Sciatic n. (L4, 5, S1, 2, 3)

Common fibular (peroneal) division of sciatic n. (L4, 5, S1, 2)

Short head of biceps femoris m.

Long head *(cut)* of biceps femoris m.

Common fibular (peroneal) n.

Articular branch

Lateral sural cutaneous n.

Sural communicating branch

Lateral calcaneal branches

Lateral dorsal cutaneous n.

Cutaneous innervation

Posterior femoral cutaneous n.

Common fibular (peroneal) n. via lateral sural cutaneous n.

Medial sural cutaneous n.

Superficial fibular (peroneal) n.

Sural n.

Tibial n. via medial calcaneal branches

From sciatic n.

Fig. 4.14 Sciatic nerve (L4, L5; S1, S2, S3) and posterior femoral cutaneous nerve (S1, S2, S3): sciatic nerve and posterior cutaneous nerve of thigh.

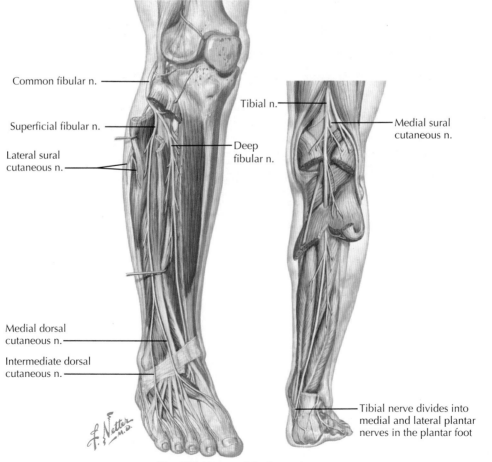

Common fibular n.

Superficial fibular n.

Lateral sural cutaneous n.

Tibial n.

Deep fibular n.

Medial sural cutaneous n.

Medial dorsal cutaneous n.

Intermediate dorsal cutaneous n.

Tibial nerve divides into medial and lateral plantar nerves in the plantar foot

Fig. 4.15 Nerves of the Lower Leg.

CLINICAL CORRELATION 4.14   Damage to the Sciatic, Tibial, and Fibular Nerves

The signs of damage to branches of the sciatic nerve will depend a great deal on the exact site of the injury. Damage to the deep fibular nerve would result in paralysis of the muscles of the anterior compartment of the leg, causing weak dorsiflexion and digital extension and foot drop, as well as loss of sensation between digits 1 and 2. Damage to the superficial fibular nerve would cause weakness in everting the foot, manifesting as frequently inverting the ankle and falling, as well as loss of sensation on the anterolateral leg and dorsum of the foot (but sparing the skin between digits 1 and 2). Damage to the common fibular nerve, possibly by compression from the fibular head, would show up as a combination of deep and superficial fibular nerve loss.

Damage to the tibial neve causes weakness in plantarflexing the foot at the ankle, flexing all toes, and weakness of muscles of the plantar foot. This would make normal walking very difficult.

Damage to the sciatic nerve in the thigh manifests as common fibular and tibial nerve dysfunction, including loss of sensation on the posterior leg due to sural nerve involvement, but would spare the hamstring muscles. Damage to the proximal sciatic nerve in the gluteal region would be similar but also include profound weakness of the hamstring muscles, making forceful knee flexion and hip extension difficult. Damage to the sciatic nerve at this site would make walking nearly impossible.

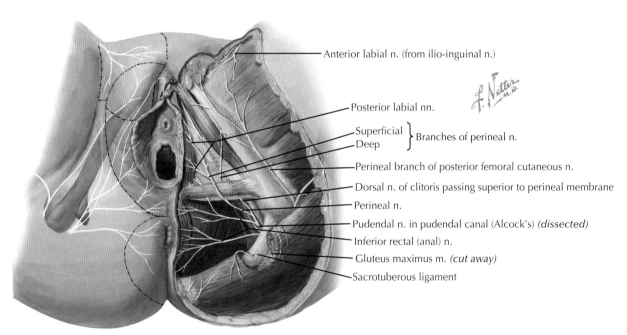

Anterior labial n. (from ilio-inguinal n.)

Posterior labial nn.

Superficial
Deep } Branches of perineal n.

Perineal branch of posterior femoral cutaneous n.

Dorsal n. of clitoris passing superior to perineal membrane

Perineal n.

Pudendal n. in pudendal canal (Alcock's) *(dissected)*

Inferior rectal (anal) n.

Gluteus maximus m. *(cut away)*

Sacrotuberous ligament

Fig. 4.16 Perineum: Nerves.

Vascular Supply of the Muscle Compartments

INTRODUCTION

This chapter will introduce the cardiovascular system and the major vessels that supply blood to the back and limbs. Unlike the nerves, which innervate specific muscles and regions of skin, vessels tend to supply blood to any structure in their immediate vicinity. The specific branching of these vessels will be discussed in Chapters 9 to 12.

BASIC CONCEPTS OF CIRCULATION

The heart is divided into four muscular chambers that receive and propel blood throughout the body (Fig. 5.1). The **right atrium** receives deoxygenated blood from veins coming from the back, limbs, and organs. Blood is then pumped through a three-leafed **tricuspid valve** into the **right ventricle**. The muscular wall of the right ventricle contracts to pump blood past three **pulmonary semilunar valves** into the **pulmonary arteries**. These carry deoxygenated blood to the lungs where the red blood cells exchange carbon dioxide for oxygen. **Pulmonary veins** carry the oxygenated blood to the **left atrium** of the heart where it is pumped past a two-leafed, **bicuspid (mitral) valve** into the **left ventricle**. The incredibly thick muscle of the left ventricle propels blood past three **aortic semilunar valves** into the **ascending aorta**, the largest artery of the body. The pumping of the left ventricle into the arteries creates **pulses** that can be felt at various locations of the body. The blood vessels to the heart itself, the **right and left coronary arteries**, are very proximal branches of the ascending aorta.

From the aorta, red blood cells in the **arteries** carry oxygen to the tissues and organs throughout the body. Large arteries branch into smaller arteries and eventually become microscopic, thin-walled **capillaries** that allow oxygen to enter the nearby tissues. Carbon dioxide from the tissues enters the bloodstream and is carried away. Capillaries fuse to create small **veins,** which also fuse, to create larger veins that eventually reach the heart. The process then begins again.

MAJOR ARTERIES OF THE BODY

Arch of the Aorta—Head, Neck, Upper Limbs, and Thorax

Blood is pumped into the ascending aorta by contraction of the muscles of the left ventricle. It then travels into the arch of the aorta, which has three branches: the **brachiocephalic trunk** (which splits to form the right common carotid and right subclavian arteries), the **left common carotid artery**, and the **left subclavian artery** (Figs. 5.2 and 5.3A). The arteries on each side will be treated as symmetrical unless specifically noted, but please note that variation in blood vessel branching patterns are very common, even between the left and right sides of a single person's body.

Common Carotid Arteries—The Head and Neck

The **common carotid arteries** (see Figs. 5.2 and 5.3A) on each side ascend into the anterior neck surrounded by the fascia of the carotid sheath. The pulse of the common carotid arteries can be taken on the lateral neck, just anterior to the sternocleidomastoid muscle. Near the level of the mandible, the common carotid artery splits into the external carotid and internal carotid arteries. The **external carotid artery** (see Fig. 5.3A) gives off many branches to the anterior neck, face, scalp, oral cavity, nasal cavities, and dura mater. These branches will not be addressed in detail in this volume.

The **internal carotid artery** does not branch until it enters the skull. It gives off the **ophthalmic artery** to the eye and orbit before reaching the neurocranium (see Fig. 5.3A). Here the right and left internal carotid arteries contribute to the **circle of Willis** (see Fig. 5.3B), a vascular ring at the base of the brain. The internal carotid arteries provide blood to the **anterior cerebral artery**, which supplies the medial anterior aspect of the cortex. The right and left anterior cerebral arteries are connected by the **anterior communicating artery**. The internal carotid artery also supplies the majority of blood to the **middle cerebral artery**, which supplies blood to the lateral aspect of the cortex.

Subclavian Arteries—The Head, Neck, and Upper Limb

The **subclavian artery** gives rise to several branches to the neck and proximal upper limb (Fig. 5.4, see also Figs. 5.2 and 5.3A). One of these major branches is the **vertebral artery**. It ascends in the neck, typically travelling through the transverse foramina of C6 up to C1. It then travels across the posterior arch of the atlas before piercing the dura mater. Inside the skull each vertebral artery ascends along the anterior brainstem (see Figs. 5.3 and 5.4). Each vertebral artery gives off a left and right **posterior**

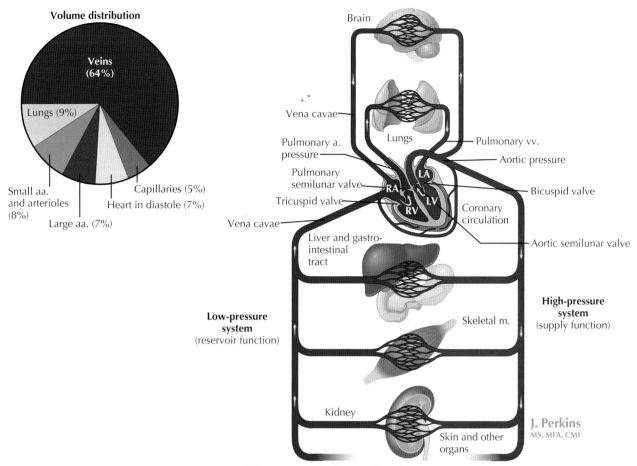

Volume distribution

Veins (64%)

Lungs (9%)

Small aa. and arterioles (8%)

Large aa. (7%)

Capillaries (5%)

Heart in diastole (7%)

Brain

Vena cavae

Pulmonary a. pressure

Pulmonary semilunar valve

Tricuspid valve

Vena cavae

Lungs

Pulmonary vv.

Aortic pressure

Bicuspid valve

Coronary circulation

Aortic semilunar valve

RA   LA   LV   RV

Liver and gastro-intestinal tract

Skeletal m.

Kidney

Skin and other organs

Low-pressure system (reservoir function)

High-pressure system (supply function)

J. Perkins
MS, MFA, CMI

Fig. 5.1 Cardiovascular System Overview.

spinal artery (sometimes from a branch of the vertebral) and both contribute to a single **anterior spinal artery** that descend on their respective sides of the spinal cord. Each also gives off a **posterior inferior cerebellar artery** before fusing with its fellow vertebral artery to form the **basilar artery**. The single basilar artery ascends toward the midbrain, giving off the **anterior inferior cerebellar arteries** and **superior cerebellar arteries**. These cerebellar arteries supply not only the cerebellum but also the rest of the brainstem. The basilar artery terminates when it splits into the right and left **posterior cerebral arteries**, which supply blood to the medial and lateral sides of the posterior cerebral cortex. Disruption of blood flow through the cerebral or cerebellar arteries can cause profound problems in the musculoskeletal system, which will be elaborated on in Chapter 8.

The subclavian artery supplies a branch that runs down the lateral aspect of the sternum, the **internal thoracic artery** (see Fig. 5.4). In addition to supplying the sternum itself, these arteries give off anterior intercostal arteries that supply blood to the intercostal muscles and overlying tissues. Muscles in the posterior portion of the 1st and 2nd intercostal spaces are supplied by the **supreme intercostal artery**, which also arises from the subclavian artery.

For the upper limb, the subclavian artery gives off the **transverse cervical** and **suprascapular arteries** (see Fig. 5.4), which will supply blood to the posterior scapula, including the supraspinatus, infraspinatus, and rhomboid muscles. Once it crosses the first rib, the subclavian artery is renamed the **axillary artery.**

Axillary and Brachial Arteries—The Upper Limb

The axillary artery supplies blood to the muscles, bones, and skin of the proximal upper limb, lateral thoracic wall, and breast (Fig. 5.5). One of its early branches is the **thoracoacromial trunk**, which subdivides to supply the acromion, clavicle, pectoral, and deltoid muscles. The nearby **lateral thoracic artery** supplies the serratus anterior muscle and other tissues on the lateral thoracic wall. A bit further along are two vessels that wrap around the surgical neck of the humerus and supply nearby tissues, the **anterior** and **posterior circumflex humeral arteries**. Next, the large **subscapular artery** branches into the **circumflex scapular artery**, which wraps around the lateral border of the scapula to supply rotator cuff muscles, as well as the **thoracodorsal artery** that supplies blood to the latissimus dorsi muscle.

As the axillary artery crosses the inferior border of the teres major muscle, its name changes to the **brachial artery** (see Fig. 5.5). It passes parallel to the medial aspect of the humerus, giving off the **deep brachial artery** to provide blood to the posterior arm. In the cubital fossa, the brachial artery splits into the radial and ulnar arteries, which travel through the forearm and hand (see Fig. 5.5). They supply blood to muscles, bones, and skin of the anterior and posterior compartments of the forearm and the hand. Several collateral and recurrent branches from these arteries form an anastomotic network around the elbow.

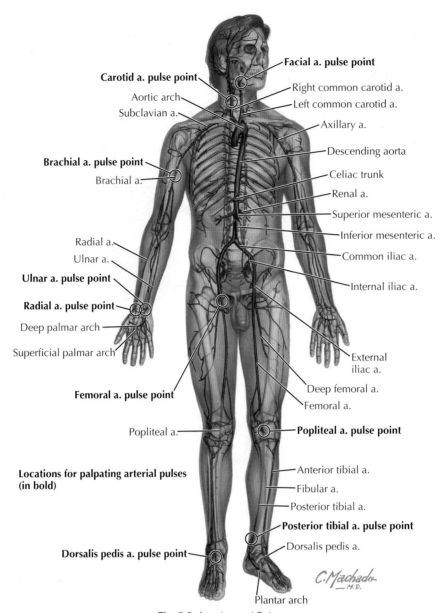

Carotid a. pulse point

Aortic arch

Subclavian a.

Brachial a. pulse point

Brachial a.

Radial a.

Ulnar a.

Ulnar a. pulse point

Radial a. pulse point

Deep palmar arch

Superficial palmar arch

Femoral a. pulse point

Popliteal a.

Locations for palpating arterial pulses (in bold)

Dorsalis pedis a. pulse point

Facial a. pulse point

Right common carotid a.

Left common carotid a.

Axillary a.

Descending aorta

Celiac trunk

Renal a.

Superior mesenteric a.

Inferior mesenteric a.

Common iliac a.

Internal iliac a.

External iliac a.

Deep femoral a.

Femoral a.

Popliteal a. pulse point

Anterior tibial a.

Fibular a.

Posterior tibial a.

Posterior tibial a. pulse point

Dorsalis pedis a.

Plantar arch

C. Machado
—M.D.

Fig. 5.2 Arteries and Pulses.

The **ulnar artery** gives off **interosseous arteries** that travel on the anterior and posterior sides of the interosseous membrane between the radius and ulna. It then travels along the medial aspect of the anterior forearm, crossing the wrist just lateral to the pisiform bone. Thereafter it provides the majority of blood to the **superficial palmar arch**. The **radial artery** travels along the lateral aspect of the anterior forearm but crosses dorsally in the vicinity of the scaphoid bone. It then travels to the palmar aspect of the hand by passing between the 1st and 2nd metacarpals, where it provides the majority of blood to the **deep palmar arch**. The superficial and deep palmar arches each give off a variety of vessels to the digits, which will be discussed in Chapter 10 (see Fig. 5.5).

Descending Aorta—Thorax, Abdomen, Abdominal Organs

After giving off the left subclavian artery, the aortic arch moves posteriorly to become the descending aorta within the thorax

(Fig. 5.6A, see also Fig. 5.2). It gives off arteries to the esophagus and bronchi as well as **posterior intercostal arteries**. Left and right posterior intercostal arteries leave the aorta at each intercostal space and run anteriorly to anastomose with anterior intercostal arteries from the internal thoracic artery. As it passes into the abdomen, the aorta gives off arteries to the superior and inferior surface of the diaphragm (see Fig. 5.6).

Within the abdomen the aorta gives off three unpaired vessels (see Fig. 5.6B). The **celiac trunk** supplies blood to the foregut (stomach, liver, gall bladder, spleen, proximal duodenum, part of pancreas), the **superior mesenteric artery** gives blood to the midgut (distal duodenum, part of pancreas, small intestine, proximal large intestine), and the **inferior mesenteric artery** supplies the hindgut organs (distal large intestine and rectum).

The abdominal aorta also gives off several paired arteries (see Fig. 5.6B). Like the intercostal arteries in the thorax,

A. Arteries to brain and meninges

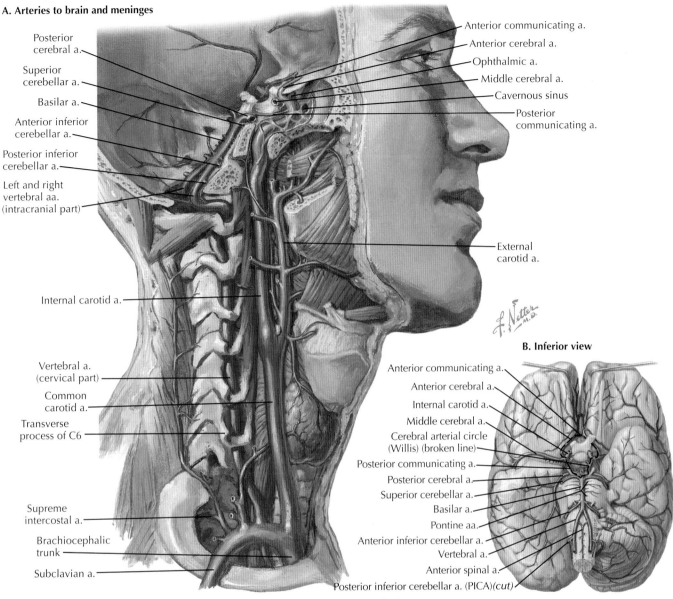

Fig. 5.3 Arteries to the Brain.

B. Inferior view

lumbar segmental arteries at each level provide blood to the body wall. **Renal arteries** travel to the right and left kidneys, supplying them and nearby structures such as the ureter and suprarenal (adrenal) glands. A bit lower are the **gonadal arteries** that descend into the pelvis (ovarian arteries) or scrotum (testicular arteries) to supply those reproductive organs. The descending aorta terminates as it splits into the left and right **common iliac arteries** (Clinical Correlation 5.1).

Iliac Arteries—Pelvis and Lower Limb

On each side the **common iliac artery** descends between the ilium and the sacrum, traveling inferolaterally before splitting into an **external and internal iliac artery** (see Fig. 5.6B). The internal iliac artery travels medially to supply the muscles and organs within the pelvis. Among the many arteries that arise from it are the **superior gluteal and inferior gluteal** (gluteal muscles), **obturator** (medial compartment of thigh), and

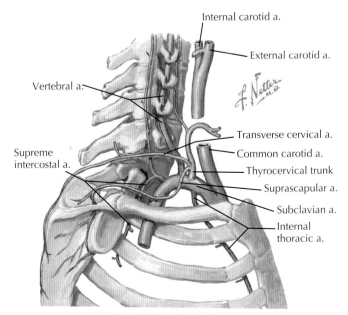

Fig. 5.4 Subclavian Artery.

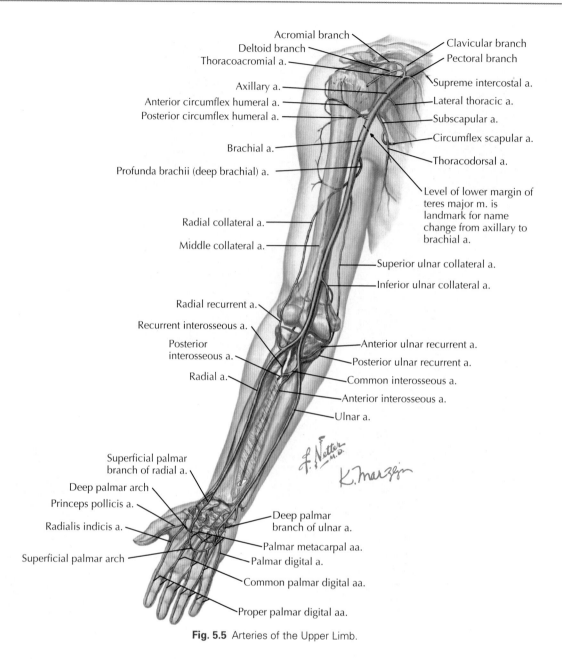

Acromial branch
Deltoid branch
Thoracoacromial a.
Clavicular branch
Pectoral branch
Axillary a.
Supreme intercostal a.
Anterior circumflex humeral a.
Lateral thoracic a.
Posterior circumflex humeral a.
Subscapular a.
Circumflex scapular a.
Brachial a.
Thoracodorsal a.
Profunda brachii (deep brachial) a.
Level of lower margin of
teres major m. is
landmark for name
change from axillary to
brachial a.
Radial collateral a.
Middle collateral a.
Superior ulnar collateral a.
Inferior ulnar collateral a.
Radial recurrent a.
Recurrent interosseous a.
Posterior
interosseous a.
Radial a.
Anterior ulnar recurrent a.
Posterior ulnar recurrent a.
Common interosseous a.
Anterior interosseous a.
Ulnar a.
Superficial palmar
branch of radial a.
Deep palmar arch
Princeps pollicis a.
Radialis indicis a.
Superficial palmar arch
Deep palmar
branch of ulnar a.
Palmar metacarpal aa.
Palmar digital a.
Common palmar digital aa.
Proper palmar digital aa.

Fig. 5.5 Arteries of the Upper Limb.

internal pudendal arteries (anal region and external genitalia). The external iliac artery gives off the large **inferior epigastric artery** that supplies the rectus abdominis muscle, before it continues descending through the abdominal wall to become the **femoral artery** (Fig. 5.7, see also Fig. 5.6B).

Femoral and Popliteal Arteries—Lower Limb

The **femoral artery** is located fairly superficially in the upper anterior thigh (see Figs. 5.6B and 5.7). Proximally it gives rise to the **deep femoral artery** (note that there is no superficial femoral artery, although some clinicians call the femoral artery by that name), which supplies blood to the medial thigh, as well as the posterior compartment of the thigh via perforating branches. It also gives off the **lateral and medial circumflex femoral arteries** that wrap around the proximal femur, supplying the bone and nearby tissues (Clinical Correlation 5.2).

The femoral artery moves medially as it descends (see Fig. 5.7) and becomes covered by the sartorius muscle. It passes through the adductor magnus muscle in a channel called the **adductor hiatus**. It exits the adductor hiatus into the popliteal fossa. At this point it changes its name to become the **popliteal artery**, which gives off a network of five **genicular arteries** that surround and nurture the tissues of the knee and patella. The popliteal artery terminates inferior to the knee as the **anterior and posterior tibial arteries**.

Tibial and Fibular Arteries—The Leg and Foot

After branching from the popliteal artery, the **anterior tibial artery** (see Fig. 5.7) travels through the interosseous space between the tibia and fibula to reach the anterior compartment of the leg. It provides blood to the structures in this compartment while it descends. After it passes the talus, it is called the **dorsalis pedis artery** and

CLINICAL CORRELATION 5.1   Aortic Aneurysms

Weakening of an artery can result in a ballooning outward, called an **aneurysm**. The arch of the aorta is particularly prone to developing aneurysms due to the volume of blood in the aorta, the pressures it must withstand with every heartbeat, and the U-turn the blood must make as it travels through the arch. If the aneurysm bursts or dissects the layers of the vessel itself, massive

hemorrhage can kill in a very short time. Like the aortic arch, the distal portion of the aorta is also prone to aneurysm due to the turbulence created when the aorta splits into the left and right common iliac arteries. An abdominal aortic aneurysm can occasionally be palpated as a large pulsatile mass in the lower abdomen.

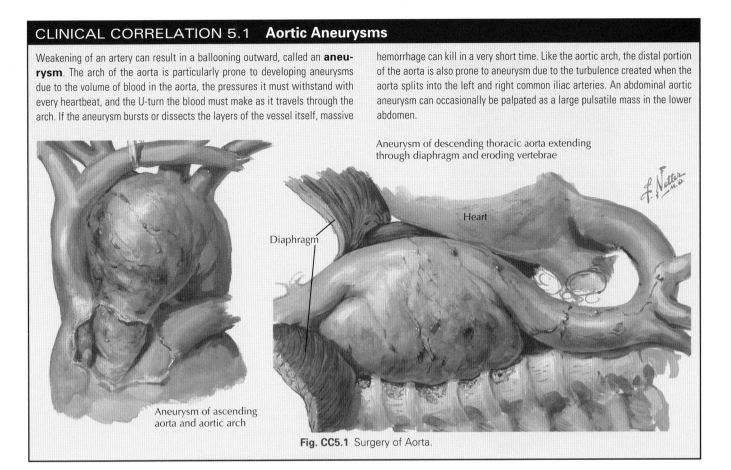

Aneurysm of descending thoracic aorta extending through diaphragm and eroding vertebrae

Heart

Diaphragm

Aneurysm of ascending aorta and aortic arch

Fig. CC5.1 Surgery of Aorta.

supplies blood to the dorsum of the foot with a **deep plantar** branch passing inferiorly between the 1st and 2nd metatarsals.

The **posterior tibial artery** continues inferiorly in the posterior compartment of the leg, supplying nearby structures as it does so (see Fig. 5.7). It gives off a lateral branch, the **fibular artery,** which also supplies the posterior compartment but has several perforating branches to the lateral compartment of the leg. The posterior tibial artery crosses inferior to the medial malleolus to reach the plantar foot. Here it splits into the **medial and lateral plantar arteries** that supply their respective sides of the plantar foot. They anastomose to create a single **plantar arch**, which gives off vessels to the digits and anastomoses with the deep plantar artery from the dorsalis pedis.

MAJOR VEINS OF THE BODY

By and large, veins run antiparallel to the arteries and drain deoxygenated blood from approximately the same areas to which their corresponding arteries supply oxygenated blood, eventually reaching the right atrium of the heart (Fig. 5.8A). There are some arteries that do not have a vein of the same name that accompanies them, such as the aorta, carotid arteries, and celiac trunk. Sometimes veins are single vessels; at other times the veins form a network around their corresponding artery. Blood in veins is not propelled by contraction of the heart and it tends to accumulate inferiorly due to gravity. Fortunately, contraction of nearby muscles can squeeze the blood proximally

and valves in the walls of the veins prevent it from returning to the area it just left (see Fig. 5.8B).

Veins of the Head and Neck

Blood from the brain drains into special veins located inside the dura mater lining the skull. Most of the blood in these **dural venous sinuses** exits the skull into the **internal jugular vein**, which descends alongside the common carotid artery just deep to the sternocleidomastoid muscle. Blood from the face and neck can also drain into the internal jugular vein but may also flow into the **external jugular** or **anterior jugular veins**, which are located superficial to the sternocleidomastoid muscle (Fig. 5.9, see also Fig. 5.8A).

Veins of the Upper Limb

In the upper limb, **deep veins** run from distal to proximal, alongside arteries of the same name (see Fig. 5.8A). Digital veins drain to the veins of the palmar arches, which then drain into **radial and ulnar veins**. These fuse to create the **brachial vein**, which then receives blood from the **deep brachial vein** before becoming the **axillary vein**. Blood from numerous smaller veins (circumflex humeral, subscapular, lateral thoracic) empties into the axillary vein. As it crosses the first rib it becomes the **subclavian vein**, which receives additional blood from the **internal thoracic vein** and **suprascapular veins**, among others.

There are also some superficial veins within the subcutaneous tissues of the upper limb that have no corresponding artery (Fig. 5.10). Many veins exist in the subcutaneous tissues of the upper

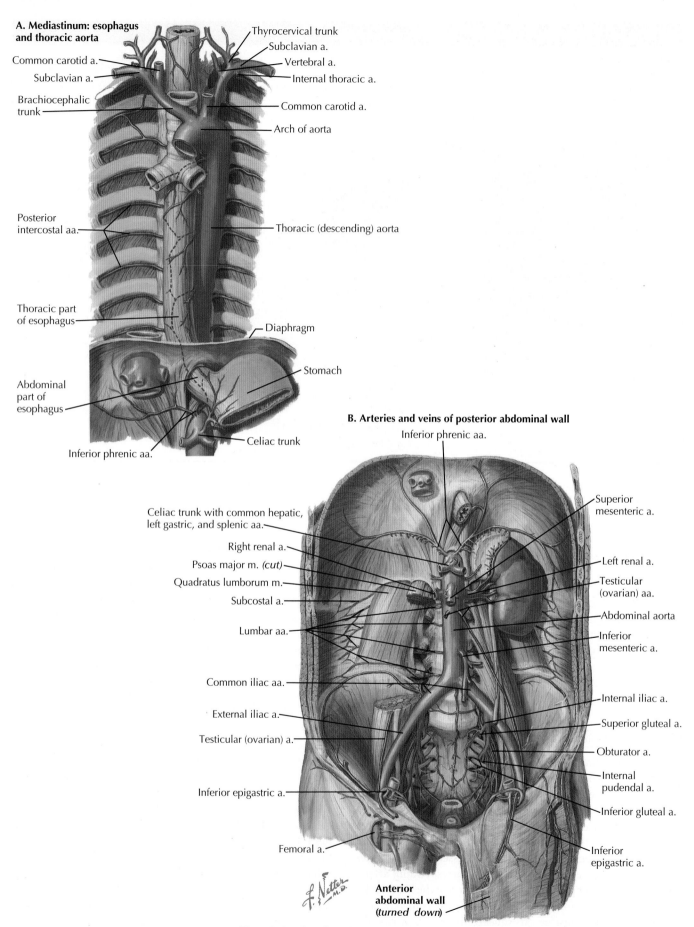

A. Mediastinum: esophagus and thoracic aorta

Common carotid a.

Subclavian a.

Brachiocephalic trunk

Thyrocervical trunk

Subclavian a.

Vertebral a.

Internal thoracic a.

Common carotid a.

Arch of aorta

Posterior intercostal aa.

Thoracic (descending) aorta

Thoracic part of esophagus

Diaphragm

Stomach

Abdominal part of esophagus

Inferior phrenic aa.

Celiac trunk

B. Arteries and veins of posterior abdominal wall

Inferior phrenic aa.

Celiac trunk with common hepatic, left gastric, and splenic aa.

Right renal a.

Psoas major m. *(cut)*

Quadratus lumborum m.

Subcostal a.

Lumbar aa.

Common iliac aa.

External iliac a.

Testicular (ovarian) a.

Inferior epigastric a.

Femoral a.

Superior mesenteric a.

Left renal a.

Testicular (ovarian) aa.

Abdominal aorta

Inferior mesenteric a.

Internal iliac a.

Superior gluteal a.

Obturator a.

Internal pudendal a.

Inferior gluteal a.

Inferior epigastric a.

Anterior abdominal wall (*turned down*)

Fig. 5.6 Arteries of the Thorax and Abdomen.

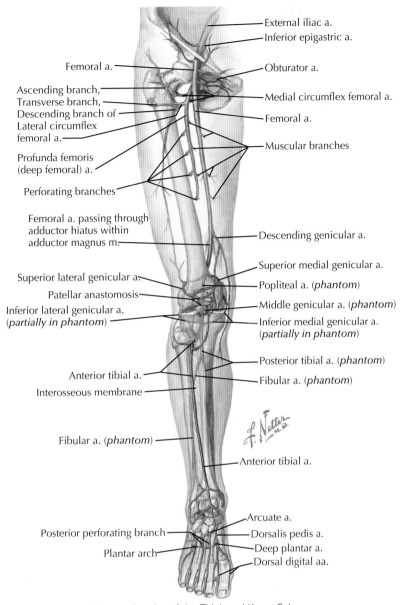

External iliac a.
Inferior epigastric a.
Femoral a.
Obturator a.
Ascending branch,
Transverse branch,
Descending branch of
Lateral circumflex
femoral a.
Medial circumflex femoral a.
Femoral a.
Muscular branches
Profunda femoris
(deep femoral) a.
Perforating branches
Femoral a. passing through
adductor hiatus within
adductor magnus m.
Descending genicular a.
Superior medial genicular a.
Superior lateral genicular a.
Popliteal a. (*phantom*)
Patellar anastomosis
Middle genicular a. (*phantom*)
Inferior lateral genicular a.
(*partially in phantom*)
Inferior medial genicular a.
(*partially in phantom*)
Posterior tibial a. (*phantom*)
Anterior tibial a.
Fibular a. (*phantom*)
Interosseous membrane
Fibular a. (*phantom*)
Anterior tibial a.
Arcuate a.
Posterior perforating branch
Dorsalis pedis a.
Deep plantar a.
Plantar arch
Dorsal digital aa.

Fig. 5.7 Arteries of the Thigh and Knee: Schema.

limb (and their branching pattern varies tremendously) but they tend to drain into the large basilic and cephalic veins. The **basilic vein** drains the anteromedial aspect of the hand and forearm before dumping its blood into the brachial vein on the medial side of the distal arm. The **cephalic vein** drains the posterolateral aspect of the hand, forearm, and lateral aspect of the arm. It ascends along the lateral arm, running in a groove between the deltoid and pectoralis major muscles before diving deep to empty into the subclavian vein. The prominent **median cubital vein** connects the basilic and cephalic veins in the cubital fossa.

Veins of the Thorax

On each side, the subclavian and internal jugular veins fuse to become the **right and left brachiocephalic veins** (Fig. 5.11). These veins fuse to create the **superior vena cava**, which carries venous blood from the head, neck, and upper limbs into the right atrium of the heart. In the thorax, **posterior intercostal veins** collect blood from the vicinity of each intercostal space and carry it

posteriorly. On the right side, this blood enters the **azygos vein**. On the left side, it typically enters the **hemiazygos** and **accessory hemiazygos veins**. While there is variation in this system, the hemiazygos and accessory hemiazygos veins tend to pass anterior to the thoracic vertebrae to empty into the azygos vein (see Fig. 5.11), which then carries blood into the superior vena cava.

Veins of the Lower Limb

In the lower limb, **deep veins** run from distal to proximal, alongside arteries of the same name (see Fig. 5.8A). **Medial and lateral plantar veins** drain to the **posterior tibial vein**, which also receives blood from the **fibular vein**. The **dorsalis pedis vein** ascends across the talus and becomes the **anterior tibial vein** within the anterior compartment of the leg and ascends and passes into the posterior compartment of the leg near the knee. The anterior and posterior tibial veins fuse to create the **popliteal vein**, which also receives blood from a network of **genicular veins** before passing into the anterior compartment of the thigh

CLINICAL CORRELATION 5.2   Avascular Necrosis of the Femoral Head

A fracture of the femoral neck can lacerate the medial circumflex femoral artery, which is the major blood supply to the head of the femur. Even after the bone is repaired, insufficient blood supply to the femoral head can cause its tissues to die. This is called **avascular necrosis**.

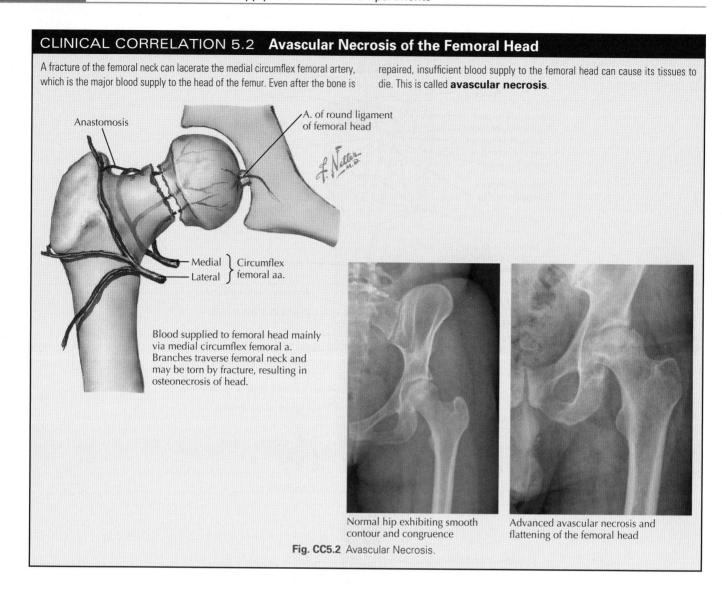

Anastomosis

A. of round ligament of femoral head

Medial ⎫ Circumflex
Lateral ⎭ femoral aa.

Blood supplied to femoral head mainly via medial circumflex femoral a. Branches traverse femoral neck and may be torn by fracture, resulting in osteonecrosis of head.

Normal hip exhibiting smooth contour and congruence

Advanced avascular necrosis and flattening of the femoral head

Fig. CC5.2 Avascular Necrosis.

to become the **femoral vein**. Within the anterior compartment the **medial** and **lateral circumflex femoral veins** drain blood into the **deep femoral vein**, which in turn drains from the posterior and medial compartments of the thigh. The deep femoral vein joins the already massive femoral vein and ascends to pierce the abdominal wall just inferior to the inguinal ligament.

Like the upper limb, there are superficial veins within the subcutaneous tissues of the lower limb that have no corresponding artery (Fig. 5.12, see also Fig. 5.8A). The **small saphenous vein** drains the superficial plantar foot and posterolateral leg before dumping its blood into the popliteal vein. The **greater saphenous vein** drains the dorsal foot, anteromedial ankle, leg, and medial thigh. It ascends along the medial aspect of the entire lower limb, before emptying into the femoral vein just inferior to the inguinal ligament and abdominal wall.

Veins of the Pelvis and Abdomen

After entering the abdomen, the femoral vein changes its name, becoming the **external iliac vein;** it travels proximally and medially. It fuses with the **internal iliac vein**, which drains blood from the **pelvic organs**, as well as the **superior and inferior**

gluteal veins. Once the external and internal iliac veins fuse with each other, they create the **common iliac vein**. The right and left common iliac veins fuse to create the **inferior vena cava** that ascends to the right of the vertebral bodies and transports blood from the lower limbs and abdominopelvic organs to the right atrium of the heart (Fig. 5.13, Clinical Correlation 5.3).

Within the abdomen, the inferior vena cava receives blood from **lumbar segmental veins**, the **right gonadal vein**, and the **left and right renal veins**. The **left gonadal vein** drains into the left renal vein instead of directly to the inferior vena cava (see Fig. 5.13).

While it is not the focus of this volume, we will also briefly discuss blood drainage of the abdominal organs. Blood from the hindgut organs is drained by the **inferior mesenteric vein** into the **splenic vein**, which carries a large amount of blood, iron, and heme from the spleen. Venous blood from midgut organs is carried by the **superior mesenteric vein**, which fuses with the splenic vein to create the **hepatic portal vein**. Several branches from foregut organs empty into the hepatic portal vein, which then enters the liver where it is filtered. Blood leaving the liver through **hepatic veins** drains into the inferior vena cava immediately inferior to the diaphragm.

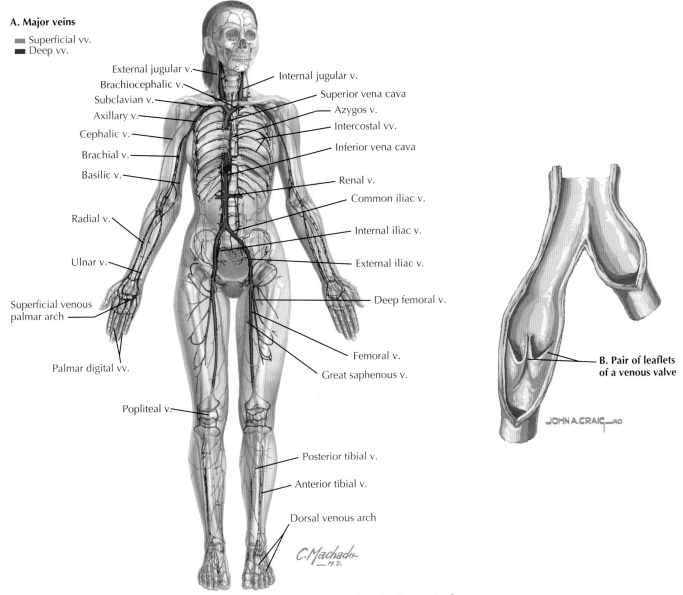

A. Major veins

▰ Superficial vv.
■ Deep vv.

External jugular v.
Brachiocephalic v.
Subclavian v.
Axillary v.
Cephalic v.
Brachial v.
Basilic v.
Radial v.
Ulnar v.
Superficial venous palmar arch
Palmar digital vv.
Popliteal v.

Internal jugular v.
Superior vena cava
Azygos v.
Intercostal vv.
Inferior vena cava
Renal v.
Common iliac v.
Internal iliac v.
External iliac v.
Deep femoral v.
Femoral v.
Great saphenous v.
Posterior tibial v.
Anterior tibial v.
Dorsal venous arch

B. Pair of leaflets of a venous valve

JOHN A. CRAIG—MD

C. Machado
—M.D.

Fig. 5.8 Major Systemic Veins of the Cardiovascular System.

LYMPHATICS OF THE MUSCULOSKELETAL SYSTEM

While many nutrients, wastes, and gasses travel through the arteries and veins, there are other substances in the extracellular spaces of the body that cannot move into the blood vessels. These include degraded fibers, cellular debris, and remnants of pathologic organisms. If these substances are allowed to accumulate in the extracellular spaces, they pull water into the area and cause swelling. To clear such substances, the body has a third set of vessels, the **lymphatics** (Fig. 5.14). These vessels are open-ended, allowing fluid and debris to move freely into their lumen. Smooth muscle in their walls and the contraction of nearby muscles propels lymphatic fluid further along the vessel. As in veins, valves in the wall of lymphatic vessels prevent back-flow.

As this fluid travels through lymphatic vessels, it enters small organs, **lymph nodes,** which are important parts of the immune system, like the spleen, bone marrow, tonsils, and thymus. As fluid travels through each lymph node, it encounters many B and T lymphocytes, which may mount an immune response to antigens carried by the fluid. Lymphatic fluid leaves each node and is likely to encounter many more nodes as small lymph vessels fuse to create larger lymph vessels that carry the fluid toward the core of the body.

In the lower limbs, **deep lymphatic vessels** parallel the large arteries and veins, carrying lymphatic fluid proximally. Superficial lymphatic vessels carry lymph from the skin and subcutaneous fat of the plantar foot and posterior leg to the popliteal fossa, where they encounter **popliteal lymph nodes** and enter the nearby deep lymphatics around the popliteal artery and vein. Superficial lymphatic vessels from

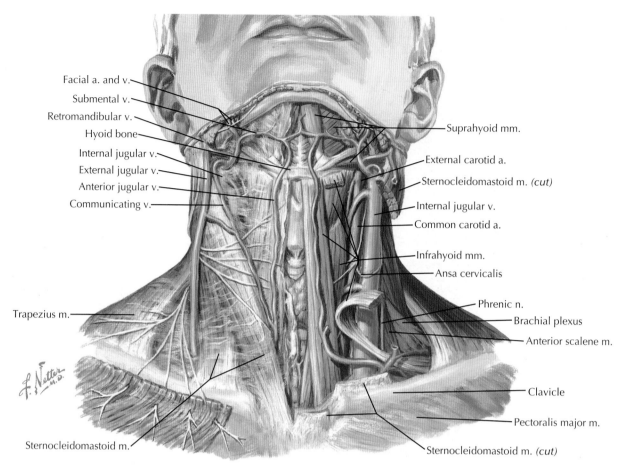

Fig. 5.9 Superficial Veins and Cutaneous Nerves of the Neck.

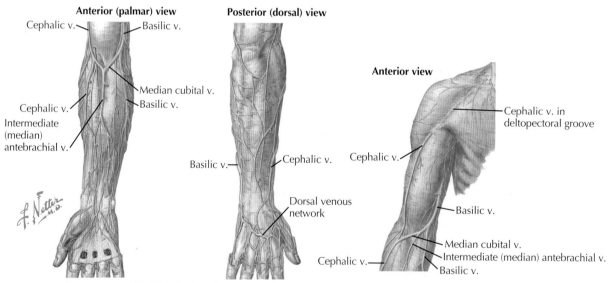

Fig. 5.10 Surface Anatomy: Superficial Veins and Nerves of the Upper Limb.

the dorsal foot, anterior leg, and thigh eventually converge on **superficial inguinal lymph nodes** near the groin (Fig. 5.15A, see also Fig. 5.14). These drain to several other lymph nodes in the pelvis and along the posterior body wall, near the aorta. Lymph from both lower limbs and the abdominopelvic organs collects in a sac, the **cisterna chyli**. From

there a single large lymphatic vessel, the **thoracic duct**, projects superiorly beside the aorta and esophagus. It then passes posterior to the arch of the aorta and drains into the left subclavian vein near the left internal jugular vein (see Fig. 5.14), where the lymphatic fluid becomes part of the blood plasma and is filtered by the kidneys and liver.

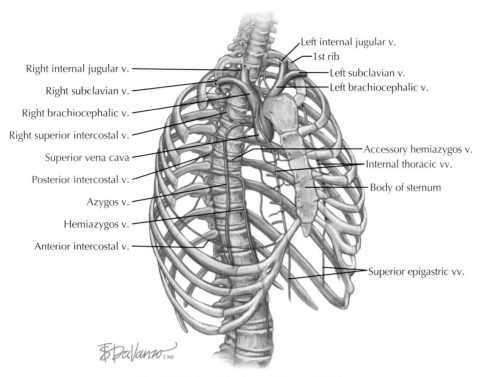

Fig. 5.11 Veins of the Internal Thoracic Wall.

In the upper limbs, deep lymphatic vessels also parallel the large arteries and veins. Superficial lymphatic vessels carry lymph from the skin and subcutaneous fat of the palmar hand and anterior forearm to converge on the cubital fossa and **cubital lymph nodes**, where they join the deep lymphatic vessels near the brachial artery and vein. Superficial lymphatic vessels from the dorsum of the hand and posterior forearm continue into the arm and eventually converge on **deltopectoral lymph nodes** or the **axillary lymph nodes** (see Fig. 5.14 and 5.15B).

The axillary lymph nodes are a large and clinically vital group of lymph **nodes** (Fig. 5.16, see also Figs. 5.14 and 5.15B). They consist of several subdivisions: **lateral (humeral) axillary lymph nodes, posterior (subscapular) axillary lymph nodes, anterior (pectoral) axillary lymph nodes, central axillary lymph nodes,** and **apical axillary lymph nodes**. The posterior axillary lymph nodes drain the region of the subscapularis muscle and the superior back. The lateral axillary lymph nodes receive lymphatic fluid from the upper limb. The anterior axillary lymph nodes get fluid from the anterior chest, including the **interpectoral lymph nodes** and most of the breast. However, lymphatic fluid from the medial breast tends to drain to **parasternal lymph nodes**, which drain to the ipsilateral subclavian vein via a broncho-mediastinal trunk.

The posterior, lateral, and anterior axillary lymph nodes send lymphatic vessels to the central axillary lymph nodes; they all send lymphatic fluid to the nodes at the top of the axilla, the apical axillary lymph nodes. From there, lymphatic fluid goes to **supraclavicular lymph nodes**. Thereafter, the lymphatic fluid drains into the right or left subclavian vein through a **subclavian lymph trunk**. On the left side, it may join the thoracic duct (Clinical Correlation 5.4).

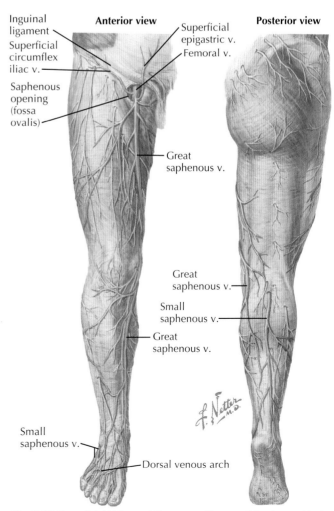

Fig. 5.12 Superficial Veins and Cutaneous Nerves of the Lower Limb.

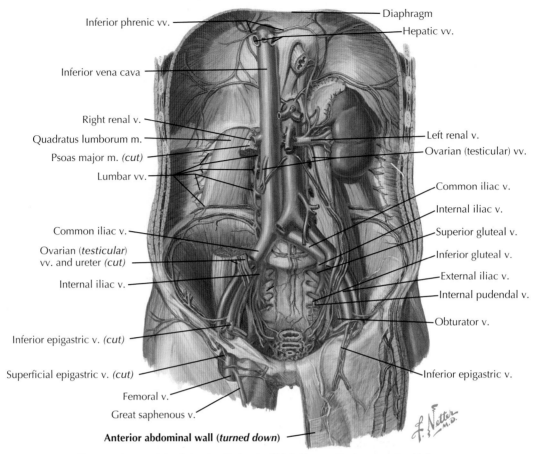

Inferior phrenic vv.

Inferior vena cava

Right renal v.

Quadratus lumborum m.

Psoas major m. *(cut)*

Lumbar vv.

Common iliac v.

Ovarian *(testicular)* vv. and ureter *(cut)*

Internal iliac v.

Inferior epigastric v. *(cut)*

Superficial epigastric v. *(cut)*

Femoral v.

Great saphenous v.

Diaphragm

Hepatic vv.

Left renal v.

Ovarian (testicular) vv.

Common iliac v.

Internal iliac v.

Superior gluteal v.

Inferior gluteal v.

External iliac v.

Internal pudendal v.

Obturator v.

Inferior epigastric v.

Anterior abdominal wall (*turned down*)

Fig. 5.13 Veins of the Posterior Abdominal Wall: Venous Drainage of the Abdomen.

CLINICAL CORRELATION 5.3   **Deep Venous Thrombosis**

Muscle contraction and the valves help propel venous blood superiorly against gravity. If blood in the veins becomes stagnant (due to inactivity or injury) the blood within them can form clots in the lumen, called **thrombi**. If these thrombi break loose, they become **emboli**. An embolus will travel through the veins until it encounters a vessel that is smaller in diameter than itself. It will lodge in that vessel and deprive the downstream areas of blood. In the case of thrombi originating in deep veins of the upper and lower limbs, they will often lodge in branches of the pulmonary arteries. These pulmonary emboli are painful and life-threatening, because they prevent blood from exchanging gasses in the lungs.

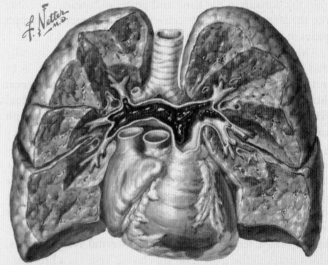

Saddle embolus completely occluding the right pulmonary artery and partially obstructing the pulmonary trunk and left pulmonary artery.

Fig. CC5.3 Massive Embolization.

Lymphatic fluid from the head and neck travels through a large number of nodes before draining into the **deep cervical lymph node group**, which sends lymphatic fluid into a **jugular lymphatic trunk**. The left and right jugular lymphatic trunks drain into the left and right subclavian veins; on the left it often joins the thoracic duct. Since the left subclavian vein receives lymphatic fluid from the left head, neck, upper limb, and thoracic duct, more than ¾ of the body's lymph enters circulation at that site (see Fig. 5.14).

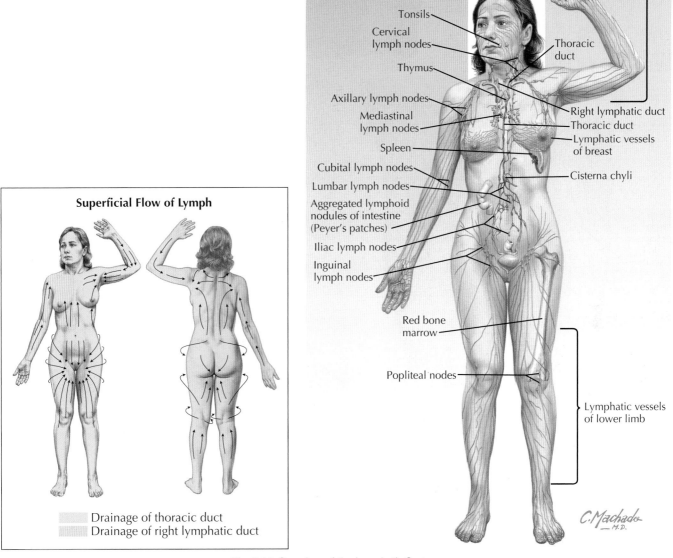

Fig. 5.14 Overview of the Lymphatic System.

A. Lymph vessels and nodes of lower limb

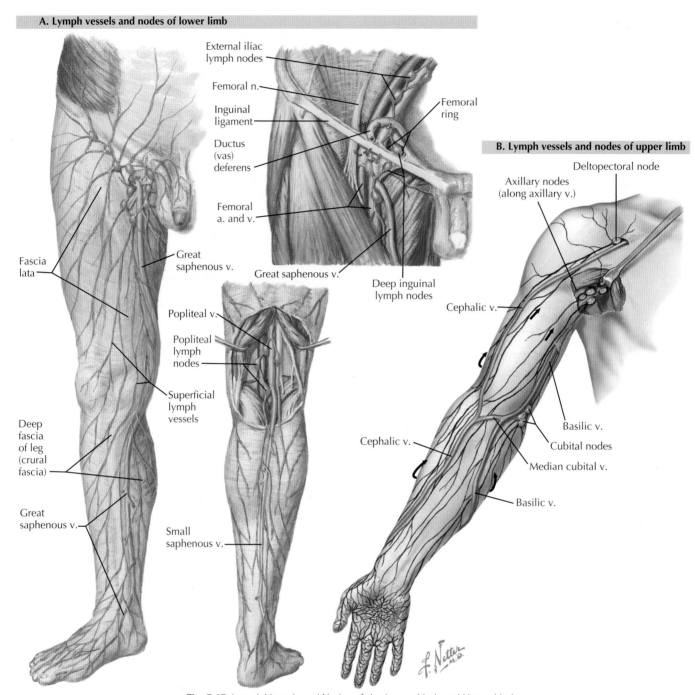

B. Lymph vessels and nodes of upper limb

Fig. 5.15 Lymph Vessels and Nodes of the Lower Limb and Upper Limb.

CLINICAL CORRELATION 5.4 Lymphatic Spread of Breast Cancer

Carcinomas, tumors that originate from epithelial cells, tend to invade nearby lymphatic vessels and spread. This is called metastasis. Carcinomas of the breast often spread into the nearby lymphatics and spread to medial parasternal lymph nodes or the interpectoral and pectoral axillary lymph nodes. If the tumor spreads to the axillary lymph nodes, it can invade others, such as the central and apical axillary lymph nodes. If it is not treated, it can then move to infraclavicular and supraclavicular lymph nodes and then into the subclavian vein. From there, tumor cells can disperse throughout the body via the bloodstream.

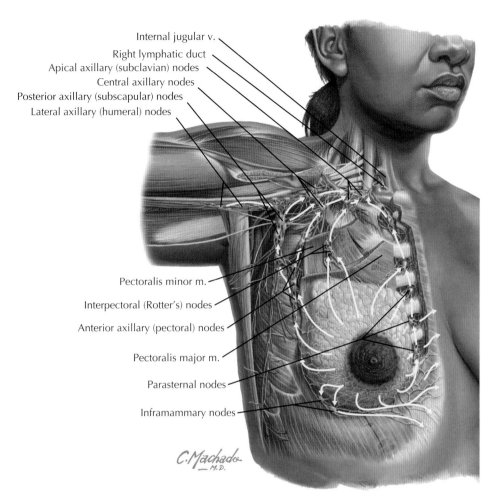

Internal jugular v.
Right lymphatic duct
Apical axillary (subclavian) nodes
Central axillary nodes
Posterior axillary (subscapular) nodes
Lateral axillary (humeral) nodes

Pectoralis minor m.
Interpectoral (Rotter's) nodes
Anterior axillary (pectoral) nodes
Pectoralis major m.
Parasternal nodes
Inframammary nodes

Fig. 5.16 Lymphatic Drainage of the Breast.

Overview of Musculoskeletal Histology, Physiology, and Biochemistry

HISTOLOGY BASICS

As we move from gross anatomy (what we can see at the macroscopic scale) to histology (microscopic anatomy), we need to use a new set of terms. When organs and tissues are cut from an organism, they are typically frozen or fixed in preservative and then stained. There are many types of stains, but the most common is **hematoxylin** and **eosin** (H&E). Cells, tissues, or other structures that preferentially bind with hematoxylin appear purple and are referred to as being "basophilic." Likewise, binding to eosin produces a pink, "eosinophilic," hue. The visual differences between stained structures allow us to distinguish and categorize them. The organs of the body are composed of multiple tissues with specialized functions. Tissues, in their turn, are composed of multiple cell types. The cells that make up the tissues of the body can be divided into four groups: **epithelium, muscle, nervous**, and **connective tissue**.

EPITHELIAL TISSUES

Epithelial cells line body cavities, vascular spaces, and any place where the body is in contact with the external environment. This includes the lining of the digestive, respiratory, urinary, and reproductive tracts. Epithelial cells create and maintain a structure on their deep surface called the **basement membrane**. This membrane anchors the cells to underlying tissues and allows oxygen and nutrients to diffuse to the epithelial layer of cells, which is otherwise avascular.

Regions of an Epithelial Cell (Fig. 6.1)

Epithelial cells have three distinct regions that allow them to carry out their specialized functions.

- The **apical domain** faces away from the basement membrane and is in contact with the vascular lumen, body cavities, or the external environment. The surface of these cells may contain other structures related to the organ in which they reside.
  - **Cilia** are long, mobile extensions of the cell that sweep material along the lumen. These are prominent in the respiratory tract.
  - **Stereocilia** are very long, immobile extensions of the cell that sense and respond to changes in the area just outside the apical domain. These are prominent in the auditory and vestibular systems.
  - **Microvilli** are tiny, immobile extensions on the surface of the apical domain that massively increase its surface area. These are prominent in the gastrointestinal tract.
- The **lateral domain** contains a variety of cell adhesion molecules that keep the epithelial layer intact and make it harder for pathogenic organisms to pass through the layer.
  - **Anchoring junctions** fuse epithelial cells to their neighbors.
  - **Occluding junctions** isolate the apical region from the rest of the epithelial layer.
  - **Communicating junctions** allow direct contact and diffusion between the cytoplasm of neighboring cells.
- The **basal domain** maintains contact with the basement membrane.
  - **Focal adhesions** and **hemidesmosomes** anchor actin and intermediate filaments within the cell to the basement membrane.

Epithelial Cell Appearance (see Fig. 6.1)

Because they exist in a wide range of tissues and have diverse functions, epithelial cells vary widely in appearance. These differences are reflected in the thickness of the cells and how many layers are stacked on each other. Epithelial cells in a single layer are called "**simple**," and each cell is in contact with the basement membrane. Epithelial tissues with two or more layers are referred to as "**stratified**" with only the most basal cells in contact with the basement membrane. "**Pseudostratified**" epithelial cells appear to be layered, but each cell is actually in direct contact with the basement membrane.

Cells can also be classified according to their shape.

- The principal characteristic of **squamous cells** is that they are flat.
  - **Simple squamous cells** are found lining the lumen of blood vessels (called **endothelial cells**), the lining of body

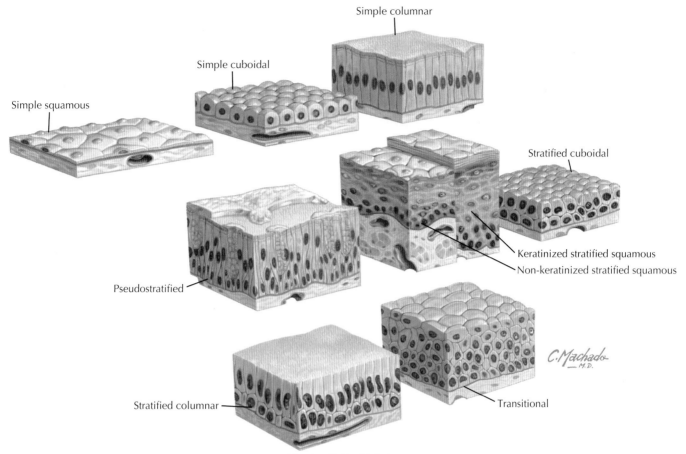

Fig. 6.1 Epithelial Cells.

cavities (**mesothelial cells**), along the outer layer of internal organs, lining the lowest part of the airway, and along the conjunctiva of the eye.

- **Stratified squamous cells** are layered squamous cells that make up the outermost layer of the skin, the lining of the oral cavity, and parts of the pharynx, esophagus, true vocal folds, and anal region.
- **Cuboidal cells** are epithelial cells that are cube-shaped and appear as squares on microscope slides. They are found almost exclusively lining the ducts of secretory glands.
  - **Simple cuboidal** cells are seen lining the lumen of secretory ducts and in the lower part of the airway.
  - **Stratified cuboidal** cells are found exclusively lining the lumen of large ducts.
- **Columnar cells** are epithelial cells that are taller than they are wide.
  - **Simple columnar** cells line the inside of the gall bladder and digestive tract from the stomach to the rectum.
  - **Stratified columnar** cells are very uncommon and are only seen lining the lumen of the largest ducts of secretory glands.
  - **Pseudostratified ciliated columnar** epithelial cells are a special type that is only seen in the respiratory tract, lining the nasal cavity, parts of the pharynx, trachea, bronchi, and bronchioles. For this reason, it is also called "**respiratory epithelium.**"
- **Transitional epithelial cells** are scallop-shaped and line the urinary spaces outside the kidney. When these cells are

relaxed, they appear to be stratified, but when distended, each cell is seen to be in contact with the basement membrane.

CONNECTIVE TISSUE

Connective tissue is essentially everything except for epithelium, nervous tissue, and muscle tissue. Because this encompasses such a broad range of bodily structures, connective tissue manifests in many ways. In general, it serves to support epithelial, muscle, or nervous tissues so they can accomplish their functions. Every type of connective tissue consists of cells, fibers, and extracellular matrix. The major types of connective tissue are connective tissue proper, cartilage, bone, and blood.

Connective tissue proper (Fig. 6.2) could be considered "typical" connective tissue, although it also has various subtypes. **Fibroblast** cells create and maintain connective tissue proper by releasing fibers and ground substance into the extracellular space. Their cytoplasm is difficult to discern in most H&E stained slides, but they have basophilic nuclei that are elongated with pointed ends. The major connective tissue fibers released by fibroblasts are **type I collagen, type III collagen**, and **elastic fibers**. The ground substance of connective tissue contains proteoglycans, multiadhesive glycoproteins, and glycosaminoglycans. The ratio of cells, fibers, and extracellular matrix creates distinctive subtypes of connective tissue proper.

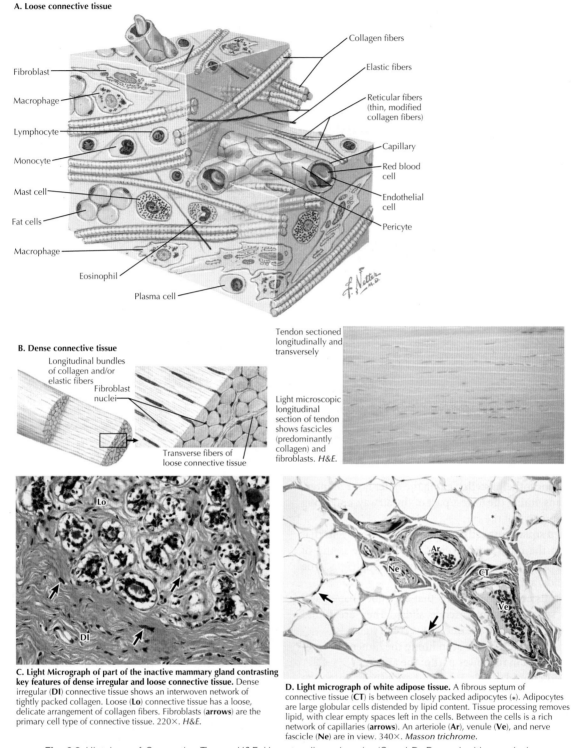

A. Loose connective tissue

Fibroblast
Macrophage
Lymphocyte
Monocyte
Mast cell
Fat cells
Macrophage
Eosinophil
Plasma cell

Collagen fibers
Elastic fibers
Reticular fibers (thin, modified collagen fibers)
Capillary
Red blood cell
Endothelial cell
Pericyte

B. Dense connective tissue

Longitudinal bundles of collagen and/or elastic fibers
Fibroblast nuclei
Transverse fibers of loose connective tissue

Tendon sectioned longitudinally and transversely

Light microscopic longitudinal section of tendon shows fascicles (predominantly collagen) and fibroblasts. *H&E.*

C. Light Micrograph of part of the inactive mammary gland contrasting key features of dense irregular and loose connective tissue. Dense irregular (**DI**) connective tissue shows an interwoven network of tightly packed collagen. Loose (**Lo**) connective tissue has a loose, delicate arrangement of collagen fibers. Fibroblasts (**arrows**) are the primary cell type of connective tissue. 220×. *H&E.*

D. Light micrograph of white adipose tissue. A fibrous septum of connective tissue (**CT**) is between closely packed adipocytes (∗). Adipocytes are large globular cells distended by lipid content. Tissue processing removes lipid, with clear empty spaces left in the cells. Between the cells is a rich network of capillaries (**arrows**). An arteriole (**Ar**), venule (**Ve**), and nerve fascicle (**Ne**) are in view. 340×. *Masson trichrome.*

Fig. 6.2 Histology of Connective Tissue. *H&E,* Hematoxylin and eosin. (C and D, Reused with permission from Ovalle W, Nahirney P. *Netter's Essential Histology.* 3rd ed. Elsevier; 2021.)

- **Mucous connective tissue** consists of a gelatinous extracellular matrix with a large proportion of ground substance and few fibroblasts or fibers. It is seen in the umbilical cord (known as Wharton jelly) and the nucleus pulposus at the core of intervertebral discs.
- **Loose connective tissue** contains a lot of ground substance and more cells than fibers. It is found in places that require quick

diffusion of substances, such as the lamina propria of the digestive system where nutrients absorbed from the lumen must quickly migrate into the blood vessels in the submucosa. Many of the cells in loose connective tissue are circulating white blood cells that migrate to the area to protect the body from pathogens.

- **Dense irregular connective tissue** consists of more fibers than cells. Type I collagen fibers in this tissue do not have any

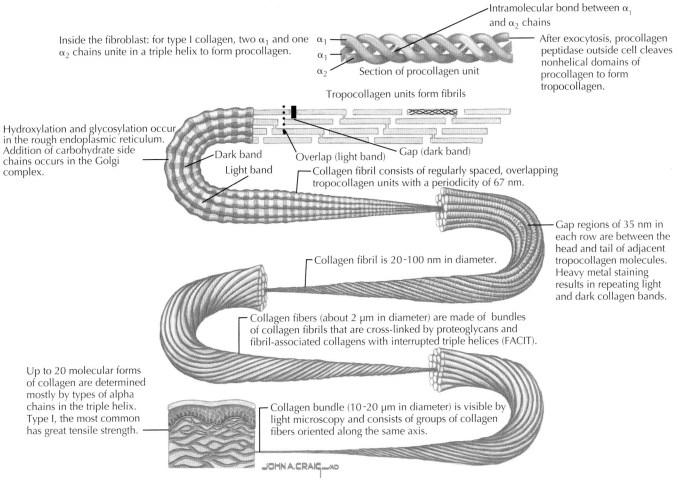

Inside the fibroblast: for type I collagen, two α_1 and one α_2 chains unite in a triple helix to form procollagen.

α_1
α_1
α_2 Section of procollagen unit

Intramolecular bond between α_1 and α_2 chains

After exocytosis, procollagen peptidase outside cell cleaves nonhelical domains of procollagen to form tropocollagen.

Tropocollagen units form fibrils

Hydroxylation and glycosylation occur in the rough endoplasmic reticulum. Addition of carbohydrate side chains occurs in the Golgi complex.

Dark band
Light band

Overlap (light band)   Gap (dark band)

Collagen fibril consists of regularly spaced, overlapping tropocollagen units with a periodicity of 67 nm.

Collagen fibril is 20-100 nm in diameter.

Gap regions of 35 nm in each row are between the head and tail of adjacent tropocollagen molecules. Heavy metal staining results in repeating light and dark collagen bands.

Collagen fibers (about 2 μm in diameter) are made of bundles of collagen fibrils that are cross-linked by proteoglycans and fibril-associated collagens with interrupted triple helices (FACIT).

Up to 20 molecular forms of collagen are determined mostly by types of alpha chains in the triple helix. Type I, the most common has great tensile strength.

Collagen bundle (10-20 μm in diameter) is visible by light microscopy and consists of groups of collagen fibers oriented along the same axis.

JOHN A.CRAIG—AD

Fig. 6.3 Collagen Synthesis.

overall orientation but provide support in multiple directions. It is found in the dermis and the submucosal layer of the gastrointestinal tract.

- **Dense regular connective tissue** consists of vastly more fibers than cells. The type I collagen fibers in this tissue are all oriented in one direction and are very good at strongly resisting force in that direction. It is found in tendons and ligaments.
- **Adipose tissue** contains fibroblasts but also many **adipocytes.** These are large "signet ring" cells that contain a large intracellular space where triglycerides are stored. These spaces appear empty in most slides because fats are removed as a by-product of the staining process.

Connective Tissue Fibers

Type I collagen is the most frequently encountered type of collagen in the body and therefore the most frequently encountered fiber. It forms pink, eosinophilic bundles that are visible with a light microscope. Each collagen molecule is formed by three α **chains** that form a triple helix. The different types of α chains are what make the different types (currently 28) of collagen.

The synthesis of collagen (Fig. 6.3) is complex and therefore has several stages at which it can be compromised, leading to connective tissue disorders.

1. The polypeptide chain that creates individual collagen α chains is translated from messenger RNA (mRNA) in the rough endoplasmic reticulum and released into intracellular cisternae.
2. The amino-terminal side of the protein is separated from the central region of the α chain.
3. Several amino acids along the length of the procollagen are hydroxylated so that each α chain can form hydrogen bonds with two other α chains.
4. The carboxy-terminal side of the procollagen molecule will help to align it with the other two α chains to form a **procollagen molecule.**
5. Other proteins prevent the procollagen molecules from binding within the cell. Instead, the procollagen molecules are moved to the Golgi apparatus and then released to the outside of the cell.
6. The procollagen is released into depressions in the cell membrane, **coves,** where it is added onto a growing **collagen fibril.**
7. Once outside, the carboxy-terminal ends of procollagen are cleaved so that the new bundles can contribute to the nearby collagen fibrils.
8. Collagen fibrils associate and bundle together to form **collagen fibers (Clinical Correlations 6.1 and 6.2).**

Reticular fibers (type III collagen) are formed in a similar way to type I collagen but are much narrower in diameter and are not visible in H&E stains, although special stains using silver can make them more noticeable. They are present throughout the body and are a minority contributor to most types of connective tissue proper. However, they are very prominent in cell-rich organs that require a great deal of blood flow over the cells of the organ, such as the liver and spleen. In these organs, type I collagen would impede the flow of blood, so the smaller type III collagen is more useful.

Elastic fibers are not a type of collagen. They consist of a core of coiled **elastin** surrounded by a meshwork of **fibrillin**. Elastin molecules bond to each other, creating a slightly random network of fibers extending through any tissues they inhabit. Fibrillin helps to guide the architecture of the elastic molecules (Clinical Correlation 6.3).

Contents of the Extracellular Space (Fig. 6.4)

In addition to fibers, the extracellular space contains ground substance, which is largely made of **proteoglycan aggregates**, large molecules formed by a core of **hyaluronic acid** bound to other **glycosaminoglycans** such as chondroitin sulfate, heparan sulfate, and keratan sulfate. These structures form large, bristled molecules that draw water into the extracellular space due to the negative charges clustered on their surface. Another cellular product, **multiadhesive glycoproteins**, such as fibronectin, anchor the extracellular matrix to the cells within it.

Fasciacytes (described by Stecco et al., 2018) are round cells with round nuclei that are located within the loose connective tissue between layers of deep fascia and on the surface of the deep

---

CLINICAL CORRELATION 6.1   Scurvy

Hydroxylation of the lysine and prolines of the collagen α chains in the rough endoplasmic reticulum requires vitamin C (ascorbic acid). Without hydroxylation, the hydrogen bonds that create the collagen triple helix cannot form. This impairs collagen formation, which makes wound healing and maintenance of the body's connective tissue difficult. This condition, **scurvy**, was frequently encountered by sailors until vitamin C–containing foods such as limes were added to their diet. The British Navy added lime juice to their rations in the 1850s, resulting in British sailors being called "Limeys."

CLINICAL CORRELATION 6.2   Osteogenesis Imperfecta

Osteogenesis imperfecta results from faulty formation of type I collagen. Although this can affect many tissues of the body, it is very noticeable in bone. Because type I collagen fibers support the mineralized bone, their absence makes bones brittle and easy to break. There are several types that correspond to mutations that affect different stages in the formation of type I collagen.

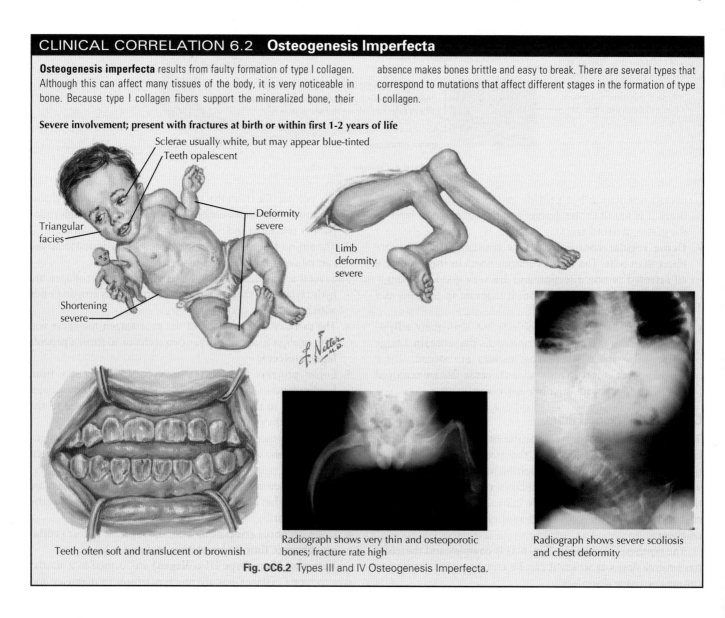

Severe involvement; present with fractures at birth or within first 1-2 years of life

Sclerae usually white, but may appear blue-tinted

Teeth opalescent

Triangular facies

Deformity severe

Limb deformity severe

Shortening severe

Teeth often soft and translucent or brownish

Radiograph shows very thin and osteoporotic bones; fracture rate high

Radiograph shows severe scoliosis and chest deformity

Fig. CC6.2 Types III and IV Osteogenesis Imperfecta.

CLINICAL CORRELATION 6.3 Marfan Syndrome

Marfan syndrome is caused by a mutation in the fibrillin gene or dysfunction in its expression. Because elastic fibers will not form properly without fibrillin, patients with **Marfan syndrome** will often have hypermobile joints, heart valve dysfunction, and problems with their large arteries, which are unable to elastically rebound from each heartbeat as readily as they might. These patients are often very tall and thin, with a wingspan (finger-to-finger length) exceeding their height.

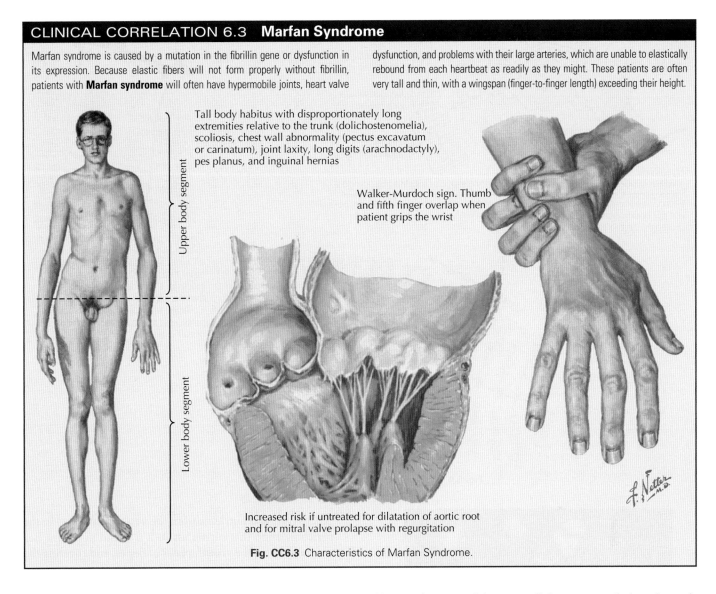

Tall body habitus with disproportionately long extremities relative to the trunk (dolichostenomelia), scoliosis, chest wall abnormality (pectus excavatum or carinatum), joint laxity, long digits (arachnodactyly), pes planus, and inguinal hernias

Upper body segment

Lower body segment

Walker-Murdoch sign. Thumb and fifth finger overlap when patient grips the wrist

Increased risk if untreated for dilatation of aortic root and for mitral valve prolapse with regurgitation

Fig. CC6.3 Characteristics of Marfan Syndrome.

fascia itself. They release proteoglycans and hyaluronic acid as part of the ground substance of connective tissue so that layers of deep fascia can glide across each other without excessive friction or irritation to the tissues. Even though they have similar functions, fasciacytes are visibly distinct from fibroblasts, which have long and spindly nuclei and are commonly seen within dense connective tissues. It appears that fibroblasts tend to maintain the fiber-rich dense connective tissues while fasciacytes tend to maintain loose connective tissue, which has a smaller number of fibers and greater amount of ground substance.

Cartilage

Cartilage (Fig. 6.5) can be conceived of as a variation on connective tissue proper with some distinctive features. Unlike other connective tissues, cartilage is (mostly) avascular and has no blood vessels within its tissues. Instead of type I collagen, cartilage contains **type II collagen**. Instead of fibroblasts, **chondroblasts** are the cells that secrete the fibers and extracellular matrix of collagen. Once they are completely surrounded by their secretory products within small islands, **lacunae**, they are called **chondrocytes**. These cells maintain the type II collagen

fibers and matrix of the extracellular space, including the multiadhesive glycoproteins in the area immediately surrounding the cell, the **territorial matrix**, which appears darkly eosinophilic on H&E stain. The area between chondrocytes, the **interterritorial matrix**, appears lighter in color and has a greater proportion of fibers.

Cartilage is surrounded by **perichondrium**, a layer of dense irregular connective tissue that contains the nerve and vascular supply to the cartilage. The inner layer of the perichondrium contains chondroblasts that can become active and release new type II collagen fibers and extracellular matrix until they are surrounded by it and become chondrocytes. This process is called **appositional growth**. Chondrocytes can also undergo **interstitial growth** during which they divide to form two or more daughter cells within a single lacuna. These daughter cells are referred to as an **isogenous group**. As each cell in the isogenous group secretes extracellular matrix and fibers, they push each other away until they are once again single chondrocytes in separate lacunae. This process is what allows bone to grow, because cartilage proliferates before transforming into bone. This process will be discussed in detail later.

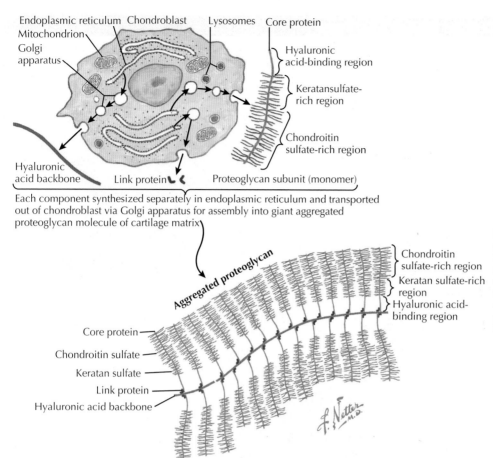

Each component synthesized separately in endoplasmic reticulum and transported out of chondroblast via Golgi apparatus for assembly into giant aggregated proteoglycan molecule of cartilage matrix

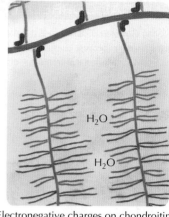

Electronegative charges on chondroitin sulfate and keratan sulfate molecules (SO_4^{2-}) cause side chains to repel each other and to attract and trap electropositive dipoles of water (H^+), thus acting as molecular sponge. Collagen fibers in matrix entangle proteoglycan aggregate, preventing its full extension.

Fig. 6.4 Formation and Composition of Proteoglycan.

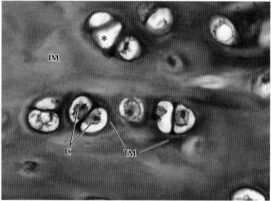

Light micrograph of hyaline cartilage from the trachea.
Groups of chondrocytes (**C**), the isogenous nests, sit in lacunae. Preparation artifact causes some lacunae to appear empty (∗). In other lacunae, chondrocytes shrank away from walls to leave a clear pericellular halo. Each cell has a slightly irregular shape and contains a single nucleus, often eccentric in location. A thin rim of basophilic territorial matrix (**TM**) is in the immediate vicinity of lacunae, which indicates a high concentration of newly synthesized sulfated GAGs. Between the chondrocytes, the interterritorial matrix (**IM**) appears more eosinophilic and has a typical glassy appearance. 480×. H&E.

Fig. 6.5 Cartilage. *H&E*, Hematoxylin and eosin. (Reused with permission from Ovalle W, Nahirney P. *Netter's Essential Histology*. 3rd ed. Elsevier; 2021.)

There are several subtypes of cartilage (Fig. 6.6), each of which has distinctive features.

- **Hyaline cartilage** has a glassy, refractory appearance and can be considered "typical" cartilage. It contains chondrocytes in lacunae, type II collagen in the matrix, and is avascular. It gets oxygen and nutrients from the vessels that travel in the perichondrium that surrounds it. It is found in the trachea and bronchi, in the growth plates of bones, and covering the articular surfaces of bones.

- **Elastic cartilage** is nearly identical to hyaline cartilage, with the only change being a substantial number of elastic fibers in the matrix alongside the type II collagen. It is found in the core of the ears, epiglottis, and nasal cartilages.

- **Fibrocartilage** is essentially an amalgam of dense irregular connective tissue and hyaline cartilage. It contains fibroblasts, chondrocytes, and type I and type II collagen in the matrix, and unlike other types of cartilage, it may be slightly vascular. It is found in the annulus fibrosis of the intervertebral discs, pubic symphysis, menisci, and other articular discs (e.g., ulnar, sternoclavicular, acromioclavicular, temporomandibular) that cushion the interactions of bones but also endure significant force.

Bone (Fig. 6.7)

Bone is a hard tissue that is more structurally supportive than cartilage due to the presence of calcium and phosphate-rich **hydroxyapatite** crystals, $Ca_{10}(PO_4)_6(OH)_2$, in the extracellular matrix that are supported by a latticework of type I collagen. Although bone can seem rocky and inert, it is a very active and resilient tissue. The outermost region of bones consists of **dense (compact) bone**. The inner portion of bone is called **trabecular (spongy) bone** and features struts of bone, **trabeculae**, within a

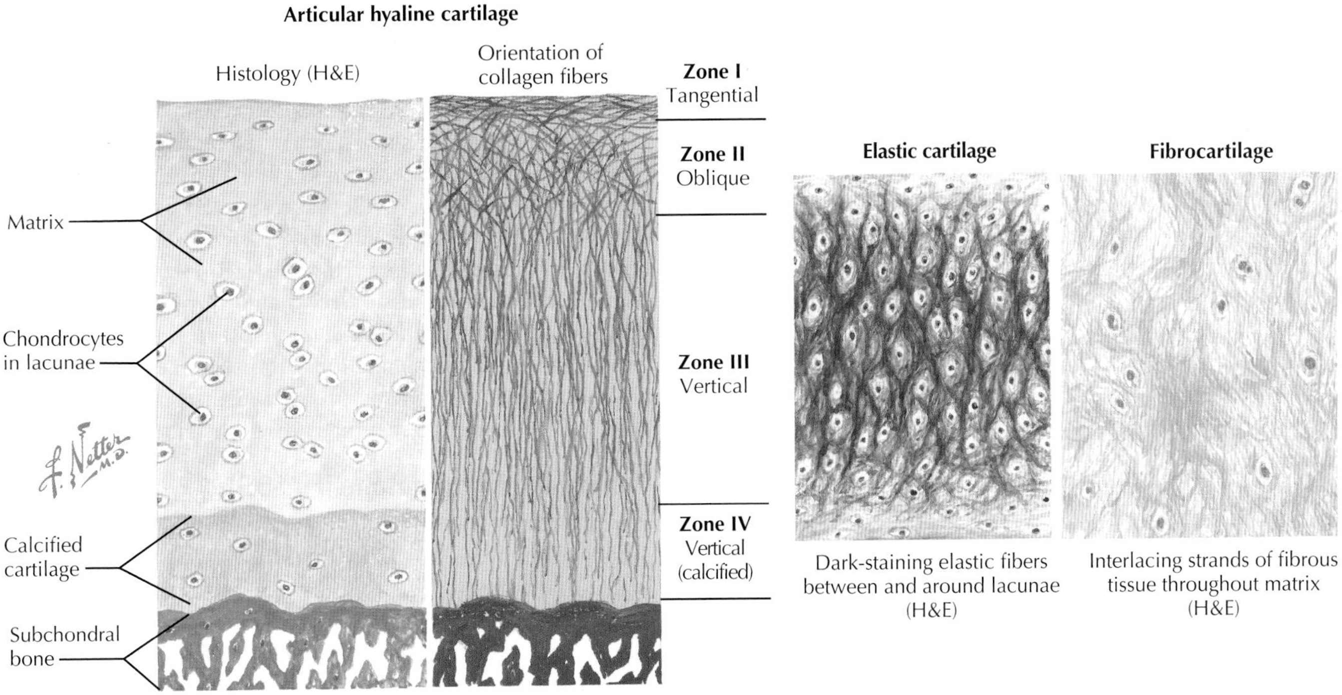

Articular hyaline cartilage

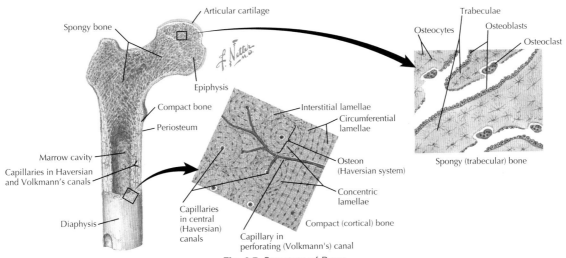

Histology (H&E)

Orientation of collagen fibers

Zone I
Tangential

Zone II
Oblique

Zone III
Vertical

Zone IV
Vertical
(calcified)

Matrix

Chondrocytes
in lacunae

Calcified
cartilage

Subchondral
bone

Elastic cartilage

Fibrocartilage

Dark-staining elastic fibers
between and around lacunae
(H&E)

Interlacing strands of fibrous
tissue throughout matrix
(H&E)

Fig. 6.6 Structure of Three Types of Cartilage. *H&E*, Hematoxylin and eosin.

Articular cartilage

Spongy bone

Epiphysis

Compact bone

Periosteum

Marrow cavity

Capillaries in Haversian
and Volkmann's canals

Diaphysis

Capillaries
in central
(Haversian)
canals

Capillary in
perforating (Volkmann's) canal

Interstitial lamellae

Circumferential
lamellae

Osteon
(Haversian system)

Concentric
lamellae

Compact (cortical) bone

Trabeculae

Osteocytes

Osteoblasts

Osteoclast

Spongy (trabecular) bone

Fig. 6.7 Structure of Bone.

cavity that contains adipose and hematopoietic (blood-forming) cells. The innermost portion of the shaft of a long bone contains a large **marrow cavity** with very few trabeculae.

Aside from a bone's articular surfaces, dense bone is covered by a layer of dense irregular connective tissue called **periosteum** (Fig. 6.8). This brings blood vessels to the bone, but unlike cartilage, these vessels actually penetrate the bone and supply its cells. The type I collagen fibers within bone are connected to the periosteum and the tendons and ligaments that attach to it. The fibers that connect the tendon, periosteum, and bone are **Sharpey fibers**. They help to prevent the tendons and ligaments avulsing from the surface of the bone during strenuous activity. The inner layer of periosteum contains **osteoprogenitor cells** that can differentiate to become osteoblasts. These osteoprogenitor cells also line the inside of the marrow cavity. Just like

chondroblasts in the inner layer of perichondrium, they can become active, secrete substances into the extracellular matrix, and become osteoblasts.

Osteoblasts release an unmineralized form of bone called **osteoid** into the extracellular space, as well as enzymes that mineralize the osteoid. **Type I collagen** fibers form a scaffold for the hydroxyapatite crystals. The presence of collagen fibers makes bone much more resilient than crystals alone. Approximately 65% of the extracellular matrix of bone is mineral, and the remaining 35% is made of fibers, glycoproteins, proteoglycans, and cells. Once osteoblasts have completely surrounded themselves in a lacuna, they are called **osteocytes**. Osteocytes maintain the mineralized bone in their immediate vicinity and can recycle a small amount of bone (osteoblastic osteolysis) or lay down more osteoid in response to the stresses they encounter.

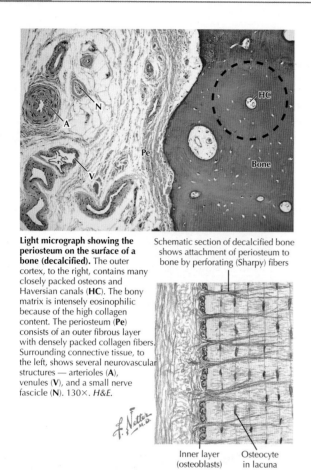

Light micrograph showing the periosteum on the surface of a bone (decalcified). The outer cortex, to the right, contains many closely packed osteons and Haversian canals (**HC**). The bony matrix is intensely eosinophilic because of the high collagen content. The periosteum (**Pe**) consists of an outer fibrous layer with densely packed collagen fibers. Surrounding connective tissue, to the left, shows several neurovascular structures — arterioles (**A**), venules (**V**), and a small nerve fascicle (**N**). 130×. H&E.

Schematic section of decalcified bone shows attachment of periosteum to bone by perforating (Sharpy) fibers

Inner layer (osteoblasts)   Osteocyte in lacuna

Fig. 6.8 Periosteum and Bone. *H&E*, Hematoxylin and eosin. (Reused with permission from Ovalle W, Nahirney P. *Netter's Essential Histology.* 3rd ed. Elsevier; 2021.)

Osteoblasts and osteocytes can deposit new bone, whereas **osteoclasts** are cells that are specialized to break down bone. Osteoclasts are large, multinucleated, phagocytic cells that are able to demineralize hydroxyapatite crystals. Actin filaments and other molecules inside an osteoclast attach it onto the surface of bone. The surface facing the bone has a **ruffled border**, consisting of many microvilli that release H+ ions. The low pH demineralizes the underlying bone and forms a depression known as a **resorptive bay** (Howship lacuna). Osteoclasts also release enzymes, such as **matrix metalloproteases**, that break apart type I collagen and other proteins in the resorptive bay. The calcium and phosphate ions from demineralized crystals are endocytosed into the osteoclast and then released into the extracellular space and eventually reach the blood.

Woven and Mature Bone (Fig. 6.9)

When osteoid mineralizes, it initially forms a uniform mass called **woven bone**. It is solid but not as stable as mature dense bone. That is because dense bone consists of organized tubes called **osteons**. These form as woven bone is destroyed by clusters of osteoclasts that move though it in a linear direction. This **cutting cone** creates an open, cylindrical channel into which waves of osteoblasts migrate. The osteoblasts lay down osteoid that mineralizes, making the cylinder slightly narrower. Then more waves of osteoblasts move in, narrowing the cylinder further until the osteocytes and their bone form concentric lamellae of mineralized bone with a **central (osteal/haversian) canal** at the center. Cutting cones also recycle and remodel older dense bone, leaving behind the remnants of older osteons, called **interstitial lamellae**. The presence of osteons in dense

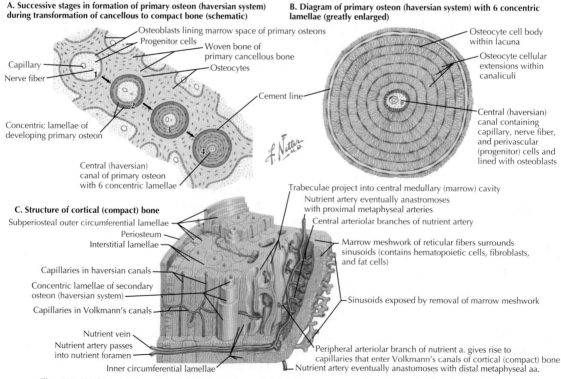

Fig. 6.9 (A) Secondary osteon and (B) microscopic structure of mature long bone: basic science of bones.

CLINICAL CORRELATION 6.4   Bone Fracture and Healing

After bone has fractured, there will be hemorrhage in the immediate area from the vessels in the bone, the periosteum, and possibly even nearby arteries and veins that are lacerated by bone edges. Within a week, macrophages will migrate into the area to phagocytose and clear cellular debris. Fibroblasts will create loose connective tissue between bone fragments, which is replaced by a soft callus of cartilage laid down by chondroblasts over the next 2–3 weeks. The soft callus is replaced by osteoid and woven bone laid done by osteoblasts over the next 4–16 weeks, which will eventually be replaced by mature bone as bone remodeling takes place and new osteons are created over the next four months or more. If a fracture is not set properly at an early stage, the healing will proceed but may lock the bone into a malformed shape.

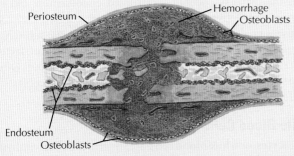

Stage of inflammation-A hematoma forms as the result of disruption of intraosseous and surrounding vessels. Bone at the edges of the fracture dies. Bone necrosis is greater with larger amounts of soft tissue disruption. Inflammatory cells are followed by fibroblasts, chondroblasts, and osteoprogenitor cells. Low pO_2 at the fracture site promotes angiogenesis.

Stage of soft callus formation Soft callus forms, initially composed of collagen; this is followed by cartilage and osteoid formation.

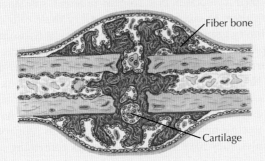

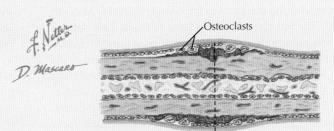

Stage of hard callus formation Osteoid and cartilage of external, periosteal, and medullary soft callus become mineralized as they are converted to woven bone (hard callus)

Stage of bone remodeling Osteoclastic and osteoblastic activity converts woven bone to lamellar bone with true haversian systems. Normal bone contours are restored; angulation may be partially or completely corrected.

Fig. CC6.4 Healing of Fracture.

bone gives it a greater degree of stability than woven bone. Some of the larger trabeculae within the spongy bone and marrow cavity may also contain osteons.

The central canal contains blood vessels that nurture the osteocytes. However, within the osteon each osteocyte is encased in a lacunae of hydroxyapatite crystals and seemingly unable to reach the vessels. Thankfully, osteocytes are good neighbors and have multiple cytoplasmic extensions that radiate out and contact the cytoplasmic extensions of neighboring osteocytes. These processes travel through very small channels in the bone, **canaliculi,** and allow the cells to transmit nutrients, O_2, and CO_2 to each other, passing them to and from the nearby vessels. **Perforating (Volkmann) canals** run at 90-degree angles to the central canals and carry blood to them. All blood in the bones comes from **nutrient arteries** that branch off larger nearby vessels, pierce the periosteum, and enter the bone. **Nutrient veins** and small periosteal veins drain the blood from the same areas.

During fetal development and childhood, the marrow cavities of most long bones contains **red marrow**, which is an active site of blood cell formation, or **hematopoiesis**. In adults, the marrow cavity in long bones is typically full of **yellow marrow**, which contains a lot of adipose tissue and is not a major site of hematopoiesis. The sternum, iliac crests, and bodies of the vertebrae retain a greater amount of red marrow and remain important sites of blood cell formation throughout life (Clinical Correlation 6.4).

Entheses

Specialized microscopic organs called **entheses** (Milz et al., 2004) are present where tendons, ligaments, and joint capsules insert onto bones. An enthesis is formed by fibrocartilage (containing types I and II collagen) that sits between the type I collagen of a tendon or ligament and the type I collagen of the periosteum and bone itself. The fibrocartilage near the ligament/tendon is unmineralized but abruptly transitions to mineralized fibrocartilage as it approaches the bone. The presence of an enthesis helps to spread out the stress experienced by bone as traction is placed on it and also allows it to resist compressive forces. Dysfunction (enthesopathy) or inflammation (enthesitis) of these structures has been associated with pain and bone spurs (enthesophytes) forming in the nearby soft tissues.

Blood (Fig. 6.10)

Blood is a very unusual type of connective tissue in that it contains no fibers but consists of circulating cells within **plasma**, a fluid that is essentially blood's extracellular matrix. Each adult human has approximately 6 L of blood circulating throughout the body, which typically has 55% plasma and 45% circulating cells. Approximately 99% of the circulating cells are red blood cells, **erythrocytes**, and the remaining 1% are white blood cells, **leukocytes**.

Blood plasma is 90% **water** and approximately 8% **plasma proteins** such as albumin, immunoglobulins, and fibrinogen. **Albumin**, which makes up nearly half of all plasma proteins, is generated in the liver and maintains the proper osmotic pressure in the blood. It also helps to transport circulating hormones, bilirubin, and some drugs. **Immunoglobulins** or antibodies are released by immune cells and can (among other things) circulate through the blood and attach to pathogenic organisms. **Fibrinogen** is a large, soluble plasma protein that can polymerize during clotting reactions to form large, insoluble fibers to close cuts. The remaining 2% of plasma is made from **solutes** such as ions, salts, amino acids, lipids, hormones, and vitamins.

Erythrocytes, or **red blood cells**, are the characteristic cells of blood. They are eosinophilic (pink), biconcave discs without a nucleus or mitochondria. Their shape gives them much elasticity that allows them to navigate through the smallest capillaries. Approximately 30% of their cytoplasm is hemoglobin, a protein with a prominent iron-heme group that can bind to O_2 and CO_2. I have not focused on the exact size of cells, but it is worthwhile to remember that erythrocytes are 7 to 8 μm in diameter. They are an excellent reference for the size of other cells and microscopic structures because they are very consistent in size and are present in almost any slide you might examine.

Erythrocytes come from stem cells in red bone marrow that are called **erythroblasts**. We will not go into the detailed development of blood cells in this volume, and a quick summary of the process will suffice. Erythroblasts are supported in the red marrow by phagocytotic cells called macrophages. These cells will endocytose the "debris" that erythroblasts jettison as they become erythrocytes. They begin by creating many ribosomes, which appear basophilic (bluish purple) on an H&E stain. These ribosomes translate a great deal of RNA for the hemoglobin molecule, which contains iron, binds to O_2 and CO_2, and appears eosinophilic (pinkish) on H&E stain. The cells become more and more eosinophilic as hemoglobin accumulates in the cytoplasm and ribosomes dwindle. Eventually the cell jettisons its nucleus and forms a **reticulocyte**, which may begin circulating. Reticulocytes have some lingering ribosomes in their cytoplasm, creating the appearance of a mesh. As the basophilic meshwork disappears, the cell becomes a mature erythrocyte, which will circulate for approximately 120 days before being destroyed in the spleen or liver.

Platelets, or thrombocytes, are small 1- to 4-μm cellular fragments that circulate for approximately 10 days before being broken down in the spleen. They are created by extremely large cells, **megakaryocytes**, which are stuck in the bone marrow. The megakaryocytes extend tendrils of their cytoplasm into the vascular spaces of the bone marrow. The tendril tips bleb off from the cell and become platelets once they begin circulating. Platelets contain several cytoplasmic granules that are released when the platelets encounter disrupted endothelium and the outlying connective tissue. These granules contain vasoconstrictive signals that narrow hemorrhaging vessels, substances that promote clumping of platelets, and coagulation factors that create a fibrinogen mesh around the cut or wound. Other factors stimulate nearby smooth muscle cells and fibroblasts to proliferate and promote healing in the damaged area.

White Blood Cells

Leukocytes, or **white blood cells**, are small in number within the circulating blood but are incredibly important in the response to pathogens, in monitoring the health of cells, and in turning over the tissues of the body when they become damaged.

- **Granulocytes** are circulating leukocytes that have granules in their cytoplasm that contain different substances that help them to combat pathogens. All of these cells contain **primary granules**, which are essentially just lysosomes that degrade endocytosed material. They are formed in red bone marrow and, once in circulation, they can no longer divide.
- **Neutrophils** are the majority of circulating leukocytes, comprising approximately 60% to 70% of the total. They are noticeably larger than red blood cells and have distinctive multilobed nuclei. In addition to primary granules, they have **secondary granules** containing reactive oxygen molecules as well as bacteriostatic and bactericidal enzymes. They also release metalloproteases and other structures that help them to migrate out of the bloodstream and into peripheral tissues. Their secondary granules do not take up eosinophil or basophil, so they appear more "neutral" in color, hence their name.
- **Eosinophils** make up only 1% to 4% of circulating leukocytes. They have a multilobed nucleus, and their secondary granules are very eosinophilic, giving their cytoplasm a distinctive red hue. They are specialized to fight parasitic infections and can release reactive oxygen molecules, neurotoxins, and substances that perforate target cell membranes, as well as proteins that cause mast cells to degranulate (see later).
- **Basophils** are very rare, less than 1% of circulating leukocytes. Their secondary granules are basophilic, giving the cytoplasm a blue hue. They release heparin, an anticoagulant, as well as histamine to dilate small vessels. Basophils also release chemotactic factors that attract eosinophils and neutrophils. **Mast cells** are very similar to basophils and are found in peripheral tissues; however, they come from separate precursors. They release histamine and heparin into the peripheral tissues, making nearby vessels leaky and thinning the blood. This causes swelling in the area but also helps neutrophils migrate into the affected tissues.

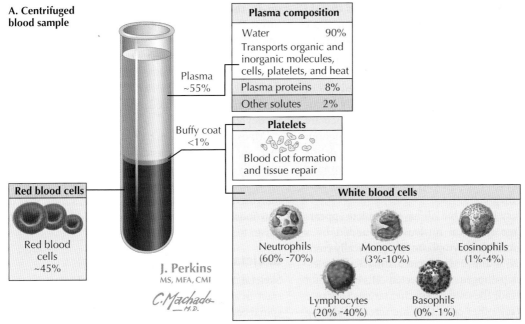

A. Centrifuged blood sample

Plasma ~55%

Plasma composition

Water	90%
Transports organic and inorganic molecules, cells, platelets, and heat	
Plasma proteins	8%
Other solutes	2%

Buffy coat <1%

Platelets

Blood clot formation and tissue repair

Red blood cells

Red blood cells ~45%

J. Perkins
MS, MFA, CMI

C. Machado
_M.D.

White blood cells

Neutrophils (60% -70%)   Monocytes (3%-10%)   Eosinophils (1%-4%)

Lymphocytes (20% -40%)   Basophils (0% -1%)

B. Formed elements of blood

Features of Erythrocytes and Platelets in Wright-Stained Blood Smears

Cells	Diameter (μm)	Life span (days)	No. of cells/ L of blood	Shape and nucleus type	Cytoplasm	Functions
Erythrocyte (red blood cell)	7–8	120	5×10^{12} in males; 4.5×10^{12} in females	Biconcave disc, anucleate	Pink because of acidophilia of hemoglobin; halo in center	Transports hemoglobin that binds O_2 and CO_2
Platelet (thrombocyte)	1–4	10	150 to 400×10^9	Oval biconvex disc, anucleate	Pale blue; central dark granulomere, peripheral less dense hyalomere	In hemostasis, promotes blood clotting; plugs endothelial damage

Features of Leukocytes in Wright-Stained Blood Smears (Total Number: 5 –10 x 10^9/L Blood)

Cells	Diameter (μm)	Differential count (%)	Nucleus	Cytoplasm	Functions
Granulocytes					
Neutrophil	9–12	60–70	Segmented, 3–5 lobes, densely stained	Pale, finely granular, evenly dispersed specific granules	Phagocytoses bacteria; increases in number in acute bacterial infections
Eosinophil	12–15	1–4	Bilobed, clumped chromatin pattern, densely stained	Large homogeneous red granules that are coarse and highly refractile	Phagocytoses antigen-antibody complexes and parasites
Basophil	10–14	0–1	Bilobed or segmented	Large blue specific granules that stain with basic dyes and often obscure nucleus	Involved in anticoagulation, increases vascular permeability
Agranulocytes					
Monocytes	12–20	3–7	Indented, kidney-shaped, lightly stained	Agranular, pale blue cytoplasm, with lysosomes	Is motile; gives rise to macrophages
Lymphocyte • Small • Medium to large	6–10 11–16	20–40	Small, round or slightly indented, darkly stained	Agranular, faintly basophilic, blue to gray	Acts in humoral (B cell) and cellular (T cell) immunity

Fig. 6.10 (A) Centrifuged blood sample and (B) formed elements of blood.

- **Nongranular leukocytes** are circulating leukocytes that do not have any visible granules within their cytoplasm. They originate in the red bone marrow but retain the ability to divide.
  - **Monocytes** are very large cells with a kidney-shaped nucleus that typically make up between 3% and 7% of circulating leukocytes. Monocytes are essentially circulating stem cells for a variety of **macrophages**, which are immune cells located in a variety of tissues throughout the body. They phagocytose pathogens and cellular debris and take that material and present it to other immune cells using major histocompatibility compatibility (MHC) II molecules on their cell surface.
  - **Lymphocytes** vary in size, but all have a similar appearance with a large spherical nucleus surrounded by a relatively thin rim of clear cytoplasm. They typically comprise between 25% and 33% of circulating leukocytes. These cells attack pathogens and infected cells but are not phagocytic; instead, they attack specific targets. Because lymphocytes attack other cells, they are screened during development to prevent their recognizing normal self-cells and tissues within the body. If they inappropriately start to react to self, autoimmune diseases can result. There are many types of lymphocytes and we will only discuss a few of the more prominent members of this group.
    - **B lymphocytes** can recognize specific antigens that are presented to them and release an immunoglobulin that will bind to that exact antigen. Once activated, B lymphocytes can migrate into peripheral tissues to become **plasma cells** that release huge amounts of their specific immunoglobulin. These have a characteristic "clock face" nucleus and (often) visible Golgi apparatus. Once the infection has passed, an activated B lymphocyte can become a **memory B cell**, which will reside in lymph tissues throughout the body waiting to encounter the same antigen and become active once again.
    - **T lymphocytes** undergo additional development in the thymus. They can become **cytotoxic (killer) T cells**, which can recognize the antigens that are on MHC molecules of the various antigen presenting cells (e.g., macrophages). They release several molecules to attack their targets, including perforins to create holes in the target cell's membrane. **Helper T cells** also recognize antigens presented on MHC molecules. They divide and recruit other lymphocytes to the area.
    - **Natural killer cells** are preprogrammed to destroy cells that no longer present normal structures on their surface due to infection and transformation by viruses or cancer.

MUSCLE TISSUE

The hallmark of muscle tissue is its ability to contract. Each type of muscle tissue contains cells called **myocytes** that are able to actively contract themselves and pass that contraction on to the surrounding connective tissues and other structures. There are two major types of muscle tissue, **striated** and **smooth muscle**.

Under the microscope, striated muscle cells appear striped due to the regular arrangement of actin and myosin molecules that make up the majority of their cytoplasm. Striated muscle is further subdivided into **cardiac myocytes** and **skeletal myocytes**.

Myosatellite cells are small cells with minimal cytoplasm that are located alongside the skeletal myocytes. They are typically quiescent but can become active and proliferate to form additional myosatellite and myocyte cells in response to increased exercise or muscle trauma. In adults, they do not form new muscle from scratch but fuse to add their nuclei and cytoplasm to nearby myocytes.

Skeletal Muscle (Fig. 6.11)

Skeletal muscles are generally under voluntary control and contract in response to signals from lower motor neurons in the spinal cord. Each skeletal muscle cell, or **muscle fiber**, is shaped like an elongated cylinder that sits side by side with neighboring muscle fibers. Each muscle fiber (individual cell) is surrounded by a thin layer of connective tissue, the **endomysium**, that is largely composed of reticular fibers. Several muscle fibers and their surrounding endomysium are bundled together into **muscle fascicles** that are surrounded by a thicker layer of connective tissue, the **perimysium**. The outermost layer of connective tissue covering an entire muscle is called the **epimysium**. All the connective tissues within a muscle are continuous with each other, the muscle tendon, periosteum, and collagen fibers within the bone onto which they insert.

Before we get rolling, please note that the prefix "*sarco-*" is derived from the Greek "*sarx*" for "*flesh*" and is used extensively when describing the features of skeletal muscle cells. For example, **sarcopenia** refers to the loss of muscle mass (approximately 3% per decade) that tends to occur due to decrease in muscle activity with age. The cell membrane of skeletal muscle cells is called the **sarcolemma**, and it surrounds the cell's cytoplasm, or **sarcoplasm**. One peculiar aspect of the sarcolemma is that it forms deep channels called **T tubules** (or transverse tubules if you are not into the whole brevity thing) through the sarcoplasm, extending from one side of the sarcolemma to the other. Because of this, the inside of each T tubule is actually filled with extracellular fluid. Each muscle fiber also contains many nuclei (hundreds in a single fiber), mitochondria that produce copious amounts of adenosine triphosphate (ATP), myoglobin to store O_2, and glycogen and triglycerides as a source of energy. The majority of the sarcoplasm is taken up by **myofibrils**, the functional organelles of each myocyte. Each myofibril is approximately 1 μm in diameter and extends through the entire length of the muscle fiber. Because all the myofibrils are aligned in parallel, their contraction shortens the length of the muscle fiber in that single direction.

The sarcoplasm surrounds the myofibrils and is rich in magnesium, phosphate, and potassium ions, as well as some specialized proteins. Also located within the sarcoplasm is a specialized smooth endoplasmic reticulum, the **sarcoplasmic reticulum**.

The muscular system

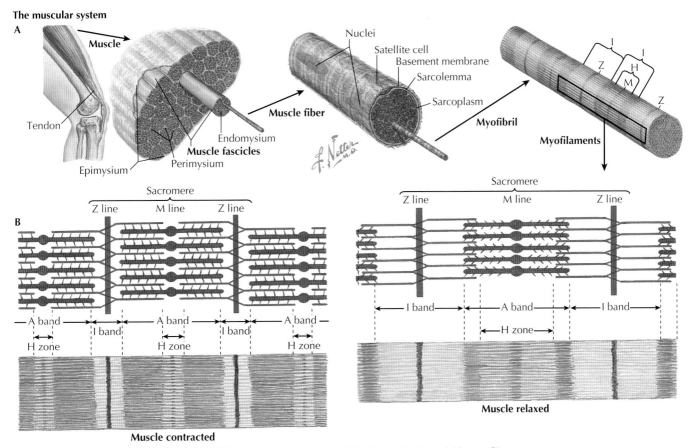

Fig. 6.11 (A) The muscular system and (B) sliding of thick and thin myofilaments.

It contains, releases, and recovers calcium ions, which are vital in the process of translating depolarization into contraction.

The Sarcomere (Figs. 6.11 and 6.12)

The myofibrils that fill the sarcoplasm are composed of thick and thin **myofilaments** that slide across each other during muscular contraction and relaxation. These myofilaments are lined up in a pattern, called a **sarcomere**, that gives it a striped (striated) pattern. These sarcomeres have a very characteristic appearance that reflects the organization of actin, myosin, and other molecules that allow contraction to occur. Because we need to start somewhere, we will begin with the sarcomere and then go into detail regarding how its subcomponents function.

Each individual sarcomere is bounded by a **Z line** on each of its ends. At the middle of each sarcomere is a single **M line**. The **thin filaments** are all anchored to the Z lines. The light-colored portion of each sarcomere that extends from each Z line contains only thin filaments and is called the **I band**. Because I bands extend from each side of the Z line, each I band is shared by two neighboring sarcomeres. The **thick filaments** are anchored at the M line. The portion of each sarcomere extending from each M line that contains any thick filaments is called the **A band**, while the portion that contains *only* thick filaments is called the **H zone**. As muscles contract the thick and thin filaments slide across each other, causing the sarcomere to shorten. The A band, containing thick filaments, never visibly shortens.

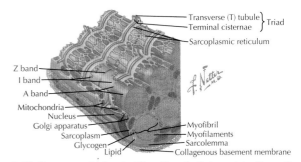

Fig. 6.12 Segment of Muscle Fiber Greatly Enlarged to Show Sarcoplasmic Structures and Inclusions.

However, as the thin filaments glide in-between the thick filaments, the I and H bands appear to shrink.

Molecular Basis of the Sarcomere (Fig. 6.13)

Individual actin molecules, **G actin**, each have a myosin-binding site and polymerize to form a long linear form, called **F actin**. Two F actin polymers wrap around each other to create a double helix that has its myosin-binding sites facing outward. From now on when I use the word "actin," I am referring to this double-helical polymer, which forms thin myofilaments seen in the sarcomere. Several specialized molecules associate with actin and control access to its myosin-binding site. **Tropomyosin** is a long molecule that covers the myosin-binding sites of seven adjacent G actin monomers. It is linked

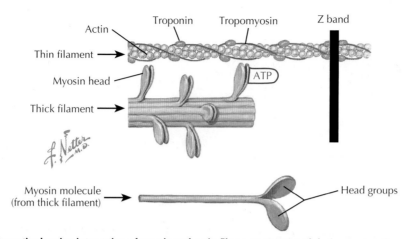

Schematic showing interaction of myosin and actin filaments at rest and during contraction.
The Z band is drawn closer to the edge of the A band by the sliding of filaments, and the I band region narrows.

Fig. 6.13 Schematic Showing Interaction of Myosin and Actin Filaments at Rest and During Contraction. *ATP,* Adenosine triphosphate.

to a trio of other molecules, the **troponin complex. Troponin I** binds to the actin molecule, **troponin T** binds to tropomyosin, and **troponin C** binds to (and releases) Ca^{2+} ions. This cadre of molecules are what controls the binding of actin and myosin molecules to each other.

The thick myofilaments are made from **myosin.** As with actin, when I say "myosin" later in the text, I am referring to an entire complex of molecules, in this case two **heavy chains** and four **light chain** myosin subunits. The two heavy chain molecules have long intertwining **tails** that form a double helix while their enlarged **heads** are connected to the tails by a flexible **hinge region.** The heads extend from each hinge region at a steep angle but are able to change the angle at which they project. The myosin heavy chain dimers cluster together so that the tails form large bundles (like a tree trunk) with the heads projecting outward (like very short limbs). Near the M line is a "bare area" consisting of myosin tails without projecting heads. Each myosin head has an **actin-binding site** and an **ATPase site.** Each head also associates with two light chains, the **essential light chain** and **regulatory light chain.** The light chains ensure that each head is positioned correctly relative to its neighboring myosin molecules.

Muscle Contraction at the Molecular Level (Fig. 6.14)

During muscle contraction, myosin heads repeatedly change the angle of their heads so they can "walk" along the F actin polymers, forming cross bridges that bind strongly and then release. Their actin-binding sites bind and release the myosin-binding sites of the individual G actin monomers and pull the light chains closer to the sarcomere's M line. This is an energetically demanding process that uses much ATP from the mitochondria within the myocytes.

1. When Ca^{2+} binds to troponin C (we will discuss where the calcium comes from shortly), it causes the troponin complex and the attached tropomyosin molecule to shift off of the myosin-binding sites of the F actin polymer, which then bind to the actin-binding site of a nearby myosin head at

a 90-degree angle. It is important to note that at this time, the ATPase site of the myosin head is bound to adenosine diphosphate (ADP) and an inorganic phosphate (Pi) ion. In this state, the myosin heads have a great affinity for binding to actin.

2. When the Pi is released, the hinge region of the myosin changes conformation so that the head shifts into a 45-degree angle and the actin polymer is pulled one unit further along the heavy chain. This is known as the **power stroke.** Note that it occurs when the Pi is released, NOT when the ATP is hydrolyzed.

3. ADP is released at the end of the power stroke, and the myosin head is left tightly bound at a 45-degree angle to the G actin monomer it just shifted. This is called the **rigor state** and normally does not last very long.

4. The open ATPase site binds to ATP, and this causes the myosin head to detach from the unit of G actin it had just moved.

5. The ATPase site on the myosin head now lives up to its name and hydrolyses the ATP into ADP and Pi, which both remain bound to the myosin head. This process releases energy from the ATP, and some of that energy shifts the myosin head from 45 degrees back to 90 degrees.

6. The myosin head (including the ADP and Pi) is now ready (perhaps even eager) to bind to a new G actin subunit just a bit further along the actin myofilament. If the actin's myosin-binding site remains available, we return to step 2, and muscle contraction continues.

Different myosin heads in a thick filament are each in a different state of this process at any given time during muscle contraction. One useful metaphor is a large group of people pulling on a long rope. They succeed in moving the rope (light filament) along even though their hands (myosin heads) each pull and release specific regions of the rope (G actin subunits) at different times. In addition, the amount of stretch a muscle experiences prior to contraction affects the amount of force it can generate. To contract strongly, a sarcomere must start near its resting length (Fig. 6.15). If it is overcontracted, the thin actin filaments override each other, making it difficult to establish

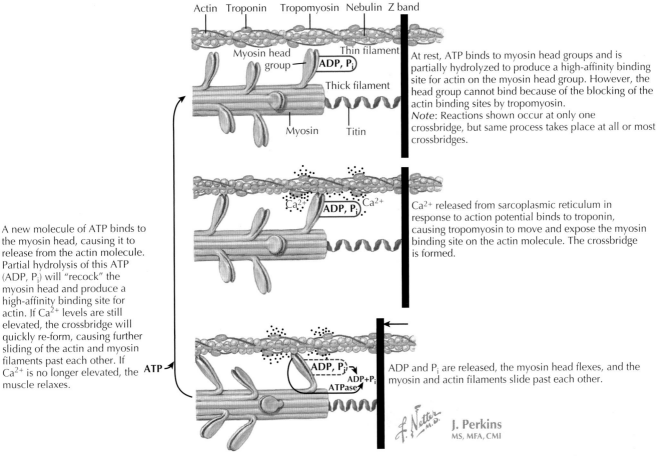

At rest, ATP binds to myosin head groups and is partially hydrolyzed to produce a high-affinity binding site for actin on the myosin head group. However, the head group cannot bind because of the blocking of the actin binding sites by tropomyosin.
Note: Reactions shown occur at only one crossbridge, but same process takes place at all or most crossbridges.

Ca^{2+} released from sarcoplasmic reticulum in response to action potential binds to troponin, causing tropomyosin to move and expose the myosin binding site on the actin molecule. The crossbridge is formed.

A new molecule of ATP binds to the myosin head, causing it to release from the actin molecule. Partial hydrolysis of this ATP (ADP, P_i) will "recock" the myosin head and produce a high-affinity binding site for actin. If Ca^{2+} levels are still elevated, the crossbridge will quickly re-form, causing further sliding of the actin and myosin filaments past each other. If Ca^{2+} is no longer elevated, the muscle relaxes.

ADP and P_i are released, the myosin head flexes, and the myosin and actin filaments slide past each other.

J. Perkins
MS, MFA, CMI

Fig. 6.14 Biochemical Mechanics of Muscle Contraction. *ADP,* Adenosine diphosphate; *ATP,* adenosine triphosphate.

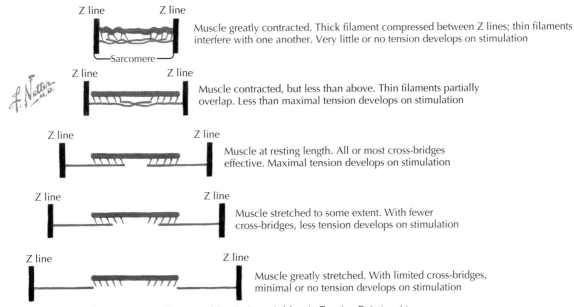

Muscle greatly contracted. Thick filament compressed between Z lines; thin filaments interfere with one another. Very little or no tension develops on stimulation

Muscle contracted, but less than above. Thin filaments partially overlap. Less than maximal tension develops on stimulation

Muscle at resting length. All or most cross-bridges effective. Maximal tension develops on stimulation

Muscle stretched to some extent. With fewer cross-bridges, less tension develops on stimulation

Muscle greatly stretched. With limited cross-bridges, minimal or no tension develops on stimulation

Fig. 6.15 Muscle Length-Muscle Tension Relationships.

actin and myosin cross bridges and to contract further. If it is overstretched, fewer myosin heads are in the vicinity of the actin filaments and cannot generate significant force until the filaments are pulled closer to the resting state to engage more cross bridges (Clinical Correlation 6.5).

Transmission of Contraction From Sarcomere to Tendon (Fig. 6.16)

The M lines of parallel sarcomeres are formed by **myomesin** and **M protein** molecules, which bind to the midpoint of the myosin molecules. Actin polymers are anchored to α-**actinin** dimers, which form the Z line on each side of the sarcomere. Another molecule, **nebulin**, is anchored to α-actinin at the Z line and extends along each F actin polymer. The free end of each F actin polymer is capped by **tropomodulin** molecules, which regulate their length. Large, coiled **titin** molecules (the largest known protein!) anchor the myomesin molecules of the thick myosin chains to the α-actinin molecules at the Z line and act as springs that prevent excessive stretching of the sarcomere and also help to return the sarcomere to its resting position. Also at the Z line are telethonon and myotilin molecules.

As a sarcomere contracts and shortens, the contraction is passed to the neighboring sarcomeres by their mutual attachments at the Z line. **Desmin** molecules form a network of filaments running between the Z discs of nearby sarcomeres as well as the sarcolemma (cell membrane). As the myofibers shorten, the whole skeletal muscle cell shortens along its long axis. If this occurred in isolation, we would just have individual muscle cells contracting like an accordion but not passing that contraction to the outside. The filamin proteins are thought to anchor the actin filaments and myotilin to the sarcolemma. In turn, the sarcolemma is anchored to the endomysium surrounding each muscle cell by a complex of proteins. This complex, called the **dystrophin glycoprotein complex**, includes proteins such as **dystrophin**, the four transmembrane **sarcoglycans**, and the

---

CLINICAL CORRELATION 6.5   Rigor Mortis

At the time of death, respiration ceases and ATP is no longer produced by the mitochondria of the body. Without ATP to bind the myosin heads, they remain firmly (and immovably) attached to actin in the rigor state. This results in **rigor mortis** (stiffness of death) when the body becomes rigid and stiff. Rigor mortis ceases when decay sets in and the muscle proteins begin breaking down.

---

two **dystroglycans**. Dystrophin is a massive protein that links desmin, Z lines, and their associated actin filaments to the sarcolemma. The sarcoglycans anchor the complex to the sarcolemma, and the dystroglycans attach the complex to **laminin** on the outside of the cell and the endomysium that surrounds each myofiber. This is what allows the intracellular contraction of the sarcomere to put traction on the connective tissue fibers on the outside of the cell. The pull on the endomysium is passed to the perimysium and eventually the epimysium. The connective tissue fibers of the epimysium, primarily type I collagen, bundle together to become tendons. Tendons insert into the periosteum, or connective tissue around bones. The collagen fibers also pierce the bone itself to anchor the attachment site strongly in place (Clinical Correlation 6.6).

Biochemistry of Muscle Contraction (Figs. 6.12 and 6.17)

We have explored the process of muscle contraction but have left a few questions lingering: where does all the ATP come from? Why do muscles get sore and irritated when they are fatigued? What makes some muscles faster or slower than others?

There is typically some ATP in the sarcoplasm of a resting muscle fiber. However, this supply runs out very quickly during activity. During muscle contraction, the level of ADP in each cell rises, and this stimulates oxidative phosphorylation and substrate-level phosphorylation to make ATP. However, this process takes a long time (in cellular timescales) and would leave the muscle without adequate energy. To span the gap in time, muscle cells contain **creatine phosphate**, a molecule that has a high-energy phosphate ion. It "donates" its phosphate to ADP to create ATP and **creatine**. This reaction is catalyzed by **creatine kinase**, an enzyme that can oversee this reaction in both directions. Thus the enzyme generates ATP and creatine

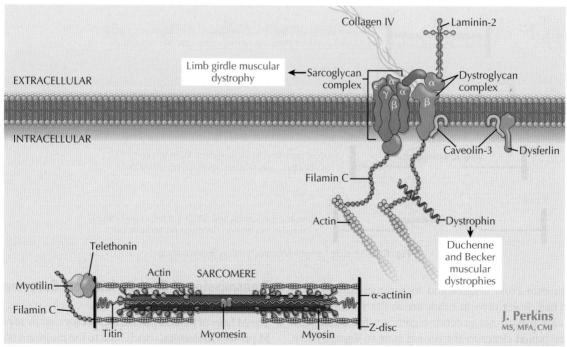

Fig. 6.16 Sarcoglycan Complex and Sarcomere Proteins.

during muscle contraction but builds up a supply of creatine phosphate during relaxation.

Glycogen is a form of sugar that is stored in many organs but especially muscle cells. **Glucose** that is brought to the muscle cells in the bloodstream can be stored as glycogen until it is

needed. When the muscle cell requires energy, glycogen is converted back to glucose, and the process of **glycolysis** produces ATP and **pyruvate**. Pyruvate can be converted into **acetyl coenzyme A (CoA)**, which enters the **Krebs cycle** to produce CO_2 and ATP in mitochondria. **Coenzyme-2H** is another product of the citric acid (Krebs) cycle, and it assists with the process of **oxidative phosphorylation**. In short, this process takes O_2 that is delivered by hemoglobin in the blood and creates ATP and H_2O. Note that both acetyl CoA and coenzyme-2H can also be generated by fatty acids or ketones that are brought to the muscle cell by the blood.

If O_2 levels in the cell get too low to support the ATP-rich process of oxidative phosphorylation, then **anaerobic glycolysis** begins. This converts pyruvate into lactate, harvesting only two ATP molecules per glucose but doing so quickly.

During moderate activity, a short burst of glycolysis followed by oxidative phosphorylation is sufficient to supply ATP to the muscle. As moderate activity continues, muscles rely increasingly on glucose and fatty acids that are brought to the cell by the blood to undergo β-**oxidation**. During intense exercise, oxidative phosphorylation cannot keep up with the cells' demands and glycolysis increases, as does substrate-level phosphorylation. Increased glycolysis produces more pyruvate than the Krebs cycle can accommodate, and the excess pyruvate is converted to lactate (lactic acid) by the enzyme **lactate dehydrogenase**. Lactate is removed from the muscle cells into the blood, but during intense

CLINICAL CORRELATION 6.6 Muscular Dystrophies

Many different molecules are needed to transfer the force of sarcomere shortening to the surface of a skeletal myocyte and manifest as a forceful contraction. Mutations of these molecules result in a wide variety of muscular dystrophies or myopathies. Mutations affecting the dystrophin gene can result in **Duchenne muscular dystrophy**, in which the protein is not functional, and **Becker muscular dystrophy**, in which the protein is somewhat functional. Patients with these diseases will accumulate damage to their muscle cells at a rapid rate, resulting in muscular weakness that is pronounced in the large muscles such as the gluteus maximus and quadriceps but eventually affects muscles throughout the body. The dystrophin gene is located on the X chromosome, so these diseases almost exclusively affect males. Symptoms manifest in early childhood (Duchenne) or later childhood or teen years (Becker). The muscle wasting will cause an inability to move and eventual death as the heart weakens and the diaphragm is unable to contract during inhalation, causing respiratory failure.

Dysfunction of the sarcoglycan complex and other molecules that enable muscle contraction will result in a variety of **limb girdle muscular dystrophies** that primarily (but not exclusively) affect the proximal limb muscles.

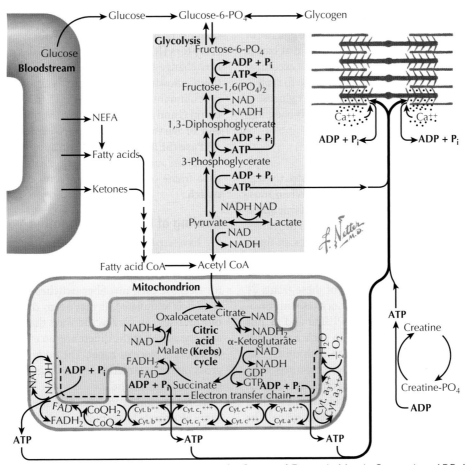

Fig. 6.17 Regeneration of Adenosine Triphosphate for Source of Energy in Muscle Contraction. *ADP*, Adenosine diphosphate; *ATP*, adenosine triphosphate; *NEFA*, nonesterified fatty acid.

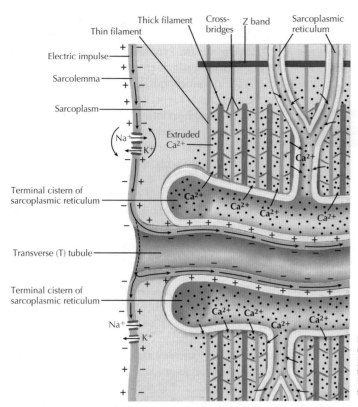

Electric impulse traveling along muscle cell membrane (sarcolemma) from motor endplate (neuromuscular junction) and then along transverse tubules affects sarcoplasmic reticulum, causing extrusion of Ca^{2+} to initiate contraction by "rowing" action of crossbridges, sliding filaments past one another.

Fig. 6.18 Initiation of Muscle Contraction by Electric Impulse and Calcium Movement.

exercise, it can build up at a rate that exceeds the cells' ability to clear it. Lactate in the blood can be converted to blood glucose or stored as glycogen in the liver. It has been theorized that lactate irritates the muscles, creating the sense of soreness that accompanies intense muscular effort. However, it may also help to replenish stores of NAD^+, which is converted to NADH as glucose is converted to pyruvate. Lactate can also be converted back into pyruvate once oxygen levels rise in the muscle cells.

Initiation of Contraction (Fig. 6.18)

To work on command, skeletal muscle cells must strictly regulate when Ca^{2+} is allowed to bind to troponin C. When muscle cells are not contracting, the intracellular level of calcium is very low because Ca^{2+} ions are actively pumped into the sarcoplasmic reticulum. The sarcoplasmic reticulum forms an interwoven network around the myofibrils of the cell and expands to form elongated **terminal cisternae** on either side of the T tubules that permeate the sarcoplasm. Each of these triads (T tubule flanked by two terminal cisternae) associates with myofibrils at the place where each sarcomere's I line and A line meet. Neighboring myofibrils are lined up in such a way that their sarcomeres are all arrayed in parallel to each other. The rest of the sarcoplasmic reticulum's interwoven channels wrap around the myofibril until they reach the next terminal cisterna. Recall that the T tubules are part of the sarcolemma and their lumen is actually in contact with the extracellular space. The significance of this fact is that when acetylcholine release from a lower motor neuron causes depolarization of the sarcolemma, the T tubules participate in this depolarization. They are linked to the sarcoplasmic reticulum by voltage-gated receptors called

dihydropyridine (DHP) receptors that, in turn, are bound to calcium channels in the terminal cisternae called **ryanodine receptors (RYRs)**. When the T tubules depolarize, DHP receptors change the conformation of the RYRs that are bound to them, allowing them to dump calcium from the sarcoplasmic reticulum into the sarcoplasm. The Ca^{2+} ions associate with troponin C and initiate sarcomere contraction. Within 30 ms of the end of nerve stimulation, **sarcoendoplasmic reticulum Ca^{2+} ATPase (SERCA) pumps** return Ca^{2+} ions to the sarcoplasmic reticulum and restore the resting balance. This incredibly short time frame of maximal contraction and relaxation is called a **twitch**.

Scaling of Muscle Contraction

We have covered how muscles contract at the molecular level, but there is a great deal of regulation that goes into translating these tiny movements into willful and appropriate motor activity. Because each myofiber twitches at maximum intensity any time it is stimulated, it may seem difficult to understand how our muscles can contract in ways that allow very precise motor activity, as well as the differences in effort required to lift a heavy weight or a piece of paper. The body is able to scale the level of gross motor contraction by varying the size of motor units and the speed of the twitch.

A **motor unit** consists of all the myofibers that are innervated by a single lower motor axon. When that axon depolarizes, it stimulates the **motor end plates** of its myofibers, and contraction will occur in ALL those myofibers. Some lower motor neurons innervate many myofibers (large motor units), and some innervate very few (small motor units).

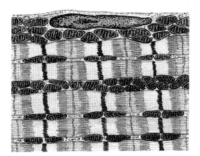

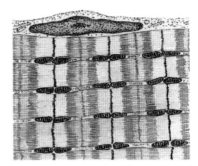

Type I: Dark or red fiber. Large profuse mitochondria beneath sarcolemma and in rows as well as paired in interfibrillar regions. Z lines wider than in type II.

Type II: Light or white skeletal muscle fiber in longitudinal section on electron microscopy. Small, relatively sparse mitochondria, chiefly paired in interfibrillar spaces at Z lines.

Histochemical classification Fiber type	ATPase stain	SDH stain
1. Fast-twitch, fatigable (IIb) Stain deeply for ATPase, poorly for succinic acid dehydrogenase (SDH), a mitochondrial enzyme active in citric acid cycle. Therefore fibers rapidly release energy from ATP but poorly regenerate it, thus becoming fatigued.		
2. Fast-twitch, fatigue-resistant (IIa) Stain deeply for both ATPase and SDH. Therefore fibers rapidly release energy from ATP and also rapidly regenerate ATP in citric acid cycle, thus resisting fatigue.		
3. Slow-twitch, fatigue-resistant (I) Stain poorly for ATPase but deeply for SDH. Therefore fibers only slowly release energy from ATP but regenerate ATP rapidly, thus resisting fatigue.		

Fig. 6.19 Muscle Fiber Types. *ATP*, Adenosine triphosphate.

Action potentials cause muscle depolarization, calcium is released from the sarcoplasmic reticulum to initiate a twitch, and calcium is pumped back into the sarcoplasmic reticulum, stopping the twitch. If action potentials come faster than the calcium can be returned to the sarcoplasmic reticulum, the muscle approaches its absolute maximum tension as the thick and thin myofilaments shorten to their limit with each stimulus. If the action potentials come so fast that each twitch never has the opportunity to finish, **tetanus** occurs. In this state, calcium is always present in the sarcoplasm and contraction plateaus as the myofilaments shorten to their limit and stay locked in that position. Unfused tetanus occurs when some degree of relaxation occurs between twitches but not enough to allow it to return to a resting state. In a state of fused tetanus, action potentials occur so quickly that no relaxation can occur and the force of contraction plateaus at the absolute maximum possible by the myocyte.

Slow Twitch and Fast Twitch Fibers (Fig. 6.19)

When a myofiber contracts, it generates a twitch at 100% effort and (under normal circumstances) each myofiber will twitch with the same intensity every time it is stimulated. However, individual myofibers twitch at different speeds and intensities. These differences are due to different types of ATPase located on the myosin heads that can act at a relatively fast or slow pace.

Type I fibers, also known as slow-oxidative fibers, cleave ATP at a slower pace than the other types; therefore they generate a smaller maximum force. They are "slow twitch." These muscles contain large numbers of mitochondria because the ATP in these muscles primarily comes aerobically from oxidative phosphorylation of glucose and triglycerides that are brought to the muscle cells from the blood. They tend to have smaller fiber diameters and appear reddish due to the large amount of **myoglobin** in the cells and the prevalence of capillaries surrounding them. Myoglobin is a red-pigmented molecule that binds O_2 within muscle cells and transfers it quickly to the mitochondria. Slow twitch muscles typically do not store a lot of glycogen in their cytoplasm, and the creatine kinase enzyme in these fibers is slower than in other fiber types. They are commonly seen in large postural muscles that are frequently active and need to be fatigue resistant.

Type IIa fibers are considered to be "fast twitch" fibers but are actually somewhat intermediate in their speed and diameter. The myosin ATPase in these fibers operates 3 to 5 times faster than in type I fibers, allowing these fibers to generate a greater maximal force of contraction. They have a fair number of mitochondria and a moderate amount of both myoglobin and glycogen in their cytoplasm. Therefore they are able to operate effectively both aerobically (using O_2-dependent oxidative phosphorylation to create ATP) and anaerobically (ATP production coming from glycolysis without the need for O_2). The creatine kinase found in these muscles operates at a moderate rate. They are most frequently used during high-intensity, short-duration activities.

Type IIb fibers are the far extreme of "fast twitch" fibers. Their myosin ATPase operates very quickly, allowing these large-diameter fibers to generate very strong contraction forces for a brief period. They rely on having substantial glycogen stores for anaerobic, glycolysis-based contraction and have relatively few mitochondria and little myoglobin. The creatine kinase in these

---

CLINICAL CORRELATION 6.7 Creatine Kinase

Large quantities of the enzyme creatine kinase are present in skeletal muscle and cardiac muscle cells. When either skeletal or cardiac muscles are damaged, the levels of this enzyme in the blood increase and can be detected clinically.

CLINICAL CORRELATION 6.8 Dark Meat and White Meat

A chicken dinner can help to teach muscle biochemistry because differences between slow-twitch and fast-twitch muscles are visible in cooked poultry. Type I fibers are seen in muscles that are frequently used, such as the leg and thigh muscles of these birds that spend a lot of their time walking around a farmyard. "Dark meat" appears dark because it contains a lot of red-colored myoglobin and many small vessels. Type II fibers are easily fatigued but are able to generate a great deal of force over a short period of time. Chickens do not have to fly often and cannot fly very far, so their breast muscles are "white meat," containing more type II fibers, with less myoglobin, and fewer blood vessels.

---

fibers works very quickly to supply ATP during contraction. They have relatively few capillaries permeating them (Clinical Correlations 6.7 and 6.8).

Types of Contraction

Isotonic contractions occur when the force of a muscle contraction is greater than the load it is working against, so the muscle is able to shorten as the load is lifted. In this case the sarcomeres shorten and pass their contraction to the connective tissues around the muscle, which is caught between the contracting myofibers and the load. The connective tissues stretch in response but are eventually able to move the load. Imagine pulling a heavy door closed, which moves with difficulty but eventually does close. Your arm's flexor muscles were contracting isotonically. An **isometric contraction** occurs when the force of contraction is not enough to move the load it is working against. So even though it is contracting, the muscle remains the same length. In this situation the sarcomeres shorten but the connective tissues that surround the myofibers are stretched by the load but are unable to lift (or shift) the load itself. So even though the muscle remains the same length, it is because of the elastic nature of the connective tissues surrounding the myofibers. Imagine trying to close a door that has been (unbeknownst to you) locked in place and will not move. In this instance, your arm's flexors are contracting isometrically. An **eccentric contraction** occurs when the sarcomeres are shortening but the muscle as a whole, especially its connective tissues, are lengthening. In this case, imagine trying to close a door that someone else is successfully pulling open. The flexor muscles of your arm would be contracting eccentrically.

Stretch Receptors (Fig. 6.20)

When discussing muscle activity, we tend to focus on their motor actions; however, muscles are also sensory organs that constantly update the central nervous system regarding stretch, tone, and position. The two sensory receptors that accomplish this are **muscle spindles** and **Golgi tendon organs**.

Muscle spindles are small sensory organs made of a few specialized myofibers, **intrafusal fibers**, lying in parallel to the **extrafusal fibers** of a large muscle. The intrafusal fibers are enclosed within a **capsule** of connective tissue that separates them (somewhat) from the surrounding extrafusal fibers (Fig. 6.21). Within each capsule there are typically two intrafusal **nuclear bag fibers**, muscle fibers with an expanded central region containing many nuclei. Several smaller, intrafusal **nuclear chain fibers** are also within the capsule and get their name from a chain of nuclei in their central region. **Annulospiral endings** wrap around the body of each intrafusal fiber and project back to the spinal cord while **flower-spray endings** stretch along the fibers to insert along their ends. The intrafusal fibers are innervated by **gamma (γ) motor neurons**. For the purpose of understanding muscle spindle activity, the motor neurons that innervate the surrounding extrafusal fibers are referred to as **alpha (α) motor neurons**.

The major role of muscle spindle fibers is to sense stretch and adjust muscle tone. When muscles are at their resting length, there is a baseline level of activity from the annulospiral and flower-spray endings projecting from the central fibers. When the extrafusal fibers are stretched, the intrafusal fibers are also stretched; this causes an increase in activity of the sensory endings. Likewise, if the extrafusal fibers relax, the intrafusal fibers will also relax. Dynamic nuclear bag fibers (bag 1 fibers) sense the rate of stretch. Static nuclear bag fibers (bag 2 fibers) sense the onset of a stretch but not its magnitude. Finally, the nuclear bag fibers sense sustained stretch. Gamma motor neurons will activate the contractile intrafusal fibers surrounding the central fibers to shorten the entire muscle spindle so that it can continue sensing changes in muscle tone. When muscles contract, the alpha and gamma motor neurons fire in tandem so that the tone of extrafusal and intrafusal fibers remain similar.

As an example of how muscle spindles affect muscle tone, picture filling a glass of water that is held in your hand. As the glass fills, it becomes heavier and stretches your biceps brachii and brachialis muscles. If these muscles do not increase their tone, the water will spill. Fortunately, the stretch is sensed by the annulospiral and flower-spray endings of the central intrafusal fibers. They project back to the spinal cord and increase activity of the alpha motor neurons in the same agonist muscles to increase tone. Being clever, they also decrease the activity of the antagonist muscles (in this case the triceps brachii) to make this easier. Gamma motor neurons also increase the tone of the intrafusal fibers accordingly so they can remain sensitive to further changes in muscle tone.

Golgi tendon organs are also stretch receptors that affect muscle tone, but their sensory nerve endings (axon ends) are wrapped around the collagen fibers at the muscle-tendon interface. They are active only during extreme contractions or passive stretches that might damage the muscle or tendon in which they reside. These axons project back to the spinal cord and act in an opposite manner to muscle spindles. They will decrease the tone of the agonist muscles and increase the tone of the antagonist muscles.

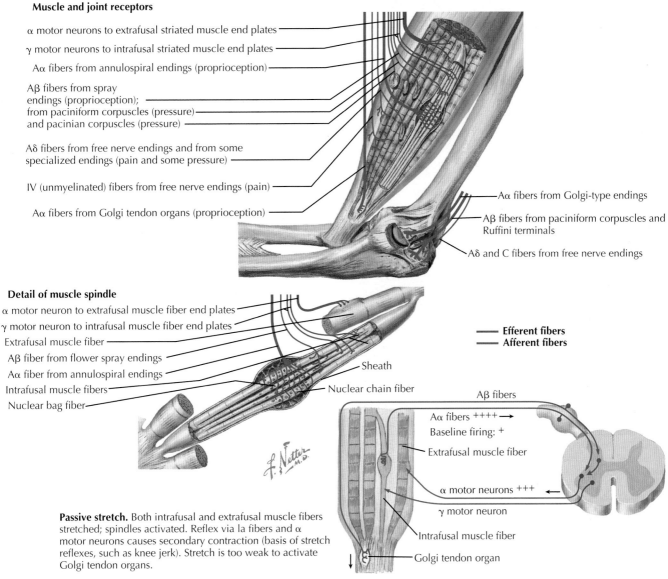

Muscle and joint receptors

α motor neurons to extrafusal striated muscle end plates

γ motor neurons to intrafusal striated muscle end plates

Aα fibers from annulospiral endings (proprioception)

Aβ fibers from spray
endings (proprioception);
from paciniform corpuscles (pressure)
and pacinian corpuscles (pressure)

Aδ fibers from free nerve endings and from some
specialized endings (pain and some pressure)

IV (unmyelinated) fibers from free nerve endings (pain)

Aα fibers from Golgi tendon organs (proprioception)

Aα fibers from Golgi-type endings

Aβ fibers from paciniform corpuscles and
Ruffini terminals

Aδ and C fibers from free nerve endings

Detail of muscle spindle

α motor neuron to extrafusal muscle fiber end plates

γ motor neuron to intrafusal muscle fiber end plates

Extrafusal muscle fiber

Aβ fiber from flower spray endings

Aα fiber from annulospiral endings

Intrafusal muscle fibers

Nuclear bag fiber

Sheath

Nuclear chain fiber

— Efferent fibers
— Afferent fibers

Aβ fibers

Aα fibers ++++ →

Baseline firing: +

Extrafusal muscle fiber

α motor neurons +++ ←

γ motor neuron

Intrafusal muscle fiber

Golgi tendon organ

Passive stretch. Both intrafusal and extrafusal muscle fibers
stretched; spindles activated. Reflex via Ia fibers and α
motor neurons causes secondary contraction (basis of stretch
reflexes, such as knee jerk). Stretch is too weak to activate
Golgi tendon organs.

Fig. 6.20 Muscle and Joint Receptors and Muscle Spindles.

As an example of how Golgi tendon organs work, picture yourself aggressively stretching to touch your toes on a day when your hamstrings are particularly tight. The hamstrings are stretched to their limit, and you risk avulsing the muscles from the ischial tuberosity. Fortunately, the Golgi tendon organs will sense the stretch and signal back to the spinal cord to decrease tone in the hamstring (agonist) and increase tone in the quadriceps (antagonist) muscles. You may have experienced this "release" during a stretching or yoga routine. The decreased agonist tone may alleviate the problem, but if the stretch continues to take up the slack, there will eventually be an injury to the hamstrings.

Cardiac Muscle (Fig. 6.22)

Cardiac muscle is not the focus of this text, so we will not deal with it at the same level of detail as skeletal muscle. However, **cardiac myocytes** are remarkably similar to skeletal muscle in many ways. Both use calcium ions from the sarcoplasmic reticulum to control the sliding of myofilaments across each other. Both use the same light and heavy myofilaments of the sarcomere to generate contractions that are spread to their neighbors and the surrounding endomysium. Because of this, **cardiac myocytes** have the same striated appearance as skeletal myocytes.

However, there are some definite differences. Cardiac myocytes branch from each other and connect in parallel to neighboring cardiac myocytes. At the point where two cardiac myocytes meet, there are visible lines that attach myocytes to their neighbors, called **intercalated discs**. Each disc's visible, **transverse component** runs at a 90-degree angle to the fibrils within the cell. A **lateral component**, which is not distinguishable during visible microscopy, runs parallel to the fibrils in adjacent cells. The transverse components of intercalated discs contain many **adhering junctions**. This is where the thin filaments (actin) of cardiac myocytes are anchored to the cell membrane. **Desmosomes** bind the ends of adjacent myocytes

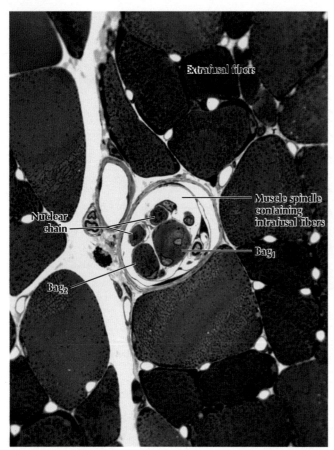

Fig. 6.21 Light Micrograph of a Muscle Spindle in the Equatorial Region. (Reused with permission from Ovalle W, Nahirney P. *Netter's Essential Histology*. 3rd ed. Elsevier; 2021.)

to each other. They are found in both the transverse and lateral components of the intercalated discs. The lateral component also contains numerous **gap junctions** that connect the cytoplasm of neighboring cells, which allows depolarization to spread from cell to cell. Once cardiac myocytes begin contracting, the contraction spreads inevitably to all downstream cells.

At a smaller scale, the sarcoplasmic reticulum, transverse tubules, and sarcomeres of cardiac myocytes are similar to those found within skeletal muscle but with a few differences. The sarcoplasmic reticulum does not form large terminal cisternae; instead they associate more loosely with the transverse tubules. In addition, the T tubules extend along the Z line of the sarcomeres within the cell, instead of the A to I junction. In cardiac muscle, depolarization of the cell membrane continues into the T tubules and causes voltage-gated calcium channels to open, allowing calcium to enter the cytoplasm of the cardiac myocyte. However, instead of having voltage-sensitive receptors linked directly to the sarcoplasmic reticulum, the calcium must diffuse into the cytoplasm of cardiac myocytes, where it activates channels in the sarcoplasmic reticulum, which then open to release a much larger amount of calcium into the cytoplasm, causing sarcomere contraction.

Unlike skeletal muscle, which contracts only when acetylcholine is released by the synaptic bulb of a lower motor neuron, cardiac muscle has an inherent rhythmic contractility. Modified cardiac myocytes, the **pacemaker cells** (e.g., the sinoatrial [SA] and atrioventricular [AV] nodes), initiate contractions at a faster rate than cardiac myocytes would do by default. Once these nodes initiate contraction, the depolarization spreads by means of the gap junctions at the intercalated discs. Specialized cardiac myocytes, such as **Purkinje cells**, have a large quantity of glycogen in their cytoplasm and appear more translucent than normal cardiac myocytes. They depolarize quickly and speed the depolarization from the AV node, down the interventricular septum to the apex of the heart, where other typical myocytes initiate depolarization and contraction. This allows the ventricles to contract from the apex and propel blood toward the large arteries.

Even though cardiac myocyte pacemaker cells contract automatically, they can be made to speed up and strengthen their contraction by norepinephrine and epinephrine. These neurotransmitters come to the heart through axons of the sympathetic nervous system or via the bloodstream when it is released by the adrenal glands. Acetylcholine released by axons of the parasympathetic nervous system slows the rate of contraction of the pacemaker cells.

Smooth Muscle (Fig. 6.23)

Smooth muscle cells are very different from cardiac and skeletal muscle cells. Smooth muscle cells do not have visible striations. Instead of having sarcomeres that strongly contract in a single direction, smooth muscle cells contract more globally, transitioning from an elongated state to a rounded state when contracted. This shrinks the perimeter of the cell and puts traction on the nearby connective tissue. Smooth muscle is found throughout the body, including the iris, respiratory tract, gastrointestinal tract, and genitourinary structures. The major impact of the smooth muscle on the musculoskeletal system is its ability to regulate the blood flow to the skeletal muscles and skin as **precapillary sphincters**. During exercise, precapillary sphincters to skeletal muscles, cardiac muscles, and the skin will relax and allow more blood flow to enter those tissues. This allows more blood and oxygen to reach the muscles and also permits heat to radiate from the skin. Smooth muscle lining the airway will relax, allowing faster movement of oxygen and carbon dioxide to and from the lungs. At the same time, precapillary sphincters to the gastrointestinal and reproductive organs will contract, limiting their blood supply and shunting that blood to the muscles. At rest, the situation reverses and blood flow to skeletal muscles, cardiac muscle, and skin will decrease as the capillary sphincters contract. The airways will constrict, and precapillary sphincters to the gastrointestinal and reproductive organs will relax, increasing their blood supply and activity.

Their cytoplasm appears uniformly eosinophilic (pink), and their nuclei, when the cell is viewed longitudinally, are elongated and have a slight corkscrew appearance but with rounded ends. When viewed in cross-section, the nuclei appear circular. The cytoplasm also contains a sarcoplasmic reticulum, glycogen granules, mitochondria, a Golgi apparatus, and distinctive (on electron microscopy) **dense bodies** scattered in a network throughout the cell.

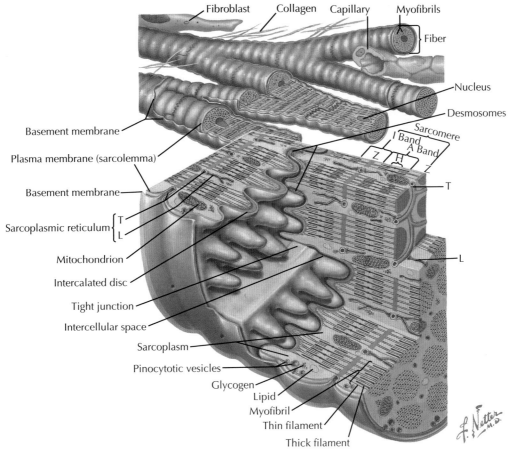

Fig. 6.22 Histology of the Myocardium.

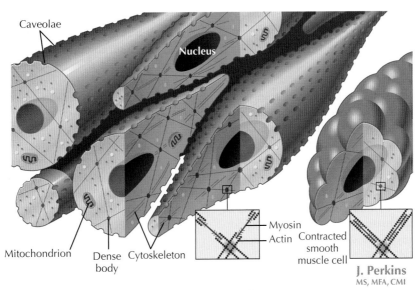

Fig. 6.23 Smooth Muscle Structure.

Contraction and Relaxation of Smooth Muscle (Fig. 6.24)

Smooth muscle cells' thin filaments, made of actin, are bound to dense bodies that are scattered throughout the cytoplasm. These dense bodies are also present along the plasma membrane as **attachment plaques**. The myosin-heavy filaments lie in parallel to the thin filaments. Interestingly, the individual myosin molecules are similar to those seen in skeletal and cardiac muscles but are bundled together in a different way. Myosin molecules in skeletal and cardiac muscles are bundled together with the heads extending radially outward on either end of the thick filament with a bare area in the middle. In smooth muscle they are laid out with their heads extending outward in a single row on both sides of the heavy chain. As a result, it lacks a bare area,

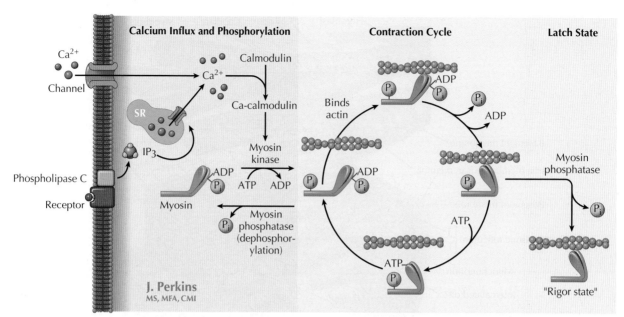

Fig. 6.24 Excitation and Contraction Coupling of Smooth Muscle. *ADP,* Adenosine diphosphate; *ATP,* adenosine triphosphate.

and therefore the myosin molecules can pull themselves along actin molecules for a much longer distance than they would be able to do in a sarcomere.

Like skeletal muscle, smooth muscle contracts in response to neurotransmitters released by axons but also in response to hormonal signals and mechanical stretch. In all cases the muscle contracts as calcium concentration in the cytoplasm rises. If calcium levels remain constant, the smooth muscle will continue to contract; the greater the amount of calcium, the stronger the contraction.

Neurotransmitters and hormones bind to surface receptors, some of which are calcium transmembrane channels that allow calcium to flow into the cell to initiate contraction. Mechanical stretch of the smooth muscle can also cause these transmembrane channels to open. Other receptors increase the level of **inositol triphosphate (IP3)** in the cell, which will bind to an **IP3-activated receptor channel** in the sarcoplasmic reticulum (not as well developed as in striated muscle), releasing calcium into the cytoplasm.

Once in the cytoplasm, calcium binds to (and dephosphorylates) **calmodulin**. The **Ca^{2+}-calmodulin complex** activates an enzyme, **myosin light chain kinase**. This kinase then phosphorylates light chains on the myosin heads, increasing the activity of the **myosin ATPase**, leading to cross-bridge formation and consumption of ATP as the myosin heads climb along their associated actin thin filaments. There is a competing **myosin phosphatase** enzyme that dephosphorylates the myosin light chain and slows cross-bridge formation. The balance between the myosin light chain kinase and myosin phosphatase is what truly determines the degree to contraction at any given time. Smooth muscle myosin ATPase operates at a much slower pace than the ATPase of skeletal muscle, making smooth muscle cross-bridge cycling slower and lengthening the time of contraction.

Because the actin and myosin filaments crisscross the smooth muscle cell and are anchored to dense bodies within the

cell and anchored to the membrane at attachment plaques, contraction causes the cell to become rounded. In smooth muscle the myosin thick filaments have no bare area and the actin thin filaments are very long. This allows thick and thin filaments to slide over a longer distance and to relax over a longer distance while still maintaining tone.

Smooth muscle relaxes as intracellular calcium levels fall. The sarcoplasmic reticulum contains calcium-ATPase pumps that move calcium back into the sarcoplasmic reticulum. As calcium leaves the cytoplasm, less of it is available to form the Ca^{2+}-calmodulin complex, which leaves calmodulin in its inactive state. Without the Ca^{2+}-calmodulin complex, the myosin light chain kinase is inactivated, reducing the activity of the myosin ATPase. The myosin phosphatase enzyme gains the upper hand, dephosphorylating the myosin light chain, reducing ATPase activity, and stopping contraction.

One interesting aside is that deactivation of the myosin ATPase does not necessarily cause relaxation. The myosin and actin may enter a state akin to the rigor state seen in skeletal muscle. In this way, the smooth muscle can stay contracted over extended periods of time without any energy expenditure. This is frequently seen in smooth muscle sphincters that stay contracted until they are triggered to relax.

Innervation of Smooth Muscle (Fig. 6.25)

Smooth muscle can be innervated by parasympathetic (acetylcholine) and sympathetic (norepinephrine) axons. Unlike skeletal muscle cells, which are each innervated by an axon motor end plate, smooth muscle cells are not typically in direct contact with their axon terminals. Instead, the autonomic nerve axons in the vicinity of their target smooth muscle have multiple **neuron varicosities** running along the length of their axons. These bulges in the axons release neurotransmitters into the extracellular space around the smooth muscle rather than at a synapse. The neurotransmitter then has to diffuse to nearby smooth

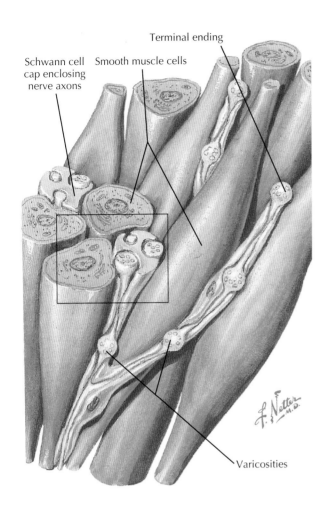

Fig. 6.25 Electron Micrograph of Smooth Muscle Cells Close to Nerve Axon in Transverse Section.

muscle cells. As those cells depolarize in response to the signal, **gap junctions** between the cells spread the depolarization to neighboring smooth muscle cells.

The smooth muscle found in the precapillary sphincters is innervated by the sympathetic nervous system. The norepinephrine from these nerves can bind to a variety of receptors, causing a variety of responses. Binding to an α1 or α2 **receptor** results in contraction and vasoconstriction. Binding to a β2 **receptor** will typically cause relaxation, leading to vasodilation and more blood flow to the vessels downstream from the sphincter.

NERVOUS TISSUE

Nervous tissue creates the structures of the central nervous system and peripheral nervous system. It allows the brain to sense changes in the external and internal environment and to effect changes that help it to deal with those changes. Although there are many cell types in nervous tissue, **neurons** (Fig. 6.26) are the functional cells of the nervous system. They form tremendously complex interconnected networks that make sensation, movement, thought, memory, personality, and all other mental activities possible.

Neuron cell bodies, or **soma**, tend to be large and round; they contain the nucleus, Golgi apparatus, and most other organelles of the cell. The neurotransmitters that are specific to each nerve cell are created here and sent to a long extension of the cytoplasm, the **axon**.

Typically, each nerve cell has a cone-shaped region, an **axon hillock**, that leads to a narrow, single axon extending from the body towards its target tissue. The length of an axon is variable, but some lower motor neurons can stretch more than a meter away from their cell bodies in the spinal cord before reaching their target muscle. Each axon contains microtubules that carry neurotransmitters along the length of the axon. There are voltage-gated, transmembrane channels present along the length of the axon. These depolarize and then pass this depolarization down the length of the axon to other voltage-gated channels. The end of an axon is an enlarged **synaptic bulb**, which interacts with another neuron or a target tissue via a small space between the two, the **synapse**. The synaptic bulb contains different voltage-gated channels that trigger the release of synaptic vesicles that contain **neurotransmitters**. Each neuron releases only one neurotransmitter, which may be excitatory or inhibitory.

Dendrites are the cytoplasmic extensions off the neuron cell body that typically interact with the axons of other neurons. Dendrites contain the receptors that bind with the neurotransmitters released by other neurons. The sum of the inputs (excitatory and inhibitory) to each neuron through these dendrites determine whether or not that neuron will depolarize.

Types of Neurons (Fig. 6.27)

- **Multipolar neurons** are "typical" neurons that have one long axon and multiple dendrites radiating off the cell body. Motor neurons and **interneurons**, which connect with other neurons within the central nervous system, are multipolar.
- **Pseudounipolar neurons** have a single axon extending from the cell that divides into two axonal extensions. They do not have dendrites per se. Sensory neurons are pseudounipolar, with their cell bodies clustered in peripheral structures called ganglia (singular: ganglion). One axonal extension extends from the ganglion toward skin and muscles (somatosensory) or to organs (viscerosensory). The other side of the axon extends from the ganglion toward the spinal cord or brainstem. This allows peripheral stimuli to be conveyed to the central nervous system.
- **Bipolar neurons** have a single axon and a single dendrite. These are found only in the retina and inner ear.

Support Cells of the Nervous System (see Fig. 6.27)

- **Satellite cells** surround and support nerve cell bodies in the peripheral nervous system.
- **Schwann cells** surround and protect the axons of the peripheral nervous system. Schwann cells can form **myelin sheaths** around a short segment of a single axon that insulate it to cause faster depolarization. In this case the plasma membrane of a single Schwann cell wraps around an axon segment, forming multiple layers that have very little cytoplasm

Structure of a neuron (pyramidal cell of cerebral motor cortex)

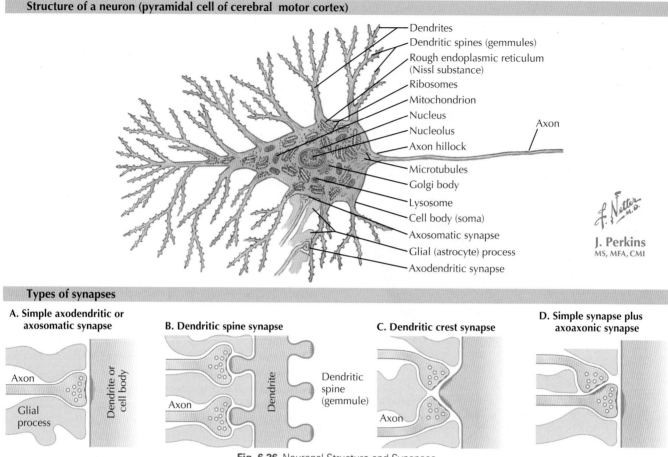

Types of synapses

A. Simple axodendritic or axosomatic synapse

B. Dendritic spine synapse

C. Dendritic crest synapse

D. Simple synapse plus axoaxonic synapse

Fig. 6.26 Neuronal Structure and Synapses.

within. These **myelin sheaths** of adjacent Schwann cells meet at a **node of Ranvier**, where the axon itself is exposed. **Unmyelinated nerves** are also protected by Schwann cells, but in this case the cells do not form myelin sheaths and a single Schwann cell's cytoplasm may surround nearby segments of multiple axons.

- **Oligodendrocytes** are the cells that support and protect the axons of the central nervous system. They are similar to Schwann cells in that they can create myelin sheaths to insulate axons. However, a single oligodendrocyte can create multiple myelin sheaths around segments of multiple axons, while a Schwann cell can form a myelin sheath around only a short segment of a single axon.
- **Astrocytes** are found only in the central nervous system. These cells maintain the environment of the central nervous system and pass nutrients and gasses to and from neurons. They also tightly surround the blood vessels of the central nervous system, creating the blood-brain barrier, which prevents most substances from reaching the delicate neurons of the central nervous system.
- **Ependymal cells** line the fluid-filled spaces of the ventricular system. They appear like cuboidal epithelial cells but lack a basal lamina and are therefore not epithelial.
- **Microglial cells** are phagocytic cells that are derived from early-embryonic monocytes that populate the central nervous system. They take up cellular debris and degrade

damaged neurons and other cells. They can act as antigen-presenting cells, helping the immune system respond to infection.

Electrochemical Properties of Neurons (Figs. 6.28–6.30)

Like other cells, neurons contain a variety of membrane-bound **leak (open) channels** that are open between the external and internal environment, as well as **gated channels**. Gated channels allow specific ions or other substances to pass in or out of the cell when they are opened. **Ligand-gated channels** open/close when a substance binds to them and changes their conformation. **Mechanically gated channels** open/close as physical forces cause deformation or changes to the structure of the channel or cell membrane. **Voltage-gated channels** open/close in response to changes in the neuron's electrical state. Metabotropic receptors bind to extracellular ligands, but instead of opening a channel, they mediate changes to the activity of intracellular enzymes, often via a G protein and other second messengers.

The various charged ions that are located inside and outside of a neuron give it a distinctive electrical **resting potential**. For most neurons, the inside of the cell is more negatively charged (**−70 mV**) compared with the extracellular space. Maintaining and manipulating this **polarized** state are what allow neurons to pass along signals from one place

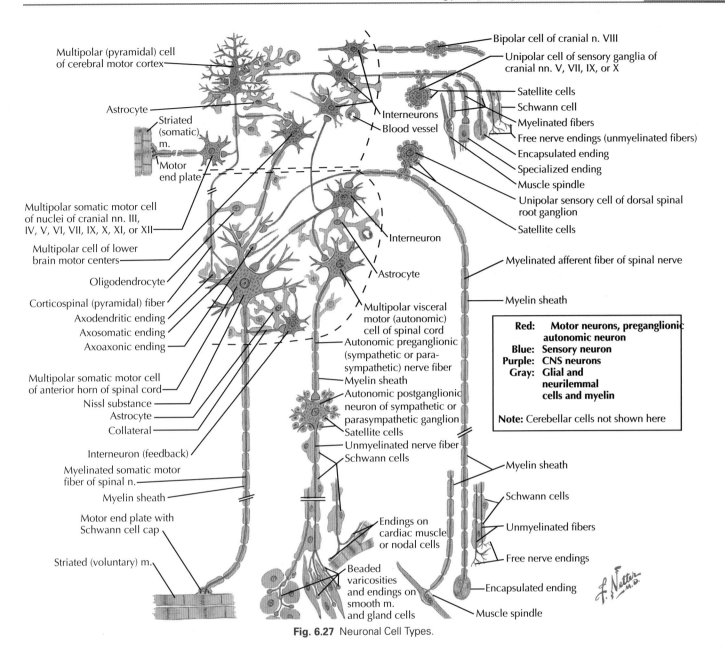

Fig. 6.27 Neuronal Cell Types.

to another. The nerve cell manipulates the concentrations of each ion by allowing them to move in and out of the cell via ion channels (which can be opened or closed) or by using ATP to actively pump ions in or out of the cell. To begin, note that K⁺ is typically far more concentrated inside cells and Na⁺, Ca⁺, and Cl⁻ are more highly concentrated outside of cells.

Nerve cells have leak channels in their plasma membrane that freely allow K⁺ and Na⁺ to pass in or out of the cell. Because ions will naturally diffuse from areas of high concentration to areas of lower concentration, K⁺ tends to exit the cell and Na⁺ tends to enter the cell. Because there are many more K⁺ channels than Na⁺ channels, the rate of K⁺ exit quickly out-paces Na⁺ inflow. This causes the inside of the cell to become more negatively charged than the outside. Because the negative interior of the cell exerts an attractive affect on positive ions, ion exchange finds a steady state around −70 mV and the rate of Na⁺ entry

is equal to the rate of K⁺ departure. It is **negatively polarized**. To maintain this state, the cell membrane also contains Na⁺/K⁺ pumps that use ATP to actively pump two K⁺ ions into the cell and three Na⁺ ions out of the cell. This maintains the **concentration gradients** of the two ions and, as a direct result, the −70 mV resting potential.

Before we proceed, note that the neuron has created a situation where K⁺ moves down its concentration gradient to exit the cell through open channels, making the neuron more negative. Na⁺ moves down its concentration gradient to enter the cell at a slower rate through open channels, making the neuron more positive but not enough to counteract the effect of K⁺. The neuron has a negatively polarized interior that exerts an electrical attraction to positive ions outside the cell, but that attraction is balanced by their migration down their chemical concentration gradients. This complex situation would be fairly pointless if we were not planning to put it to use in some way. Fortunately,

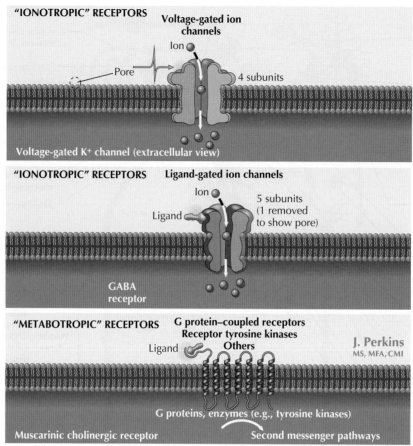

Fig. 6.28 Mechanisms of Molecular Signaling in Neurons. *GABA*, γ-Aminobutyric acid.

nerve cells are able to make rapid changes to this state in a way that allows them to rapidly **depolarize** and send action potentials along their axons to reach other nerves or target tissues, such as muscle.

Nerve Cell Depolarization (Fig. 6.31)

Starting from its −70 mV resting potential, the opening or closing of channels can put a neuron into a more negatively charged, **hyperpolarized** state or more positively charged, **depolarized** state. If a neuron depolarizes to reach its **threshold** of approximately −55 mV, then a large-scale **action potential** will occur and spread down the axon. The leak channels and Na⁺/K⁺ pumps will eventually return the neuron to its resting potential, called **repolarization**. When gated ion channels open, they can hyperpolarize the neuron, which **inhibits** it and makes it more difficult to reach threshold. They can also depolarize it, which **stimulates** it and makes it easier to reach the threshold of −55 mV.

Typically, the opening or closing of these channels will elicit a **graded potential** that changes the polarization state of the neuron by only a small amount that affects the immediate vicinity of the channel. If these graded potentials occur in isolation, they are unlikely to cause enough depolarization to result in an action potential. However, if many graded potentials occur together in one location or during a brief period, they may depolarize the neuron to its threshold state and cause an action potential.

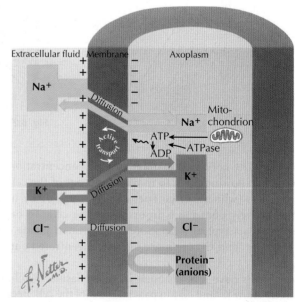

Fig. 6.29 Neuronal Resting Potential: Resting Membrane Potential. *ADP*, Adenosine diphosphate; *ATP*, adenosine triphosphate.

Action Potentials (See Figs. 6.30 and 6.31)

Once a set of graded potentials brings a portion of a neuron (or muscle cell) to its threshold level, it will typically produce a large, fast depolarization called an **action potential**. Starting at the axon hillock, this action potential will spread down the

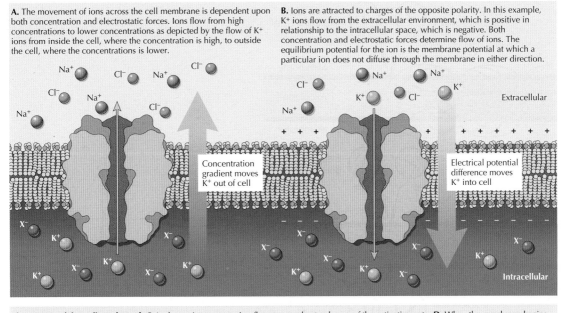

A. The movement of ions across the cell membrane is dependent upon both concentration and electrostatic forces. Ions flow from high concentrations to lower concentrations as depicted by the flow of K+ ions from inside the cell, where the concentration is high, to outside the cell, where the concentrations is lower.

B. Ions are attracted to charges of the opposite polarity. In this example, K+ ions flow from the extracellular environment, which is positive in relationship to the intracellular space, which is negative. Both concentration and electrostatic forces determine flow of ions. The equilibrium potential for the ion is the membrane potential at which a particular ion does not diffuse through the membrane in either direction.

Concentration gradient moves K+ out of cell

Electrical potential difference moves K+ into cell

Extracellular

Intracellular

Three states of the sodium channel. C. In the resting state, no ion flow occurs due to closure of the activation gate. **D.** When the membrane begins to depolarize, the activation channel opens and ion flow occurs. **E.** As the cell becomes depolarized, the inactivation gate closes and no further ion flow occurs. Only when the cell repolarizes does the sodium channel return to the resting state.

J. Perkins
MS, MFA, CMI

C. Resting (closed)

D. Activated (open)

E. Inactivated (closed)

Activation gate

Inactivation gate

Depolarization

Inactivation gate closes

Repolarization

Fig. 6.30 Neuronal Membrane Potential and Sodium Channels.

entire length of an axon without diminishing in magnitude until it reaches the axon terminal. The action potentials rapidly change the polarized resting state of the neuron before slightly overcorrecting and then returning to the polarized resting state. This occurs in three stages: (1) depolarization, (2) repolarization, and (3) hyperpolarization, after which it returns to the resting state.

1. **Depolarization**: this process relies on the opening of voltage-gated Na+ channels. These channels appear to have two gate systems that are linked to changes in membrane potentials. These channels will allow Na+ to enter the cell only if both gates are open. During the resting state of −70 mV, their **activation gate** is closed and their **inactivation gate** is open. However, once the plasma membrane reaches the threshold of −55 mV, the activation gate will open, allowing a massive influx of Na+ down both chemical and electrical gradients. The opening of these channels makes the membrane temporarily far more permeable to Na+ than to K+ ions, depolarizing the neuron. The inactivation gate responds to depolarization by closing, but it does so more slowly than

the activation gate. This stops the influx of Na+ as the neuron reaches approximately +30 mV. This tremendous change in membrane potential will open nearby voltage-gated Na+ channels and continue the propagation of the action potential down the axon.

2. **Repolarization**: once the inactivation gate of the voltage-gated Na+ channels are closed, Na+ ions move out of the cell through leak channels and Na+/K+ pumps. At the same time, voltage-gated K+ channels open in a delayed response to the recent action potential. This allows K+ ions to leave the cell, lowering its membrane potential back towards the resting state.

3. **Hyperpolarization**: K+ channels close as the membrane potential becomes more negative, but before that happens, the membrane potential will decrease to less than the resting state of −70 mV, toward the maximum allowed by K+ outflow (approximately −85 mV). Once the voltage-gated K+ channels close, leak channels and the Na+/K+ pumps will help the neuron to depolarize slightly and reach the resting state.

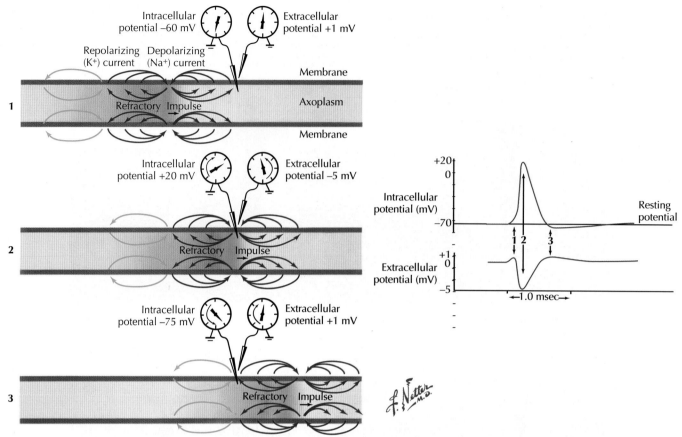

Fig. 6.31 Propagation of the Action Potential.

Refractory Periods and Propagation of Action Potentials (see Fig. 6.31)

After an action potential has traveled down a bit of the axon, it enters a state of lowered excitability, the **refractory period**. The portion of an axon that is undergoing an action potential will have the inactivation gates of its voltage-gated Na^+ channels close as the depolarization stage nears its end. These will not be able to reopen again until the membrane potential becomes more negative. Without the ability to open these channels, another action potential cannot occur. This period is called the **absolute refractory period**. As the membrane potential becomes more negatively charged, the voltage-gated Na^+ channels are able to open again. Even then, not all voltage-gated Na^+ channels are available immediately, and the voltage-gated K^+ channels remain open, which makes it possible but more difficult to initiate another action potential. This is the **relative refractory period**.

The relative refractory period is important in allowing the body to gauge the extremity of a stimulus. No matter how strong the graded potentials are that bring a neuron to its threshold to cause an action potential, the action potential itself is always the same strength. A graded potential that reaches the threshold will cause a single action potential. A stronger set of graded potentials will cause an action potential immediately and another one as soon as its intensity is enough to trigger opening of the voltage-gated Na^+ channels during the repolarization phase. An even stronger graded potential will cause even more

CLINICAL CORRELATION 6.9
Tetrodotoxin

Blowfish express tetrodotoxin, which blocks and inactivates voltage-gated Na^+ channels in axons. This will stop action potentials from propagating and can lead to death due to paralysis of the thoracic diaphragm. Paradoxically, the less-toxic portions of blowfish are served as sushi, called *fugu*. Typically, this does not contain enough toxin to kill but will cause tingling of the lips and tongue as sensory conduction from the oral region is temporarily impeded. The same sort of process is used to deliberately numb the mouth and teeth during dental procedures. Novocaine and other injected local anesthetics also block nearby voltage-gated Na^+ channels so that sensation cannot reach the central nervous system until the effect wears off and the procedure is finished.

action potentials because it will reopen the voltage-gated Na^+ channels even more quickly.

Only one segment of an axon undergoes action potential depolarization at a time. The positive membrane potential will cause downstream voltage-gated Na^+ channels to open and pass the action potential along like a row of dominoes falling (or if you prefer, a compression wave being passed down a slinky). The action potential does not move in a retrograde manner, because the upstream segments of the axon are in their absolute refractory period (Clinical Correlation 6.9).

Speed of Propagation (Fig. 6.32)

The speed at which an action potential propagates is affected in several ways. The larger the axon, the more rapidly the changes

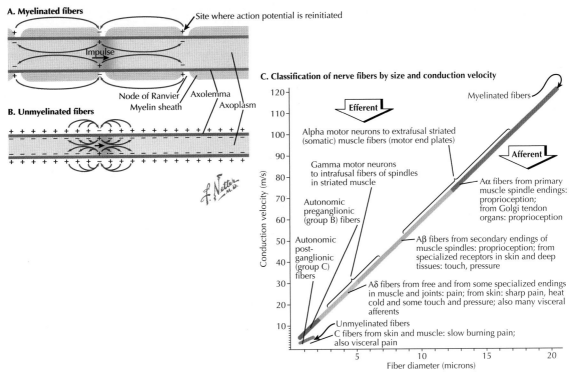

Fig. 6.32 Conduction Velocity.

in membrane potential are transmitted along its length due to decreased resistance. The axons with the widest diameter are those that innervate skeletal muscle, followed by axons transmitting the sensations of fine touch, pressure, and vibration. Smaller axons innervate the muscle spindle fibers and convey the sensations of pain and temperature. The smallest-diameter axons innervate the smooth muscle and glands of the sympathetic and parasympathetic nervous systems.

Another way in which the nervous system can change the speed of propagation is by myelinating axons. **Myelin sheaths** are produced by **Schwann cells** (peripheral nervous system) and **oligodendrocytes** (central nervous system), and they insulate a portion of the axon. Each myelinated segment meets an adjacent segment at a less insulated area, a **node of Ranvier**. This allows the neuron to cluster the voltage-gated Na^+ and K^+ channels at the nodes to maintain the action potential. In between the nodes, the positive membrane potential spreads as an electrical current underneath the axon membrane. This current is not strong enough to travel down the entire length of an axon, but it is strong enough to hop between two neighboring nodes. This is called **saltatory conduction** (Clinical Correlation 6.10).

Unmyelinated axons are protected by Schwann cells or oligodendrocytes but do not have myelin sheaths or nodes of Ranvier. The speed of propagation in these neurons is slower because, instead of saltatory conduction, the action potential must spread progressively down the entire length of the axon, opening and closing voltage-gated Na^+ and K^+ channels until it reaches the axon terminal.

Myelination and Speed of Action Potential

Myelin sheathes make depolarization move more quickly along an axon. However, the thickness of the myelin sheath makes a significant impact, with depolarization moving quickly along thickly myelinated axons and slowly along lightly myelinated or nonmyelinated axons.

- **A-alpha (Aα) fibers** have the thickest myelin sheaths and surround lower motor neurons and proprioceptive inputs to the spinal cord.
- **A-beta (Aβ) fibers** have relatively thick myelin sheaths and convey fine touch and vibration inputs to the spinal cord.
- **A-gamma (Aγ) fibers** have less stout myelin sheaths and surround lower motor neurons to intrafusal muscle spindle fibers.
- **A-delta (Aδ) fibers** are lightly myelinated fibers that convey pain and temperature sensations from the skin to the spinal cord.
- **B fibers** have a very slight myelin sheath and surround preganglionic autonomic visceromotor axons.
- **C fibers** denote nonmyelinated, postganglionic autonomic visceromotor axons, although they are still surrounded by Schwann cells. They also convey pain and temperature sensations from the skin to the spinal cord.

Synaptic Transmission of the Action Potential (Figs. 6.26 and 6.33)

Each neuron in the central or peripheral nervous system releases a neurotransmitter from its axon terminal. In general, the neurotransmitters are synthesized in the soma and transported down the axon to be stored in **synaptic vesicles** within the cytoplasm of the axon terminal. The axon terminal may contact another neuron at its dendrites (**axodendritic**), cell body (**axosomatic**), or axon (**axoaxonic**). It may also meet skeletal muscle at the myoneural junction, also known as a **motor end plate.**

CLINICAL CORRELATION 6.10   Demyelinating Diseases

Any disruption of the myelin sheaths can impair the ability of neurons to transmit an action potential. If the myelin sheathes become so damaged that they can no longer allow saltatory conduction, the muscles or other tissues innervated by the nerves will become dysfunctional. Some demyelinating diseases are caused by an autoimmune reaction to molecules in the myelin sheath, others result from infection, and others do not yet have a clear underlying cause. Some affect the central nervous system (e.g., multiple sclerosis, tabes dorsalis/syphilitic myelopathy) and others affect the peripheral nervous system (Guillain-Barré).

— **Pathogenesis** —

Stage I. Lymphocytes migrate through endoneural vessels and surround nerve fiber, but myelin sheath and axon not yet damaged.

Stage II. More lymphocytes extruded and macrophages appear. Segmental demyelination begins; however, axon not yet affected.

Stage III. Multifocal myelin sheath and axonal damage. Central chromatolysis of nerve cell body occurs and muscle begins to develop denervation atrophy.

Stage IV. Extensive axonal destruction. Some nerve cell bodies irreversibly damaged, but function may be preserved because of adjacent less-affected nerve fibers.

Clinical phase 1
Tingling of hands and feet

Phase 2
Difficulty in arising from chair

Phase 3
Areflexia, weakness, distal sensory loss

From Ashbury, Arnason, and Adams

Fig. CC6.10 Acute Inflammatory Demyelinating Polyneuropathy (Guillain-Barré Syndrome).

As the action potential reaches the axon terminal, the depolarization will open a new set of channels in the bulbous end of the axon, **voltage-gated Ca^{2+} channels**. These channels will open and allow extracellular Ca^{2+} to enter the cell, flowing down its electrochemical gradient. This is important because there are numerous synaptic vesicles packed into the axon terminal that contain neurotransmitters. The increased level of Ca^{2+} ions will cause the synaptic vesicles to fuse with the axon's plasma membrane and to release the neurotransmitter into the narrow space between the axon terminal and the target, the **synapse** or **synaptic cleft**. Each time an action potential reaches the axon terminal, more synaptic vesicles empty their neurotransmitters into the synapse. Therefore the more frequent the action potentials, the greater the effect from the neurotransmitters. To prevent continual stimulation from one action potential, the voltage-gated Ca^{2+} channels close shortly after opening as the axon terminal repolarizes and Ca^{2+} is actively pumped out of the cell by means of a Na^+/Ca^{2+} exchange pump that moves one Ca^{2+} ion out of the cell for three Na^+ ions moving into the cell, down their electrochemical gradient.

Receptors in the target cell will bind to the neurotransmitter and can respond in several ways. A **channel-linked receptor** is a ligand-gated channel that will bind to a neurotransmitter (ligand) and then open briefly to allow ions to flow into or out

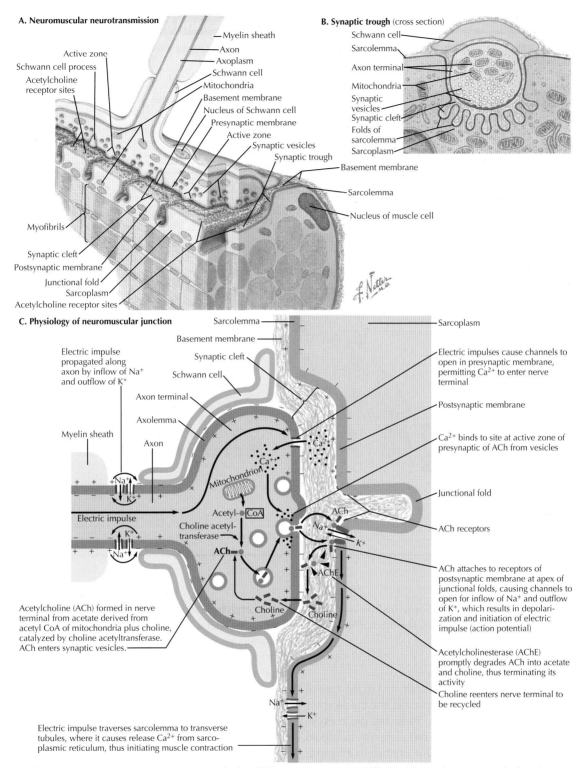

Fig. 6.33 (A) Neuromuscular neurotransmission; (B) synaptic trough; and (C) physiology of neuromuscular junction.

of the cell. The channel will close as the neurotransmitter disassociates from it. This is typically a very fast process, and the target cell will quickly be depolarized (excited) or hyperpolarized (inhibited). If it reaches threshold, it may generate its own action potential. Other receptors are metabotropic receptors that bind to the neurotransmitter and activate an intracellular G protein. This G protein may then open ion channels or work through other second messenger systems to change the state of

various ion channels. Because it involves multiple intracellular steps, this process is slower than the response from a channel-linked receptor.

If neurotransmitters stayed in the synaptic cleft indefinitely, they would cause continuous activation of the receptor. To prevent this, the neurotransmitters are sometimes inactivated by enzymes and then actively transported back into the neuron that released them to recycle them for another round of use or

CLINICAL CORRELATION 6.11 Lambert-Eaton Syndrome and Myasthenia Gravis

In this autoimmune condition, the body produces antibodies that bind and deactivate the voltage-gated Ca^{2+} channels at the axon terminal near a myoneural junction. It frequently occurs alongside small-cell lung cancer.

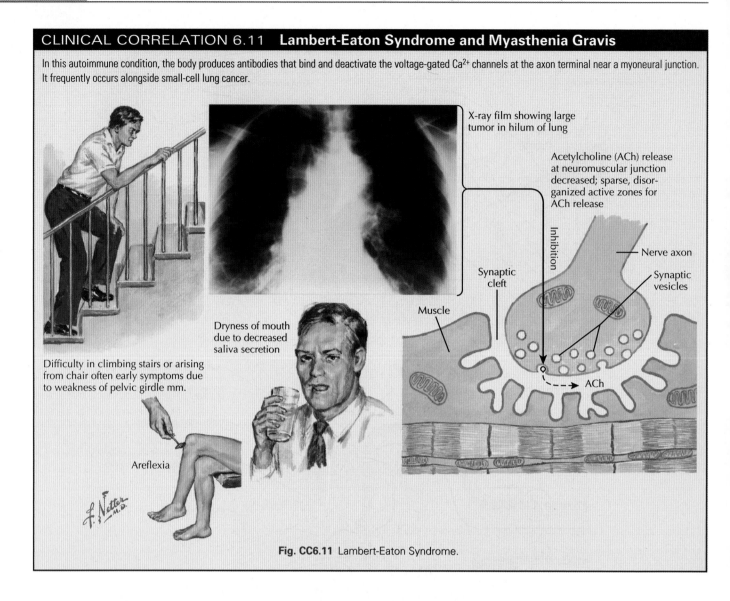

X-ray film showing large tumor in hilum of lung

Acetylcholine (ACh) release at neuromuscular junction decreased; sparse, disorganized active zones for ACh release

Inhibition

Nerve axon

Synaptic cleft

Synaptic vesicles

Muscle

ACh

Difficulty in climbing stairs or arising from chair often early symptoms due to weakness of pelvic girdle mm.

Dryness of mouth due to decreased saliva secretion

Areflexia

Fig. CC6.11 Lambert-Eaton Syndrome.

broken down into their components. Some neurotransmitters drift out of the area and become part of the extracellular fluid (Clinical Correlation 6.11).

Neurotransmitters

The activity of a nerve cell is very intimately tied to the type of neurotransmitter released by its axon terminal and the receptor on the other side of the synaptic cleft. These can cause **excitatory** responses that bring the target cell closer to threshold and may initiate an action potential. One example is a ligand-gated channel or metabotropic receptor that opens a channel that allows Na^+ into the cell, slightly depolarizing it. Conversely, neurotransmitters can cause an **inhibitory** response that hyperpolarizes the target cell, making an action potential more difficult to generate. This might occur if neurotransmitter binding resulted in opening a channel that allows more K^+ to exit the cell. Therefore the responses that are seen when a neuron action potential reaches its target rely on the neurotransmitter that is released and the activity of the receptor that binds to the neurotransmitter.

Acetylcholine is an important neurotransmitter for the musculoskeletal system because it is released by lower motor neurons at motor end plates to innervate skeletal muscle and varicosities to reach smooth muscle. It is also released by pre- and postganglionic parasympathetic neurons, preganglionic sympathetic neurons, and (very specifically) postganglionic sympathetic neurons innervating sweat glands. It is synthesized in cholinergic neurons from acetyl CoA and choline by the enzyme **choline acetyl transferase** (CAT). When released from synaptic vesicles into the synaptic cleft, it can bind to a variety of cholinergic receptors. To prevent overstimulation by acetylcholine, there is an enzyme in the space called **acetylcholinesterase** (AChE) that breaks it into acetate and choline. The acetate leaves the synaptic cleft while the choline can be actively transported back into the presynaptic neuron and used to make new acetylcholine molecules (see Fig. 6.33C).

Acetylcholine receptors fall into two main categories, **nicotinic** (nicotine-binding) and **muscarinic** (muscarine-binding) receptors.

CLINICAL CORRELATION 6.12   **Dysfunctions of Synaptic Muscle Activity**

Different drugs or toxins act to increase the activity of neurotransmitters by keeping them in the synaptic cleft longer, mimicking the activity of neurotransmitters, preventing their degradation, or inhibiting their reuptake. Other drugs decrease the effect of neurotransmitters by binding to their receptors without triggering the receptors appropriately.

Curare is a plant-derived alkaloid that competitively binds to the nicotinic acetylcholine receptor but does not open the Na^+/K^+ ion channel. This causes muscle paralysis and may result in death if the thoracic diaphragm is affected.

Myasthenia gravis presents in a similar way to Lambert-Eaton syndrome but is due to an autoimmune attack on the postsynaptic acetylcholine receptors. This causes the cell to destroy the affected receptors, leaving fewer functional receptors to respond to acetylcholine, causing muscle weakness. Muscles affected by myasthenia gravis become more fatigued with effort and recover somewhat with rest.

Tetanus is caused by infection by the anaerobic bacterium *Clostridium tetani* as it releases tetanospasmin toxin into the surrounding extracellular space. This toxin migrates to the neuromuscular junctions and will then move along the axon in a retrograde motion to reach the central nervous system. Once there, tetanospasmin will block the release of inhibitory neurotransmitters (glycine and γ-aminobutyric acid), causing prolonged and violent muscle spasms.

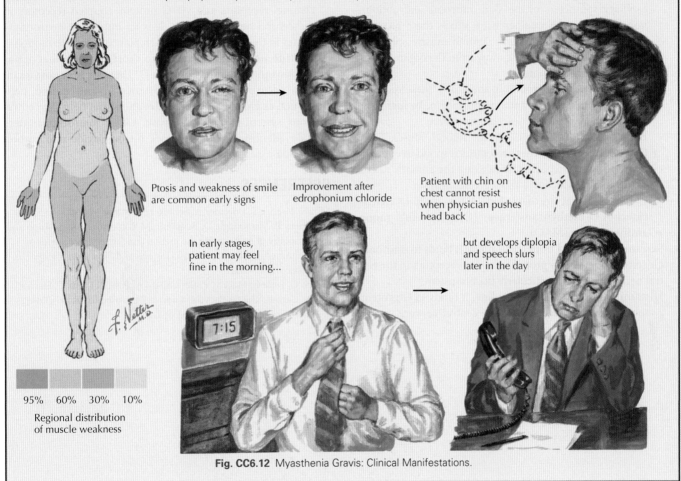

Ptosis and weakness of smile are common early signs

Improvement after edrophonium chloride

Patient with chin on chest cannot resist when physician pushes head back

In early stages, patient may feel fine in the morning...

but develops diplopia and speech slurs later in the day

95%   60%   30%   10%
Regional distribution of muscle weakness

Fig. CC6.12 Myasthenia Gravis: Clinical Manifestations.

- **Nicotinic receptors** are ion-channel receptors found on skeletal muscle, on postganglionic autonomic neurons, and within the central nervous system. When two acetylcholine molecules bind to the two binding sites on the nicotinic receptor, the channel opens to allow inflow of Na^+ and outflow of K^+. Because Na^+ inflow exceed the outflow of K^+, there is a net depolarization of the neuron or target tissue, making it more likely to generate an action potential.
- **Muscarinic receptors** are G protein–coupled receptors found on the surface of smooth muscle cells, cardiomyocytes, endocrine glands, and exocrine glands and within the central nervous system. The binding of a single acetylcholine molecule to the binding site will activate a coupled G protein

that can then activate a variety of second messenger systems or open other ion channels (Clinical Correlation 6.12).

Amines are neurotransmitters that are modified amino acids.
- **Catecholamines** are amines that are derived from tyrosine and contain a six-carbon ring with two hydroxyl groups, a catechol.
  - **Dopamine** binds to dopaminergic, G protein–coupled receptors in the central nervous system. It is an important neurotransmitter in the basal ganglia, nerve cells that plan and initiate motion. They will be discussed in detail in Chapter 8.
  - **Norepinephrine** (noradrenaline) binds to alpha- and beta-adrenergic receptors throughout the body. It is

released by postganglionic sympathetic neurons and within the central nervous system.

- **Epinephrine** (adrenaline) is similar to norepinephrine but is primarily released into the bloodstream by the medulla of the suprarenal/adrenal glands.
- **Adrenergic receptors** are G protein–coupled receptors found on smooth muscle, cardiac myocytes, endocrine glands, and exocrine glands and within the central nervous system. Only the receptors with major effects on the musculoskeletal system are listed.
  - **Alpha 1 receptors** are found in the smooth muscles of capillary sphincters of the skin, mucosae and abdominopelvic organs. Norepinephrine affects these receptors strongly, causing precapillary smooth muscle sphincters to contract and shunt blood away from the organs during a fight or flight reaction.
  - **Beta 1 receptors** are found in the heart. These receptors respond to epinephrine and norepinephrine by increasing the rate and strength of heart contraction.
  - **Beta 2 receptors** are found in the smooth muscle lining the respiratory tract. These receptors respond to epinephrine and norepinephrine by relaxing the smooth muscle of the airway, which will allow greater airflow.
  - **Catecholamines** are degraded in the synaptic cleft by **catechol-O-methyltransferase** (COMT) and **monoamine oxidase** (MAO).
- **Serotonin** is derived from tryptophan. It binds to serotonergic ion channel and G protein–coupled receptors in the central nervous system, particularly the brainstem.
- **Histamine** is derived from histidine. It binds to G protein–coupled histamine receptors in the central nervous system, particularly the hypothalamus. It is also released peripherally by mast cells and basophils.

Amino acid neurotransmitters are active in the central nervous system.

- **Glutamate** and **aspartate** are major excitatory neurotransmitters that open Na^+/K^+ ion channel receptors and depolarize target cells.
- **Glycine** tends to act in an inhibitory manner by opening Cl^- ion channel receptors and hyperpolarizing the target cell.
- **GABA** (γ-aminobutyric acid) is derived from glutamate and is a major inhibitory neurotransmitter that opens Cl^- ion channel receptors and via G protein–coupled receptors in the central nervous system. It is an important neurotransmitter in the basal ganglia, which plan and initiate motion.

Peptide neurotransmitters are short proteins that act as neurotransmitters and hormones. They include oxytocin, thyroid-releasing hormone, substance P, and opioid peptides such as enkaphalin and endorphins that help the central nervous system to modulate pain. Other neurotransmitters include adenosine and the gases nitrous oxide and carbon monoxide.

REFERENCES

Milz S, Tischer T, Buettner A, Schieker M, Maier M, Redman S, Emery P, McGonagle D, Benjamin M. Molecular composition and pathology of entheses on the medial and lateral epicondyles of the humerus: a structural basis for epicondylitis. *Ann Rheum Dis.* 2004;63:1015–1021.

Stecco C, Fede C, Macchi V, Porzionato A, Patrelli L, Biz C, Stern R, De Caro R. The fasciacytes: a new cell devoted to fascial gliding regulation. *Clin Anat.* 2018;31:667–676.

Development of the Musculoskeletal System

QUICK SUMMARY OF EARLY DEVELOPMENT (FIG. 7.1)

Like every other body system, the musculoskeletal system begins with the fertilization of an **oocyte** by a **spermatocyte**. When the two germ cells fuse, they create a single-celled **zygote** that develops further to become a genetically distinct individual. Approximately 30 hours after fertilization, the zygote begins to divide without growing in size. When it reaches the 16-cell stage, it is referred to as a **morula**. Each morula consists of an **outer cell mass** surrounding an **inner cell mass**, which will become the **placenta** and the **embryo**, respectively. In this chapter we will focus exclusively on the inner cell mass and ignore the (interesting but off-topic) development of the placenta from the outer cell mass, cytotrophoblast, and syncytiotrophoblast.

The oocyte and zygote are surrounded by a protective covering called the zona pellucida that gradually disappears and is gone by the morula stage. Once it is gone, approximately 4 days after fertilization, fluid penetrates the morula and creates a space between inner and outer cell masses. The fluid-filled space between the two cell masses is called the blastocyst cavity, and the entire structure is now called a **blastocyst**. The inner cell mass remains in contact with the outer cell mass in one section, which will form the **connecting stalk**. Normally, the blastocyst implants into the uterine lining sometime on the 6th day and further development occurs there.

By the 8th day, another space, the **amniotic cavity**, forms within the inner cell mass on the opposite side from the blastocyst cavity, which is now called the **primary yolk sac**. Even though it is very small at this time, the amniotic cavity will eventually enlarge to surround the entire embryo. The portion of the inner cell mass in contact with the amniotic cavity is called the **epiblast**. The portion that is in contact with the blastocyst cavity is now called the **hypoblast**. The epiblast cells are tall columnar cells, while the hypoblast cells are cuboidal or squamous (flat).

The oval sheets of epiblast and hypoblast cells lay in contact with each other forming a **bilaminar disc**. For that reason, this stage is referred to as the **bilaminar embryo**.

By the 9th day, the embryo has fully implanted into the uterus. The cells surrounding the primary yolk sac have proliferated to form a distinctive layer, the **extraembryonic mesoderm**, which separates the developing embryo (primary yolk sac, bilaminar disc, and amniotic cavity) from the developing placenta. As the extraembryonic mesoderm enlarges, additional, small fluid-filled spaces appear within it too. By the 12th day, the fluid-filled spaces within the extraembryonic mesoderm converge to create a large spherical space surrounding the entire embryo, the **extraembryonic coelom** (cavity). As this coelom expands, the embryo is suspended within it only by the connecting stalk (eventually becoming the **umbilical cord**) that allows it to communicate with the placenta. Like seemingly everything else in this chapter, the extraembryonic coelom changes its name to become the **chorionic cavity** as it expands to surround the embryo.

As we move into the 13th and 14th days (Figs. 7.1 and 7.2), the primary yolk sac is pinched by the expanding chorionic cavity. The larger portion remains in contact with the hypoblast and is now called the **secondary yolk sac**, and it becomes lined by cells derived from the proliferating hypoblast. In one small region, these hypoblast cells enlarge and form the **prechordal plate**, a structure that will fuse tightly to the overlying ectoderm, creating the **oropharyngeal membrane**, the eventual location of the mouth. This is exciting because it is the first evidence of the body's eventual orientation from superior to inferior. Opposite the prechordal plate, the proliferating epiblast cells near the embryo's caudal/inferior pole form a furrow called the **primitive streak**. This will allow the process of **gastrulation**, when the bilaminar disc is replaced by a **trilaminar disc** consisting of three new germ cell layers, the **embryonic ectoderm**, **intraembryonic mesoderm**, and **embryonic endoderm**.

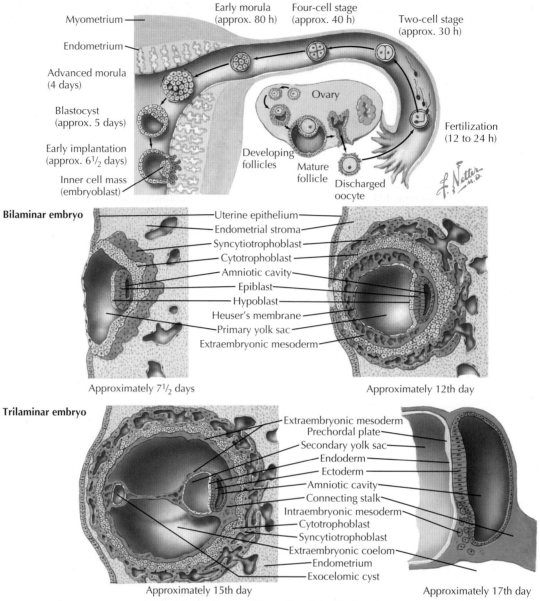

Fig. 7.1 Development From Oocyte to Blastocyst.

GASTRULATION AND THE TRILAMINAR EMBRYO (FIGS. 7.2 AND 7.3)

To form the trilaminar disc, the primitive streak extends from the caudal end of the epiblast toward the prechordal plate but does not quite reach it. As it extends cranially, epiblast cells replicate rapidly and involute into the furrow, creating a deep fissure called the **primitive groove** as they push into and invade the space between the epiblast and hypoblast. Caudally, the primitive streak stops before reaching another area where the ectoderm and endoderm are tightly fused, the **cloacal membrane**.

As gastrulation proceeds, the hypoblast layer is entirely replaced by cells that migrate through the primitive streak and along the inside of the secondary yolk sac. This new layer is the **embryonic endoderm** and will produce the cells that line the respiratory, urogenital, and gastrointestinal tracts as well as many of the body's glands. The cells of the former epiblast are now referred to as **embryonic ectoderm**, and this layer will produce the epidermis, central nervous system, and the migratory **neural crest cells**. Between the endoderm and ectoderm is the **intraembryonic mesoderm** that produces everything else: the kidneys and gonads, as well as the vascular, muscular, and most connective tissue structures of the body.

The migration of epiblast cells occurs along the entire length of the primitive groove, but there are some important features that occur at its cranial end, an area called the **primitive node**. The epiblast cells that migrate through the primitive node move directly toward the prechordal plate, forming an important signaling structure called the **notochordal process**. The notochordal process initially forms a flat line of cells in contact with the fluid in the secondary yolk sac. It folds in on itself to create a tube within the mesoderm called the **notochord**, an important structure in directing further development of the three germ cell layers (Clinical Correlation 7.1).

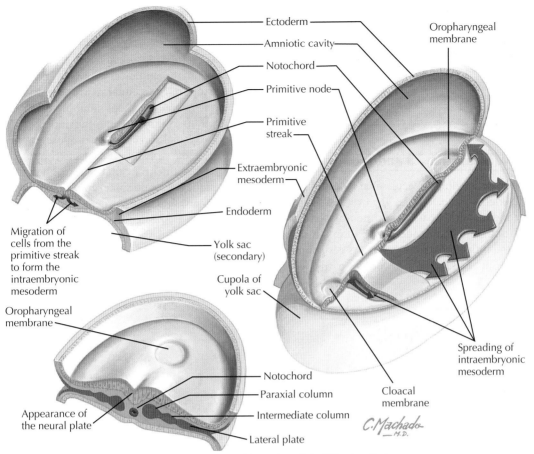

Fig. 7.2 Gastrulation and Formation of the Trilaminar Embryo.

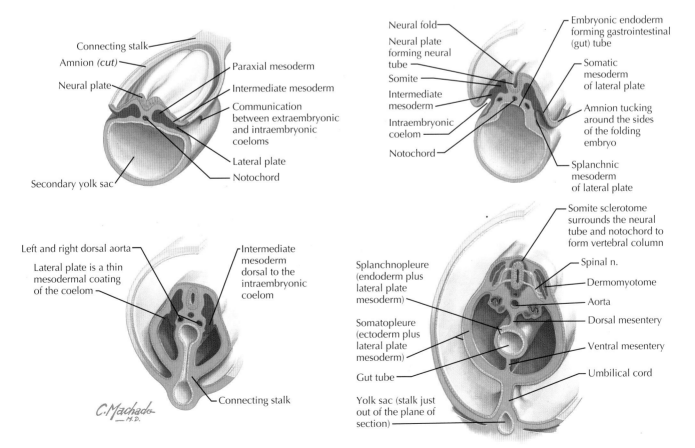

Fig. 7.3 Further Development of the Trilaminar Embryo and Neurulation.

NEURULATION (SEE FIGS. 7.3 and 7.4)

The notochord releases signaling molecules that induce changes in the nearby mesoderm and ectoderm. The overlying, central region of the ectoderm thickens to form a **neural plate** that pinches together to invade the mesoderm and form a midline **neural groove** on the 14th day of development. As development proceeds from the 16th to 18th day, the two sides of the neural plate approach each other as **neural folds** and come together as the **neural tube** inside the mesoderm, which will form the spinal cord, brainstem, and cerebral cortex. The central portion of the neural tube pinches together at or around day 21, leaving openings into the amnion at its cranial and caudal ends, the **cranial neuropore** and **caudal neuropore**. Starting in its central region, the neural tube "zips" shut in both the cranial and caudal directions as it moves into the underlying mesoderm. This causes the cranial and caudal neuropores to shrink and eventually close on days 24 and 27, respectively. The core of the neural tube contains a **neural canal** that will become the ventricular system of the brain and spinal cord (Clinical Correlation 7.2).

After the neural tube has detached from the ectoderm, other ectodermal cells, the **neural crest cells**, leave the neural folds and migrate into the mesoderm just posterior to the tube. They will form the posterior root ganglia and the sensory ganglia of the cranial nerves. Neural crest cells also migrate to form the Schwann

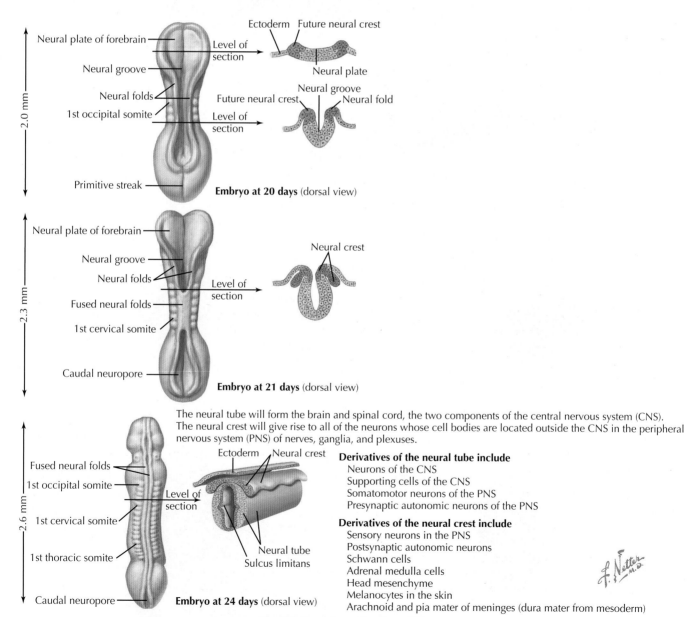

The neural tube will form the brain and spinal cord, the two components of the central nervous system (CNS). The neural crest will give rise to all of the neurons whose cell bodies are located outside the CNS in the peripheral nervous system (PNS) of nerves, ganglia, and plexuses.

Derivatives of the neural tube include
Neurons of the CNS
Supporting cells of the CNS
Somatomotor neurons of the PNS
Presynaptic autonomic neurons of the PNS

Derivatives of the neural crest include
Sensory neurons in the PNS
Postsynaptic autonomic neurons
Schwann cells
Adrenal medulla cells
Head mesenchyme
Melanocytes in the skin
Arachnoid and pia mater of meninges (dura mater from mesoderm)

Fig. 7.4 Formation of the Neural Tube.

CLINICAL CORRELATION 7.2   Spina Bifida

The cranial and caudal neuropores close to create a complete spinal cord within the mesoderm. Because the caudal neuropore is the last to close, delays in closure can prevent the sclerotomal mesenchyme in that region from migrating posterior to the spinal cord. In addition, the spinous processes are typically the last segment of a vertebra to chondrify and ossify. Because of all this, there are a variety of malformations wherein the spinous processes and laminae fail to fuse, called **spina bifida**.

- **Spina bifida occulta** occurs when the defect is very minor and there is no displacement of the underlying meninges or spinal cord. It is often discovered incidentally but is sometimes notable for inducing the growth of a tuft of hair over the affected region.

- **Meningocele** results from failure of the spinous processes and laminae to form properly. The affected newborn will have a "bubble" of cerebrospinal

fluid (CSF)-filled meninges (dura and arachnoid mater) extending from the vertebral canal to the back. This is evident at birth and can be detected during prenatal ultrasound screening.

- **Meningomyelocele** is an even more severe form of this malformation. The affected newborn will have a bubble of CSF-filled meninges extending from the vertebral canal that also includes the spinal cord or nerve roots. There are frequently neurologic deficits below the malformation. This is also evident at birth and can be detected during prenatal ultrasound screening.

- **Rachischisis** is the most severe form of spina bifida. In this condition, neurulation fails to occur and the neural tube does not form in the affected area. Instead, the potential nervous tissue is still located on the back (which is also derived from the ectoderm) and the body below the lesion is completely deinnervated.

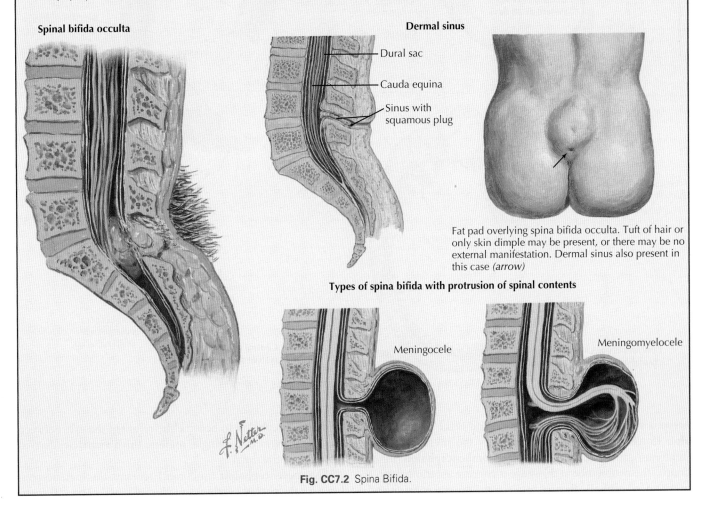

Spinal bifida occulta

Dermal sinus

Dural sac

Cauda equina

Sinus with squamous plug

Fat pad overlying spina bifida occulta. Tuft of hair or only skin dimple may be present, or there may be no external manifestation. Dermal sinus also present in this case *(arrow)*

Types of spina bifida with protrusion of spinal contents

Meningocele

Meningomyelocele

Fig. CC7.2 Spina Bifida.

and satellite cells that protect peripheral nerves. If that were not enough, they also differentiate into sympathetic ganglia, cells of the adrenal medulla, postsynaptic parasympathetic ganglia in the head and organs, connective tissue structures of the face, and the melanocytes throughout the skin, hair, and iris.

The epiblast-derived **neuroepithelial cells** that line the neural canal proliferate extensively, expanding outward from the **ventricular zone** into the **intermediate** and **marginal zones** of the thickening neural tube. There is a functional division of the neural tube called the **sulcus limitans** that splits it into a

posterior **alar plate**, which will develop into sensory neurons, and an anterior **basal plate** that will develop into motor neurons. The dividing line between the two plates is called the **sulcus limitans**.

DIFFERENTIATION OF THE NERVOUS SYSTEM AND VENTRICLES (FIG. 7.5)

The neural tube and accompanying neural canal develop expansions that will eventually become distinct regions of the central

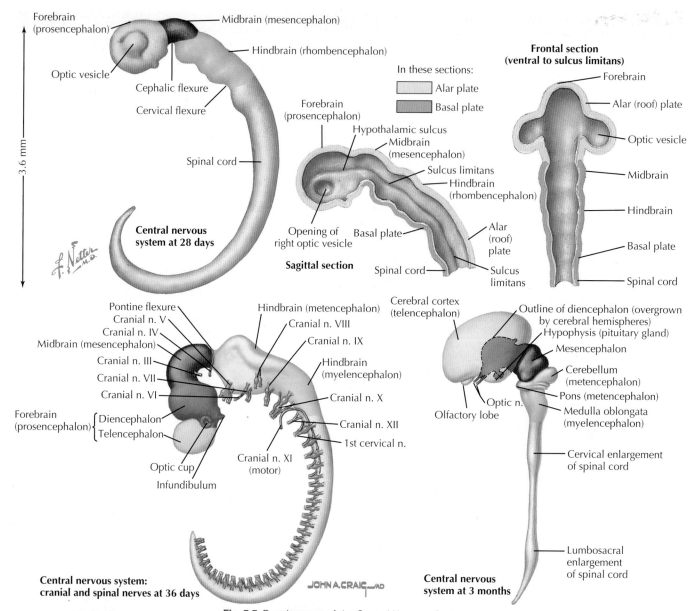

Fig. 7.5 Development of the Central Nervous System.

nervous system. The expanded cranial end is the **prosenceph-alon** (forebrain), the middle portion is the **mesencephalon** (midbrain), and the caudal end is the **rhombencephalon** (hind-brain). The neural tube at this stage is concave anteriorly with a pronounced **cephalic flexure** between the prosencephalon and mesencephalon that gives the human brain its characteristic "tilted forward" appearance. A similar **cervical flexure** is pres-ent between the rhombencephalon and spinal cord.

The prosencephalon differentiates into the bulbous **telen-cephalon** and the smaller **diencephalon**. The telencephalon expands outward to the left and right, eventually forming the lobes of the left and right **cerebral cortices** and is associated with cranial nerve I (olfactory). The left and right **lateral ven-tricles** are present in the telencephalon and are derived from the neural canal. The diencephalon forms the **thalamus** on the left and right sides, part of the pituitary gland, the **hypothalamus**, and **epithalamus/pineal gland**. Cranial nerve II (optic) projects

off the diencephalon to become the retina of the eye. Between the two thalami is the single, midline **third ventricle**, derived from the neural canal.

The **mesencephalon** (midbrain) remains the mesencepha-lon with the narrow cerebral aqueduct. Cranial nerves III (ocu-lomotor) and IV (trochlear) project off its ventral and dorsal sides, respectively. The rhombencephalon differentiates into the **metencephalon** and **myelencephalon**. Anteriorly, the meten-cephalon becomes the pons, with cranial nerves V (trigemi-nal) and VI (abducens) exiting its ventral surface. Posteriorly, the metencephalon develops into the **cerebellum**. The myelen-cephalon becomes the **medulla oblongata**, with cranial nerves VII (facial), VIII (vestibulocochlear), IX (glossopharyngeal), X (vagus), and XII (hypoglossal) projecting off its lateral and ventral surfaces. The **spinal cord** extends inferiorly thereafter, with cranial nerve XI (spinal accessory) leaving its lateral sides. A **pontine flexure** develops between the metencephalon and

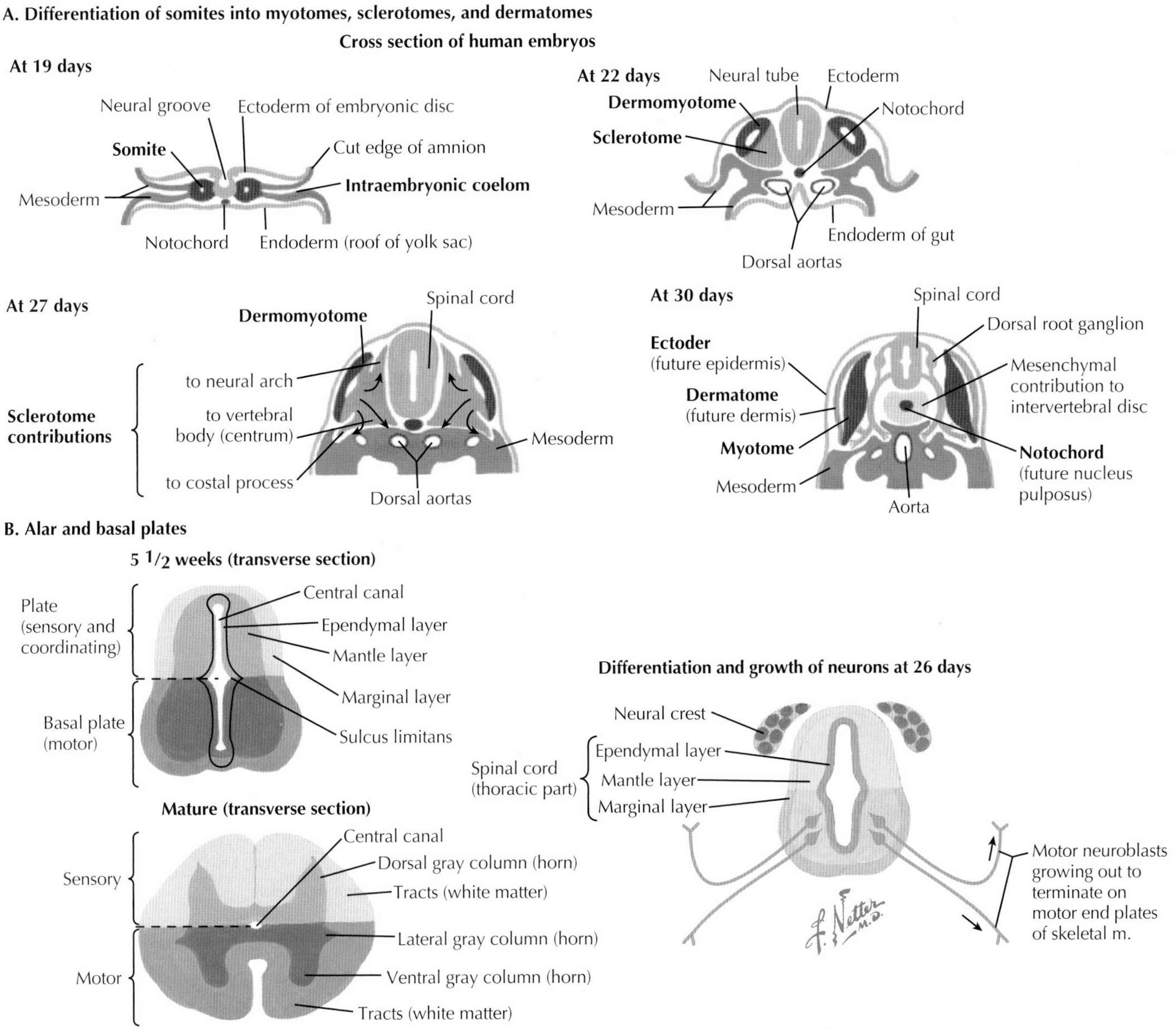

A. Differentiation of somites into myotomes, sclerotomes, and dermatomes

Cross section of human embryos

At 19 days

Neural groove
Ectoderm of embryonic disc
Somite
Cut edge of amnion
Mesoderm
Intraembryonic coelom
Notochord
Endoderm (roof of yolk sac)

At 22 days Neural tube Ectoderm
Dermomyotome Notochord
Sclerotome
Mesoderm
Endoderm of gut
Dorsal aortas

At 27 days
Dermomyotome Spinal cord

Sclerotome contributions
to neural arch
to vertebral body (centrum)
Mesoderm
to costal process
Dorsal aortas

At 30 days Spinal cord
Dorsal root ganglion
Ectoder (future epidermis)
Mesenchymal contribution to intervertebral disc
Dermatome (future dermis)
Myotome **Notochord** (future nucleus pulposus)
Mesoderm
Aorta

B. Alar and basal plates

5 1/2 weeks (transverse section)

Plate (sensory and coordinating)
Central canal
Ependymal layer
Mantle layer
Marginal layer
Basal plate (motor)
Sulcus limitans

Differentiation and growth of neurons at 26 days

Neural crest
Ependymal layer
Spinal cord (thoracic part)
Mantle layer
Marginal layer
Motor neuroblasts growing out to terminate on motor end plates of skeletal m.

Mature (transverse section)

Central canal
Dorsal gray column (horn)
Sensory
Tracts (white matter)
Lateral gray column (horn)
Ventral gray column (horn)
Motor
Tracts (white matter)

Fig. 7.6 Differentiation of Somites Into the Myotome, Sclerotome, and Dermatome.

the myelencephalon, with its concavity facing posteriorly. The **fourth ventricle** sits between the pons and medulla anteriorly and the cerebellum posteriorly. The rest of the neural tube caudal to the myelencephalon will become the spinal cord with a central canal at its core.

DIFFERENTIATION OF THE MESODERM (FIGS. 7.3 AND 7.6)

The notochord releases molecular signals that induce changes in the neural tube and nearby mesoderm. This allows the mesoderm to differentiate into many distinctive structures. **Paraxial mesoderm** is found immediately lateral to the neural tube and notochord. It will differentiate into **somites**, large blobs of mesoderm that form visible bumps on either side of the neural tube. Somites will develop into the axial skeleton and its muscles as well as the dermal layer of skin. Just lateral to the paraxial

mesoderm is the **intermediate mesoderm**, which differentiates into urogenital organs. Because the intermediate mesoderm does not contribute to the musculoskeletal system, this is the last we will hear of it in this volume. Lateral to the intermediate mesoderm is the **lateral plate mesoderm**, which will split into two sheets, one that surrounds the gut tube, and the other that forms the anterior body wall and limbs. At this stage, we can follow the development of any organ system but will focus on the nervous and musculoskeletal systems.

PARAXIAL MESODERM AND SOMITES

The somites in the paraxial mesoderm form as distinctive pairs on either side of the neural tube. They begin appearing on day 25 and gradually increase in number as development proceeds. This progression is so well characterized that many of developmental events are described using the number of somites as a reference. There will eventually be 4 occipital, 8 cervical, 12 thoracic, 5 lumbar, 5 sacral, and a variable (but small) number of coccygeal somites.

The mesenchyme (undifferentiated stem cells) that makes up somites will proliferate and eventually subdivide into specialized regions, the **sclerotome, meningotome,** and **dermomyotome**. The notochord and ventral neural tube release an important signaling molecule, **Sonic Hedgehog (Shh)**, which induces the proliferating mesenchyme of the sclerotome to surround the notochord and neural tube, forming a loose model of the vertebrae that will become cartilage and then bone. The dorsal portion of the sclerotome will eventually become the spinous process and lamina; the central sclerotome becomes the pedicles and articular processes; the ventral sclerotome turns into the vertebral bodies and annulus fibrosus of the intervertebral disc; and the lateral sclerotome forms the transverse processes and ribs.

Medial to the sclerotome is the **meningotome**, which becomes the dura, arachnoid, and pia mater. The dorsal neural tube and overlying ectoderm release a different signaling molecule Wnt, which induces the formation of the **dermomyotome** lateral to the sclerotome. It subdivides into the dermatome and myotome. The **myotome** is made of mesenchymal cells that migrate around the torso and limbs as it differentiates to form skeletal muscles. Lateral to the myotome is the **dermatome**, which will form the inner part of the skin, the **dermis**. The dermis contains the blood vessels and nerves that nurture the outmost **epidermis**, which is derived from the ectoderm that surrounds the entire developing embryo.

LATERAL PLATE MESODERM AND BODY WALL FORMATION (FIGS. 7.3, 7.6, AND 7.7)

Lateral to the paraxial and intermediate mesoderm is the **lateral plate mesoderm**, which is continuous with the extraembryonic

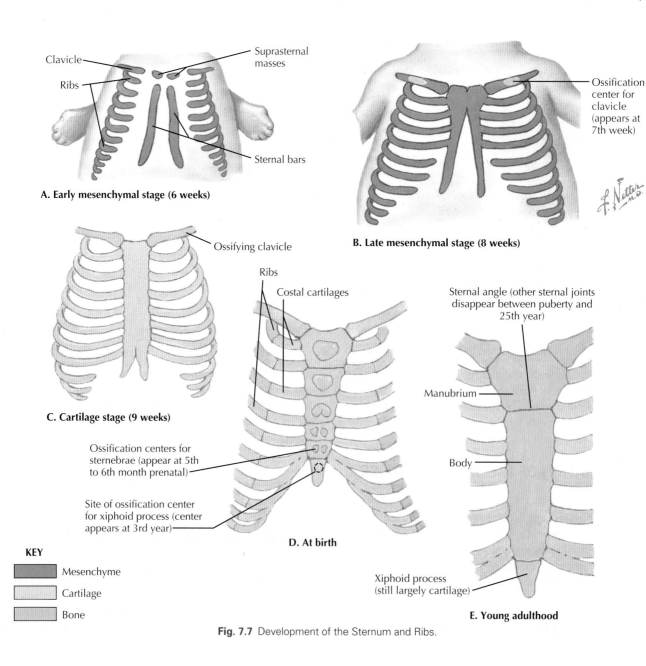

A. Early mesenchymal stage (6 weeks)

Clavicle
Ribs
Suprasternal masses
Sternal bars

B. Late mesenchymal stage (8 weeks)

Ossification center for clavicle (appears at 7th week)

C. Cartilage stage (9 weeks)

Ossifying clavicle

Ribs
Costal cartilages

Ossification centers for sternebrae (appear at 5th to 6th month prenatal)

Site of ossification center for xiphoid process (center appears at 3rd year)

D. At birth

Sternal angle (other sternal joints disappear between puberty and 25th year)

Manubrium

Body

Xiphoid process (still largely cartilage)

E. Young adulthood

KEY

Mesenchyme
Cartilage
Bone

Fig. 7.7 Development of the Sternum and Ribs.

mesoderm as it reaches the boundaries of the trilaminar embryo. It is in contact with the ectoderm on its dorsal/posterior side and the endoderm on the ventral/anterior side. Small, fluid-filled gaps begin to form inside the lateral plate mesoderm that enlarge and fuse to create a new space, the **intraembryonic coelom** (cavity). It does not look like much initially, but it will eventually form all the body cavities. As the intraembryonic coelom enlarges, it splits the lateral plate mesoderm into two sheets. The **visceral layer of lateral plate mesoderm** is in contact with the endoderm, and the group name for this combined structure (visceral layer + endoderm) is the **splanchnopleure**. The right and left splanchnopleure move closer to each other and eventually meet, fuse, and create the gut tube. The endoderm forms the lining of the gastrointestinal tract while the visceral layer will become the mesentery that connects it to the posterior body wall. As this happens, the cylindrical gut tube pushes the secondary yolk sac away, remaining attached to it in one place called the vitelline duct.

The **parietal layer of lateral plate mesoderm** is in contact with the ectoderm. The group name for this structure (parietal layer + ectoderm) is the **somatopleure**. Starting on day 22, the somatopleure begins to elongate and expand laterally (like a manta ray's wings). By the 24th day, it is lateral to the developing gut tube, and by the 26th day the left and right somatopleure meet each other on the midline and fuse. Thus they form the anterior body wall and enclose the gut tube within the intraembryonic coelom, which will eventually form the peritoneal, pericardial, and pleural cavities.

Inside the leading edge of the somatopleure are mesenchymal condensations called the **sternal bars**. They fuse as the body wall becomes continuous and "zips shut" from superior to inferior. The mesenchyme of the developing ribs fuses with the sternal bars. The mesenchyme becomes cartilage and eventually ossification centers develop in the cartilage of the sternal body shortly before birth. The sternum finishes ossifying during young adulthood, although a synovial joint remains between the manubrium and sternal body and the xyphoid process does not ossify until much later in life.

DEVELOPMENT OF THE BACK (FIGS. 7.8–7.10)

The skeletal muscles of the back, torso, and limbs come from the mesenchymal cells of the myotome. Undifferentiated myoblast cells fuse to create long, multinucleated **myotube** cells that start producing myofilaments. As they enlarge and migrate to their final positions, myofilaments take up most of the cytoplasm, pushing the nuclei to the periphery of the cell. For muscles to become functional, they must be innervated by a motor neuron from the spinal cord. Lower motor neurons in the ventral/anterior horn of the spinal cord extend their axons to reach the myotome. They have difficulty doing this due to the dense sclerotome mesenchyme between the neural tube and the myotome. The body's solution to this problem is rather interesting. The sclerotome from each somite splits into a superior and anterior division at a **fissure of Von Ebner**. This creates a cleft in

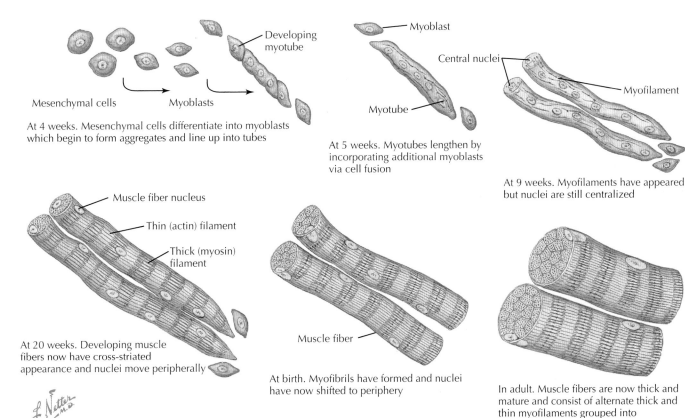

Developing myotube

Mesenchymal cells   Myoblasts

At 4 weeks. Mesenchymal cells differentiate into myoblasts which begin to form aggregates and line up into tubes

Myoblast

Central nuclei

Myotube

At 5 weeks. Myotubes lengthen by incorporating additional myoblasts via cell fusion

Myofilament

At 9 weeks. Myofilaments have appeared but nuclei are still centralized

Muscle fiber nucleus

Thin (actin) filament

Thick (myosin) filament

At 20 weeks. Developing muscle fibers now have cross-striated appearance and nuclei move peripherally

Muscle fiber

At birth. Myofibrils have formed and nuclei have now shifted to periphery

In adult. Muscle fibers are now thick and mature and consist of alternate thick and thin myofilaments grouped into longitudinal bundles as myofibrils with nuclei located at periphery (satellite cells are not shown)

Fig. 7.8 Development of Skeletal Muscle Fibers.

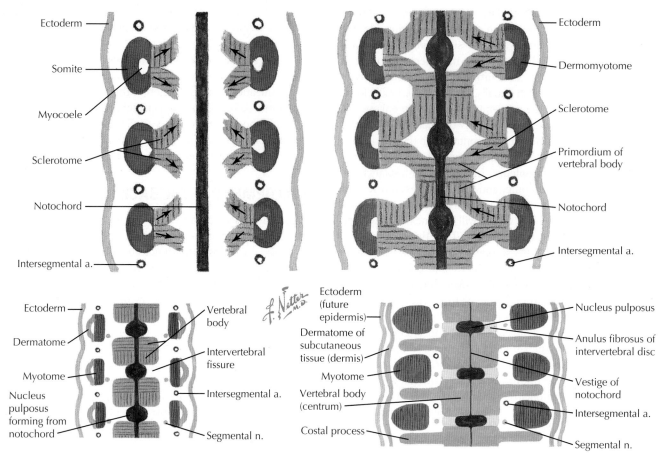

Fig. 7.9 Stages in Formation of the Vertebral Column, Dermatomes, and Myotomes.

the middle of the (formerly intact) somite that allows the motor axons to migrate laterally and reach the myotome. The location of the cleft will eventually be marked by the intervertebral foramen between two vertebrae.

As for the sclerotome, the superior division will fuse with the inferior division of its superior neighbor (I wish there were an easier way to say that) to create a vertebra, leaving some sclerotome tissue between each vertebral body that will become the annulus fibrosus of the intervertebral disc. In this way, each vertebra comes from half of two different, but adjacent, sclerotomes. There are a few exceptions: the occipital sclerotomes and the superior division of C1 form part of the occipital bone, C1 has part of its sclerotome "stolen" by C2 to create the dens. The sacral sclerotomes will split normally but then fuse to neighboring sacral vertebrae.

The loose mesenchyme model of each vertebra will transition to become cartilage at **chondrification centers** in the **centrum** (developing vertebral body), pedicles, and laminae. Cartilage provides rigidity along with an ability to grow as the body elongates. Eventually **primary centers of ossification** develop in the centrum and pedicle and begin to replace cartilage with bone. Thereafter **secondary centers of ossification** develop within the transverse processes and spinous process and at the annular epiphysis along the superior and inferior rim of the vertebral body. The final area of the vertebra to chondrify and ossify is the spinous process.

So far, the development of the vertebrae has been relatively general; however, each vertebra and vertebral region has distinctive features that distinguish it from the others. The differences seen between vertebrae are the result of the expression of the homeobox (*Hox*) gene family. In the occipital region, only two *Hox* gene family members are expressed in the developing vertebrae. As we move inferiorly, those genes continue to be expressed but additional Hox genes are added. The further inferiorly we travel, the more *Hox* genes are being expressed, with approximately 24 *Hox* family members expressed at the tip of the coccyx (Clinical Correlations 7.3).

Each myotome subdivides into **hypaxial muscles** and **epaxial muscles** (see Fig. 7.10). The hypaxial muscles are innervated by **anterior rami** and become the muscles of the anterior neck, torso, limbs, and perineum. As they migrate through the body wall and limbs, they drag their anterior rami behind them, creating the various plexuses in each region of the body. Epaxial muscles form the intrinsic muscles of the back. The spinal nerve branches to the epaxial muscles become **posterior rami** and will be pulled posteriorly as the epaxial muscles divide into a lateral epaxial muscle column and medial epaxial muscle column and attach to the vertebrae and other bony features related to the back.

The neural crest cells positioned posterior to the neural tube at each level will differentiate to become the posterior root ganglia, containing sensory nerve cells. They extend a

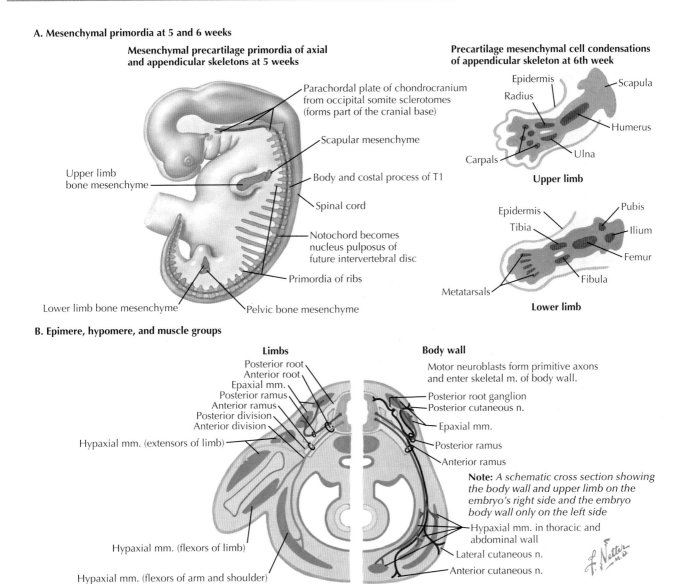

A. Mesenchymal primordia at 5 and 6 weeks

Mesenchymal precartilage primordia of axial and appendicular skeletons at 5 weeks

Parachordal plate of chondrocranium from occipital somite sclerotomes (forms part of the cranial base)

Scapular mesenchyme

Body and costal process of T1

Spinal cord

Upper limb bone mesenchyme

Notochord becomes nucleus pulposus of future intervertebral disc

Primordia of ribs

Lower limb bone mesenchyme

Pelvic bone mesenchyme

Precartilage mesenchymal cell condensations of appendicular skeleton at 6th week

Epidermis

Radius

Scapula

Humerus

Ulna

Carpals

Upper limb

Epidermis

Tibia

Pubis

Ilium

Femur

Fibula

Metatarsals

Lower limb

B. Epimere, hypomere, and muscle groups

Limbs

Posterior root
Anterior root
Epaxial mm.
Posterior ramus
Anterior ramus
Posterior division
Anterior division

Hypaxial mm. (extensors of limb)

Hypaxial mm. (flexors of limb)

Hypaxial mm. (flexors of arm and shoulder)

Body wall

Motor neuroblasts form primitive axons and enter skeletal m. of body wall.

Posterior root ganglion
Posterior cutaneous n.

Epaxial mm.

Posterior ramus

Anterior ramus

Note: *A schematic cross section showing the body wall and upper limb on the embryo's right side and the embryo body wall only on the left side*

Hypaxial mm. in thoracic and abdominal wall

Lateral cutaneous n.

Anterior cutaneous n.

Somatic nervous system innervates somatopleure (body wall).

Fig. 7.10 Mesenchymal Primordia at 5 and 6 Weeks.

pseudounipolar axon that splits into a medial and lateral division. Because the motor axons have already migrated across the split sclerotome, the lateral division of these sensory axons follow them to reach the myotome and overlying dermatome. The lateral division of each nerve then conveys sensory input from the muscle spindle fibers, Golgi tendon organs, and sensations from the skin to the posterior root ganglia. The medial division of these neurons then extends toward other nerve cells developing in the posterior horn of the spinal cord so that they can convey sensations from the muscles and skin back to the central nervous system.

After neurulation and the early formation of the vertebrae, the spinal cord extends through the entire length of the vertebral canal with spinal nerves exiting their respective foramina. At this time the spinal cord segments are at the corresponding level of the vertebral canal (i.e., the L3 spinal cord segment is enclosed by the L3 vertebra). However, the rapid growth of the rest of the fetal body outpaces the ability of the spinal cord to

elongate. Thankfully the spinal cord remains firmly attached to the brainstem, and its tapered end, the **conus medullaris**, remains tethered to the coccyx by a thin cord, the **filum terminale**. By the end of the 5th month in utero, the conus medullaris has "ascended" (it does not really ascend, it just does not elongate as quickly as the vertebral column) to the S2 vertebral level, and by the time we are born it is at L3. Elongation of the body proceeds far more slowly after birth, and by the time we reach adulthood the conus medullaris is typically encountered at the L2 vertebral level. In all, the adult vertebral column is approximately 22 times its fetal length, whereas the adult spinal cord is only approximately 12 times its fetal length.

Because each spinal nerve is linked to a specific intervertebral foramen before the cord "ascends," they are stretched as the vertebral column elongates considerably before birth. The anterior and posterior spinal nerve roots elongate between the cord and their exit from the vertebral canal. The collection of paired nerve roots seen between L2 and the coccyx is called

CLINICAL CORRELATION 7.3   Sacralization and Lumbarization

Because the differences between vertebrae are caused by their expression of related members of the *Hox* gene family, the vertebrae near each other tend to be similar. One interesting manifestation of this is sacralization, in which the L5 vertebra fuses with S1, effectively forming an enlarged sacrum and foreshortened lumbar region. Not surprisingly, lumbarization occurs when the S1 vertebra fails to fuse with S2, forming a shortened sacrum and lengthened lumbar region.

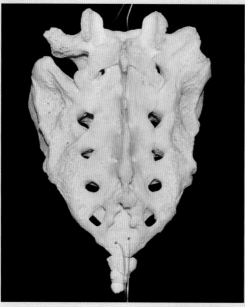 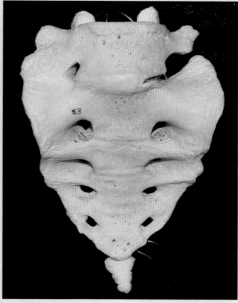

This specimen demonstrates partial sacralization of the L5 vertebra. The right side is completely fused to S1 but the left side retains the typical appearance of a lumbar vertebra.

Fig. CC7.3 Partial Sacralization of L5 on the Right Side.

the **cauda equina** (horse's tail) and runs in parallel to the single filum terminale.

Because of this differential growth, spinal cord segments are not necessarily located at the corresponding vertebral level (Fig. 9.1):

- The upper cervical spinal levels tend to be close to the same vertebral levels.
- The lower lumbar spinal cord segments are in close association with the T12 vertebral body.
- All sacral spinal cord segments are in close association with the L1 vertebral body.

DEVELOPMENT OF THE LIMBS (FIGS. 7.10 AND 7.11)

The upper and lower limb buds start to extend outward and laterally from the somatopleure after the anterior body wall has formed. The **upper limb bud** forms first, after 30 days of development, and the lower limb bud follows at day 34. The cells at the tip of the limb bud proliferate wildly and cause the bud to grow outward and create distinctive regions such as the shoulder, arm, forearm, wrist, and hand. At the core of each limb bud are **mesenchymal condensations** that form a rough model of the eventual bones in each region. A **hand plate** is formed after 35 days, and the extension of the limb bud ceases. **Digital rays** form in the hand plate, marking the eventual location of fingers. The fingers are formed as the cells of the hand plate between

each digital ray undergo programmed cell death, **apoptosis**. The fingers are distinct by the 52nd day. The **lower limb bud** forms similarly but begins later on day 39, forms the gluteal, thigh, leg, ankle, and foot regions, and has distinct toes by the 56th day. The lower limb buds develop on either side of a tail segment with its own vertebrae and somites. Normally this tail segment will rescind with only the coccyx marking its location (Clinical Correlations 7.4 and 7.5).

The bones of the upper limb form via endochondral ossification, which will be described in detail at the end of this chapter. In this process, mesenchyme at the core of the limbs condenses to form a loose model of the bones in each region. These mesenchymal cells will transition into hyaline cartilage before transitioning yet again to become bone by forming ossification centers. Cartilage cells between the ossification centers form growth plates that proliferate and allow elongation of the bones during childhood and adolescence. The cartilage cells in the growth plates proliferate in response to growth hormone (GH), Indian Hedgehog (IHH), and insulin-like growth factor 1 (IGF1). Eventually the ossification centers meet and close the growth plates, and the bone reaches its mature length. A higher circulating proportion of estrogen compared with testosterone will tend to close growth plates. Because women tend to have a higher estrogen/testosterone ratio than men, the growth plates of women tend to fuse earlier. Please note that this is a generality and that many factors (genetics, nutrition, stress) influence growth, not just hormones (Clinical Correlations 7.6–7.8).

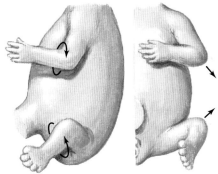

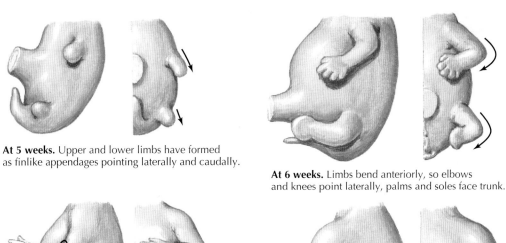

At 5 weeks. Upper and lower limbs have formed as finlike appendages pointing laterally and caudally.

At 6 weeks. Limbs bend anteriorly, so elbows and knees point laterally, palms and soles face trunk.

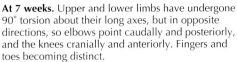

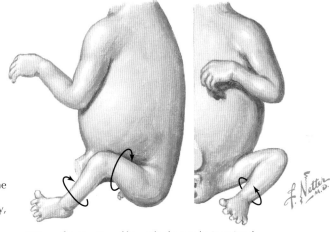

At 7 weeks. Upper and lower limbs have undergone 90° torsion about their long axes, but in opposite directions, so elbows point caudally and posteriorly, and the knees cranially and anteriorly. Fingers and toes becoming distinct.

At 8 weeks. Torsion of lower limbs results in twisted or "barber pole" arrangement of their cutaneous innervation.

Fig. 7.11 Limb Bud Rotation.

The spinal nerve branches to hypaxial muscles are the **anterior rami** that become the cervical plexus, brachial plexus, intercostal nerves, lumbar plexus, and lumbosacral plexus. The hypaxial muscles themselves have several divisions. A prevertebral division forms muscles along the anterior aspect of the vertebrae. Others will migrate around the body wall to form muscles of the trunk such as intercostal and abdominal muscles. Hypaxial muscles and anterior rami also migrate into the developing limb buds. Within the limb buds, the hypomere and its anterior ramus split yet again to form a **dorsal muscle mass** and **ventral muscle mass** on either side of the developing bones. The dorsal muscle masses migrate along the posterior sides of the developing limbs to form extensor muscles. In the upper limb the dorsal muscle masses are innervated by branches of the **posterior division of the brachial plexus**, such as the radial and axillary nerves. The dorsal muscle masses of the lower limb are innervated by branches of the **gluteal, femoral, and common fibular nerves**.

Likewise, the ventral muscle masses migrate along the anterior sides of the developing limbs to form flexor and adductor muscles. In the upper limb, they are innervated by branches of the **anterior division of the brachial plexus**, such as the median, ulnar, and musculocutaneous nerves. In the lower limb, they are innervated by branches of the obturator and tibial nerves. In the next section we will investigate how the innervation of the body wall and limbs connects with structures in the central nervous system.

By the 56th day of development, the upper limb rotates in a way that brings the point of the elbow (olecranon) posteriorly. This is why the extensors of the upper limb are posterior and the flexors are anterior. The lower limb rotates in the opposite direction so that the knee (patella) points anteriorly. This is why the extensors of the lower limb are anterior and the flexors are posterior.

Signals Related to Limb Patterning

Fibroblast growth factor 8 (FGF8) is expressed in the mesenchyme of the somatopleure at the locations where limb buds will form. As the buds grow outward, the lateral-most extent of the bud is called the **apical epidermal ridge (AER)** and is where the FGF8 is expressed. FGF8 not only initiates limb development, but it maintains the outgrowth of the limb buds. If it is not expressed, no limb will form; if the AER is removed, the limb will cease growing; and if FGF8-soaked beads are implanted at the right time, additional limbs will form in those locations.

Earlier, we discussed how members of the *Hox* gene family are expressed along the developing vertebrae and result in the differences in each region. Members of the same family of genes are involved in patterning the limbs as well. *Hox 9* is expressed in the shoulder, and as the AER grows outward to form the arm, *Hox 9* and *10* are expressed. *Hox 9* to *11* members are expressed in the forearm and proximal carpals, and *Hox 12* is added in the distal carpus. Finally, in the mesenchyme that will

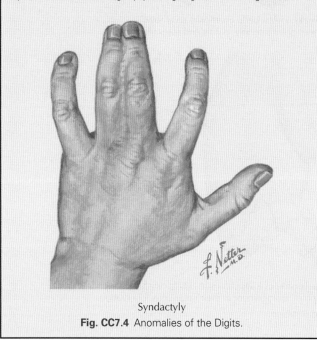

Syndactyly
Fig. CC7.4 Anomalies of the Digits.

become the hand, *Hox* genes *9* to *13* are expressed. This differential expression creates the differences between regions of the upper limb.

The inferior-most area of the growing limb bud is known as the **zone of polarizing activity (ZPA)**, and it expresses an important signaling molecule, **Sonic Hedgehog (Shh)**. Shh is most highly concentrated in the medial hand area, where the fifth digit will form, and least concentrated in the lateral region around the first digit. If Shh is experimentally placed in the lateral area of the developing hand, instead of a thumb, another fifth and fourth digit will form. Conversely, removal of the ZPA from the medial hand will result in thumbs on both sides of the developing hand (Clinical Correlation 7.9).

ENDOCHONDRAL OSSIFICATION (FIGS. 7.12 AND 7.13)

In the vertebrae and limb bones, we have seen that mesenchyme forms a rough model of the eventual bone as the limb develops. These mesenchymal cells are not strong enough to support the body in the way the bone does; however, if we formed mineralized bones at this early stage of development, they could not enlarge quickly enough to keep pace with growth of the body. So, to provide structural support along with the ability to grow quickly, mesenchymal cells proliferate rapidly before becoming hyaline cartilage, which will eventually transition to bone. This process is called **endochondral ossification**, and we will describe how it occurs in a typical long bone. The same process occurs in other bones, but their irregular shape makes the process somewhat less intuitive to understand.

Cells in the mesenchymal model of the bone differentiate to become chondroblasts that create a hyaline cartilage model of the bone. The chondrocytes proliferate and produce extracellular matrix. As one cell divides, it creates an isogenous group of daughter cells that push away from each other as they release extracellular matrix (interstitial growth), which causes cartilage to grow. Chondroblasts lining the perichondrium also become active and proliferate (appositional growth). Eventually the enlarging cartilage model becomes too large for diffusion of gasses and nutrients from the perichondrium to supply it. Some of the most central chondrocytes hypertrophy (enlarge) and begin secreting alkaline phosphatase to calcify their extracellular matrix. The cartilaginous model develops a mineralized **bone collar** around the perimeter of its shaft and deep to the perichondrium.

A nutrient artery will pierce the bone collar and infiltrate the cartilage of the shaft, bringing additional mesenchymal osteoprogenitor cells that take up residence in the mineralized cartilage. These cells begin to secrete osteoid and create the **primary center of ossification** in the middle of the **shaft**. This ossification center will expand outward, replacing cartilage with bone as it goes. In time, the central portion of the shaft, the **diaphysis**, will become somewhat hollow and will host hematopoietic (blood-forming) cells in its **marrow cavity**. Ossification also occurs at the proximal and distal ends of the cartilage model, with new arteries piercing the perichondrium and creating **secondary centers of ossification** during the first 2 years of life. The ends of bones are called the **epiphyses** (sing. epiphysis), and as ossification proceeds, it eventually replaces all the cartilage with bone, except along the articular surfaces of the bones.

As the primary and secondary centers of ossification approach each other, a strip of cartilage remains between them. This **epiphyseal plate** (growth plate) is what allows our bones to lengthen during childhood and adolescence. The region on the opposite side of the epiphysis is called the **metaphysis**. It is connected to the diaphysis but does not contain a hollow marrow cavity. The chondrocytes in the epiphyseal plate arrange themselves into several zones that allow them to push the primary and secondary centers of ossification away from each other.

- **Zone of reserve cartilage**: this region is full of quiescent chondroblasts that can become active and begin proliferating.

CLINICAL CORRELATION 7.6   Achondroplasia

Dwarfism is a classification for those who reach a mature height of 147 cm (4 feet, 10 inches) or less. One cause of this is a mutation in the fibroblast growth factor receptor 3 gene that impairs the proliferation of chondrocytes in growth plates during endochondral ossification. As a result of the mutation, growth plates close prematurely and bones will fuse earlier than typical. This is called **achondroplasia** or **disproportionate dwarfism**, and the affected person will tend to have a shorter stature because the limb bones do not lengthen as much as would be expected if the growth plates were unaffected. The facial bones also undergo endochondral ossification, so those with achondroplasia tend to have shorter

faces, making the cranium appear comparatively larger. Spinal stenosis is commonly associated with achondroplasia and may cause signs related to compression of the spinal cord. It is important to note that achondroplasia does not result in any intellectual disabilities. A similar condition, **pseudoachondroplasia**, is due to a mutation in the cartilage oligomeric matrix protein (*COMP*) gene, which helps to keep chondrocytes viable during the process of endochondral ossification. This presents in a similar way to achondroplasia but has more pronounced joint laxity and spinal curvatures and does not typically cause foreshortening of the facial bones. As before, no intellectual delays are associated with this condition.

Patients of various ages with body disproportion (short limbs, relatively long trunk, large head) and limited flexion of elbows and hips

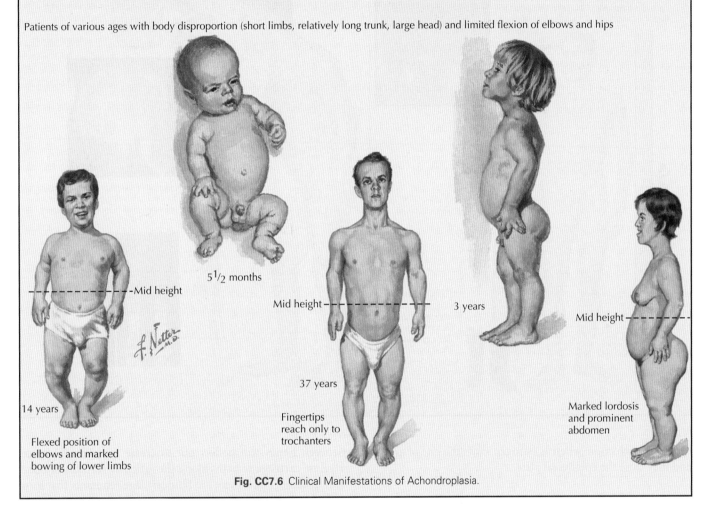

Fig. CC7.6 Clinical Manifestations of Achondroplasia.

CLINICAL CORRELATION 7.7   Proportionate Dwarfism

A different condition, **proportionate dwarfism**, occurs when there is too little GH to cause a pubertal growth spurt. In such cases, the limbs, face, and body retain typical proportions but will simply be smaller and shorter. Please note that the term "midget" has been used in the past for people fitting this description but is considered offensive and should not be used by health professionals (or others), with "little people" being considered an acceptable term at the time this was written.

- **Zone of proliferation**: as chondrocytes from the zone of reserve cartilage become active, they start to divide and form linear, **isogenous groups.** This is where the elongation of the epiphyseal plate occurs.

- **Zone of hypertrophy**: as the chondrocytes enter this region they enlarge and release alkaline phosphatase.
- **Zone of calcification**: the dead and dying chondrocytes are now encased in mineralized extracellular matrix.
- **Zone of resorption**: the calcified cartilage is broken down and replaced by bone as osteoblasts move in and begin to release osteoid using the calcified cartilage as a framework.

Eventually chondrocyte division slows down, the ossification centers of the epiphyses and metaphysis meet, and then fuse to create a single bone. At this moment the bone reaches its full length. Different epiphyseal plates close at different times, but the process is largely complete during the late teen years (Clinical Correlations 7.10 and 7.11). Hormonal signals affect the rate of cartilage proliferation. GH increases activity of

CLINICAL CORRELATION 7.8   Gigantism and Acromegaly

On the other side of the spectrum is an excess of GH (or IGF1) that causes extreme activity of the growth plates. This **gigantism** will often manifest in height well beyond the norm for the affected person's demographic background. This condition often results from a tumor of the GH-producing somatotrope cells of the anterior pituitary gland. If a person begins producing too much GH after reaching his or her mature height, he or she will have **acromegaly**. This condition causes the body to enlarge, with the forehead, jaw, neck, feet, and hands seeming to swell over time. As the jaw expands, the teeth become separated from each other. The voice may deepen as the larynx, which is made of cartilage, enlarges. However, the affected person does not gain any height because the cartilage growth plates are gone. As with gigantism, this is commonly due to a pituitary tumor.

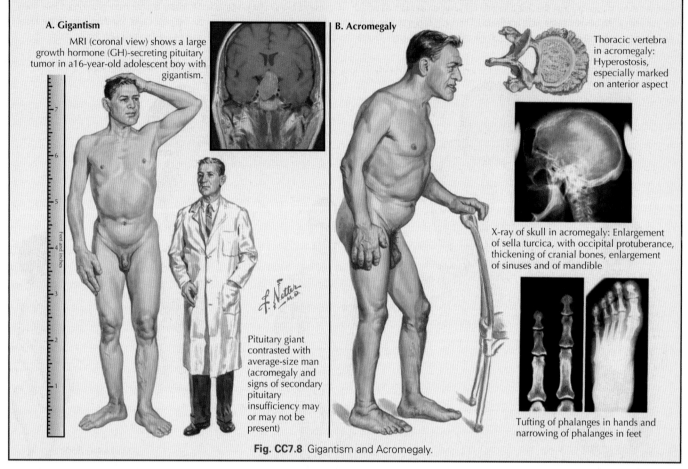

A. Gigantism

MRI (coronal view) shows a large growth hormone (GH)-secreting pituitary tumor in a16-year-old adolescent boy with gigantism.

Pituitary giant contrasted with average-size man (acromegaly and signs of secondary pituitary insufficiency may or may not be present)

B. Acromegaly

Thoracic vertebra in acromegaly: Hyperostosis, especially marked on anterior aspect

X-ray of skull in acromegaly: Enlargement of sella turcica, with occipital protuberance, thickening of cranial bones, enlargement of sinuses and of mandible

Tufting of phalanges in hands and narrowing of phalanges in feet

Fig. CC7.8 Gigantism and Acromegaly.

cartilage production, whereas estrogen slows the rate of growth and may close the epiphyseal plate.

DEVELOPMENT OF THE JOINTS (FIG. 7.14)

The early mesenchymal condensations at the core of each limb bud are initially all connected. As the limb elongates, the mesenchyme becomes less dense in the areas where synovial joints will form. The denser mesenchyme on either side of these areas will become cartilage and eventually bone; the loose mesenchyme between bones will hollow out to create the synovial space. Hyaline cartilage remains along the articular surfaces of bone, and in some joints, there are fibrocartilage remnants that form articular discs or menisci.

Initially, the fibrous outer lining of a joint is continuous with the periosteum of the ossifying bones. As development continues, the vascular synovial layer inside of the fibrous layer of the joint capsule will develop and secrete true synovial fluid. This is typically complete by the third month of development; the muscles become active, and the fetus starts moving (Clinical Correlation 7.12).

CLINICAL CORRELATION 7.9   Amelia, Meromelia, and Phocomelia

Disruption of the limb bud's growth can result in a variety of growth defects. If FGF8 is not expressed in the limb mesoderm and the AER does not form, there will be no limb in the affected area, called **amelia**. Disruption of *Hox* expression in the lengthening limb can result in a variety of malformations. Although there is some disagreement with this definition, **meromelia** is the failure of a portion of the limb to form while the hands or feet are present at the end of the shortened limb. A specific subtype of meromelia is called **phocomelia**, in which the hands and feet project from the shoulder without the arm and forearm in between.

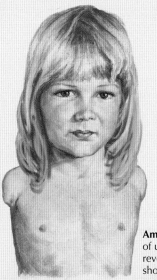

Phocomelia. Five-fingered hands attached directly to trunk. Arms and forearms absent. Fingers functional but may have some degree of motor deficit.

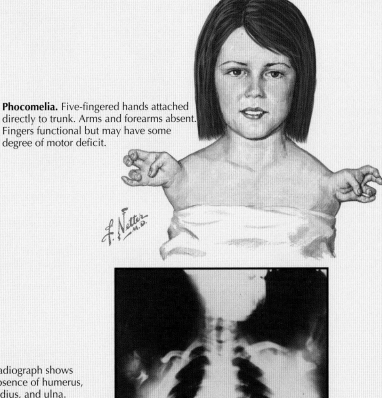

Amelia. Complete deficit of upper limbs. Radiograph reveals well-formed shoulder girdle.

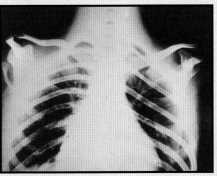

Radiograph shows absence of humerus, radius, and ulna. Rudimentary bone proximal to metacarpals cannot be identified.

Fig. CC7.9 Upper Limb Malformations.

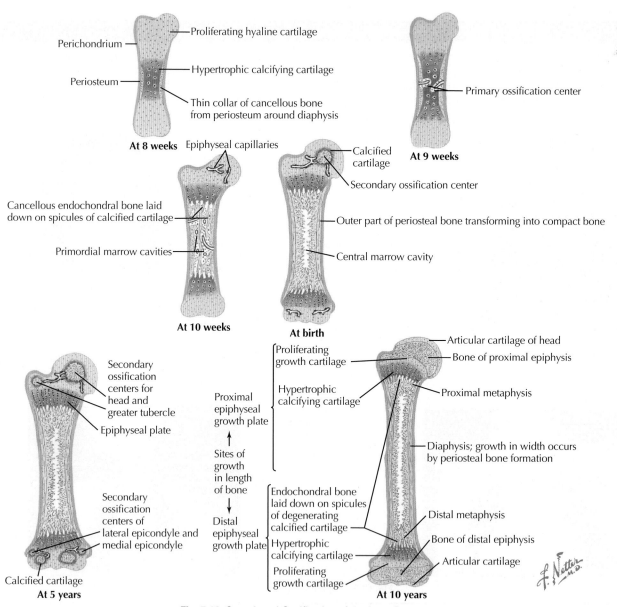

Perichondrium

Proliferating hyaline cartilage

Periosteum

Hypertrophic calcifying cartilage

Thin collar of cancellous bone from periosteum around diaphysis

At 8 weeks

Epiphyseal capillaries

Primary ossification center

At 9 weeks

Cancellous endochondral bone laid down on spicules of calcified cartilage

Primordial marrow cavities

At 10 weeks

Calcified cartilage

Secondary ossification center

Outer part of periosteal bone transforming into compact bone

Central marrow cavity

At birth

Secondary ossification centers for head and greater tubercle

Epiphyseal plate

Secondary ossification centers of lateral epicondyle and medial epicondyle

Calcified cartilage

At 5 years

Proliferating growth cartilage

Hypertrophic calcifying cartilage

Proximal epiphyseal growth plate

↑

Sites of growth in length of bone

↓

Distal epiphyseal growth plate

Endochondral bone laid down on spicules of degenerating calcified cartilage

Hypertrophic calcifying cartilage

Proliferating growth cartilage

Articular cartilage of head

Bone of proximal epiphysis

Proximal metaphysis

Diaphysis; growth in width occurs by periosteal bone formation

Distal metaphysis

Bone of distal epiphysis

Articular cartilage

At 10 years

Fig. 7.12 Growth and Ossification of the Long Bones.

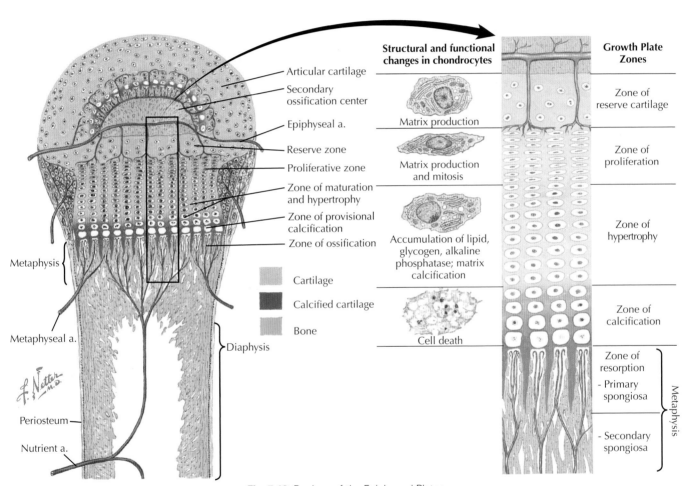

Fig. 7.13 Regions of the Epiphyseal Plates.

CLINICAL CORRELATION 7.10 Salter-Harris Fractures

Fractures involving growth plates, called **Salter-Harris fractures**, can be very serious because disruption of the plate can stall subsequent growth.

- **Type I Salter-Harris fracture:** No bony fracture but a shearing injury through the cartilaginous growth plate only.
- **Type II Salter-Harris fracture:** The facture line passes through the growth plate and some portion of the metaphysis.
- **Type III Salter-Harris fracture:** The fracture line passes through the growth plate and some portion of the epiphysis.

- **Type IV Salter-Harris fracture:** The fracture line passes through the epiphysis, growth plate, and metaphysis.
- **Type V Salter-Harris fracture:** Crush injury of the growth plate caused by compression by the epiphysis and metaphysis. This can occur without any bony fracture.
- **Type VI Salter-Harris fracture:** This involves a chip fracture on one side involving the metaphysis, epiphyseal plate, and epiphysis. When it heals, the new bone forms a pinch-point that will not grow. The rest of the plate continues to grow, causing deformation of the bone.

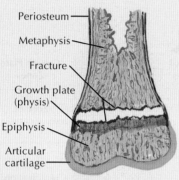

Periosteum
Metaphysis
Fracture
Growth plate (physis)
Epiphysis
Articular cartilage

Type I. Complete separation of epiphysis from shaft through calcified cartilage (growth zone) of growth plate. No bone actually fractured; periosteum may remain intact. Most common in newborns and young children

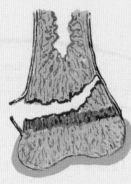

Type II. Most common. Line of separation extends partially across deep layer of growth plate and extends through metaphysis, leaving triangular portion of metaphysis attached to epiphyseal fragment

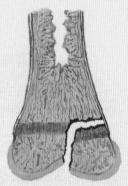

Type III. Uncommon. Intra-articular fracture through hepiphysis, across deep zone of growth plate to periphery. Open reduction and fixation often necessary

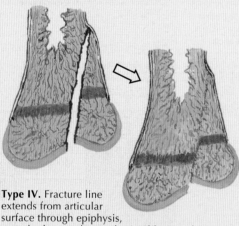

Type IV. Fracture line extends from articular surface through epiphysis, growth plate, and metaphysis. If fractured segment not perfectly realigned with open reduction, osseous bridge across growth plate may occur, resulting in partial growth arrest and joint angulation

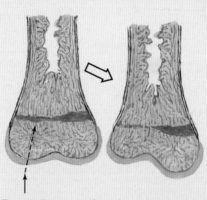

Type V. Severe crushing force transmitted across epiphysis to portion of growth plate by abduction or adduction stress or axial load. Minimal or no displacement makes radiographic diagnosis difficult; growth plate may nevertheless be damaged, resulting in partial growth arrest or shortening and angular deformity

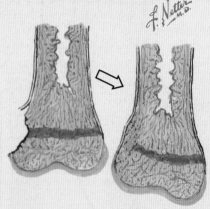

Type VI. Portion of growth plate sheared or cut off. Raw surface heals by forming bone bridge across growth plate, limiting growth on injured side and resulting in angular deformity

Fig. CC7.10 Injury to Growth Plate (Salter-Harris Classification, Rang Modification).

CLINICAL CORRELATION 7.11 False Fractures

Because cartilage is much less dense than bone, it allows x-rays to pass through its tissues and may appear dark on radiographs. Because of this, radiographs of infants, children, and adolescents may appear odd, with bone fragments appearing separate from the rest of the bones. Physicians occasionally misdiagnose fractures as a result. In fact, the spaces between these ossification centers are full of cartilage that has not yet transitioned to become bone.

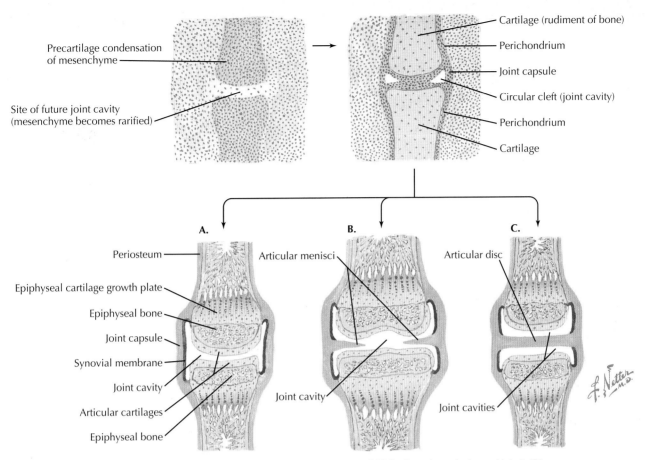

Precartilage condensation of mesenchyme

Site of future joint cavity (mesenchyme becomes rarified)

Cartilage (rudiment of bone)

Perichondrium

Joint capsule

Circular cleft (joint cavity)

Perichondrium

Cartilage

A.

B.

C.

Periosteum

Epiphyseal cartilage growth plate

Epiphyseal bone

Joint capsule

Synovial membrane

Joint cavity

Articular cartilages

Epiphyseal bone

Articular menisci

Joint cavity

Articular disc

Joint cavities

Fig. 7.14 Development of the Synovial Joints. (A) Typical synovial joint (e.g., interphalangeal joint); (B) synovial joint with menisci (e.g., knee); (C) synovial joint with articular disc (e.g., sternoclavicular joint).

CLINICAL CORRELATION 7.12   Clubfoot/Talipes Varus

If there is too little amniotic fluid in the uterus or the fetus is compressed (perhaps by a sibling sharing the uterus), he or she may be unable to move freely and help the synovial joints to develop at the correct angles. This can sometimes force the ankles to develop in a highly inverted/supinated position, called **clubbed feet** or **talipes varus**. This condition can also occur because of genetic causes, not exclusively positional ones. Prior to surgical correction, this caused life-long deformity. Fortunately, now we are able to brace the feet and reconnect the tendons in a way that allows the bones to develop properly during early childhood before they become fully ossified.

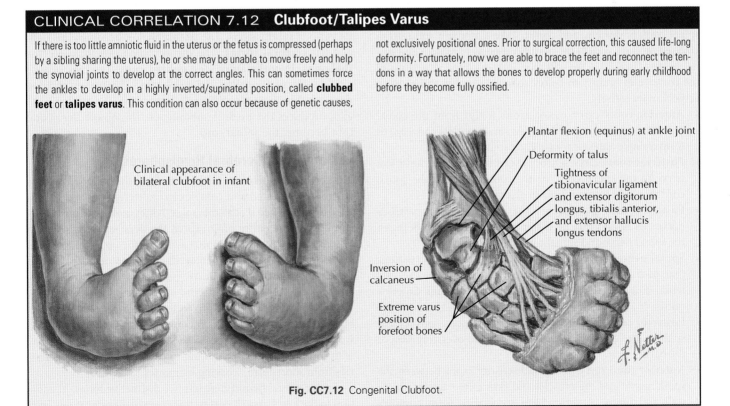

Clinical appearance of bilateral clubfoot in infant

Plantar flexion (equinus) at ankle joint

Deformity of talus

Tightness of tibionavicular ligament and extensor digitorum longus, tibialis anterior, and extensor hallucis longus tendons

Inversion of calcaneus

Extreme varus position of forefoot bones

Fig. CC7.12 Congenital Clubfoot.

The Central Nervous System in Relation to the Musculoskeletal System

INTRODUCTION

In Chapter 4 we discussed the peripheral nervous system in relation to the muscular compartments of the body. We will now go the other direction and examine the central nervous system and how it plans, executes, and edits motor activity of the skeletal muscles. We will also examine how information from the skin and muscles travels along sensory axons to reach targets in the spinal cord, brainstem, and cortex. Take a moment and refresh yourself on the basics of the peripheral nervous system and spinal nerves (Fig. 8.1). We will then introduce the structures of the cortex and brainstem before following motor and sensory activity in its entirety.

- **Anterior roots** carry motor axons (only) from the spinal cord to the spinal nerve. Multiple small rootlets converge to form a single anterior root at each spinal level.
- **Posterior roots** carry sensory axons (only) from the spinal nerve to the spinal cord. As the roots approach the spinal cord they split into multiple small rootlets.
- **Posterior root ganglia** are the pseudounipolar sensory nerve cell bodies that lie within the posterior root between the spinal nerve and spinal cord.
- **Spinal nerves** are combined motor and sensory structures that pass through the intervertebral foramina of the vertebral column. They later split into posterior and anterior rami.
- **Posterior rami** carry motor and sensory axons between the spinal nerve and the intrinsic muscles and overlying skin of the back.
- **Anterior rami** carry motor and sensory axons between the spinal nerve and the muscles and skin of the anterior body wall and limbs. Anterior rami sometimes form complex nervous structures (cervical, brachial, lumbar, and lumbosacral plexi) or they may remain separate (intercostal and subcostal nerves).

COMPONENTS OF THE CENTRAL NERVOUS SYSTEM

The central nervous system is derived from the neural tube and its various subdivisions. The telencephalon becomes the right and left **cerebral cortex**. The diencephalon develops into the **thalamus**, **hypothalamus**, and **epithalamus**. The mesencephalon produces (remains) the **midbrain**. The metencephalon develops into the **pons** and **cerebellum**, while the myelencephalon produces the **medulla oblongata**. The rest of the neural tube becomes the **spinal cord**.

Left and Right Cerebral Hemispheres

The cerebral **hemispheres**, "the brain," are the enlarged regions where sophisticated and complex neural activity takes place. It used to be believed that all mental activities took place uniformly throughout the entire brain. Later, the detailed study of brain lesions made scientists' opinion swing to the opposite extreme; it was thought that each mental function was tied explicitly to a specific region of the brain. We now know that both perspectives have some validity. Specific mental activities like speech, vision, and movement are linked to specific nervous locations but all these activities rely on connections to other regions to work optimally. Some processes like memory are very diffuse, with multiple areas contributing to creating long-term memories from short-term, working memories.

Each cerebral hemisphere has five distinctive **lobes**. In addition to the lobes of each cortex, there are smaller elevations, **gyri**

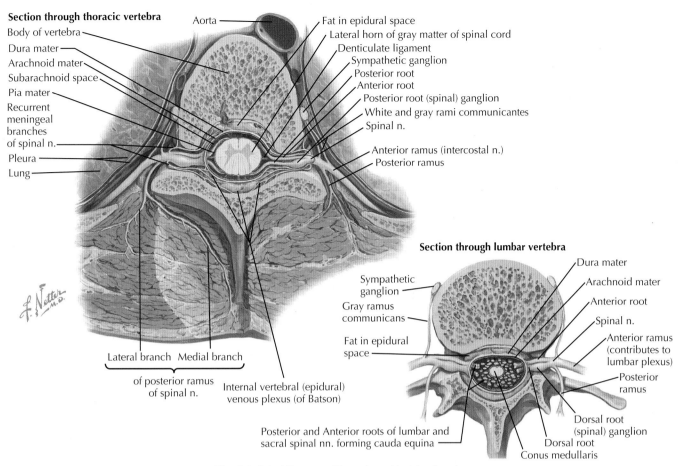

Section through thoracic vertebra
Body of vertebra
Dura mater
Arachnoid mater
Subarachnoid space
Pia mater
Recurrent meningeal branches of spinal n.
Pleura
Lung

Aorta

Fat in epidural space
Lateral horn of gray matter of spinal cord
Denticulate ligament
Sympathetic ganglion
Posterior root
Anterior root
Posterior root (spinal) ganglion
White and gray rami communicantes
Spinal n.
Anterior ramus (intercostal n.)
Posterior ramus

Lateral branch   Medial branch
of posterior ramus of spinal n.
Internal vertebral (epidural) venous plexus (of Batson)

Section through lumbar vertebra
Sympathetic ganglion
Gray ramus communicans
Fat in epidural space

Dura mater
Arachnoid mater
Anterior root
Spinal n.
Anterior ramus (contributes to lumbar plexus)
Posterior ramus
Dorsal root (spinal) ganglion
Dorsal root
Conus medullaris

Posterior and Anterior roots of lumbar and sacral spinal nn. forming cauda equina

Fig. 8.1 Spinal Nerves at Thoracic and Lumbar Levels.

(singular: gyrus) on the surface of the cortex, as well as grooves, **sulci** (singular: sulcus), between the gyri. The outside of each hemisphere consists of **gray matter**, called the **cortex**, which is composed of several layers of neuron cell bodies and axons. Deep to the gray matter is **white matter**, which is composed of large bundles of axons. White matter is "white" due to the fatty myelin sheathes that surround these axons. There are many structures in the central nervous system and we will be focusing on those that are related to musculoskeletal activity and sensations from the back and limbs. We will begin with some of the major landmarks in the cortex (Figs. 8.2 and 8.3).

- **Interlobar sulcus (longitudinal fissure):** this large gap separates the right and left hemispheres from each other. A large sickle-shaped fold of dura mater, the **falx cerebri**, sits in this space.
- **Frontal lobe:** involved in executive function, self-control, personality, motor planning, and the initiation of motor activity. The most anterior point of the frontal lobe is the **frontal pole.**
- **Parietal lobe:** where various types of sensory information are interpreted
- **Temporal lobe:** involved in auditory processing, generating memory, and emotions. The most anterior point of the temporal lobe is the **temporal pole.**
- **Lateral sulcus (Sylvian fissure):** a large cleft that separates the frontal and parietal lobes from the temporal lobe.

- **Occipital lobe:** receives and processes visual input from the retina. The most posterior point of the occipital lobe is the **occipital pole.**
- **Insular lobe:** involved in hearing, speech, and the perception of pain. It is normally covered by the temporal, frontal, and parietal lobes. If the lateral fissure is opened, the insular lobe can be seen.

From a lateral view, we can see the following features of the cortex (see Fig. 8.2).

- **Superior frontal gyrus, middle frontal gyrus,** and **inferior frontal gyrus:** these three gyri are located on the anterolateral aspect of the frontal lobe. They are separated from each other by the **superior frontal sulcus** and **inferior frontal sulcus.** The inferior frontal gyrus has a triangular region near the temporal pole that is subdivided into an orbital part, a triangular part, and an opercular part.
- **Precentral sulcus:** separates the superior, middle, and inferior frontal gyri from the precentral gyrus
- **Precentral gyrus:** this gyrus is the **primary motor cortex** and contains the **upper motor neurons (UMNs)** that project to the **lower motor neurons (LMNs)** within the anterior horn of the spinal cord. It is found on the lateral and superior cortex, extending onto the upper medial aspect of the cortex.
- **Central sulcus:** separates the precentral gyrus of the frontal lobe from the postcentral gyrus of the parietal lobe.

Lateral view of Cerebral Cortex and Lobes

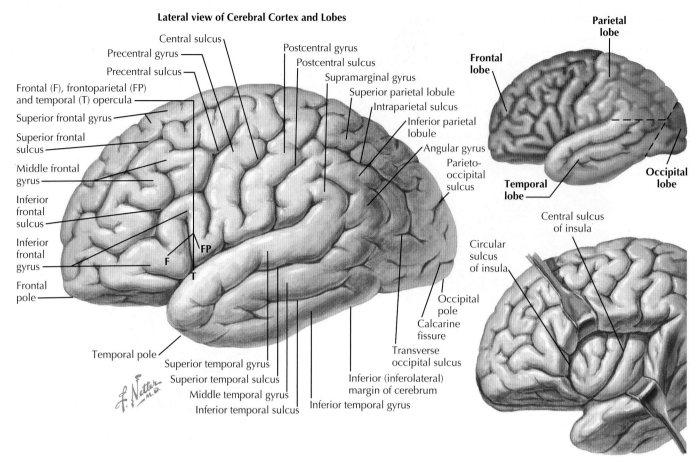

Fig. 8.2 Lateral View of Cerebral Cortex and Lobes.

- **Postcentral gyrus**: this gyrus is the **primary somatosensory cortex.** Sensory inputs from all over the body arrive here after passing through nuclei in the thalamus. It runs parallel to the precentral gyrus and covers the lateral, superior, and medial sides of the cortex.
- **Postcentral sulcus**: separates the postcentral gyrus from the rest of the parietal lobe
- Superior parietal lobule and inferior parietal lobules: located posterior to the postcentral gyrus and separated from each other by the interparietal sulcus.
- Parieto-occipital sulcus: this sulcus is barely visible on the lateral aspect of the brain but is much better pronounced on the medial side.
- Superior temporal gyrus, middle temporal gyrus, and inferior temporal gyrus: these are seen on the lateral aspect of the temporal lobe and are separated from each other by the superior temporal sulcus and inferior temporal sulcus.

    From a medial view of the cortex we can appreciate the following (see Fig. 8.3).
- **Corpus callosum**: the most distinct feature of the medial view is this massive, C-shaped structure located at the base of the longitudinal fissure and it is made from many axons that connect the right and left hemispheres. It is concave inferiorly.
  - **Genu**: the most anterior part of the corpus callosum.
  - **Rostrum**: continues posteriorly from the genu, quickly becoming much smaller. It is close to another bundle of

axons passing between the right and left sides of the cortex, the anterior commissure.
- **Body**: the largest portion of the corpus callosum runs from anterior to posterior.
- **Splenium**: the most posterior portion of the corpus callosum sits just superior to the pineal gland and midbrain.
- **Fornix**: this bundle of axons originates from the inferior aspect of the temporal lobe and is visible on the medial view of the brain, just inferior to the corpus callosum. Axons within the two structures do not connect but they are bridged by a thin sheet of pia mater, the **septum pellucidum**, which separates the two lateral ventricles.
- **Cingulate gyrus**: this large gyrus runs parallel to the corpus callosum crossing from the frontal lobe to the parietal lobe. It is separated from the corpus callosum by the **callosal sulcus.**
- Medial frontal gyrus: this huge gyrus parallels the cingulate gyrus and is separated from it by the cingulate sulcus.
- **Paracentral lobule**: this area is located at the posterior end of the medial frontal gyrus and contains the extensions of the precentral and postcentral gyri. It is bounded anteriorly by the precentral sulcus and posteriorly by the postcentral sulcus; therefore, its anterior and posterior parts are shared by the frontal and parietal lobes, respectively. The central sulcus can be seen on its superior aspect but does not extend through the lobule.

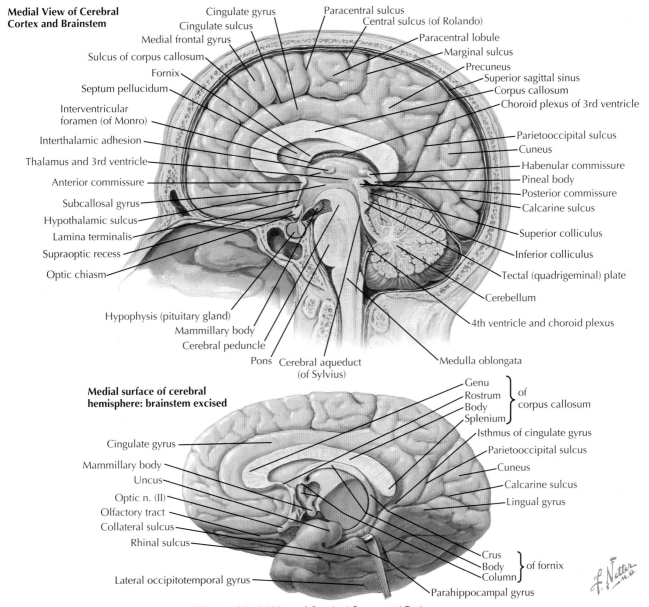

Medial View of Cerebral Cortex and Brainstem

Cingulate gyrus
Cingulate sulcus
Medial frontal gyrus
Sulcus of corpus callosum
Fornix
Septum pellucidum
Interventricular foramen (of Monro)
Interthalamic adhesion
Thalamus and 3rd ventricle
Anterior commissure
Subcallosal gyrus
Hypothalamic sulcus
Lamina terminalis
Supraoptic recess
Optic chiasm

Paracentral sulcus
Central sulcus (of Rolando)
Paracentral lobule
Marginal sulcus
Precuneus
Superior sagittal sinus
Corpus callosum
Choroid plexus of 3rd ventricle
Parietooccipital sulcus
Cuneus
Habenular commissure
Pineal body
Posterior commissure
Calcarine sulcus
Superior colliculus
Inferior colliculus
Tectal (quadrigeminal) plate
Cerebellum
4th ventricle and choroid plexus

Hypophysis (pituitary gland)
Mammillary body
Cerebral peduncle
Pons   Cerebral aqueduct (of Sylvius)
Medulla oblongata

Medial surface of cerebral hemisphere: brainstem excised

Cingulate gyrus
Mammillary body
Uncus
Optic n. (II)
Olfactory tract
Collateral sulcus
Rhinal sulcus
Lateral occipitotemporal gyrus

Genu
Rostrum } of
Body   } corpus callosum
Splenium
Isthmus of cingulate gyrus
Parietooccipital sulcus
Cuneus
Calcarine sulcus
Lingual gyrus
Crus
Body } of fornix
Column
Parahippocampal gyrus

Fig. 8.3 Medial View of Cerebral Cortex and Brainstem.

White Matter Structures of the Cortex (see Figs. 8.3–8.5)

Commissures or **commissural fibers** pass contralaterally between the two sides of the cortex. The massive **corpus callosum** on the medial aspect of the cortex sits just superior to the diencephalon and forms the roof of the lateral ventricles. The left and right frontal lobes are interconnected by axons passing through the genu of the corpus callosum; likewise, the left and right occipital lobes connect through the splenium of the corpus callosum.

Other commissures are much smaller than the corpus callosum.

- Anterior commissure: this bundle connects parts of the frontal and temporal lobes as well as the olfactory tracts.
- Hippocampal commissure: these fibers originate in the hippocampal formation of the temporal lobe, enter the fornix, and cross to the opposite fornix, creating a thin sheet of axons.

- Posterior and habenular commissures: these two, small bundles connect the structures of the epithalamus and midbrain tectum.

Projections or **projection fibers** connect the cortex to other regions of the central nervous system. These projection fibers form a large, V-shaped structure called the **internal capsule**. It has an **anterior limb** that is sandwiched between the caudate nucleus of the basal ganglia medially and the putamen and globus pallidus of the basal ganglia laterally. The **posterior limb** is similarly pressed between the thalamus medially and the lenticular nuclei of the basal ganglia laterally. The **genu** of the internal capsule connects both limbs.

Fibers and functions of the regions of the internal capsule:

- **Anterior limb**: contains axons that are traveling from the frontal lobe to the pons (**frontopontine fibers**) as well as axons from the thalamus to the frontal lobe (**anterior thalamic radiations**).

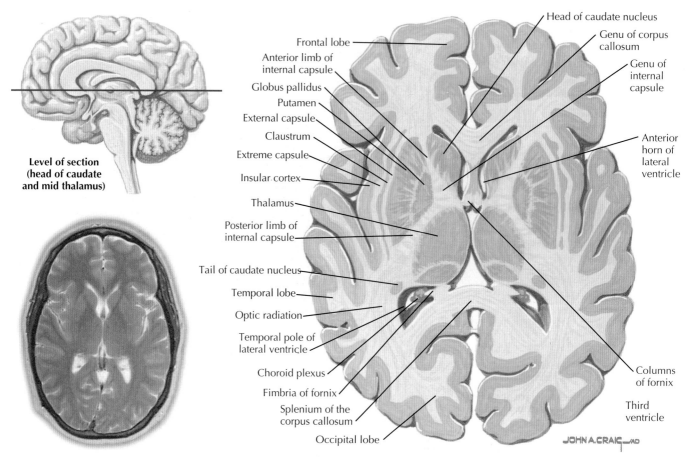

Level of section (head of caudate and mid thalamus)

Frontal lobe
Anterior limb of internal capsule
Globus pallidus
Putamen
External capsule
Claustrum
Extreme capsule
Insular cortex
Thalamus
Posterior limb of internal capsule
Tail of caudate nucleus
Temporal lobe
Optic radiation
Temporal pole of lateral ventricle
Choroid plexus
Fimbria of fornix
Splenium of the corpus callosum
Occipital lobe

Head of caudate nucleus
Genu of corpus callosum
Genu of internal capsule
Anterior horn of lateral ventricle
Columns of fornix
Third ventricle

JOHN A. CRAIG—MD

Fig. 8.4 Horizontal Sections Through the Forebrain: Anterior Commissure and Caudal Thalamus.

- **Genu:** contains upper motor axons (**corticonuclear** or **corticobulbar tract**) from the frontal lobes, particularly the precentral gyrus and nearby areas, that innervate LMNs in the cranial nerve nuclei of the brainstem.
- Posterior limb: this large structure contains upper motor axons (**corticospinal tracts**) from the frontal lobes to LMNs in the spinal cord. The central thalamic radiations contain axons travelling between the cortex and thalamus.

The axons of the various **association fibers** connect different parts of the cortex to each other ipsilaterally. **Short association fibers** form small bundles that interconnect adjacent gyri, while **long association fibers** connect more widely separated areas of each hemisphere. There are some important long association fibers to consider.

- Superior longitudinal (arcuate) fasciculus: connects frontal, parietal, and occipital lobes, located close to the surface of the cortex.
- Occipitofrontal fasciculus: connects frontal, temporal, and occipital lobes.
- Inferior longitudinal fasciculus: connects temporal and occipital lobes.
- Uncinate fasciculus: connects frontal and temporal lobes anteriorly.
- Cingulum: this fiber bundle runs from the cingulate gyrus (immediately superior to corpus callosum) to the hippocampus in the temporal lobe.

DIENCEPHALON—THALAMUS, HYPOTHALAMUS, AND PINEAL GLAND

Thalamus (Fig. 8.6)

The thalami are egg-shaped structures at the superior end of the brainstem and are surrounded by the lobes of the cerebral hemispheres. They act as a "switchboard" for the central nervous system, routing sensory information to a variety of other cortical locations.

Midline thalamic nuclei are found adjacent to the third ventricle. A Y-shaped white matter tract, the **internal medullary lamina**, divides the thalamus into **anterior, medial**, and **lateral nuclear groups**. Some **intralaminar nuclei** are located within the lamina itself. The lateral thalamus is covered by a diffuse network of nerve cells, the **thalamic reticular nucleus**, immediately medial to the posterior limb of the internal capsule.

Most thalamic nuclei can be described as **relay nuclei** since they receive inputs and route them to distinct regions of the cortex. There are many of these relay nuclei scattered throughout the thalamus. I will only list those that directly impact the musculoskeletal system.

- **Ventral lateral (VL):** receives inputs from the basal ganglia, a collection of neurons that organize and initiate movement, as well as the deep cerebellar nuclei, which are the main outputs of the cerebellum and help to make movements smooth and organized. VL axons project to the precentral gyrus

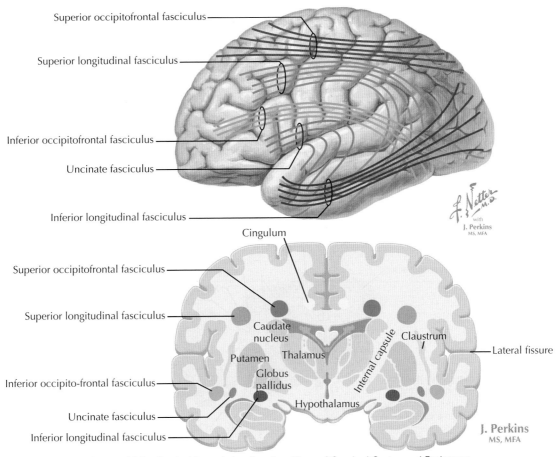

Superior occipitofrontal fasciculus

Superior longitudinal fasciculus

Inferior occipitofrontal fasciculus

Uncinate fasciculus

Inferior longitudinal fasciculus

Cingulum

Superior occipitofrontal fasciculus

Superior longitudinal fasciculus

Caudate nucleus

Putamen   Thalamus

Globus pallidus

Claustrum

Internal capsule

Lateral fissure

Hypothalamus

Inferior occipito-frontal fasciculus

Uncinate fasciculus

Inferior longitudinal fasciculus

Fig. 8.5 Major Cortical Association Bundles: View of Cerebral Cortex and Brainstem.

and premotor areas of the frontal lobe and tend to stimulate motor activity.

- **Ventral posterior lateral (VPL)**: this nucleus receives somatosensory input from afferent tracts of the body: medial lemniscus and spinothalamic tract. Neurons from the VPL then project to medial, superior, and superolateral regions of the postcentral gyrus of the parietal lobe.
- **Ventral posterior medial (VPM)**: this nucleus receives somatosensory input from the major afferent tracts of the head: the trigeminal lemniscus and trigeminothalamic tract. Neurons from the VPM then project to the lateral region of the postcentral gyrus of the parietal lobe.

The **intralaminar nuclei** also act to relay information but receive inputs from the basal ganglia and relay these inputs back to the basal ganglia and the cerebral cortex. This system will be discussed in detail at the end of the chapter with the rest of the basal ganglia. The **thalamic reticular nucleus** acts to inhibit the activity of other thalamic nuclei.

Hypothalamus and Pituitary Gland (Fig. 8.7)

The thalamus and **hypothalamus** are separated from each other by the **hypothalamic sulcus**. The posterior hypothalamus has two large bumps that are visible on the inferior surface of the brain, the **mammillary bodies**. Just anterior to the mammillary bodies is the **pituitary gland**. The hypothalamus and pituitary gland are intimately linked to control endocrine

functions that affect growth, sexual development, and water balance.

The hypothalamic nuclei can be grouped (from medial to lateral) into a periventricular nucleus, medial hypothalamic area, and lateral hypothalamic area. However, they can also be grouped (from anterior to posterior) into a preoptic area, anterior (supraoptic) area, middle (tuberal) area, and posterior (mammillary) area.

The **paraventricular nucleus** and **lateral area** contain neurons that supply axons to the descending autonomic tracts in order to modulate the activity of the parasympathetic and sympathetic systems. The lateral and medial areas regulate appetite; lateral lesions result in over-satiety and refusal to eat, while medial lesions cause insatiable eating and obesity. Nuclei in the anterior and posterior areas help regulate wakefulness with anterior lesions causing insomnia (inability to sleep) and posterior lesions causing hypersomnia (persistent sleep). Anterior and posterior area nuclei also control thermoregulation with anterior lesions causing hyperthermia and posterior lesions resulting in a "cold-blooded" status, where body temperature fluctuates with the external environment (Clinical Correlation 8.1).

The pituitary gland acts as the conductor for the endocrine system of the body and therefore affects many systems. It has a posterior lobe that develops as a down-growth of the hypothalamus and remains functionally linked to it. It releases antidiuretic hormone to influence water balance in the body as well as oxytocin, to stimulate uterine contraction and milk release.

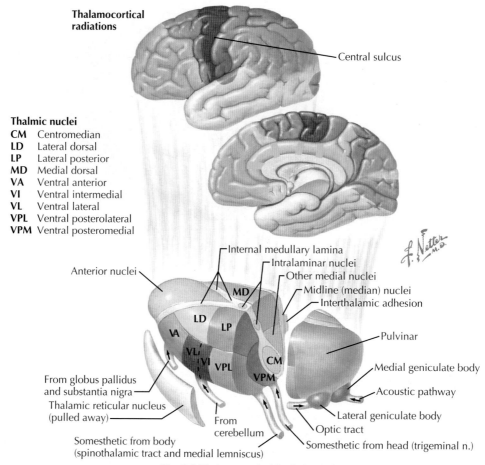

Fig. 8.6 Thalamocortical Radiations.

The anterior lobe of the pituitary gland develops from the roof of the oral cavity and migrates upward to meet the posterior lobe. It releases many hormones that affect reproductive development as well as **thyrotropic** hormone, which will stimulate the release of thyroid hormones. The anterior lobe hormone with the most direct effect on the musculoskeletal system is **growth hormone (GH)**, which is released by acidophilic (pink) **somatotrope cells**. GH promotes the release of insulin-like growth factor, which then stimulates the growth of skeletal muscle and the division of cartilage cells in the epiphyseal (growth) plates of developing bones.

Epithalamus (see Fig. 8.3)

The **epithalamus** sits posterosuperior to the thalamus and consists of Habenular nuclei and the **pineal gland**. The latter structure receives visual input from the optic nerve via intermediary neurons and helps to regulate seasonal cycles of activity based on ambient light levels. It often develops calcified regions with age and can serve as a radiographic landmark. It has little direct impact on the musculoskeletal system, so we will leave it for now.

MESENCEPHALON—MIDBRAIN (FIG. 8.8)

The midbrain has an anterior **tegmental region** and a posterior **tectum**, or "roof," that is also sometimes called the **quadrigeminal plate**. The cerebral aqueduct is located between the tegmentum and tectum and is surrounded by a distinctive tube

of neurons, the periaqueductal gray matter, which is involved in pain modulation. Some structures that impact the function of the musculoskeletal system are listed.

Tegmentum of Midbrain

- Oculomotor nucleus (cranial nerve III): provides motor innervation to four of the six extraocular muscles, the superior rectus, inferior rectus, medial rectus, and inferior oblique, as well as a muscle of the upper eyelid, the levator palpebrae superioris.
- Edinger-Westphal nucleus (cranial nerve III): provides preganglionic parasympathetic innervation to the oculomotor nerve
- Trochlear nucleus (cranial nerve IV): provides motor innervation to one extraocular muscle, the superior oblique muscle.
- Mesencephalic trigeminal nucleus (cranial nerve V): receives proprioceptive sensory input from the teeth and temporomandibular joint.
- **Red nucleus**: seen in the superior portion of the midbrain, it contains UMNs that project through the **rubrospinal tract** to innervate (primarily) flexor muscles of the upper limb. In humans, this tract is secondary to the more prominent lateral corticospinal tract.
- **Substantia nigra**: part of the basal ganglia, which help to plan and initiate movement.
- **Crus cerebri/cerebral peduncles**: Large white matter bundles that carry UMNs from the cortex to the pons, medulla,

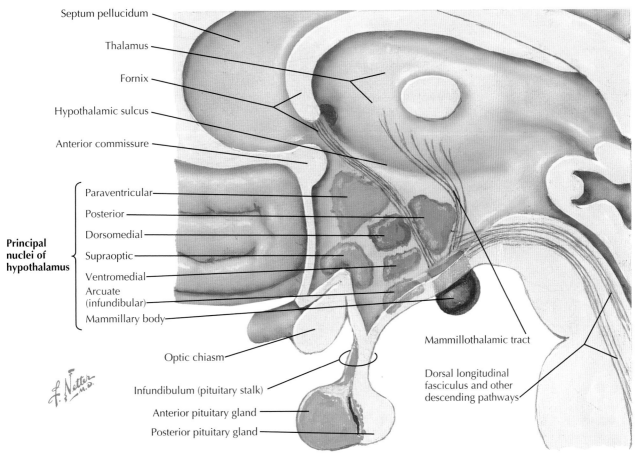

Septum pellucidum

Thalamus

Fornix

Hypothalamic sulcus

Anterior commissure

Principal nuclei of hypothalamus

Paraventricular

Posterior

Dorsomedial

Supraoptic

Ventromedial

Arcuate (infundibular)

Mammillary body

Optic chiasm

Infundibulum (pituitary stalk)

Anterior pituitary gland

Posterior pituitary gland

Mammillothalamic tract

Dorsal longitudinal fasciculus and other descending pathways

Fig. 8.7 Hypothalamus and Hypophysis.

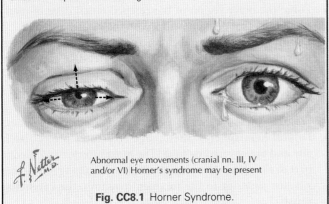

CLINICAL CORRELATION 8.1   Horner Syndrome

Horner syndrome consists of a droopy eyelid (ptosis), persistently constricted pupil (myosis), facial redness and flushing, and lack of sweat (anhydrosis) on the affected side. This constellation of neurologic signs is caused by disruption of the sympathetic nerve supply to the head. This can occur peripherally if the sympathetic (paravertebral) chain or superior cervical ganglia are damaged. It can also occur centrally if the descending sympathetic tract from the hypothalamus to the spinal cord is damaged.

Abnormal eye movements (cranial nn. III, IV and/or VI) Horner's syndrome may be present

Fig. CC8.1 Horner Syndrome.

- **Medial lemniscus**: conveys vibration, proprioception, and fine touch sensation from the body to the VPL thalamus.
- **Anterolateral system (ALS)**: conveys pain and temperature sensation from the body to sites in the brainstem, particularly the VPL thalamus.
- **Decussation of the superior cerebellar peduncles**: these are large white matter tracts that connect the midbrain to the cerebellum
- Reticular formation: a collection of nuclei near the midline that are involved in a variety of functions, including wakefulness.

Tectum of Midbrain

- Superior colliculus: helps coordinate the body's responses to visual input
- Inferior colliculus: involved in processing auditory input

METENCEPHALON—PONS AND CEREBELLUM (FIGS. 8.9 AND 8.10)

The **pons** and medulla sit anterior to the **fourth ventricle** while the **cerebellum** is posterior to it.

Pons

- **Pontine nuclei**: these neuron cell bodies are present in the anterior pons, the **pontine basis.** Their axons project laterally

and spinal cord. The **corticonuclear tract** provides UMNs to innervate cranial nerve nuclei and **corticospinal tract** axons will innervate LMNs in the anterior horn of the spinal cord.

A. Level of the Superior Colliculus

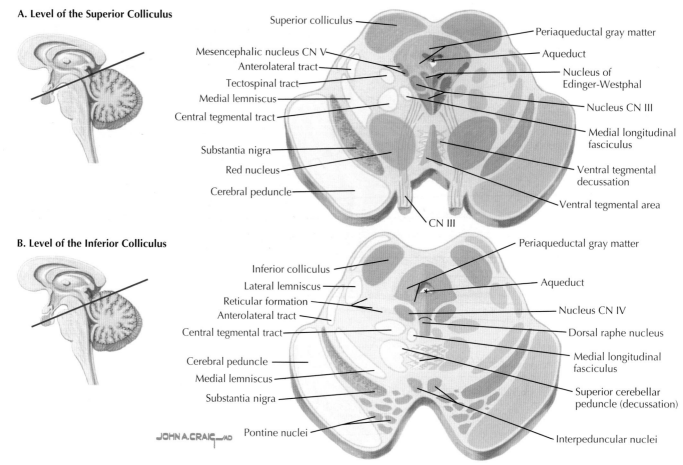

B. Level of the Inferior Colliculus

JOHN A. CRAIG—AD

Fig. 8.8 Cross Sections of the Midbrain.

and posteriorly as **pontocerebellar fibers** to create the middle cerebellar peduncle.

- **Middle cerebellar peduncle**: connects and conveys axons from the pons to the cerebellum.
- **Trigeminal motor nucleus (cranial nerve V)**: provides motor innervation to the muscles of mastication and related muscles from the first pharyngeal arch.
- Chief sensory trigeminal nucleus (cranial nerve V): receives fine touch sensory input from the head.
- Abducens nucleus (cranial nerve VI): provides motor innervation to one extraocular muscle, the lateral rectus.
- **Facial motor nucleus (cranial nerve VII)**: provides motor innervation to the muscles of facial expression and related muscles of the second pharyngeal arch.
- Superior salivatory nucleus (cranial nerve VII): provides preganglionic parasympathetic innervation to the facial nerve
- **Vestibular nuclei** and cochlear nuclei (cranial nerve VIII): receive balance and auditory inputs from the inner ear and project them to other sites in the brainstem and cortex.
- **Corticonuclear and corticospinal tracts**: these tracts continue from the crus cerebri of the midbrain and travel inferiorly, passing between the pontine nuclei.
- **Medial lemniscus**: conveys vibration, proprioception, and fine touch sensation from the body to the VPL thalamus.

- **Anterolateral system**: conveys pain and temperature sensation from the body to sites in the brainstem, particularly the VPL thalamus.
- Reticular formation: a collection of nuclei near the midline that are involved in a variety of functions, including wakefulness.

The **cerebellum** is involved in coordinating ongoing motor activity to make it smooth and precise. Its functions will be described in detail at the end of this chapter.

- **Folia**: the outer region of the cerebellum consists of many small **folia** that contain neurons on their outer surface.
- **Lobules**: when the cerebellum is cut in the sagittal plane, its white matter core has a distinctive tree-like appearance and is poetically called the "**arbor vitae**" or "tree of life." Each branch of this tree plus the associated folia is called a lobule.
- **Fissures**: these are the spaces that separate adjacent lobules.
- **Lateral hemispheres**: these large structures project laterally and are covered by folia. The most inferior and medial part of each lateral hemisphere ends as a bulging lobule that sits just superior to the foramen magnum, the **cerebellar tonsils.**
- **Vermis**: a midline collection of lobules that runs across the superior surface of the cerebellum and inferiorly, terminating as the **nodule.**

A. Level of Trigeminal Motor and Main Sensory Nuclei

B. Level of the Genu of the Facial Nerve

C. Level of the Facial Nucleus

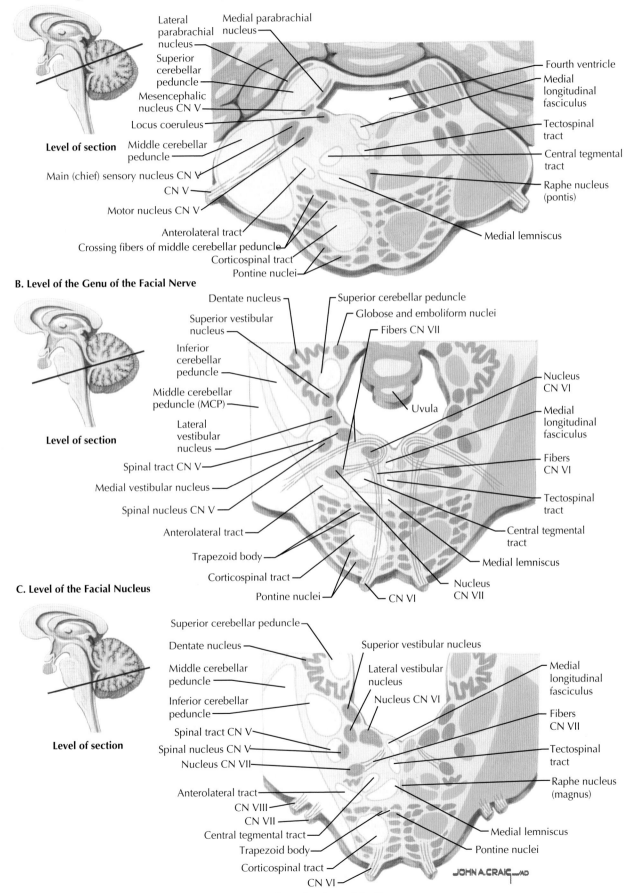

JOHN A.CRAIG—AD

Fig. 8.9 Cross Sections of the Pons.

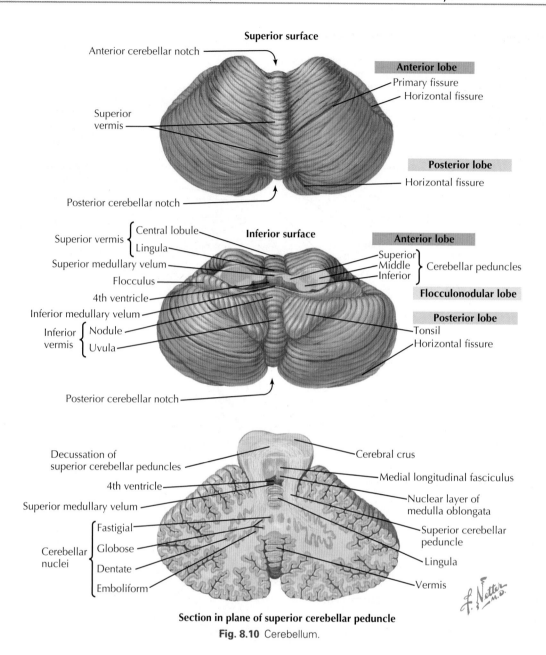

Superior surface

Anterior cerebellar notch

Anterior lobe
Primary fissure
Horizontal fissure

Superior vermis

Posterior lobe
Horizontal fissure

Posterior cerebellar notch

Inferior surface

Superior vermis { Central lobule
Lingula

Anterior lobe

Superior medullary velum

Superior
Middle } Cerebellar peduncles
Inferior

Flocculus

4th ventricle

Flocculonodular lobe

Inferior medullary velum

Posterior lobe

Inferior vermis { Nodule
Uvula

Tonsil
Horizontal fissure

Posterior cerebellar notch

Decussation of superior cerebellar peduncles

Cerebral crus

Medial longitudinal fasciculus

4th ventricle

Superior medullary velum

Nuclear layer of medulla oblongata

Cerebellar nuclei { Fastigial
Globose
Dentate
Emboliform

Superior cerebellar peduncle

Lingula

Vermis

Section in plane of superior cerebellar peduncle
Fig. 8.10 Cerebellum.

- **Anterior lobe**: formed by lobules 1 to 5 of the vermis and lateral hemispheres.
- **Posterior lobe**: formed by lobules 6 to 9 of the vermis and lateral hemisphere.
- **Primary fissure**: a cleft between lobules on the superior side of the cerebellum that separates its anterior and posterior lobes.
- **Flocculus**: a left and right flocculus is located lateral to the nodule on the anterior side of the cerebellum. The nodulus and flocculus are made from the 10th lobule of the cerebellum. They are functionally linked and sometimes are referred to as the **flocculonodular lobe.**
- **Posterolateral fissure**: separates the flocculonodular lobe from the rest of the cerebellum.
- **Deep cerebellar nuclei**: within the white matter of the cerebellum are the four deep cerebellar nuclei, the **dentate, emboliform, globose**, and **fastigial**. These receive inputs

from the spinal cord, medulla, and cerebellar folia; their outputs pass through the superior cerebellar peduncle to targets in the brainstem. The circuitry related to these nuclei will be discussed later in the chapter.
- **Inferior cerebellar peduncle**: connects the medulla to the cerebellum. It contains axons travelling to the cerebellum from the spinal cord, the **restiform body**, as well as fibers connecting the cerebellum to the vestibular nuclei, the **juxtarestiform body.**
- **Middle cerebellar peduncle**: connects the pons to the cerebellum and unsurprisingly contains pontocerebellar fibers that originate from pontine nuclei.
- **Superior cerebellar peduncle**: connects the midbrain to the cerebellum. It mostly contains axons leaving the deep cerebellar nuclei that decussate in the tegmentum of the midbrain. Some axons from the spinal cord enter the cerebellum via the superior cerebellar peduncle.

MYELENCEPHALON—MEDULLA OBLONGATA (FIG. 8.11)

Like the pons, the medulla sits anterior to the **fourth ventricle** and the **cerebellum**.

- **Inferior cerebellar peduncle**: connects the medulla to the cerebellum (see above).
- Spinal trigeminal nucleus (cranial nerves V, VII, IX, X): receives pain and temperature sensory input from the head and parts of the neck via several cranial nerves.
- Solitary nucleus and tract (cranial nerves VII, IX, X): receives taste sensation from the tongue and viscerosensory input from the organs of the body.
- **Vestibular nuclei** and cochlear nuclei (cranial nerve VIII): receive balance and auditory inputs from the inner ear and project them to other sites in the brainstem and cortex.
- **Vestibulospinal tracts**: several vestibulospinal tracts project from the vestibular nuclei to the spinal cord to coordinate movement as the body shifts position.
- Dorsal vagal motor nucleus (cranial nerve X): provides preganglionic parasympathetic innervation to the vagus nerve.
- **Nucleus ambiguus (cranial nerves IX and X)**: provides motor innervation to muscles of the palate, pharynx, and larynx.
- Inferior salivatory nucleus (cranial nerve IX): provides preganglionic parasympathetic innervation to the glossopharyngeal nerve
- **Hypoglossal nucleus (cranial nerve XII)**: provides motor innervation to the muscles of the tongue.
- **Medullary pyramids**: these large structures are present on the anterior surface of the medulla and contain the corticospinal tract axons that are travelling to the spinal cord. Most fibers in this structure decussate to the opposite side at the **pyramidal decussation** just before the medulla transitions into the spinal cord.
- **Medial lemniscus**: conveys vibration, proprioception, and fine touch sensation from the body to the VPL thalamus.
- **Anterolateral system**: conveys pain and temperature sensation from the body to sites in the brainstem, particularly the VPL thalamus.
- **Reticular formation**: a collection of nuclei near the midline that are involved in a variety of functions, including wakefulness and motor activity.
- **Inferior olivary nucleus**: located lateral to the medullary pyramids, this structure relays information between itself and the cerebellum.

SPINAL CORD (FIG. 8.12)

The interior of the spinal cord is made of nerve cell bodies, called gray matter, with the central canal at its core. The gray matter appears as a roughly butterfly-shaped structure in cross section, with the "wings" formed by an anterior horn and posterior horn on each side.

- **Posterior horn**: contains sensory neurons as well as interneurons that connect with other regions of the spinal gray matter.

- **Anterior horn**: contains LMNs that project their axons out through the anterior spinal roots to innervate skeletal muscle.
- **Intermediate zone**: contains:
  - **Interneurons**: present at all levels of the spinal cord, these neurons allow communication between different regions of the spinal cord.
  - **Spinal accessory nucleus (cranial nerve XI)**: present in upper cervical levels only, these LMNs innervate the trapezius and sternocleidomastoid muscles.
  - **Nucleus dorsalis of Clarke**: present from T1 to L2 levels, projects proprioceptive input from the body to the cerebellum.
  - **Intermediolateral cell column**: present from T1 to L2, supplies preganglionic sympathetic axons to innervate visceral structures of the body.

The white matter on the outside of the gray matter consists of sensory (afferent) axons ascending toward the brainstem or cortex as well as motor (efferent) axons travelling from the cortex and brainstem to the gray matter of the cord. The large white matter regions of the spinal cord are called **columns** or **lemnisci** and contain multiple functional tracts:

- **Dorsal columns**: contains ascending sensory tracts conveying proprioceptive, vibration, and fine touch stimuli (dorsal column-medial lemniscal system) that synapse with nuclei in the medulla.
- **Lateral columns**: contains descending motor tracts to control willful motion (lateral corticospinal and rubrospinal tracts) that synapse with nerves in the anterior horn. It also contains ascending sensory tracts (dorsal and ventral spinocerebellar tracts) to the cerebellum.
- **Anterior columns**: the anteromedial white matter of the spinal cord contains descending motor tracts (anterior corticospinal, medial and lateral vestibulospinal, reticulospinal, and tectospinal tracts) that synapse with nerve cells in the anterior horn. More laterally (where it overlaps with the lateral column) is the ALS, an ascending sensory tract that conveys pain, temperature, and crude touch to nuclei in several regions of the brainstem and VPL thalamus.
- As sensory axons from the posterior root ganglia enter the spinal cord, they may briefly ascend in a tract just superficial to the posterior horn of the spinal cord, called **Lissauer tract.** Once inside the cord, sensory axons can travel to one of several white matter columns or into gray matter.

The spinal cord is visibly enlarged in the regions that innervate the upper and lower limbs, called the **cervical** and **lumbosacral enlargements**, respectively. The white matter tracts are much thicker in the superior cervical region since the most descending tract axons that have not yet reached their targets in the gray matter and almost all ascending tract axons have already entered the spinal cord.

FLOW OF CEREBROSPINAL FLUID (FIG. 8.13)

The ependymal cells that line the lateral, third, and fourth ventricles develop vascular tufts, called the **choroid plexus**. The choroid plexus filters blood to release **cerebrospinal fluid** (CSF)

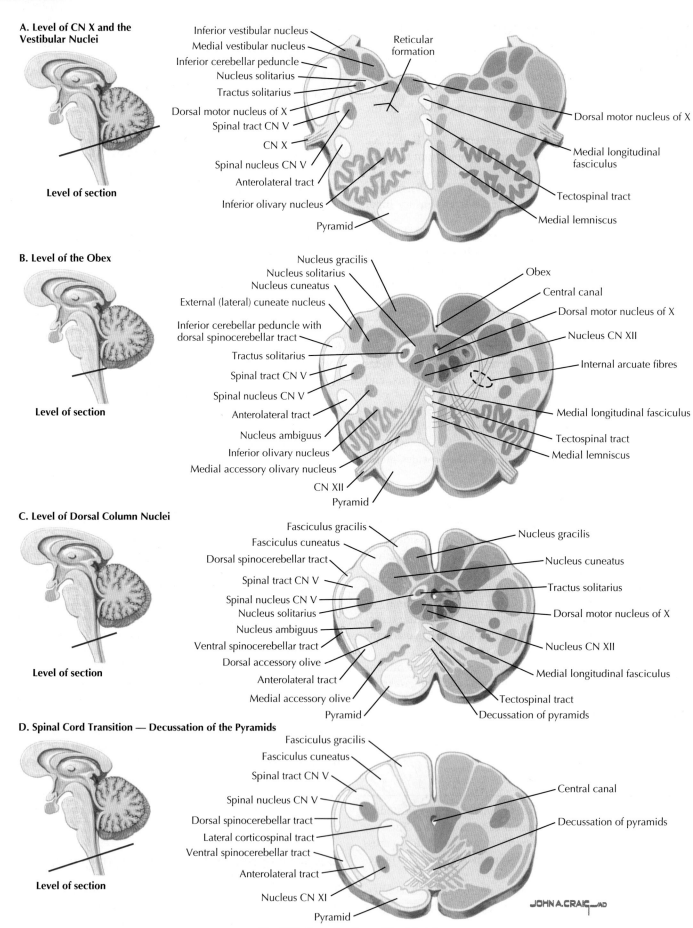

A. Level of CN X and the Vestibular Nuclei

Level of section

Inferior vestibular nucleus
Medial vestibular nucleus
Inferior cerebellar peduncle
Nucleus solitarius
Tractus solitarius
Dorsal motor nucleus of X
Spinal tract CN V
CN X
Spinal nucleus CN V
Anterolateral tract
Inferior olivary nucleus
Pyramid

Reticular formation
Dorsal motor nucleus of X
Medial longitudinal fasciculus
Tectospinal tract
Medial lemniscus

B. Level of the Obex

Level of section

Nucleus gracilis
Nucleus solitarius
Nucleus cuneatus
External (lateral) cuneate nucleus
Inferior cerebellar peduncle with dorsal spinocerebellar tract
Tractus solitarius
Spinal tract CN V
Spinal nucleus CN V
Anterolateral tract
Nucleus ambiguus
Inferior olivary nucleus
Medial accessory olivary nucleus
CN XII
Pyramid

Obex
Central canal
Dorsal motor nucleus of X
Nucleus CN XII
Internal arcuate fibres
Medial longitudinal fasciculus
Tectospinal tract
Medial lemniscus

C. Level of Dorsal Column Nuclei

Level of section

Fasciculus gracilis
Fasciculus cuneatus
Dorsal spinocerebellar tract
Spinal tract CN V
Spinal nucleus CN V
Nucleus solitarius
Nucleus ambiguus
Ventral spinocerebellar tract
Dorsal accessory olive
Anterolateral tract
Medial accessory olive
Pyramid

Nucleus gracilis
Nucleus cuneatus
Tractus solitarius
Dorsal motor nucleus of X
Nucleus CN XII
Medial longitudinal fasciculus
Tectospinal tract
Decussation of pyramids

D. Spinal Cord Transition — Decussation of the Pyramids

Level of section

Fasciculus gracilis
Fasciculus cuneatus
Spinal tract CN V
Spinal nucleus CN V
Dorsal spinocerebellar tract
Lateral corticospinal tract
Ventral spinocerebellar tract
Anterolateral tract
Nucleus CN XI
Pyramid

Central canal
Decussation of pyramids

JOHN A. CRAIG—AD

Fig. 8.11 Cross Sections of the Medulla.

Sections through spinal cord at various levels

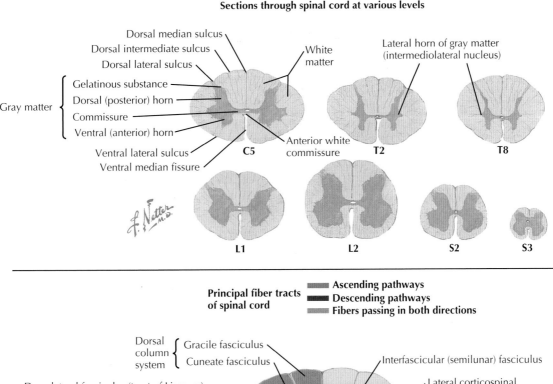

Principal fiber tracts of spinal cord

▬ Ascending pathways
▬ Descending pathways
▬ Fibers passing in both directions

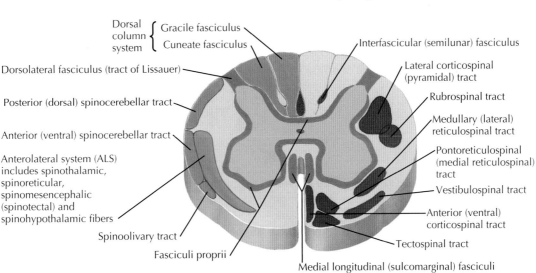

Fig. 8.12 Spinal Cord Cross Sections and Fiber Tracts.

that flows from the **lateral ventricles** through paired **interventricular foramina** (of Monro) to reach the **third ventricle**. From there it passes through the narrow **cerebral aqueduct** to reach the **fourth ventricle**, which is connected to the **central canal** of the spinal cord. Three openings in the pia mater surrounding the fourth ventricle, the two **lateral apertures** (of Luschka) and single **median aperture** (of Magendie), allow the CSF to leave the ventricular system and surround the central nervous system (CNS) within the **subarachnoid space** between the pia mater and arachnoid mater. The CSF in the subarachnoid space cushions the brain, preventing it from impacting nearby bones during normal movements. There are several **cisterns** surrounding parts of the CNS where a significant amount of CSF is present. The arachnoid mater extends several **arachnoid granulations** through the dura mater at the top of the falx cerebri. In this location is a large **dural venous sinus** called the **superior sagittal sinus**, which drains a great deal of the venous blood

from the brain and also receives CSF that leaves through microscopic channels in the arachnoid granulations. Thereafter the CSF becomes part of the blood plasma (Clinical Correlation 8.2).

SOMATOMOTOR ACTIVITY—MOTOR INNERVATION OF SKELETAL MUSCLE

The tracts that carry motor axons from nerve cells in the cortex, midbrain, and medulla are often referred to as **descending motor tracts**. These **upper motor neurons** (UMN) travel from their sites of origin, through all the regions of the brainstem inferior to them, and eventually reach the spinal cord where they synapse with **lower motor neurons** (LMN) in the anterior horn. Thereafter, the LMNs travel through the anterior roots, spinal nerves, and rami to innervate muscles throughout the body.

UMNs that originate in the cortex come overwhelmingly from the **precentral gyrus** of the frontal lobe, although some

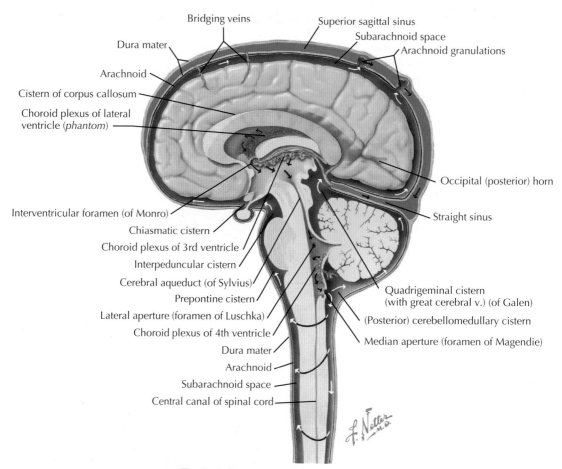

Bridging veins
Superior sagittal sinus
Subarachnoid space
Arachnoid granulations
Dura mater
Arachnoid
Cistern of corpus callosum
Choroid plexus of lateral
ventricle (*phantom*)
Occipital (posterior) horn
Interventricular foramen (of Monro)
Straight sinus
Chiasmatic cistern
Choroid plexus of 3rd ventricle
Interpeduncular cistern
Cerebral aqueduct (of Sylvius)
Prepontine cistern
Lateral aperture (foramen of Luschka)
Choroid plexus of 4th ventricle
Dura mater
Arachnoid
Subarachnoid space
Central canal of spinal cord
Quadrigeminal cistern
(with great cerebral v.) (of Galen)
(Posterior) cerebellomedullary cistern
Median aperture (foramen of Magendie)

Fig. 8.13 Circulation of Cerebrospinal Fluid.

come from nearby gyri as well. These are sometimes referred to as **giant pyramidal cells** (they are large and appear pyramid-shaped when stained) and these corticospinal and corticonuclear tracts are grouped together as the **pyramidal tracts/system**. The precentral gyrus is laid out somatotopically, with distinct regions of the body represented in different areas of the gyrus. The most lateral part of the precentral gyrus, close to the insular and temporal lobes, contains UMNs to the larynx, tongue, face, and neck. As we travel progressively more superiorly, the precentral gyrus contains UMNs for the hands, forearm, arm, thorax, abdomen, pelvis, and upper thigh. As the precentral gyrus reflects onto the medial side of the cortex (anterior part of the paracentral lobule) and then more inferiorly, it contains UMNs for the thigh, leg, and foot.

Corticospinal Tracts (Fig. 8.14)

As UMN axons leave the precentral gyrus, they first pass through a region of white matter, the **corona radiata**, before bundling together to pass through the **posterior limb of the internal capsule**. Within the internal capsule the axons to the neck are most anterior, with axons to the upper limb, torso, and lower limb located progressively more posteriorly. These axons then descend through the **crus cerebri** of the midbrain, **pontine basis**, and **medullary pyramids**. As the medulla transitions to the spinal cord, the majority of upper motor axons cross the

midline at the **pyramidal decussation** to form the contralateral **lateral corticospinal tract** in the spinal cord. A smaller number (~15%) of axons remain on the ipsilateral side as the **anterior corticospinal tract** within the anterior white matter tracts of the spinal cord.

Lateral and anterior corticospinal tract axons descend through the white matter tracts of the spinal cord. As they reach the level of the cord where they will synapse, they "peel off" or exit the tracts and synapse with nearby interneurons using the neurotransmitter glutamate. These interneurons then synapse with LMNs in the anterior horn using gamma aminobutyric acid (GABA) or glutamate. The anterior corticospinal tract tends to affect LMNs that project to axial (core) muscles of the cervical and upper thoracic regions. These are primarily located on the medial side of the anterior horn. Lateral corticospinal tract axons affect LMNs throughout the anterior horn, providing nearly all of the innervation to limb muscles, allowing precisely-controlled motor activity (Clinical Correlations 8.3–8.5).

Corticonuclear (Corticobulbar) Tract (Fig. 8.15)

The upper motor axons that innervate muscles of the head and part of the neck travel within the **corticonuclear (corticobulbar) tract**. These axons do not reach the spinal cord but synapse in cranial nerve motor nuclei within the brainstem and upper cervical spinal cord. These corticonuclear tract axons

CLINICAL CORRELATION 8.2   Hydrocephaly

The rate of CSF production may vary but it never stops. This can create problems when excessive pressure or swelling closes part of the drainage route of the ventricular system. There are several different conditions related to blocked CSF flow, or **hydrocephaly**. Congenital hydrocephaly tends to result from blockage of the cerebral aqueduct, causing the lateral and third ventricles to expand tremendously as the CSF backs up. Since the skull has not yet ossified, this can cause expansion of the cortex and skull as the brain pushes against the developing bones.

Clinical appearance in advanced hydrocephalus

Potential lesion sites in obstructive hydrocephalus

1. Interventricular foramen (of Monro)
2. Cerebral aqueduct (of Sylvius)
3. Lateral apertures (of Luschka)
4. Median aperture (of Magendie)

Section through brain showing marked dilation of lateral and 3rd ventricles

Fig. CC8.2 Hydrocephalus.

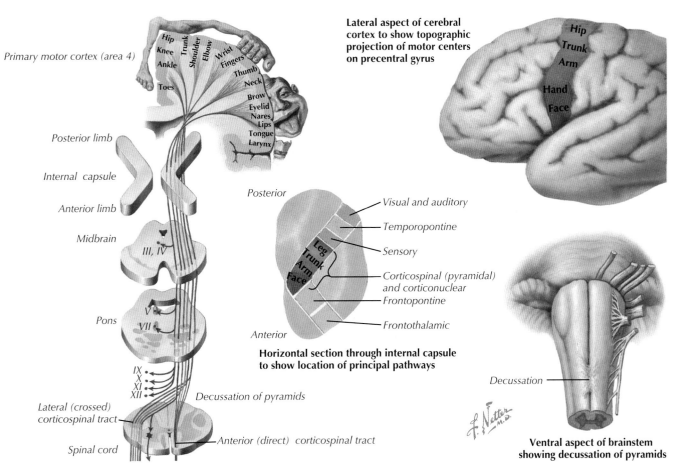

Primary motor cortex (area 4)

Posterior limb

Internal capsule

Anterior limb

Midbrain

III, IV

Pons

V
VII

IX
X
XI
XII

Lateral (crossed) corticospinal tract

Spinal cord

Decussation of pyramids

Anterior (direct) corticospinal tract

Lateral aspect of cerebral cortex to show topographic projection of motor centers on precentral gyrus

Posterior

Visual and auditory
Temporopontine
Sensory
Corticospinal (pyramidal) and corticonuclear
Frontopontine
Frontothalamic

Anterior

Horizontal section through internal capsule to show location of principal pathways

Decussation

Ventral aspect of brainstem showing decussation of pyramids

Fig. 8.14 Pyramidal System.

CLINICAL CORRELATION 8.3   Upper Motor Neuron Signs and Lower Motor Neuron Signs

Damage to the nerve cell bodies or axons of UMNs and LMNs will cause weakness and difficulty with voluntary motion. However, there are distinctive features of UMN or LMN lesions that allow clinicians to distinguish them from each other and deduce the location of the lesion.

LMN cell bodies are located in the anterior horn of the spinal cord and project their axons along the anterior roots, spinal nerves, and posterior or anterior rami (including the cervical, brachial, lumbar, and lumbosacral plexi) of each spinal level to reach skeletal muscle. If the LMN cell bodies or axons are damaged, the muscles that rely on their innervation suffer from **flaccid paralysis**. These muscles are weak (unable to generate meaningful movement), have minimal tone (resting tension), and their reflex responses will be minimal or absent. Uncoordinated fasciculations (twitches) may occur due to calcium release within the cells.

UMN cell bodies of the lateral corticospinal tract are located largely in the precentral gyrus of the cortex. Their axons descend through the corona radiata, internal capsule, crus cerebri, medullary pyramids, and lateral white matter tracts of the spinal cord before synapsing with a LMN, often via interneuron intermediaries. If the UMN cell body or axon is damaged, the muscles innervated by its LMN will suffer from **spastic paralysis**. The muscles are unable to generate meaningful movement. However, the affected muscles have increased tone (tense when at rest) and are hyper-reflexive, responding excessively to reflex testing. Since the muscles are tensed, fasciculations are typically not present. During acute UMN injury, there may be a period of flaccid paralysis that is gradually replaced by more typical UMN spastic paralysis.

The key to understanding this odd arrangement is to know that when we wish to make willful movements, the UMNs depolarize, synapse with their interneurons and associated LMNs, which then depolarize and initiate muscle contraction. However, in the absence of UMN depolarization, the UMNs and associated interneurons actually exert an inhibitory (calming) influence on the LMNs. If that is still a bit unclear, follow me through this metaphor. Think of the UMNs as a guard who is patrolling a building. The guard has a dog, representing the LMNs, on a leash. If a thief breaks into the building, the guard (UMN) will signal the dog (LMN) to attack and make a "meaningful movement" toward the thief. If there is no thief present, which is most of the time, then the guard exerts a calming influence on the dog. If some particularly vicious thief shoots the dog (my apologies, gentle reader), then no meaningful movement can occur (LMN lesion) and no motor activity is possible (flaccid paralysis). If the thief shoots the guard (UMN lesion), then the dog is let off the leash and runs around out of control, over-reacting to everything around it (spastic paralysis).

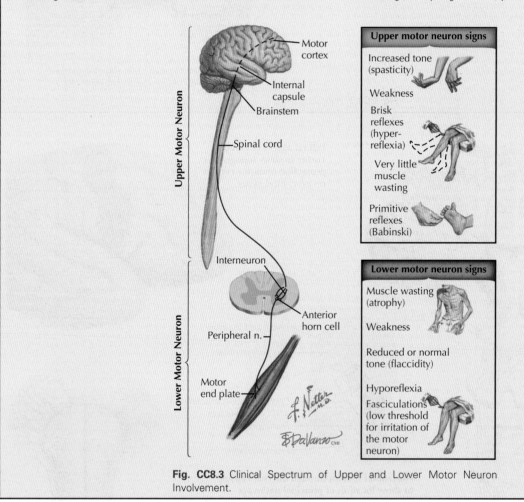

Fig. CC8.3 Clinical Spectrum of Upper and Lower Motor Neuron Involvement.

run alongside the axons that will become the corticospinal tracts but travel through the **genu of the internal capsule** and leave the tract as they reach the motor nuclei associated with cranial nerves V (trigeminal), VII (facial), IX (glossopharyngeal), X (vagus), XII (hypoglossal), and XI (spinal accessory), in that order. I am going to begin with the more inferior nuclei and work more superiorly so that all the signs associated with a lesion of this tract are clear.

The **spinal accessory nuclei** are located in the upper cervical spinal cord on the lateral side of the gray matter. They each project LMN axons through the ipsilateral spinal accessory nerve (CN XI) to innervate the sternocleidomastoid and trapezius muscles. The sternocleidomastoid is bilaterally innervated (there is some disagreement on this point) by the corticonuclear

---

CLINICAL CORRELATION 8.4
Classification of Motor Weakness

The terminology associated with motor losses is confusing. In general, *palsy* denotes some form of motor dysfunction that may include weakness or full loss of function. *Paralysis* means a complete loss of voluntary motor activity. The suffix *-plegia* has the same meaning but is added to another descriptive word to classify the area of loss (e.g., hemiplegia means complete loss of voluntary motor activity on one half of the body). *Paresis* is used to denote neurologic weakness of a muscle or group of muscles, but with some function remaining.

CLINICAL CORRELATION 8.5   Motor Neuron Diseases

There are several degenerative diseases that affect motor neurons such as **amyotrophic lateral sclerosis** (ALS), also known as Lou Gehrig disease. In this condition there is degeneration of both upper and lower motor neurons, but upper motor neuron signs may be the most noticeable during early diagnosis. **Primary lateral sclerosis** is another degenerative condition affecting upper motor neurons, while **spinal muscular atrophy** affects lower motor neurons.

---

tract while the trapezius is innervated by axons from the contralateral corticonuclear tract. A **lesion of the corticonuclear tract** will not cause outright loss of function to the **sternocleidomastoid** but it will cause weakness to the **contralateral trapezius muscle**. This is typically tested by having a patient elevate their shoulder against resistance.

The **hypoglossal nuclei** are located in the medulla oblongata. They each project axons through the ipsilateral hypoglossal nerve to innervate the **muscles of the tongue** except for the palatoglossus muscle. Each hypoglossal nucleus receives bilateral corticonuclear tract innervation BUT the LMNs that specifically innervate the **genioglossus muscle** (the only muscle to extend the tongue) are only innervated by the contralateral corticonuclear tract. This is important since a lesion of the corticobulbar tract, hypoglossal nucleus, or hypoglossal nerve will make the tongue deviate when a patient is asked to extend it. Since the genioglossus is a "push" muscle, the weak side is crowded out by the strong side. A **lesion of the hypoglossal nucleus** or nerve will affect the LMNs and cause them to deviate toward the lesioned, ipsilateral side. A **lesion of the corticonuclear tract** above the nucleus (before decussation) will affect the UMNs and result in the tongue deviating away from the lesioned, contralateral side. This is accompanied by weakness in elevating the **contralateral shoulder** since the **corticobulbar tract** is damaged superior to the **spinal accessory nucleus** (Fig. 8.16).

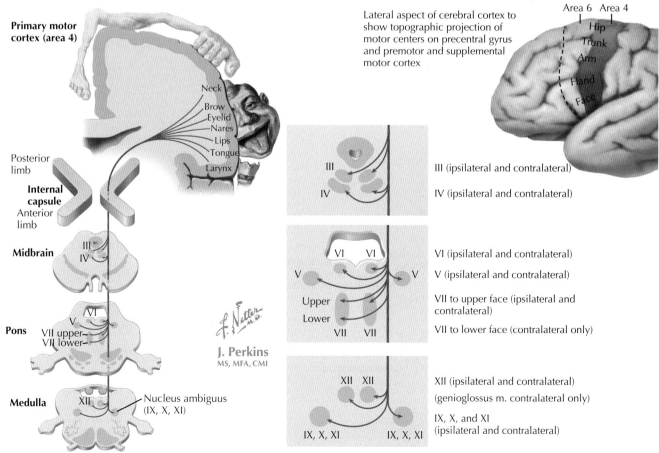

Fig. 8.15 Corticobulbar Tract.

The **nucleus ambiguus** is located on each side of the medulla oblongata and its LMNs project to the palate, pharynx, and larynx through cranial nerves IX and X. Each nucleus ambiguus receives bilateral corticonuclear tract innervation. Because of this, a lesion to this tract on only one side may result in weakness but not outright loss of function of swallowing (dysphagia) and speaking (dysphonia). However, since the lesion is cranial to the hypoglossal and spinal accessory nuclei, it would result in the tongue deviating away from the lesioned side and weakness in elevating the contralateral shoulder.

The **facial motor nuclei** are located in the cranial medulla oblongata. These LMNs each project axons through the ipsilateral facial nerve to innervate the **muscles of facial expression** and other muscles associated with the skull, hyoid bone, and ossicles. Each facial motor nucleus receives contralateral corticonuclear tract innervation except for the section that projects to the forehead, which receives bilateral corticonuclear innervation. Because of this a **lesion of the corticobulbar tract** cranial to the facial nucleus will cause **paralysis of the contralateral muscles of facial expression** except for the forehead, which is spared due to its bilateral innervation. However, since the lesion is cranial to the hypoglossal and spinal accessory nuclei, it would result in the tongue deviating away from the lesioned side and weakness in elevating the contralateral shoulder.

The **trigeminal motor nuclei** are located in the pons. These LMNs send axons along the ipsilateral mandibular branch of the trigeminal nerve (V3) to innervate the **muscles of mastication** and other muscles associated with the jaw and ossicles. Each trigeminal motor nucleus receives bilateral corticonuclear tract innervation. Thus, **unilateral lesions of the tract above the trigeminal nucleus** will not obliterate the ability to move the jaw. However, since the lesion is cranial to the facial, nucleus ambiguus, hypoglossal, and spinal accessory nuclei, the muscles of the contralateral lower two thirds of the face (inability to smile or blink completely), contralateral trapezius (weakness shrugging the shoulder), and contralateral genioglossus muscle (tongue deviates away from lesioned tract) will all have some degree of **spastic paralysis** (Clinical Correlation 8.6).

Other Descending Motor Tracts

The other descending motor tracts: rubrospinal, lateral vestibulospinal, medial vestibulospinal, reticulospinal, and tectospinal, all affect the musculoskeletal system but not to the same degree as the others mentioned above.

- **Rubrospinal tract** (Fig. 817): these UMNs originate in the magnocellular region of the **red nucleus** of the midbrain. Their axons cross to the contralateral side at the **ventral tegmental decussation** of the midbrain and descend alongside the lateral corticospinal tract axons in the lateral white matter tracts of the spinal cord. Axons of this tract preferentially synapse with excitatory interneurons that stimulate LMNs to flexor muscles in the upper limb, while other fibers stimulate interneurons that inhibit LMNs to extensor muscles. It has

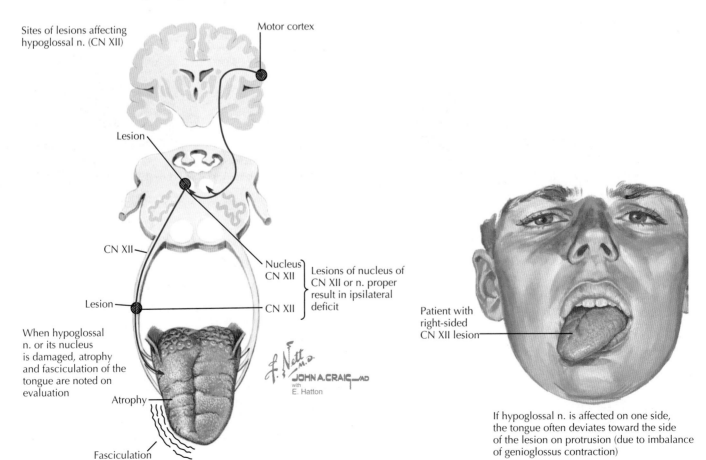

Sites of lesions affecting hypoglossal n. (CN XII)

Motor cortex

Lesion

CN XII

Lesion

Nucleus CN XII

Lesions of nucleus of CN XII or n. proper result in ipsilateral deficit

CN XII

When hypoglossal n. or its nucleus is damaged, atrophy and fasciculation of the tongue are noted on evaluation

Atrophy

Fasciculation

Patient with right-sided CN XII lesion

If hypoglossal n. is affected on one side, the tongue often deviates toward the side of the lesion on protrusion (due to imbalance of genioglossus contraction)

Fig. 8.16 Signs of Cranial Nerve XII Weakness.

CLINICAL CORRELATION 8.6 Bell Palsy Versus Corticonuclear Lesion

A lesion of the facial nucleus or the facial nerve will result in flaccid paralysis of all the ipsilateral muscles of facial expression. This is known as Bell palsy and it commonly occurs to the facial nerve as it exits the stylomastoid foramen. An affected patient will be unable to smile, blink, or wrinkle his or her forehead on the affected side. However, if all the muscles of the face are paralyzed except the forehead, that points to a lesion of the contralateral corticonuclear tract within the central nervous system. An affected patient will be unable to smile or blink on the affected side but will be able to wrinkle his or her forehead.

Left peripheral VII facial weakness

Attempt to close eye results in eyeball rolling superiorly exposing sclera (Bell phenomenon) but no closure of the lid per se

Left central facial weakness

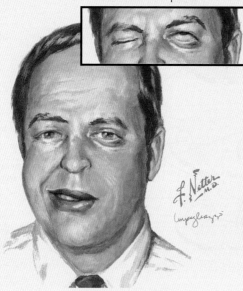
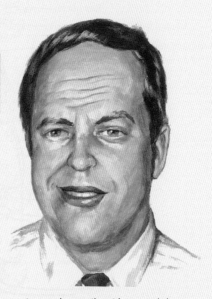

Incomplete smile with very subtle flattening of affected nasolabial fold; relative preservation of brow and forehead movement

Patient unable to wrinkle forehead; eyelid droops very slightly; cannot show teeth at all on affected side in attempt to smile; and lower lip droops slightly

Fig. CC8.6 Distinguishing Central Versus Peripheral Facial Nerve Weakness.

minimal input to the lower limbs, although a small number of axons can reach the lumbar spinal cord.

- **Lateral and medial vestibulospinal tracts** (Fig. 8.18): these UMNs originate in the **vestibular nuclei** of the medulla.
  - Axons of the lateral vestibulospinal tract do not decussate and descend in the anterior fasciculus to all levels of the spinal cord. They synapse primarily with interneurons that inhibit LMNs to flexor muscles as well as interneurons that stimulate LMNs to extensor muscles. This allows the extensor muscles to keep the body upright and balanced, even on an unstable surface. They reach all levels of the spinal cord but have their greatest effect on the lower limbs.
  - Axons of the medial vestibulospinal tract descend bilaterally (some decussate to descend contralaterally while some stay ipsilaterally) in the medial portion of the anterior fasciculus of the spinal cord, ending in the lower cervical region. They synapse primarily with LMNs that innervate muscles of the neck. This allows the neck muscles to respond automatically to movement and keep the head upright.

- **Reticulospinal tract** (Fig. 8.19): these UMNs originate from the reticular formation of the pons and medulla, under the influence of cortical inputs. They descend (mostly) in the anterior white matter tracts of the spinal cord before synapsing with interneurons that innervate LMNs. These LMNs tend to innervate core muscles of the trunk and help maintain normal posture. Axons in this tract actually tend to innervate their LMNs bilaterally.
- **Tectospinal tract** (Fig. 8.20): these UMNs originate in the **superior colliculus** of the midbrain. Their axons cross to the contralateral side at the **dorsal tegmental decussation** of the midbrain and descend in the anterior white matter tracts of the spinal cord before synapsing with LMNs in the cervical region to coordinate movements between the eyes and the head (Clinical Correlation 8.7).

Myelination and Motor Neuron Activity

As noted in Chapter 6, a myelin sheath makes depolarization move more quickly along an axon. Regarding the myelination of the motor axons:

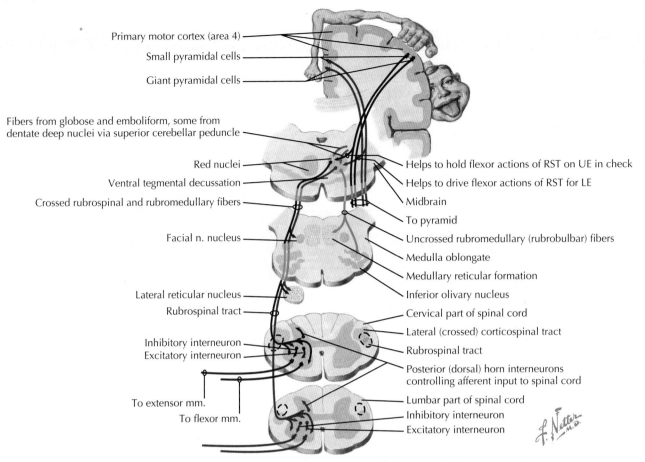

Primary motor cortex (area 4)

Small pyramidal cells

Giant pyramidal cells

Fibers from globose and emboliform, some from
dentate deep nuclei via superior cerebellar peduncle

Red nuclei

Ventral tegmental decussation

Crossed rubrospinal and rubromedullary fibers

Facial n. nucleus

Lateral reticular nucleus

Rubrospinal tract

Inhibitory interneuron

Excitatory interneuron

To extensor mm.

To flexor mm.

Helps to hold flexor actions of RST on UE in check

Helps to drive flexor actions of RST for LE

Midbrain

To pyramid

Uncrossed rubromedullary (rubrobulbar) fibers

Medulla oblongate

Medullary reticular formation

Inferior olivary nucleus

Cervical part of spinal cord

Lateral (crossed) corticospinal tract

Rubrospinal tract

Posterior (dorsal) horn interneurons
controlling afferent input to spinal cord

Lumbar part of spinal cord

Inhibitory interneuron

Excitatory interneuron

Fig. 8.17 Rubrospinal Tract. *LE*, Lower extremity; *RST*, Rubrospinal tract; *UE*, Upper extremity.

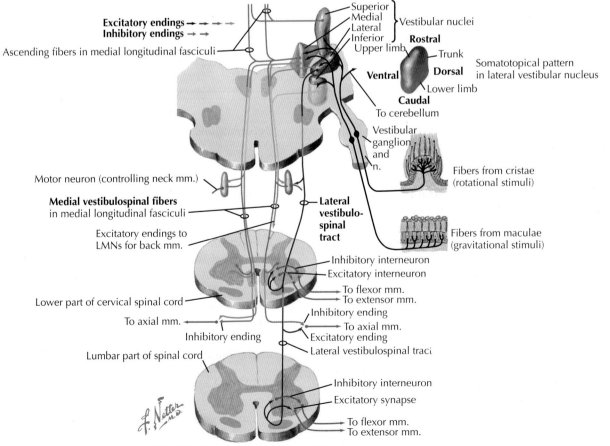

Excitatory endings → → →→ →

Inhibitory endings ⇒ → →

Ascending fibers in medial longitudinal fasciculi

Superior
Medial
Lateral
Inferior } Vestibular nuclei

Upper limb

Rostral

Trunk

Ventral **Dorsal**

Lower limb

Somatotopical pattern
in lateral vestibular nucleus

Caudal

To cerebellum

Vestibular
ganglion
and
n.

Fibers from cristae
(rotational stimuli)

Fibers from maculae
(gravitational stimuli)

Motor neuron (controlling neck mm.)

Medial vestibulospinal fibers
in medial longitudinal fasciculi

Excitatory endings to
LMNs for back mm.

Lower part of cervical spinal cord

To axial mm.

Inhibitory ending

Lumbar part of spinal cord

**Lateral
vestibulo-
spinal
tract**

Inhibitory interneuron

Excitatory interneuron

To flexor mm.
To extensor mm.

Inhibitory ending
To axial mm.
Excitatory ending

Lateral vestibulospinal tract

Inhibitory interneuron

Excitatory synapse

To flexor mm.
To extensor mm.

Fig. 8.18 Vestibulospinal Tract. *LMNs*, Lower motor neurons.

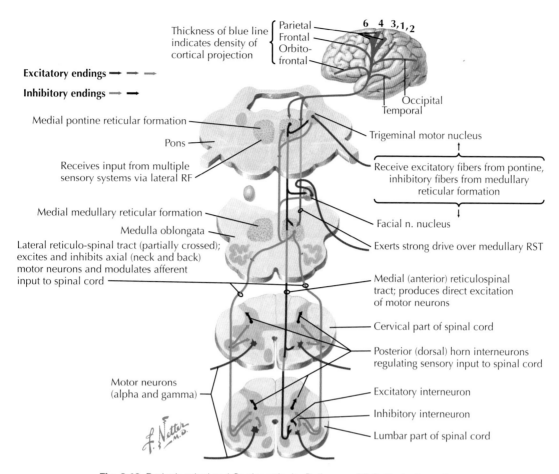

Thickness of blue line indicates density of cortical projection

Parietal
Frontal
Orbito-frontal
6 4 3,1,2
Occipital
Temporal

Excitatory endings ➤ ─ ➤ ─ ➤

Inhibitory endings ➤ ─ ➤

Medial pontine reticular formation

Pons

Receives input from multiple sensory systems via lateral RF

Trigeminal motor nucleus

Receive excitatory fibers from pontine, inhibitory fibers from medullary reticular formation

Medial medullary reticular formation

Medulla oblongata

Lateral reticulo-spinal tract (partially crossed); excites and inhibits axial (neck and back) motor neurons and modulates afferent input to spinal cord

Facial n. nucleus

Exerts strong drive over medullary RST

Medial (anterior) reticulospinal tract; produces direct excitation of motor neurons

Cervical part of spinal cord

Posterior (dorsal) horn interneurons regulating sensory input to spinal cord

Motor neurons (alpha and gamma)

Excitatory interneuron

Inhibitory interneuron

Lumbar part of spinal cord

Fig. 8.19 Reticulospinal and Corticoreticular Pathways. RF, Reticular formation.

- **A-alpha (Aα) fibers** have the thickest myelin sheaths and surround LMNs traveling to extrafusal skeletal muscle fibers. They can conduct a depolarization between 80 and 120 m/s.
- **A-gamma (Aγ) fibers** have less stout myelin sheaths and surround LMNs to intrafusal skeletal muscle fibers of the muscle spindles. Their conduction velocity drops precipitously to 15 to 30 m/s.
- **B fibers** have a very slight myelin sheath and surround preganglionic autonomic axons. The depolarization velocity drops to 3 to 15 m/s.
- **C fibers** denote non-myelinated, postganglionic autonomic axons, although they are still surrounded by Schwann cells. Their conduction velocity is approximately 0.7 to 2.3 m/s.

Somatosensory Activity—Input to the Central Nervous System From Skin and Skeletal Muscle

The nerve tracts that carry sensory information from the skin and skeletal muscles are often referred to as **ascending tracts**. These typically start with a peripheral sensory receptor and then utilize a three-neuron chain to make the trip from the periphery to their target in the cortex. Somewhere along the way they will decussate across the midline. There are two major somatosensory tracts, the **dorsal column/medial lemniscal tract** and the **anterolateral system**. As we follow the details of these tracts, pay particular attention to the location of the three neuron cell bodies (denoted as first-, second-, and third-order neurons) along

the chain and the site of decussation. Those details account for the clinical manifestations seen when these tracts are damaged.

Peripheral Sensory Receptors (Fig. 8.21)

Sensation begins with receptors within the tissues of the body. We will focus on their presence in the musculoskeletal system but please note that sensory receptors are also found in the organs of other systems but we may not be consciously aware of those stimuli. There are several ways to classify sensory receptors, but we will start by classifying them according to the thickness of their myelin sheaths and their corresponding depolarization velocity.

- **A-alpha (Aα) fibers**: thickest myelin sheath, depolarize at approximately 80 to 120 m/s.
  - **Muscle spindle fibers**: these were described in Chapter 6. In summary, the **intrafusal fibers** of these receptors are found encapsulated within the **extrafusal fibers** of the overlying muscle. They sense tension and trigger an increase in muscle tone as stretch is applied to intrafusal and extrafusal muscle fibers.
  - **Golgi tendon organs**: these were described in Chapter 6. In summary, these receptors are frequently found at the muscle-tendon juncture. They become active when intense stretch is applied to the tendon. They then trigger a decrease in tone of the stretched muscle to prevent damage or avulsion.

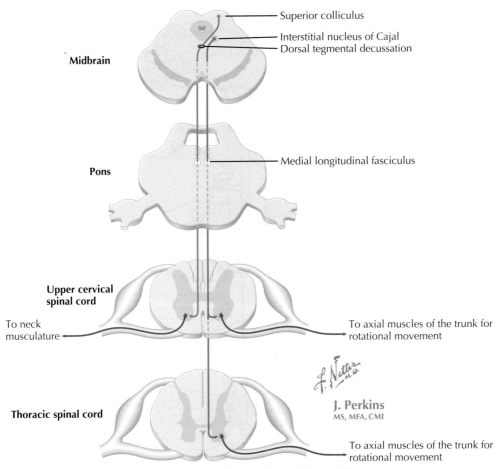

Fig. 8.20 Tectospinal Tract and Interstitiospinal Tract.

CLINICAL CORRELATION 8.7 Postural Reflexes

Massive damage to the central nervous system can result in coma with patients fixed in distinctive postures. These occur because of the loss of certain descending motor tracts.

Flexor (Decorticate) Rigidity
Damage between the thalamus and midbrain can destroy the descending corticospinal tracts at that level, which control fine motor control of the limbs. However, the red nucleus and rubrospinal tract from the midbrain remain intact and preferentially innervate flexors of the upper limb. The vestibular nuclei and vestibulospinal tracts of the upper medulla are also intact. The lateral vestibulospinal tract preferentially innervates extensors of the lower limb. Because of this, the affected person will have persistently **flexed** upper limbs and **extended** lower limbs.

Extensor (Decerebrate) Rigidity
Damage to the brainstem between the midbrain and medulla will disrupt the corticospinal and rubrospinal tracts. Thereafter the vestibulospinal tracts are the only upper motor neurons projecting to the upper and lower limbs. Because of this, the affected person will have persistently **extended** upper limbs and **extended** lower limbs.

- **A-beta (Aβ) fibers**: relatively thick myelin sheaths, depolarize at approximately 35 to 75 m/s.
  - **Meissner corpuscles**: these **fine touch** receptors are particularly good at sensing low-frequency contact and

two-point discrimination in areas like the digits, palms, plantar foot, and lips. They are **phasic**, meaning that they respond at the beginning and end of a stimulus but do not respond during the sustained period of stimulus. They are found in the dermal papillae that interface with ridges of the epidermis. The Schwann cells that surround the sensory axon give the whole structure a twisted, tornado-like appearance.

- **Merkel discs/cells**: these small cellular receptors are found within the deepest layer of the epidermis. They cover a small area and sense changes in pressure. These depolarize in a **tonic** way, remaining active during the entire duration of a stimulus.
- **Ruffini end organ/corpuscles**: these receptors consist of a branched network of axon ends encased in a capsule that is pierced by collagen fibers of the surrounding dermis. As the surrounding dermis is stretched, the collagen fibers convey that deformation to the Ruffini corpuscle. These depolarize most strongly at the beginning and end of the **stretch** stimulus in a phasic manner.
- **Pacinian corpuscles**: these large receptors are found in the deeper regions of the dermis or hypodermis and appear onion-like in cross section with multiple lamellae surrounding the sensory axon. As **vibration** or **deep pressure** reaches these corpuscles, they deform the lamellae and cause depolarization in a phasic manner.

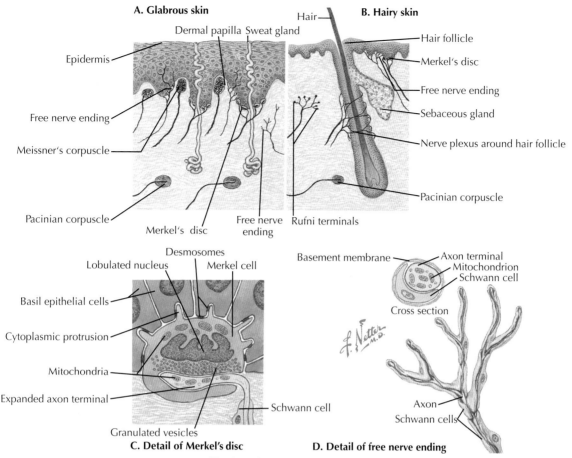

A. Glabrous skin
- Epidermis
- Dermal papilla
- Sweat gland
- Free nerve ending
- Meissner's corpuscle
- Pacinian corpuscle
- Merkel's disc
- Free nerve ending

B. Hairy skin
- Hair
- Hair follicle
- Merkel's disc
- Free nerve ending
- Sebaceous gland
- Nerve plexus around hair follicle
- Pacinian corpuscle
- Rufni terminals

C. Detail of Merkel's disc
- Desmosomes
- Lobulated nucleus
- Merkel cell
- Basil epithelial cells
- Cytoplasmic protrusion
- Mitochondria
- Expanded axon terminal
- Schwann cell
- Granulated vesicles

D. Detail of free nerve ending
- Basement membrane
- Axon terminal
- Mitochondrion
- Schwann cell
- Cross section
- Axon
- Schwann cells

Fig. 8.21 Cutaneous Receptors.

- **A-delta (Aδ) fibers** (lightly myelinated, 5 to 30 m/s) and **C fibers** (non-myelinated, 0.5 to 2 m/s) are associated with **free nerve endings.** Free nerve endings are found in the epidermis and wrap around hair follicles. They depolarize in response to being moved. Inputs from free nerve endings can be interpreted as **fine touch** (including hair follicles), **heat, cold**, or **nociception (pain).**
  - **Fine touch**: some free nerve endings in the epidermis respond to small changes in deformation of the surrounding tissue. These stimuli are conveyed by A-delta or C fibers. Inputs from nerves associated with hair follicles are conveyed more quickly by A-beta fibers and act in a phasic way.
  - **Warm receptors**: respond to temperatures between 30°C and 45°C with depolarization occurring more frequently as its upper limit is approached. These stimuli are primarily (but not exclusively) conveyed by C fibers.
  - **Cold receptors**: respond to temperatures between 20°C and 35°C with depolarization occurring most frequently around 25°C. Extreme heat (>45°C) will also cause these receptors to depolarize. These stimuli are conveyed primarily by A-delta fibers.
  - **Nociceptive (pain) receptors**: respond to intense mechanical (penetrating or blunt), thermal, or chemical stimuli and are interpreted as pain in the CNS. These

stimuli are conveyed by A-delta and C fibers. Please note that the ultra-intense input from any receptor can be interpreted as pain by the CNS.

Dorsal Columns/Medial Lemniscal System (Fig 8.22)

This sensory tract has axons ascending through two white matter structures, the dorsal columns and the medial lemniscus, thus earning its name. It conveys vibration, fine touch, and proprioceptive input to the CNS. The pathway followed by the dorsal columns/medial lemniscal (DCML) proceeds in this manner.

1. Changes in the skin or muscles are sensed by pacinian corpuscles (vibration), Meissner corpuscles, Meckel discs, Ruffini end organs (fine touch), Golgi tendon organs, and muscle spindle fibers (proprioception).
2. Depolarization occurs along each sensory receptor's axon from the periphery toward the spinal cord. These axons travel as part of the peripheral nerves of the posterior rami, anterior rami, and their various plexi.
3. The cell bodies, **first-order neurons**, of these neurons are located in the **posterior root ganglia** along each side of the vertebral column. These are pseudounipolar axons, so the depolarization continues past the ganglion without synapsing and enters the spinal cord.
4. The axons travel medially and enter the **dorsal (posterior) columns** of the spinal cord.

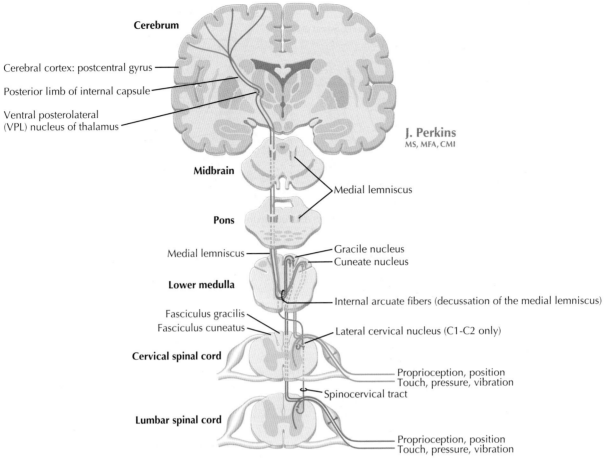

Fig. 8.22 Somatosensory System: The Dorsal Column System and Epicritic Modalities.

5. Axons from coccygeal, sacral, lumbar, and lower thoracic levels (lower limbs and inferior torso) form the most medial of the two columns, the **gracile fasciculus/fasciculus gracilis.**

6. Axons from the upper thoracic and cervical levels (superior torso and upper limbs) form a neighboring but distinct column, the **cuneate fasciculus/fasciculus cuneatus.**

7. Axons that enter the gracile or cuneate fasciculi ascend through the remaining levels of the spinal cord until they reach the inferior medulla, where they meet and synapse with **second-order neurons** located in the **gracile nucleus** and **cuneate nucleus**, respectively.

8. The axons projecting from the gracile and cuneate nuclei extend anteriorly and decussate to reach the opposite side, forming **internal arcuate fibers.**

9. After decussating, the axons from the gracile and cuneate nuclei ascend through the rest of the brainstem as the **medial lemniscus.** The medial lemniscus is laid out somatotopically along its length. In the medulla it is located very close to the midline with axons representing the feet anteriorly and the upper body posteriorly. In the pons it is located deep within the tegmentum, its axis has turned 90 degrees, with the feet represented laterally and the upper body medially. In the midbrain it has turned a few degrees further, with axons representing the feet located posterolaterally and the upper body anteromedially.

10. The axons of the medial lemniscus synapse with **third-order neurons** in the **ventral posterior lateral (VPL) thalamic nucleus.**

11. Axons from the VPL extend superiorly through the cortex via the **posterior limb of the internal capsule**, the **corona radiata**, finally reaching the **postcentral gyrus of the parietal lobe** (as well as some nearby areas). The postcentral gyrus is also arranged somatotopically in a very similar way to the precentral motor gyrus. Axons representing the genitalia, feet, and leg project to neurons on the medial side of the gyrus, the thigh, and pelvis more superiorly, with the torso, upper limbs, neck, and head continuing more laterally to the end of the postcentral gyrus.

Injuries of the DCML system will manifest as a loss of fine touch (two-point discrimination), vibration, and proprioceptive sensation. This tract decussates in the inferior medulla; therefore, injury to this tract below that level will cause ipsilateral sensory losses (fibers have not crossed over) while injuries to this tract above that level will cause contralateral losses (fibers have crossed over).

Anterolateral System (Fig. 8.23)

This ascending sensory system consists of several parallel tracts (spinoreticular, spinomesencephalic, spinohypothalamic, spinothalamic tracts) that convey pain and temperature sensation

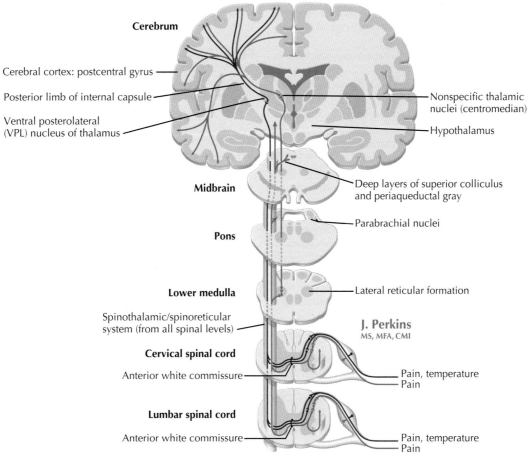

Cerebrum

Cerebral cortex: postcentral gyrus

Posterior limb of internal capsule

Ventral posterolateral
(VPL) nucleus of thalamus

Nonspecific thalamic
nuclei (centromedian)

Hypothalamus

Midbrain

Deep layers of superior colliculus
and periaqueductal gray

Parabrachial nuclei

Pons

Lower medulla

Lateral reticular formation

Spinothalamic/spinoreticular
system (from all spinal levels)

J. Perkins
MS, MFA, CMI

Cervical spinal cord

Anterior white commissure

Pain, temperature
Pain

Lumbar spinal cord

Anterior white commissure

Pain, temperature
Pain

Fig. 8.23 Somatosensory System: The Spinothalamic and Spinoreticular Systems and Protopathic Modalities.

from the periphery to a variety of targets in the CNS. This breadth of targets helps to explain why pain affects us in many different ways. In this text, we will focus on the **spinothalamic tract**, which conveys pain and temperature stimuli to the thalamus and cortex, allowing us to consciously perceive these sensations. The pathway followed by the ALS axons proceeds in this manner.

1. Free nerve endings detect changes in the skin related to heat, cold, pain, and some fine touch.
2. Depolarization occurs along each sensory receptor's axon, from the periphery toward the spinal cord. These axons travel as part of the peripheral nerves of the posterior rami, anterior rami, and their various plexi.
3. The cell bodies, **first-order neurons**, of these neurons are located in the **posterior root ganglia** along each side of the vertebral column. These are pseudounipolar axons, so the depolarization continues past the ganglion without synapsing and enters the spinal cord.
4. After a short ascent in the posterolatreal (Lissauer's) tract, the axons travel medially and enter the **posterior horn** (gray matter) of the spinal cord and synapse with **second-order neurons** located there, specifically in the **substantia gelatinosa** of the posterior horn.
5. Axons leaving the second-order neurons travel anteriorly and medially, decussating to the opposite side by passing through the **anterior white commissure** of the spinal cord.

Note that the axons typically ascend roughly two spinal levels during the process of decussation.

6. After decussating, the axons join the ALS in the anterior and lateral white matter bundle of the spinal cord. They stay in this bundle until they reach targets in the reticular formation, midbrain, hypothalamus, and the thalamus.
7. The axons of the spinothalamic tract synapse with **third-order neurons** in the **VPL thalamic nucleus.**
8. Axons from the VPL extend superiorly through the cortex via the **posterior limb of the internal capsule**, the **corona radiata**, finally reaching the **postcentral gyrus of the parietal lobe** (as well as some nearby areas). The postcentral gyrus is also arranged somatotopically. Axons representing the genitalia, feet, and leg project to neurons on the medial side of the gyrus, the thigh, and pelvis more superiorly, with the torso, upper limbs, neck, and head continuing more laterally to the end of the postcentral gyrus.

Injuries of the ALS system will manifest as a loss of pain and temperature sensation. This tract decussates continuously at all levels of the spinal cord. Therefore, injury to this tract will always cause contralateral lesions since axons do not join it until after they have decussated. Injury at the anterior white commissure of the spinal cord will cause bilateral loss of pain and temperature sensation but only at the levels that were actively decussating in the damaged area (Clinical Correlations 8.8–8.10).

Damage to the spinal cord can cause a variety of neurologic signs; here are some of the more prominent ones that can be assessed during a neurologic evaluation.

- Damage to the lateral corticospinal tract causes ipsilateral spastic paralysis below the lesion.
- Damage to the DCML causes ipsilateral loss of vibration, proprioception, and fine touch sensation below the lesion.
- Damage to the ALS causes contralateral loss of pain and temperature sensation below the lesion.
- Damage to the anterior horn of the spinal cord causes ipsilateral flaccid paralysis at the level that was damaged.
- Damage to the posterior horn of the spinal cord causes ipsilateral loss of pain and temperature sensation at the level that was damaged.
- Damage to the anterior white commissure causes bilateral loss of pain and temperature sensation to the levels that were decussating in the damaged area.

Transverse Cord Lesion

Complete transection of the spinal cord will disrupt the ascending and descending tracts as well as the gray matter at that level. All levels below the lesion will experience spastic paralysis (due to bilateral loss of the lateral corticospinal tract) as well as loss of all sensation (bilateral destruction of the ALS and DCML). Due to the ascent of sensory axons in Lissauer tract and as ALS axons ascending during their decussation, signs may manifest 1 to 2 spinal levels below the actual injury. Bilateral flaccid paralysis (due to destruction of anterior horns) at the injured level may be noted.

Hemicord Lesion/Brown-Sequard Syndrome

Destruction of one half of the spinal cord results in a unique constellation of neurologic signs that can occur during lacerations that penetrate into the spinal canal from the posterior side. Spinous processes often keep this trauma isolated to one side. Spastic paralysis (lateral corticospinal tract) as well as loss of vibration, proprioception, and fine touch sensation (DCML) will be noted ipsilaterally at all levels below the lesion since those tracts decussate in the medulla. Loss of pain and temperature sensation (ALS) will be noted contralaterally below the lesion since this tract decussates shortly after entering the spinal cord and prior to joining the

ALS in the anterior fasciculus. Destruction of the posterior and anterior horns of the spinal cord will result in loss of ipsilateral pain and temperature sensation and ipsilateral flaccid paralysis at the damaged level, respectively.

Central Cord Lesions

These lesions begin at the central canal of the spinal cord and expand outward. A frequent cause of this condition is syringomyelia in the cervical cord. This occurs when pressure in the CSF causes the central canal to expand outward. Initially this will compress the anterior white commissure, causing a bilateral loss of pain and temperature sensation at the affected levels. The typical version of this extends down to the C4 levels, creating a "cape" distribution of ALS signs bilaterally across the tops of the shoulders. If the lesion continues to expand and compromise other structures, it may cause flaccid paralysis at the affected levels (anterior horn), spastic paralysis at all levels below the lesion (lateral cortical spinal tract), loss of vibration, proprioception, and fine touch (DCML) below the lesion, and eventually loss of pain and temperature sensation below the affected level (ALS). Since these tracts are not obliterated, some function may remain.

Posterior Cord Syndrome

Lesions in this region can be due to blockage of the posterior spinal arteries, tabes dorsalis (associated with tertiary syphilis), or vitamin B12 deficiency. There will be loss of proprioception, vibration, and fine touch bilaterally below the affected level (DCML). If the lesion is especially large, there may also be some loss of pain and temperature sensation (posterior horn) at the affected level and even larger lesions may cause some spastic paralysis below the affected level (lateral corticospinal tract).

Anterior Cord Syndrome

Lesions in this region can be due to blockage of the anterior spinal arteries or trauma, such as a vertebral body fracture. These lesions will often cause bilateral loss of pain and temperature sensation (ALS) and spastic paralysis (lateral corticospinal tract) below the affected level. In addition, flaccid paralysis may occur at the affected levels (anterior horn).

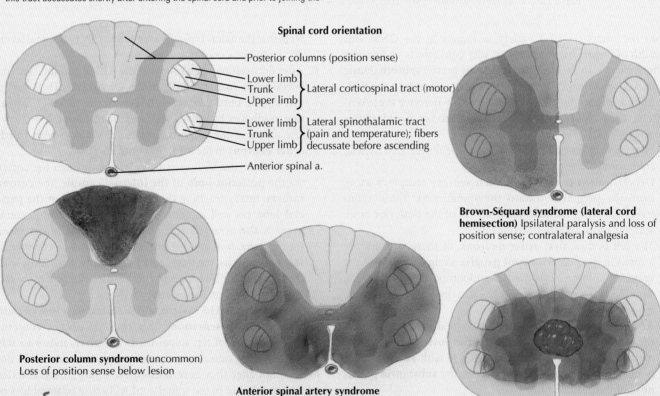

Spinal cord orientation

Posterior columns (position sense)

Lower limb ⎫
Trunk ⎬ Lateral corticospinal tract (motor)
Upper limb ⎭

Lower limb ⎫ Lateral spinothalamic tract
Trunk ⎬ (pain and temperature); fibers
Upper limb ⎭ decussate before ascending

Anterior spinal a.

Brown-Séquard syndrome (lateral cord hemisection) Ipsilateral paralysis and loss of position sense; contralateral analgesia

Posterior column syndrome (uncommon)
Loss of position sense below lesion

Anterior spinal artery syndrome
Bilateral paralysis and dissociated sensory loss below lesion (analgesia but preserved position sense)

Central cord syndrome
Parts of 3 main tracts involved on both sides; upper limbs more affected than lower limbs

Fig. CC8.8 Cervical Spine Injury: Incomplete Spinal Cord Syndromes.

CLINICAL CORRELATION 8.9 Brainstem Lesions

Damage to the brainstem can involve descending motor tracts and ascending sensory tracts. However, such lesions may also involve cranial nerve nuclei and other neurologic structures that go beyond the focus of this book. So those will be addressed briefly but accurately. There is considerable variation in the size of an infarct and some structures on the periphery of a lesion may or may not be affected.

Medulla (Fig. CC8.9A)

Medial medullary syndrome: lesions involving the blood supply to the medial medulla, primarily paramedian branches of the anterior spinal or vertebral arteries, will cause contralateral spastic paralysis (medullary pyramids/corticospinal tracts), contralateral loss of vibration proprioception, and fine touch (DCML), and ipsilateral weakness of the tongue, deviating toward the lesioned side (hypoglossal nucleus and nerve)

Lateral medullary (Wallenberg) syndrome: lesions involving the blood supply to the lateral medulla, primarily lateral branches of the vertebral arteries, will cause contralateral loss of pain and temperature sensation (ALS), losses of ipsilateral facial pain and temperature sensation (spinal trigeminal nucleus), difficulty speaking and swallowing (nucleus ambiguus), taste abnormality (solitary nucleus), ipsilateral ataxia (inferior cerebellar peduncle), and Horner syndrome (descending sympathetic tract).

Pons (Fig. CC8.9B)

Vascular infarcts of the midline pons are related to the paramedial branches of the basilar artery. These will often result in contralateral spastic paralysis

(corticospinal and corticonuclear tracts), contralateral loss of vibration, proprioception, and fine touch sensation (DCML), ipsilateral facial flaccid paralysis (facial motor nucleus and nerve), abducens nerve palsy (abducens nucleus), and contralateral ataxia (pontine nuclei, pontocerebellar fibers, and middle cerebellar peduncle).

More lateral infarcts of the pons, caused by dysfunction of the anterior inferior cerebellar artery, will often manifest with vertigo (vestibular nuclei), contralateral loss of pain and temperature sensation (ALS), ipsilateral loss of facial pain and temperature sensation (spinal trigeminal nucleus), and Horner syndrome (descending sympathetic tract).

Midbrain (Fig. CC8.9C)

Vascular infarcts that affect the tegmentum of the midbrain can manifest in a variety of ways. Paramedian branches of the posterior cerebral artery (PCA) or basilar artery can cause oculomotor nerve palsy (CN III nuclei), contralateral spastic paralysis (corticospinal, corticonuclear tracts, and the red nucleus). If the infarct is more widely spread, these signs will be joined by ataxia (superior cerebellar peduncles), contralateral loss of vibration, proprioception, and fine touch sensation (DCML), contralateral loss of pain and temperature sensation (ALS), and Horner syndrome (descending sympathetic tract).

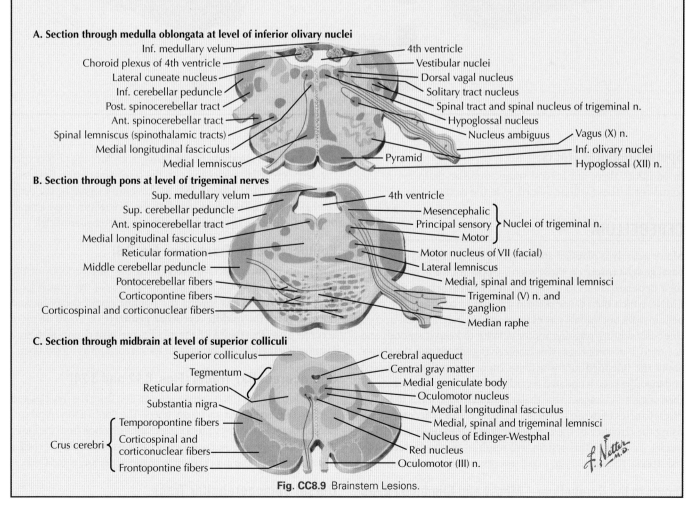

A. Section through medulla oblongata at level of inferior olivary nuclei

B. Section through pons at level of trigeminal nerves

C. Section through midbrain at level of superior colliculi

Fig. CC8.9 Brainstem Lesions.

CLINICAL CORRELATION 8.10 Cortical Lesions

The proximity of the precentral and postcentral gyri and their similar somato-topic organization makes lesions affecting the cortex relatively simple (by the standards of neurologic diagnosis) to understand. The lateral aspects of both gyri include motor and sensory activities related to the head and neck. As you travel superiorly along the gyri, regions for the hand, upper limb, torso, and upper thigh are encountered. The medial aspect of the gryi, sitting within the longitudinal fissure between cortical hemispheres, includes regions for the knee, leg, foot, and genitalia (primarily sensory).

Since the middle cerebral artery covers the lateral aspect of the cortex, disruption of blood flow through it will often result in upper motor neuron signs and profound sensory losses (DCML and ALS) of the contralateral head, neck, hand, and upper limb. On the left, this will often be accompanied by an inability to speak coherently, called Broca aphasia. The anterior cerebral artery perfuses the medial aspect of the frontal and parietal lobes. Disruption of flow through this vessel will often cause upper motor neuron signs and profound sensory losses of the contralateral lower limb.

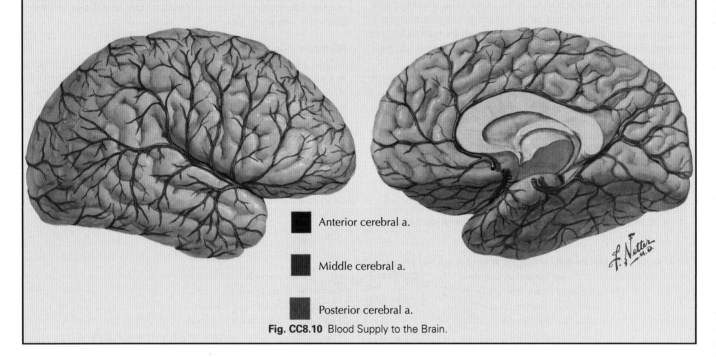

■ Anterior cerebral a.

■ Middle cerebral a.

■ Posterior cerebral a.

Fig. CC8.10 Blood Supply to the Brain.

Spinocerebellar Tracts

In addition, there are several spinocerebellar pathways in the spinal cord. These will be described in the next section.

CEREBELLUM

Motor activity is planned and organized in the frontal lobes and basal ganglia (more on those soon). Upper motor neurons carry their depolarizations to the spinal cord where they are passed to LMNs, which then cause skeletal muscles to contract. The cerebellum does not initiate any of these actions, but it is vital in continuously editing ongoing motor activity to keep it smooth and accurate. It accomplishes this by receiving input from the cortex about the intended motor activity. Inputs from the spinal cord and medulla keep it updated regarding real-time motor activity. It then suggests changes to the thalamus and frontal lobes to rectify discrepancies between intent and actuality. This is accomplished using the circuitry of the **cerebellar cortex** and **deep cerebellar nuclei**. Lesions of this system will result in motor dysfunctions like **ataxia**, the inability to make smooth, coordinated motions.

Inputs to the Cerebellum—Mossy and Climbing Fibers

All axons entering the cerebellum are called **mossy fibers** except for those coming from the inferior olivary nucleus of the medulla,

which are called **climbing fibers**. Mossy and climbing fibers excite the deep cerebellar nuclei and also the cerebellar cortex; however, the cerebellar cortex then sends an inhibitory signal to the deep cerebellar nuclei. Therefore, inputs to the cerebellum cause a rapid on/off modulation in output from the deep cerebellar nuclei.

Pontocerebellar Tracts (see Fig. 8.9)

The **pontine nuclei** receive axons from the various lobes of the cortex, including inputs from the motor areas of the frontal lobe. **Pontocerebellar axons** leaving the pontine nuclei decussate and travel through the **middle cerebellar peduncle** (it would be more accurate to say that they ARE the middle cerebellar peduncle) before distributing themselves throughout the cerebellum as mossy fibers.

Spinocerebellar Tracts (Figs. 8.12 and 8.24)

The spinocerebellar tracts convey information from the muscles and spine to the cerebellum via mossy fibers. The dorsal and ventral spinocerebellar tracts convey proprioceptive information from the lower limbs and torso while the cuneocerebellar and rostral spinocerebellar tracts covey the same information from the upper limbs and torso.

Dorsal Spinocerebellar Tract

1. Muscle spindle fibers, Golgi tendon organs, and pacinian corpuscles in the lower limbs and inferior torso send

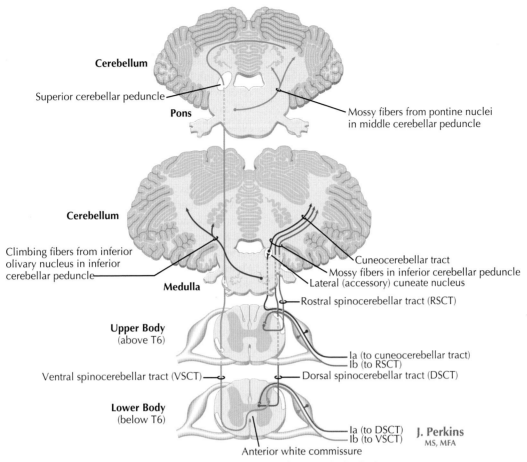

Fig. 8.24 Somatosensory System: Spinocerebellar Pathways.

proprioceptive inputs along the peripheral nerves associated with their muscles. These axons travel as part of the peripheral nerves of the posterior rami, anterior rami, and their various plexi.

2. The cell bodies of these neurons are located in the **posterior root ganglia** along each side of the vertebral column. These are pseudounipolar axons, so the depolarization continues past the ganglion without synapsing and enters the spinal cord.

3. These axons may enter the gracile fasciculus but quickly exit to synapse with neuron cell bodies in the ipsilateral **nucleus dorsalis of Clarke**, which only exists between the T1 and L2 levels of the spinal cord.

4. **Mossy fiber** axons from the nucleus dorsalis of Clarke ascend in the ipsilateral **dorsal spinocerebellar tract**, located on the posterolateral side of the spinal cord, just superficial to the lateral corticospinal tract.

5. The dorsal spinocerebellar tract ascends through the spinal cord and into the medulla before entering the cerebellum through the **inferior cerebellar peduncle**, specifically the **restiform body** within the inferior cerebellar peduncle.

6. These axons then travel to the ipsilateral cerebellar cortex. Note that this tract never decussates.

Cuneocerebellar Tract

1. Muscle spindle fibers, Golgi tendon organs, and pacinian corpuscles in the upper limbs and superior torso send proprioceptive

inputs along the peripheral nerves associated with their muscles. These axons travel as part of the peripheral nerves of the posterior rami, anterior rami, and their various plexi.

2. The cell bodies of these neurons are located in the **posterior root ganglia** along each side of the vertebral column. These are pseudounipolar axons, so the depolarization continues past the ganglion without synapsing and enters the spinal cord.

3. These axons enter the **cuneate fasciculus** and ascend within that tract to reach the inferior medulla and **external cuneate nucleus**, located alongside the cuneate nucleus.

4. The external cuneate nucleus fulfills a similar role as the nucleus dorsalis of Clarke but is located in one place rather than spread out across multiple spinal levels.

5. Axons from the external cuneate nucleus, called cuneocerebellar fibers, enter the cerebellum through the **inferior cerebellar peduncle**, specifically the **restiform body** within the inferior cerebellar peduncle.

6. These axons then travel to the ipsilateral cerebellar cortex. Note that this tract also remains ipsilateral and never decussates.

Ventral Spinocerebellar Tract

1. This tract originates from interneurons in the intermediate zone of the spinal cord's gray matter that receive afferent inputs from the lower limbs, including many types of sensory receptors.

2. Axons from these cells decussate to the contralateral side through the anterior white commissure and ascend in the ventral spinocerebellar tract, located just superficial to the ALS.
3. The ventral spinocerebellar tract ascends through the spinal cord, medulla, pons, and midbrain before entering the cerebellum through the superior cerebellar peduncle.
4. Axons of the ventral spinocerebellar tract then decussate again and travel to the contralateral cerebellar cortex. Note: this tract decussates twice as it travels from spinal cord to cerebellum.

Rostral Spinocerebellar Tract

1. This tract originates from interneurons in the intermediate zone of the spinal cord's gray matter that receive afferent inputs from the upper limbs. There is disagreement about exactly how this pathway is laid out.
2. Axons from cervical interneurons ascend near or within the ipsilateral dorsal spinocerebellar tract before entering the cerebellum through the inferior and superior cerebellar peduncles.
3. This tract is described as either remaining ipsilateral (similar to the dorsal spinocerebellar and cuneocerebellar tracts) or decussating twice (like the ventral spinocerebellar tract) as it travels from the spinal cord to the cerebellum.

Climbing Fibers and the Inferior Olivary Nucleus (see Fig. 8.11)

The **inferior olivary nucleus** (which can be subdivided into principal and accessory olivary nuclei) is in the superior medulla oblongata, just lateral to the medullary pyramid. In cross section it resembles the dentate nucleus. This nucleus receives outputs from the contralateral cerebellum. Its own axons then decussate across the midline and enter the contralateral cerebellum through the restiform body of the inferior cerebellar peduncle. These axons from the inferior olivary nucleus are called **climbing fibers**. They excite the deep cerebellar nuclei and then "climb" along the axons of several nearby Purkinje cells to reach cerebellar cortex alongside mossy fibers.

Layers and Cells of the Cerebellar Cortex (Figs. 8.25 and 8.26)

Each **lobule** of the cerebellum consists of a core of white matter that is capped by the **folium**, the three-layered cortex of the cerebellum. From outside to inside, the layers of gray matter are the **molecular layer, Purkinje cell layer**, and **granule cell layer**. The granule cell layer is densely packed with small neurons called **granule cells** as well as less numerous **Golgi cells**. The molecular layer contains granule cell axons, **stellate cells**, and **basket cells**. The large bodies of **Purkinje cells** form their own layer between the molecular and granule cell layers.

Granule cells extend their axons outward to reach the molecular layer where their axons divide into **parallel fibers** that run along the surface of the folium and excite the dendrites of Purkinje cells, stellate cells, and basket cells. The axons of stellate and basket cells travel along the nearby parallel fibers before forming inhibitory synapses on Purkinje cells. Stellate cell axons

synapse on Purkinje dendrites but basket cell axons form encasing, basket-like synapses on the Purkinje cell body. In this way, a Purkinje cell is briefly excited by granule cell axons before nearby basket and stellate cells (excited by the same granule cell axons) inhibit it. Golgi cell dendrites extend into the molecular layer where they are also excited by granule cell axons. Golgi cell axons then synapse with the dendrites of granule cells to inhibit them. This feedback loop decreases the time in which granule cells are active and makes each excitatory impulse distinct from the preceding and following impulses. If granule cells are a chatty friend, the Golgi cells are the other friend who tells them they have said enough.

Mossy fibers from the pons, spinal cord, and vestibular nuclei give off a branch axon that excites one of the deep cerebellar nuclei and another that passes into the granule cell layer of the cerebellar cortex. Here they form an enlarged terminal end, the **cerebellar glomerulus**. The glomerulus contains excitatory synapses with the dendrites of multiple granule cells. Interestingly, this is also where inhibitory synapses between Golgi cell axons and granule cell dendrites occur. Climbing fibers from the inferior olivary nucleus excite the deep cerebellar nuclei and then "climb" along the axons of several nearby Purkinje cells to reach the Purkinje and molecular cell layer. They strongly excite the Purkinje cells.

The single axon leaving each Purkinje cell is the only output from the cerebellar cortex and all the other cells in the area serve to modulate their activity. Purkinje cell axons synapse with neurons in the deep cerebellar nuclei, which will then generate the only output from the cerebellum as a whole.

Deep Cerebellar Nuclei and Cerebellar Outputs (Figs. 8.25 and 8.27)

Within the white matter tracts of the cerebellum are four collections of nerve cell bodies, the **deep cerebellar nuclei.** From lateral to medial they are the **dentate, emboliform, globose, and fastigial nuclei.** I cannot improve on the most common mnemonic to remember them, "**D**on't **E**at **G**reasy **F**ood." These nuclei receive excitatory inputs from the pons, spinal cord, and inferior olivary nuclei. Thereafter they receive inhibitory inputs from Purkinje cells from distinct regions of the cerebellar cortex. The deep cerebellar nuclei are the only outputs from the cerebellum.

Dentate Nucleus

This circuit is most active immediately before motion begins. The neurons of the dentate nucleus receive inhibitory inputs from the Purkinje cells in the **lateral cerebellar hemispheres**. The neurons of the dentate nucleus extend their axons through the ipsilateral superior cerebellar peduncle into the tegmentum of the midbrain, where they decussate. Thereafter the axons can travel to several targets, but there are two main places they project.

The first target is the contralateral (VL) thalamic nucleus. Neurons of the VL thalamus then send axons to the cortex including the premotor planning area and primary motor cortex, the precentral gyrus. This allows the cerebellum to affect motor planning and initiation. The second target is the parvocellular (small cells) portion of the contralateral red nucleus. Axons in the red nucleus then project inferiorly through the

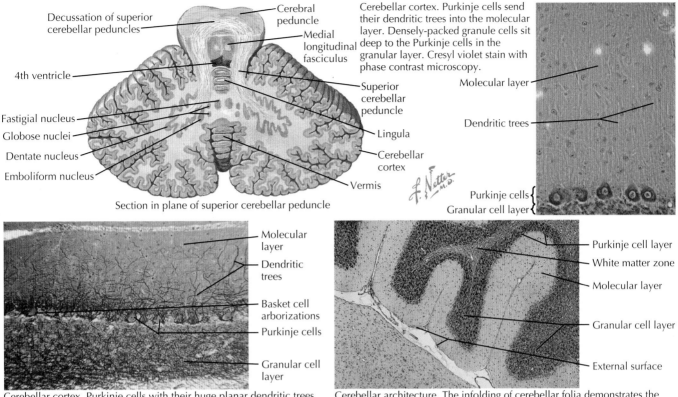

Decussation of superior cerebellar peduncles

Cerebral peduncle

Medial longitudinal fasciculus

4th ventricle

Fastigial nucleus

Globose nuclei

Dentate nucleus

Emboliform nucleus

Superior cerebellar peduncle

Lingula

Cerebellar cortex

Vermis

Section in plane of superior cerebellar peduncle

Cerebellar cortex. Purkinje cells send their dendritic trees into the molecular layer. Densely-packed granule cells sit deep to the Purkinje cells in the granular layer. Cresyl violet stain with phase contrast microscopy.

Molecular layer

Dendritic trees

Purkinje cells{

Granular cell layer{

Molecular layer

Dendritic trees

Basket cell arborizations

Purkinje cells

Granular cell layer

Purkinje cell layer

White matter zone

Molecular layer

Granular cell layer

External surface

Cerebellar cortex. Purkinje cells with their huge planar dendritic trees arborizing into the molecular layer. Basket cell arborizations surrounding the Purkinje cell bodies. Granular cell layer with granule cells and Golgi cells. The molecular layer contains outer stellate cells and basket cells. Cajal stain- fiber stain.

Cerebellar architecture. The infolding of cerebellar folia demonstrates the architecture of the cerebellar cortex. Cresyl violet stain.

Fig. 8.25 Cerebellar Anatomy: Internal Features. (Micrographs reused with permission from Felten DL, O'Banion MK, Maida MS. *Netter's Atlas of Neuroscience.* 3rd ed. Elsevier; 2016. Fig. 4.4.)

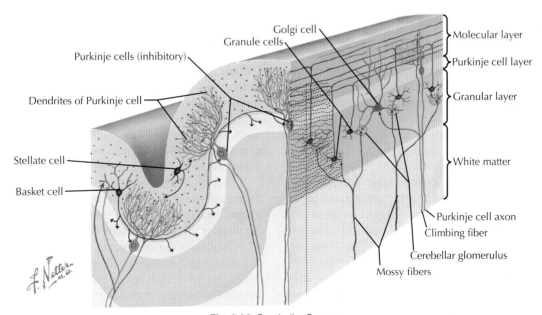

Golgi cell

Granule cells

Purkinje cells (inhibitory)

Dendrites of Purkinje cell

Stellate cell

Basket cell

Molecular layer

Purkinje cell layer

Granular layer

White matter

Purkinje cell axon

Climbing fiber

Cerebellar glomerulus

Mossy fibers

Fig. 8.26 Cerebellar Cortex.

central tegmental tract to reach the inferior olivary nucleus. Cells in the inferior olive then extend a climbing fiber axon to the contralateral cerebellum, ending on the same side where this circuit started. This circuit between the inferior olivary nucleus and the cerebellum is involved in the learning of complex motor activities and may be where muscle memory is generated. Other projections from the dentate nucleus extend to the hypothalamus and pontine nuclei.

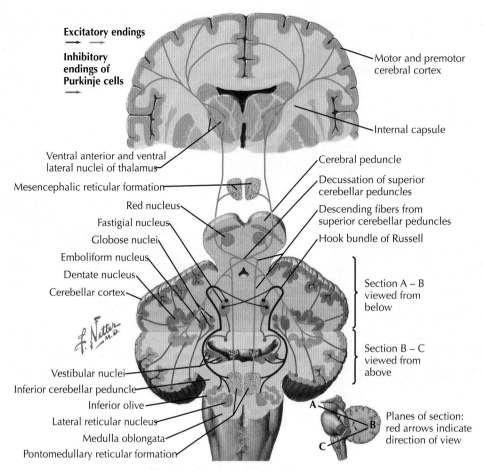

Fig. 8.27 Cerebellar Efferent Pathways.

Interposed Nuclei (Emboliform Nucleus and Globose Nucleus)

The emboliform and globose nuclei (collectively called the **interposed nuclei**) receive inhibitory inputs from Purkinje cells in the medial aspects of the cerebellar hemispheres, the **intermediate zone**. This circuit is most active during ongoing motor activity of the limbs. The neurons of the interposed nuclei extend their axons through the ipsilateral superior cerebellar peduncle into the tegmentum of the midbrain, where they decussate.

Like the dentate nucleus, the first target is the contralateral VL thalamic nucleus, leading to motor areas of the frontal lobe like the precentral gyrus. This circuit allows the cerebellum to modify the activity of the limbs by changing the activity of the lateral corticospinal tract. The lateral corticospinal tract also decussates as it descends, so the intermediate region of the cerebellar hemisphere and interposed nuclei will affect motor activity ipsilaterally due to the double decussation. The second target is the magnocellular (large cells) portion of the contralateral red nucleus. These neurons extend their axons through the ventral tegmental tract, where they decussate and form the rubrospinal tract to innervate flexor muscles of the upper limb. Other projections reach the reticular formation, inferior olivary nucleus, and anterior horn of the spinal cord.

Fastigial Nucleus

The fastigial nucleus receives inputs from Purkinje cells of the **superior vermis** and a small part of the **flocculonodular lobe**. This circuit coordinates ongoing movements of the trunk muscles. The fastigial neurons extend their axons through the ipsilateral superior cerebellar peduncle into the tegmentum of the midbrain, where they decussate before reaching the VL thalamic nucleus, leading to the precentral gyrus. This circuit allows the cerebellum to modify the activity of trunk muscles of the body by changing the activity of the lateral and anterior corticospinal tracts.

Axons from the fastigial nucleus also project inferiorly through the inferior cerebellar peduncle (this bundle is called the **juxtarestiform body**) to reach the ipsilateral **vestibular nuclei**. Simultaneously, fastigial axons decussate through a path in the white matter of the cerebellum called the **uncinate fasciculus** to reach the contralateral juxtarestiform body and vestibular nuclei. Therefore, each fastigial nucleus projects bilaterally to the left and right vestibular nuclei. Other projections reach the reticular formation, inferior olivary nucleus, and anterior horn of the spinal cord. This circuit affects movement of core muscles by changing the activity of vestibulospinal and reticulospinal tracts.

Flocculonodular Lobe and Inferior Vermis

The Purkinje cell neurons of the flocculonodular lobe and inferior vermis may extend their axons to the fastigial nucleus but

CLINICAL CORRELATION 8.11   **Cerebellar Dysfunction**

Damage to the cerebellar cortex or deep cerebellar nuclei will typically result in ataxia and other motor coordination dysfunctions on the ipsilateral side. This is because the circuits connecting the cerebellum to the cortex and spinal cord either decussate twice or not at all. However, lesions that affect the midline vermis will often result in bilateral ataxia of the trunk muscles.

- Ataxia: uncoordinated movements due to cerebellar dysfunction
  - Truncal ataxia: uncoordinated movement of the trunk muscles. May be due to damage to the vermis, spinocerebellar tracts, deep cerebellar nuclei, vestibular nuclei, or cerebellar peduncles. Affected patients will be unable to stay balanced over a narrow base and will walk with a broad, shuffling gait so they do not fall. To test, they may be asked to walk in a straight line, heel-to-toe, or to stand with their feet together and eyes closed (Romberg test). Patients tend to fall toward the affected side.

- Appendicular ataxia: uncoordinated movement of the extremities. May be due to damage to cerebellar hemispheres, spinocerebellar tracts, deep cerebellar nuclei, or cerebellar peduncles.
- Dysdiadochokinesia: the inability to perform rapid, alternating movements. This is tested by having patients set their palms on the thighs and then rapidly pronate and supinate. A lateral cerebellar lesion will make this nearly impossible.
- Dyssynergia: the breakdown of a complex movement into its individual parts
- Dysmetria: overshooting or undershooting when trying to touch moving or stationary objects
- Dysrhythmia: abnormal timing or pacing of movements
- Intention tremor: a tremor that progressively worsens as the end of an intentional motion is reached. This is often tested by having a patient extend their arm and then touch their nose. An intension tremor will grow more severe as the hand approaches the nose.

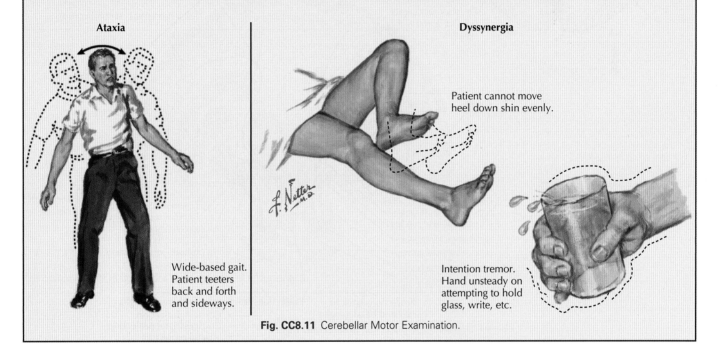

Ataxia

Wide-based gait. Patient teeters back and forth and sideways.

Dyssynergia

Patient cannot move heel down shin evenly.

Intention tremor. Hand unsteady on attempting to hold glass, write, etc.

Fig. CC8.11 Cerebellar Motor Examination.

many will bypass the deep cerebellar nuclei entirely, traveling inferiorly through the juxtarestiform body of the inferior cerebellar peduncle to synapse with the vestibular nuclei. This occurs bilaterally (possibly using the contralateral fastigial nucleus as a relay) and influences the activity of: (1) the extraocular muscles via the medial longitudinal fasciculus (a tract connecting the vestibular, abducens, trochlear, and oculomotor nuclei), (2) the medial vestibulospinal tract to coordinate movements of the head with eye movements, and (3) the lateral vestibulospinal tract to coordinate extensor movements of the lower limbs (Clinical Correlation 8.11).

BASAL GANGLIA (FIG. 8.28)

The basal ganglia are a collection of nerve cells (gray matter) nestled within the white matter tracts of the cortex. They are misnamed in that they are not true ganglia since they are not outside the CNS. They function to coordinate and initiate movement.

- **Caudate nucleus:** this tadpole-shaped gray matter structure is seen in the wall of each lateral ventricle. Its large **head** is located anteriorly and its size diminishes as it moves posteriorly to the **body** and becomes even smaller as its **tail** sits along the inferior horn of the lateral ventricle. The different regions do not have visually distinct transition points.
- **Putamen:** located deep to the insular lobe, extreme capsule, claustrum, and external capsule. It is linked by gray matter bridges with the head of the caudate nucleus. As we move posteriorly, the two become separated by the anterior limb of the internal capsule. Because of their linkage and functional similarity, the putamen and caudate nucleus are sometimes referred to together as the **striatum.**
- **Globus pallidus:** medial to the putamen is the globus pallidus. It is separated from the thalamus by the posterior limb of the internal capsule. The globus pallidus is divided into an **external** and **internal segment.** Because the putamen and globus pallidus form a lens-shaped (when viewed in an axial

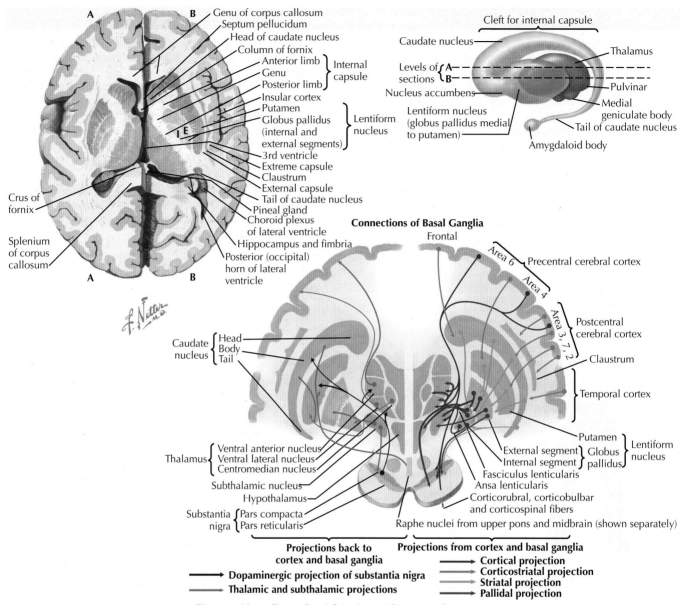

Connections of Basal Ganglia

Projections back to cortex and basal ganglia
→ Dopaminergic projection of substantia nigra
→ Thalamic and subthalamic projections

Projections from cortex and basal ganglia
→ Cortical projection
→ Corticostriatal projection
→ Striatal projection
→ Pallidal projection

Fig. 8.28 Motor Tracts, Basal Ganglia, and Dopamine Pathways.

cut) collection of gray matter, they are sometimes referred to collectively as the **lentiform or lenticular nucleus.**

- **Substantia nigra**: this is actually located in the midbrain but functions as part of the basal ganglia. It consists of two parts, the ventral **pars reticularis** and the dorsal **pars compacta.**
- **Subthalamic nucleus**: as its name suggests, it is located inferior to the thalamus but superior to the substantia nigra.

There are other nervous system structures near the basal ganglia that are not directly linked to movement but serve as worthwhile landmarks.

- **Nucleus accumbens**: found connecting the head of the caudate nucleus and the anteroinferior portion of the putamen. Involved in perception of pleasure, reward-seeking behavior, and addiction.
- **Amygdala**: located at the end of the tail of the caudate nucleus. Contributes to the limbic system and emotional processing.

Basal Ganglia Pathways That Influence Movement (Figs. 8.28 and 8.29)

The circuitry of the basal ganglia is complex. We are going to focus exclusively on how these structures affect movement but it is worth noting that the basal ganglia also influence emotion, higher-order cognition, and personality. Nearly all inputs to the basal ganglia arrive in the caudate nucleus and putamen. Since these two structures act as a unit, we will use the group term **striatum** hereafter. Outputs from the basal ganglia come almost entirely from the internal segment of the globus pallidus and the pars reticularis of the substantia nigra. These output neurons use an inhibitory neurotransmitter, GABA, to decrease the activity of neurons in the **ventral anterior (VA)** and **ventral lateral (VL)** thalamic nuclei. Since these thalamic neurons stimulate the motor regions of the frontal lobe (including the precentral gyrus), GABA inhibition from the basal ganglia will tend to decrease motor activity from the primary motor cortex.

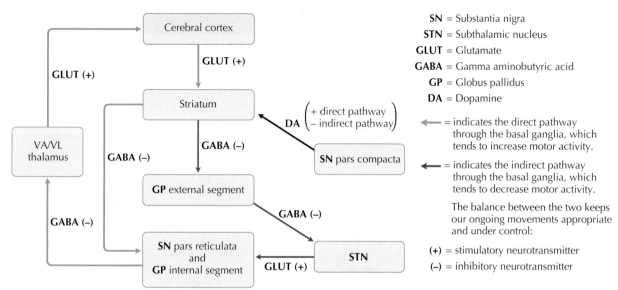

Fig. 8.29 Basic Basal Ganglia Circuitry and Neurotransmitters.

We can group basal ganglia projections into two pathways that modulate motor activity. The projections of the **direct pathway** result in a net increase in motor activity while projections of the **indirect pathway** result in a net decrease in motor activity.

Direct Pathway

In the direct pathway, the striatum receives inputs from the cortex, including the frontal premotor cortex, which stimulate its neurons with the excitatory neurotransmitter **glutamate**. Striatal neurons send inhibitory signals to neurons in the internal segment of the globus pallidus and the pars reticularis of the substantia nigra using the neurotransmitters **GABA** and **substance P**. Since these striatal neurons inhibit the inhibitory outputs of the internal segment of globus pallidus and pars reticularis of substantia nigra, the direct pathway will tend to excite motor activity in the VA and VL thalamus, which excite motor neurons in the frontal lobe. Note that **dopamine**-releasing neurons in the pars compacta of the substantia nigra also synapse with striatal neurons of the direct pathway. These striatal neurons express a receptor that binds to dopamine and stimulates the release of GABA and substance P. As a result, dopamine helps INCREASE motor activity by stimulating the direct pathway.

Indirect Pathway

In the indirect pathway, which earned its name by having additional steps, the striatum receives glutamate stimuli from the cortex just as it did in the direct pathway. In this pathway, axons from the striatum travel to the external segment of the globus pallidus and release inhibitory neurotransmitters, such as GABA and **enkephalin**. Neurons from the external segment of the globus pallidus extend GABA-releasing, inhibitory axons to the subthalamic nucleus. Neurons in the subthalamic nucleus then extend glutamate-releasing, excitatory axons to the internal segment of the globus pallidus and pars reticularis of the substantia nigra. In this way the indirect pathway inhibits neurons that inhibit neurons that excite neurons that inhibit the VA and VL thalamus and primary motor cortex. I know that last sentence is awful, but I did my best. Here is a more succinct version. The internal segment of the globus pallidus and pars reticularis of the substantia nigra inhibit the thalamus, and therefore inhibit motor activity in the frontal lobe. The indirect pathway results in a net stimulation of activity through the subthalamic nucleus. Dopamine-releasing neurons from the pars compacta of the substantia nigra also synapse with striatal neurons of the indirect pathway but via a different receptor, which actually inhibits striatal neurons of the indirect pathway. As a result, dopamine also helps INCREASE motor activity by inhibiting the indirect pathway (Clinical Correlations 8.12–8.14).

CLINICAL CORRELATION 8.12   Parkinson Disease

In Parkinson disease, the dopamine-releasing cells of the pars compacta of the substantia nigra die off. Because dopamine stimulates the direct pathway and inhibits the indirect pathway through the basal ganglia, this loss will result in a decrease in movement, called hypokinesia. People suffering from this disease tend to move with small, shuffling steps and to have a lack of facial movement and expression. Willful movement does occur, but it is constrained and minimal. When the limbs are relaxed, there will often be a resting tremor affecting the hands, upper limbs, lower limbs, or the mouth. Another classic feature of Parkinson is cogwheel rigidity; as an examiner extends a patient's elbow, the joint will extend but suddenly stop and "catch" to become immobile, after which it will extend further, catch, and repeat until the limb is extended. If the substantia nigra on one side is affected, the signs will appear primarily on the opposite side since the basal ganglia project to the ipsilateral precentral gyrus, which sends lateral corticospinal axons to the contralateral side of the body.

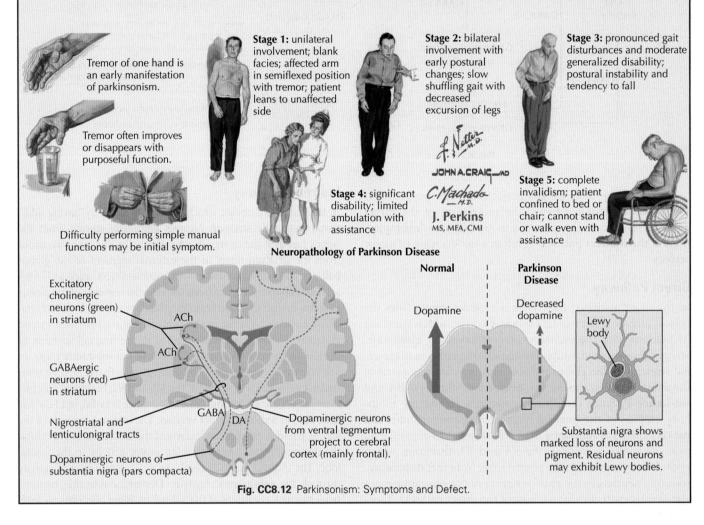

Tremor of one hand is an early manifestation of parkinsonism.

Tremor often improves or disappears with purposeful function.

Difficulty performing simple manual functions may be initial symptom.

Stage 1: unilateral involvement; blank facies; affected arm in semiflexed position with tremor; patient leans to unaffected side

Stage 2: bilateral involvement with early postural changes; slow shuffling gait with decreased excursion of legs

Stage 3: pronounced gait disturbances and moderate generalized disability; postural instability and tendency to fall

Stage 4: significant disability; limited ambulation with assistance

Stage 5: complete invalidism; patient confined to bed or chair; cannot stand or walk even with assistance

Neuropathology of Parkinson Disease

Excitatory cholinergic neurons (green) in striatum

ACh

ACh

GABAergic neurons (red) in striatum

Nigrostriatal and lenticulonigral tracts

GABA

DA

Dopaminergic neurons of substantia nigra (pars compacta)

Dopaminergic neurons from ventral tegmentum project to cerebral cortex (mainly frontal).

Normal

Dopamine

Parkinson Disease

Decreased dopamine

Lewy body

Substantia nigra shows marked loss of neurons and pigment. Residual neurons may exhibit Lewy bodies.

Fig. CC8.12 Parkinsonism: Symptoms and Defect.

CLINICAL CORRELATION 8.13　Huntington Disease

In Huntington disease or Huntington chorea, a trinucleotide repeat mutation causes the striatal cells of the caudate nucleus and putamen to die, particularly the enkephalin-releasing inhibitory neurons of the indirect pathway. As the striatal cells die, the direct pathway becomes more active and the indirect pathway becomes less active, causing an increase in uncontrolled, flinging movement, called hyperkinesia or chorea. People suffering from this disease will have unintended movements of the limbs and this is often accompanied by changes in personality. As with Parkinson disease, if one side is affected to a greater degree than the opposite side, the signs will appear primarily on the contralateral side since the basal ganglia project to the ipsilateral precentral gyrus, which sends lateral corticospinal axons to the contralateral side of the body. Because the caudate nucleus is in the lateral wall of the lateral ventricles, the ventricles themselves may appear to enlarge. This is sometimes called ventriculomegaly or *hydrocephalus ex vacuo* and should not be confused with obstructive hydrocephalus.

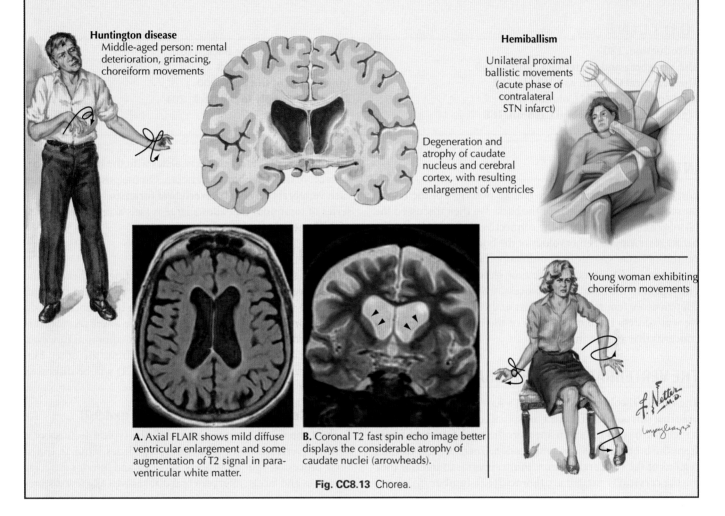

Huntington disease
Middle-aged person: mental deterioration, grimacing, choreiform movements

Hemiballism
Unilateral proximal ballistic movements (acute phase of contralateral STN infarct)

Degeneration and atrophy of caudate nucleus and cerebral cortex, with resulting enlargement of ventricles

Young woman exhibiting choreiform movements

A. Axial FLAIR shows mild diffuse ventricular enlargement and some augmentation of T2 signal in paraventricular white matter.

B. Coronal T2 fast spin echo image better displays the considerable atrophy of caudate nuclei (arrowheads).

Fig. CC8.13 Chorea.

CLINICAL CORRELATION 8.14　Hemiballismus

This condition is characterized by uncontrollable flinging of the limbs, primarily affecting the proximal segment (humerus or femur). It is often due to a lesion of the subthalamic nucleus, which typically stimulates the internal segment of the globus pallidus and pars reticularis of the substantia nigra to inhibit motor activity arising from the thalamus and precentral gyrus. Since death of the subthalamic neurons compromises the indirect pathway, it results in a net increase of uncontrolled motor activity. Neurologic signs appear primarily on the opposite side since the basal ganglia project to the ipsilateral precentral gyrus, which sends lateral corticospinal axons to the contralateral side of the body.

Clinical Anatomy of the Back

INTRODUCTION

Early on in Chapters 2 to 5 we had an overview of the bones, muscles, nerves, and vessels of the back. We then discussed the histology and physiology of the connective tissues and muscles, before reviewing the embryology of the body and the role of the central nervous system in coordinating bodily sensations and movement in Chapters 6–8. We now shift focus to investigate one region of the body. In the process, we will review the prior content as we remix it in the context of the back. Along the way, we will address the biomechanics of the back and the clinical concerns that arise in this region.

THE VERTEBRAE AND VERTEBRAL COLUMN

The **vertebral column** is made from a series of individual vertebrae that surround and protect the spinal cord and its associated structures. It supports and maneuvers the head, transmits forces from the limbs, and resists compression. There are five distinct regions of the vertebral column. From superior to inferior they are the **cervical** (7 vertebrae), **thoracic** (12), **lumbar** (5), **sacral** (5), and **coccygeal** (3 to 5) regions.

Except for the atlas, all vertebrae have a **vertebral body** on their anterior side that supports the weight of the body superior to it and transmits forces from the vertebrae inferior to it. Extending posteriorly from the vertebral body is the **vertebral arch**, which surrounds and protects the spinal cord and associated structures. The portions of the vertebral arch that connect to the vertebral body are the right and left **pedicles**. The right and left **laminae** extend from the pedicles and meet each other on the midline. The space formed by the vertebral arch and body is the **vertebral foramen**. A single **spinous process** extends posteriorly off the vertebral arch at the point where the right and left laminae meet. The right and left **transverse processes** extend laterally from the arch where the pedicles meet the laminae. Near the transverse processes are the **superior** and **inferior articular processes**. The superior articular process extends superiorly and features a **superior articular facet**. The **inferior articular process** extends inferiorly and hosts an

inferior articular facet that articulates with the superior articular facet of the neighboring vertebra. On the posterior aspect of each vertebral body is a **basivertebral foramen** (or sometimes a series of foramina) that allows large vessels access to the inside of the bone.

Cervical Vertebrae

There are seven cervical vertebrae connecting the head to the thoracic vertebrae. Their vertebral bodies are relatively small compared to those in other regions of the body since they do not support much of the body's weight. The lower cervical vertebrae (3rd to 7th) have many features in common; however, the upper cervical vertebrae are distinct from the other five. For that reason, the atlas (C1) and axis (C2) will be discussed separately.

Lower Cervical Vertebrae (Figs. 9.1 and 9.2)

Each of the C3–C7 vertebrae have all the typical features of a vertebra (vertebral body, vertebral arch, pedicles, laminae, transverse processes, spinous process, superior and inferior articular processes and facets, intervertebral disc) as well as a few distinctive features. The superior aspect of the vertebral bodies have raised lateral edges, **uncinate processes**, that cradle the nearby intervertebral disc and form synovial **uncovertebral joints** with the inferolateral aspect of the vertebral body above it. The C1–C6 vertebrae typically feature a hole in their transverse processes called **the transverse foramen** that surrounds the left and right vertebral arteries and veins as they travel from the subclavian vessels to the brainstem. The transverse processes also have raised **anterior** and **posterior tubercles** that flank the transverse foramen and are separated by a depression, the **groove for the spinal nerve**. The anterior tubercle of C6 is particularly large and is referred to as the **carotid tubercle**. The spinous processes of C3–C6 are typically **bifid**, split into two posteriorly.

Upper Cervical Vertebrae (Fig. 9.3)

The **axis** (C2) appears very much like a typical cervical vertebra but is unique in that is has a large, thumb-shaped **dens** (odontoid process) extending superiorly from the vertebral body, with

Inferior aspect of C3 and superior aspect of C4 showing the sites of the facet and uncovertebral articulations

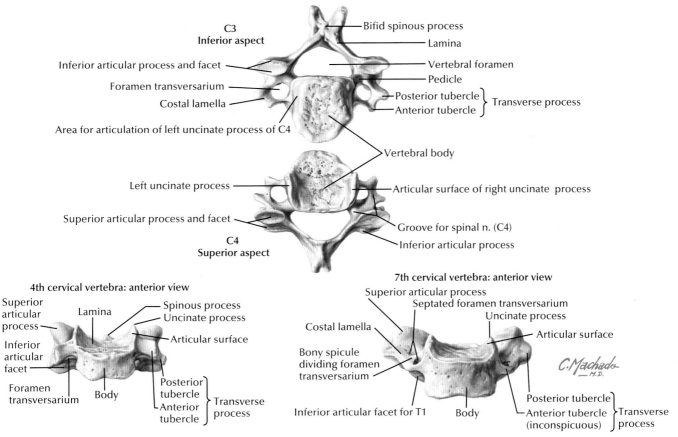

4th cervical vertebra: anterior view

7th cervical vertebra: anterior view

Fig. 9.1 Cervical Vertebrae.

Cervical vertebrae: anterior view

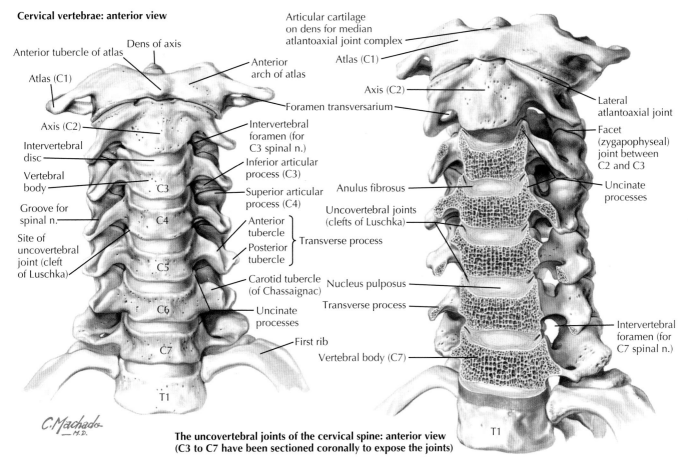

The uncovertebral joints of the cervical spine: anterior view
(C3 to C7 have been sectioned coronally to expose the joints)

Fig. 9.2 Cervical Vertebrae: Uncovertebral Joints.

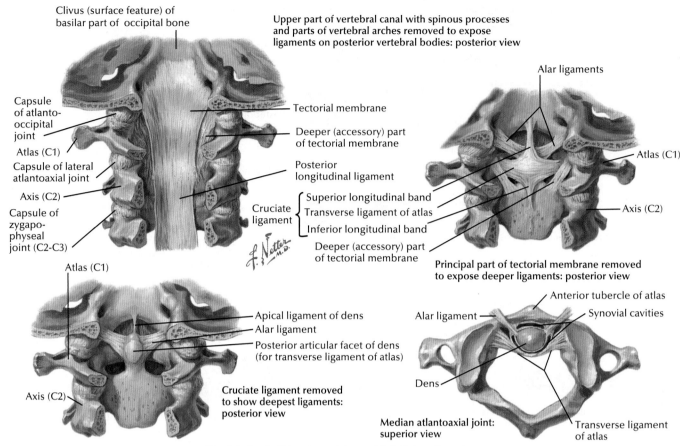

Fig. 9.3 Cervical Vertebrae: Atlas and Axis Spine: Osteology.

the pointed **apex** of the dens at the most superior point. The dens is actually the C1 vertebral body that fused with the vertebral body of C2 while the sclerotomes were separating during development. The dens has **anterior** and **posterior articular facets** that allow it to articulate with the atlas (anterior) and the transverse ligament of the atlas (posterior) as the atlas rotates with the dens as its fulcrum. The axis interacts with the atlas via its superior articular facet and the dens; there is no intervertebral disc between them.

The **atlas** (C1) is an oval-shaped bone that lacks a vertebral body; however, the atlas has large **lateral masses** that host the transverse processes, transverse foramina, as well as superior and inferior articular facets. The superior articular facets articulate with occipital condyles while the inferior articular facets articulate with the superior articular facets of the axis. Anteriorly, the lateral masses are connected by a short **anterior arch**, which has a distinct **anterior protuberance** at its midpoint. The inner surface of the anterior arch has the **articular facet for the dens**. The large **posterior arch** extends from the lateral masses to enclose the vertebral foramen. It has a **posterior protuberance** on its posterior midline as well as a notable **groove for the vertebral artery** running along its superior aspect.

Thoracic Vertebrae (Fig. 9.4)

The twelve thoracic vertebrae have all the typical features of a vertebra as well as a few distinctive features that relate to their interaction with the ribs. Each thoracic vertebra articulates with

one or two **ribs** via a **costal facet**, or **inferior** and **superior costal demifacets**. Costal facets (T1, T11, and T12) are seen when the head of a rib articulates with a single vertebral body, whereas superior and inferior demifacets (T1–T10) are seen when a rib head straddles two adjacent vertebral bodies and the intervertebral disc between them. The ribs also articulate with the anterior aspect of vertebral transverse processes at the **transverse costal facet**. The transverse costal facets are generally not present on T11 and T12. Immediately posterior to the costal facets of the T1 vertebral body are stunted left and right **uncinate processes** that interact with C7. None of the other thoracic vertebrae have uncinate processes.

From a lateral view, the upper and middle spinous processes are long and angled inferiorly, especially the middle (T4–T9) thoracic spinous processes. The lower thoracic spinous processes are smaller and square-shaped.

Lumbar Vertebrae (Fig. 9.5)

The five lumbar vertebrae have very large vertebral bodies to support the body's weight. The transverse processes of the lumbar vertebrae are elongated and flat in the coronal plane. The spinous processes of the lumbar vertebrae are very large and square-shaped. There are some special landmarks on the posterior lumbar vertebrae for muscle attachment. **Mammillary processes** project posteriorly from the superior articular processes, and notable **accessory processes** are located on the posterior aspect of the lumbar transverse

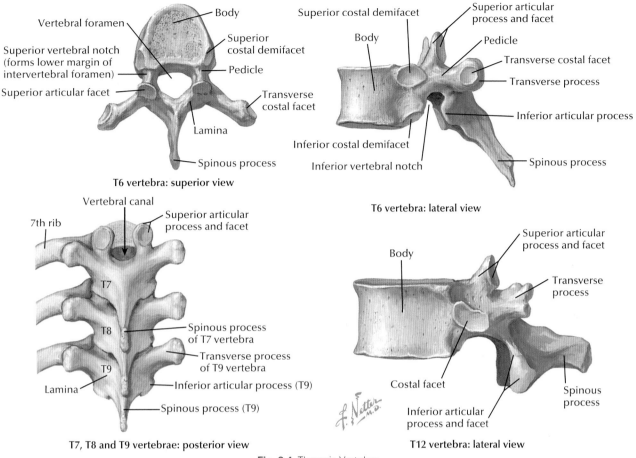

T6 vertebra: superior view

T6 vertebra: lateral view

T7, T8 and T9 vertebrae: posterior view

T12 vertebra: lateral view

Fig. 9.4 Thoracic Vertebra.

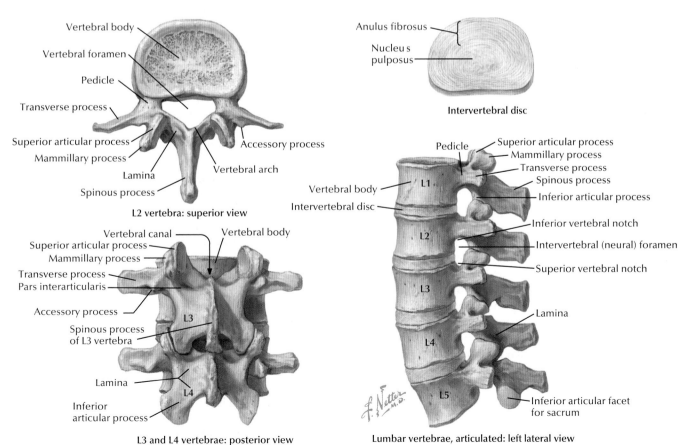

Intervertebral disc

L2 vertebra: superior view

L3 and L4 vertebrae: posterior view

Lumbar vertebrae, articulated: left lateral view

Fig. 9.5 Lumbar Vertebrae and Intervertebral Disc Spine: Osteology.

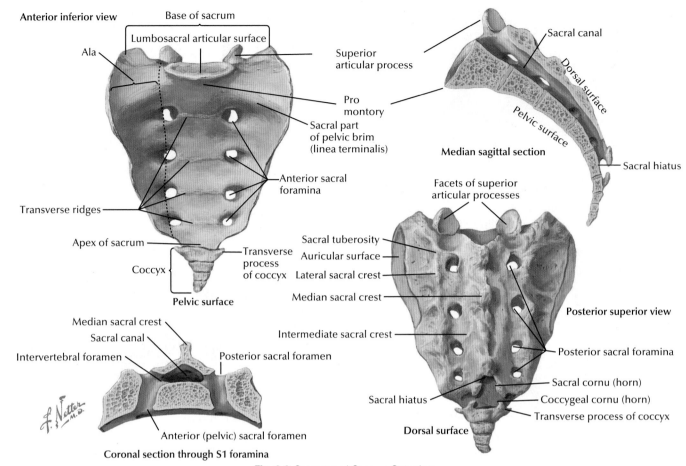

Fig. 9.6 Sacrum and Coccyx: Osteology.

processes. The accessory processes actually mark where the transverse processes would normally have stopped; the rest of the lumbar transverse processes are actually stunted ribs, called **costal processes** when spoken of as a distinct structure. However, most clinicians and anatomists call the whole assembly of accessory process and costal process the **transverse process**.

Sacral Vertebrae (Fig. 9.6)

The **sacrum** consists of five bones that fuse during development. The sites of fusion, marking where intervertebral discs would have been, are the **transverse ridges** on the anterior surface of the sacrum. At the lateral limits of each transverse line are large **anterior sacral foramina** for the anterior rami leaving the sacrum and travelling to the pelvic organs and lower limbs. The large superior portion of the sacrum is the **sacral base**, which terminates anteriorly as the **sacral promontory**. The inferior tip of the sacrum that articulates with the coccyx is called the **apex of the sacrum**. The large bony wings, **alae** (singular **ala**), that extend laterally from the sacral vertebral bodies articulate with the ilium at the sacrum's **auricular surface**.

Because the sacral vertebrae are fused, the vertebral foraminae create a continuous **sacral canal** that surrounds anterior and posterior nerve roots extending from the spinal cord. Its inferior opening is the **sacral hiatus**, which is bounded by two **sacral cornua**. The posterior aspect of the sacrum has a large

ridge of bone that covers the midline of the sacral canal, the **median sacral crest**. It is formed by the spinous processes of the fused vertebrae but only extends to S3 or S4. On either side of the median sacral crest are right and left **intermediate sacral crests**, which are formed by fused articular processes and also cover the sacral canal. The intermediate sacral crests terminate superiorly as **superior articular processes** and **facets** that articulate with the inferior articular facets of L5. Further laterally are the right and left **lateral sacral crests**, formed by fusion of the sacral transverse processes. Between the intermediate and lateral sacral crests are the **posterior sacral foramina**, which transmit posterior rami from the sacrum to the lower back. In between the lateral sacral crest of S1–S3 and the auricular surface are a series of three depressions and **three sacral tuberosities** that mark where the posterior sacroiliac ligament attaches to the sacrum.

Coccygeal Vertebrae (See Fig. 9.6)

The **coccyx** (tailbone) is a series of 3 to 5 fused and vestigial vertebrae. These conjoined vertebral bodies have lost all the other characteristic features of vertebrae aside from a stunted **transverse process** on each side of the first coccygeal vertebra. The posterosuperior aspect of the first coccygeal vertebra may also have left and right **coccygeal horns**, or **cornua**, extending superiorly. These nearly insignificant bones serve as an attachment point for muscles of the pelvic diaphragm and anus. They do not seem insignificant when they are fractured, since acute pain is caused by sitting and defecating, activities no one is able to postpone indefinitely (Clinical Correlation 9.1).

Intervertebral Foramen (See Fig. 9.5)

When viewed laterally, the pedicles have small indentations on their superior and inferior surfaces, the **superior vertebral notch** and the larger **inferior vertebral notch**. The inferior and superior vertebral notches of adjacent vertebrae create an **intervertebral foramen** that allows a spinal nerve to exit at each vertebral level. The cervical and upper thoracic intervertebral foramina are narrow, while the lumbar and lower thoracic intervertebral foramina are quite large. Side-bending can narrow the intervertebral foramina on the concave side of the curvature. Bony overgrowth around the intervertebral foramen or osteophytes around the facet joints can also narrow the space (Clinical Correlation 9.2).

Intervertebral Discs (Fig. 9.7, See Also Fig. 9.5)

Neighboring vertebral bodies, except for C1–C2 and the sacral vertebrae, are connected by **intervertebral discs**. These discs serve as shock absorbers for the forces that are transmitted along the vertebral column. They have a gelatinous core, the **nucleus pulposus**, consisting of mucous connective tissue that is rich in proteoglycans and loosely arranged fibers. The nucleus pulposus is the only remnant of the notochord, which occupied the same position at a much earlier stage of development. Surrounding each nucleus pulposus is the **annulus fibrosus**, which is formed by many concentric rings of fibrocartilage. Each ring has laminae of collagen fibers (types I and II) running perpendicular to their neighboring rings. The annulus fibrosus and vertebral bodies are both derived from the sclerotome, but the annulus does not ossify. The annulus surrounds the nucleus and keeps it in a central location. This allows the disc to rebound when it experiences compressive forces.

The interface between the vertebral body and intervertebral disc is the **vertebral endplate**. This fascinating structure also comes from sclerotomal mesenchyme but remains as hyaline cartilage even after the vertebral bodies have ossified. The endplates are fused with the inner rings of the annulus fibrosus as well as the raised superior and inferior rims of the vertebral bodies, the **annular epiphyses**. Small vessels within the endplates allow nutrients to diffuse from the trabecular bone of the vertebral bodies to reach the intervertebral discs, which are otherwise avascular. In dry bone specimens the endplates are not present and this gives the flat surfaces of the vertebral body a spongy appearance. The ossification of the endplates with age and loss of vessels passing through them to the discs may be one factor that contributes to degenerative disc disease (Biomechanics Box 9.1 and Clinical Correlation 9.3).

CLINICAL CORRELATION 9.1   Stable and Unstable Spinal Injuries

Injuries of the vertebral (spinal) column are classified as stable, not requiring immobilization, or unstable, requiring immobilization. To make these designations, the vertebrae are conceptualized as having three columns: (1) the anterior ½ of the vertebral body; (2) the posterior ½ of the vertebral body and pedicles; and (3) the laminae, articular processes, and spinous processes. Injury that involves only one column is classified as stable and unlikely to damage the spinal cord. Injury involving 2 or 3 columns is unstable and the patient must be restrained to minimize the potential for neurologic trauma.

Compression and Burst Fractures (Fig. CC9.1A)

Osteoporosis is the loss of bone density, which is one of several things that can lead to **osteopenia**, bone weakness. Vertebral bodies are particularly vulnerable, since they bear the weight of the body above their level. If they become too weak, they may undergo a **compression fracture** in which the vertebral body collapses in on itself. Since the posterior aspect of the vertebrae are supported by the pedicles and articular processes, the anterior sides become more severely compressed, resulting in a wedge-shaped vertebral body with the narrow end pointing anteriorly. This is one cause of increased thoracic kyphosis with age. In a burst fracture, massive compressive force causes the vertebral body to explode outward, possibly impinging on structures in the vertebral canal and causing neurologic signs.

Fracture of the Atlas and Axis (Fig. CC9.1B)

Sudden compression of the head from above can put tremendous pressure on the articular facets of the atlas. When the atlas is compressed violently, it pushes the lateral masses laterally and can result in snapping of the anterior and posterior arches of the atlas. Like the pelvis, the atlas is a ring of bone and almost always fractures in more than one place.

The articular processes of the axis are stouter than those in the atlas. They are characteristically prone to fracture through the area between superior and inferior articular processes (pars interarticularis) when the head is forcibly extended relative to the upper cervical vertebrae. This is famously (and horrifyingly) used during a hanging, when the knot of the noose is placed alongside the jaw so that when the rope goes taut, the head is jerked into extension, fracturing the axis and destroying the upper spinal cord, causing nearly instantaneous death. More horrendously, if this is not done properly the victim will gradually asphyxiate as the airway and vessels of the neck are compressed.

Spondylolysis and Spondylolisthesis (Fig. CC9.1C)

Fractures of the pars interarticularis are known as **spondylolysis**. This is a relatively common injury in young athletes and tends to occur when the vertebrae are compressed during forceful extension. If this fracture occurs bilaterally, the arch of the affected vertebra remains attached to its inferior neighbor and the vertebral body is attached to its superior neighbor. This instability can result in the vertebral body shifting anteriorly as the supporting ligaments and intervertebral disc weaken and stretch. Fracture of the pars interarticularis, spondylolysis, coupled with displacement is **spondylolisthesis**. It can gradually worsen as the affected vertebral body slides anteriorly, relative to its inferior neighbor. As this condition worsens, the spinal cord posterior to the affected vertebra can become compressed. This can occur at any level but is most common in the lumbar and cervical levels, due to their lordotic (concave posteriorly) curvature, which makes hyperextension injuries more likely. When imaged using a posterior oblique view, this condition has a classic "Scotty dog" sign. The dog's head is formed by the pedicle, superior articular facet, and transverse process. The neck is formed by the pars interarticularis. The foreleg is formed by the inferior articular facet, while the body and hindlimbs are formed by the spinous process and opposite inferior articular process. If the Scotty dog appears well, then the pars interarticularis is intact. If he is wearing a dark collar, there is a spondylolysis. If the dog has been decapitated (sorry, gentle readers) then the pars interarticularis is fractured and there has been significant displacement, a spondylolisthesis. This description is still used although CT scans are being used more frequently to diagnose this condition.

Continued

A. Trauma of the Spine

Three-Column Concept of Spinal Stability

| Posterior column | Middle Anterior columncolumn | Posterior column | Middle Anterior columncolumn | Burst fracture |

Three-column concept. If more than one column involved in fracture, then instability of spine usually results

Lateral view. Note that lateral facet (zygapophyseal) joints in posterior column, with intervertebral foramina in middle column

Burst fracture of unstable vertebral body involving both anterior and middle columns resulted in instability and spinal cord compression

Flexion
Distraction results in complete transverse fracture through entire vertebra. Note hinge effect of anterior longitudinal ligament

B. Fractures of cervical vertebrae

Fracture of dens

Type I. Fracture of tip

Type II. Fracture of base or neck

Superior articular facet

Inferior articular facet

Type III. Fracture extends into body of axis

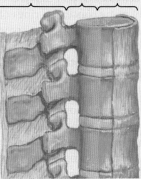

Jefferson fracture of atlas (C1)
Each arch may be broken in one or more places

Fracture of anterior arch

Superior articular facet

Fracture of posterior arch

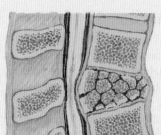

Superior articular facet

Inferior articular process

Inferior articular facet

Hangman fracture
Fracture through neural arch of axis (C2), between superior and inferior articular facets

Superior articular facet

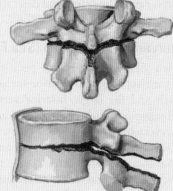

C. Spondylolysis and spondylolisthesis

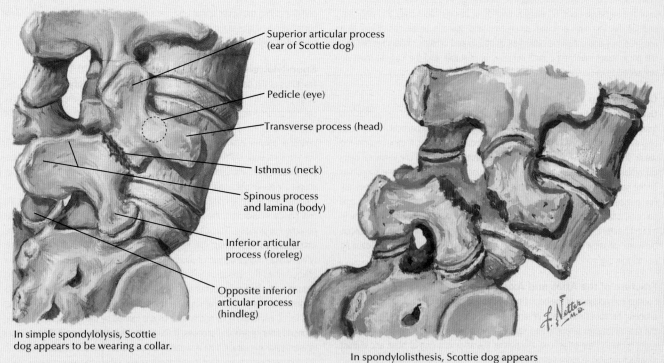

Superior articular process (ear of Scottie dog)

Pedicle (eye)

Transverse process (head)

Isthmus (neck)

Spinous process and lamina (body)

Inferior articular process (foreleg)

Opposite inferior articular process (hindleg)

In simple spondylolysis, Scottie dog appears to be wearing a collar.

In spondylolisthesis, Scottie dog appears decapitated.

Fig. CC9.1 Stable and Unstable Spinal Injuries (Trauma, Cervical Vertebral Fractures, Spondylolysis).

CLINICAL CORRELATION 9.2   Palpating the Back and Topographical Anatomy

Palpating the spinous processes of the vertebral column is commonly done to identify the exact level of a complaint or vertebral dysfunction. The vertebra prominens (most prominent spinous process) extends the most posteriorly and is usually either C7 or T1. If you wish to determine which, you can palpate it and ask your patient to flex his or her neck. If it moves, the vertebra prominens is C7; if it is stable, it is T1.

However, since the spinous processes do not project perfectly horizontally, it is a bit confusing to identify which spinous process corresponds to which vertebral body.

Clinicians have created the **rule of threes** to keep track of these relationships in the thoracic spine.

- T1–T3: the spinous process of each vertebra is at the same level as its vertebral body
- T4–T6: the spinous process of each vertebra is ½ level inferior to its vertebral body
- T7–T9: the spinous process of each vertebra is 1 level below its vertebral body
- T10: the spinous process of each vertebra is 1 level below its vertebral body (like T7–T9)
- T11: the spinous process of each vertebra is ½ level inferior to its vertebral body (like T4–T6)
- T12: the spinous process of each vertebra is at the same level as its vertebral body (like T1–T3)

However, recent studies have demonstrated that the rule of threes is not as accurate as we might hope and an alternative, **Geelhoed's rule**, has been proposed. This rule states that the spinous processes of all thoracic vertebrae lie in the same horizontal plane as the transverse processes of their inferior neighboring vertebra.

There are a few landmarks of note below the thoracic region. The L4 spinous process is palpable at the same level as the superior-most aspect of the iliac crest, while the S2 spinous process (of the median sacral crest) is palpable at the level of the posterior superior iliac spine. The S3 spinous process is palpable at the superior limit of the gluteal cleft.

THE VERTEBRAL COLUMN AS A WHOLE (FIG. 9.8)

When the entire vertebral column is viewed from the side, the different regions have distinctive curves. The cervical and lumbar regions appear concave (scooped out) posteriorly and convex (bulging) anteriorly; this type of curvature is called a **lordosis.** Conversely, the thoracic and sacral regions appear concave anteriorly and convex posteriorly; this type of curvature is called a **kyphosis.** The thoracic and sacral kyphoses are **primary curvatures** as they are present at birth and are an intrinsic feature of the way these bones develop. The cervical and lumbar lordoses are **secondary curvatures** since they only develop after birth as our body learns to cope with gravity. Since the cervical and lumbar vertebrae are not fused or restricted by the ribcage, these lordotic curvatures can vary considerably from person to person. **Scoliosis** (also called rotoscoliosis) refers to a lateral curvature of the spine. These lateral curves are not a normal feature of the vertebral column but can develop due to poor posture or can be caused by degenerative diseases. Their severity can vary considerably, depending upon their cause.

JOINTS OF THE VERTEBRAL COLUMN (SEE FIGS. 9.2, 9.3, 9.5, AND 9.8)

In addition to the intervertebral discs, vertebrae interact as the facets on their inferior articular processes meet the articular facets on the superior articular processes of the vertebra immediately inferior to it. The interaction creates a vertebral **facet joint** (a.k.a. **zygapophyseal joint**) on each side. Despite the differences in their orientation, the facet joints of the vertebrae from C1 to S1 share several features in common. Like other synovial joints, the facet joints have an outer fibrous layer and an inner, synovial layer that filters blood to create the synovial fluid within the capsule. Within the capsule, the articular surfaces of the bones are typically covered by hyaline (often called "articular") cartilage. This allows their motions to be smooth and minimizes friction and irritation.

The **atlantooccipital joints**, formed by the superior articular facet of the atlas and the occipital condyles, allow a great deal of flexion/extension and are responsible for the majority of the flexions/extension in the cervical region (nod your head "yes" if you understand) as well as a small amount of side-bending. Rotation is limited. There are thickened capsular ligaments on their anterior, posterior, and lateral aspects.

There are several **atlantoaxial joints**. The **median atlantoaxial joint** is formed as the anterior and posterior articular surfaces of the dens articulate with the anterior arch of the atlas and the transverse ligament of the atlas. The inferior articular facet of the atlas connects to the superior articular facet of the axis in a way that is very similar to the lower cervical facet joints, forming the **lateral atlantoaxial joints**. These joints allow a tremendous amount of rotation (shake your head "no" if this is unclear) but limited side-bending and flexion/extension.

The superior and inferior articular facets of the **lower cervical facet joints** are oriented somewhat in the horizontal plane but become more vertically oriented (in the coronal plane) as they get closer to the thoracic vertebrae. On their own, these facet joins would allow a considerable amount of movement. However, the uncinate processes severely limit the amount of rotation and lateral displacement of the lower cervical vertebrae, allowing some flexion/extension, anterior/posterior translation, and a small amount of side-bending in this region. Contact of the spinous processes limits the amount of extension that is possible in the neck; however, the bifid spinous processes of the cervical vertebrae straddle the spinous process of their inferior neighbor, allowing just a bit more extension than would otherwise be possible. Superior and inferior articular facets of the **thoracic facet joints** are largely vertical in the coronal plane. On their own, these would allow a tremendous amount of movement, but the ribcage constrains them considerably, limiting (but not eliminating) flexion/extension, side-bending, and rotation. The overlapping thoracic spinous processes limit extension severely. **Lumbar facet joints** are largely oriented vertically in the sagittal plane with the inferior articular facets surrounded by their neighbor's superior articular facets. They allow a large amount of flexion/extension and side-bending but limit rotation. The **lumbosacral facet joint** is similar to the lumbar facet joints. Finally, the **sacrococcygeal joint** is a small synovial

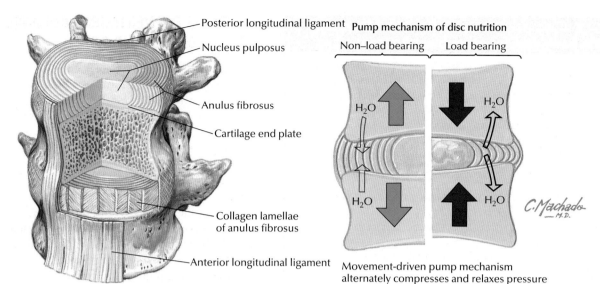

Intervertebral disc composed of central nuclear zone of collagen and hydrated proteoglycans surrounded by concentric lamellae of collagen fibers

Movement-driven pump mechanism alternately compresses and relaxes pressure on disc, pumping water and waste products out and water and nutrients in.

Fig. 9.7 Intervertebral Disc.

BIOMECHANICS BOX 9.1 Intervertebral Disc Function

When standing or sitting upright, the intervertebral discs are compressed and flattened in a uniform manner. Compression of the intervertebral disc creates increased pressure on the nucleus pulposus, which is held within the layers of the anulus fibrosus. As the vertebral column flexes (becomes concave anteriorly) the nucleus pulposus is pinched anteriorly and pushes posteriorly. Conversely, as the vertebral column extends (becomes concave posteriorly), the nucleus pulposus is pushed anteriorly. As one bends to one side, such as leaning to the left, the nucleus pulposus is pushed toward the convexity, in this case, to the right.

joint (not a facet joint since there are no superior or inferior articular facets at this level) between the S5 apex of the sacrum and the body of the Co1 vertebra. The **sacroiliac joint** will be discussed in Chapter 11.

LIGAMENTS OF THE VERTEBRAL COLUMN (FIG. 9.9)

The facet joints and intervertebral discs stabilize the vertebrae and help to prevent excessive motion. However, they are not strong enough on their own to keep the vertebral column stable. Many vertebral ligaments and muscles assist in this endeavor.

Ligaments of the Vertebral Arch

Medial to the facet joints and posterior to the vertebral canal, the laminae of adjacent vertebrae are connected by **ligamenta flava** that allow flexion to occur while keeping the vertebral arches connected. These ligaments are slightly yellow in appearance due to a large number of elastic fibers within them. Since these ligaments are elastic, they do not fold on themselves during extension of the back, which would potentially impinge on the spinal cord. It has been held that since these connect adjacent laminae, they are not present on the midline; however,

recent work has shown that they often do cover the midline of the vertebral arch. The ligamenta flava of the atlantoaxial space (C1–C2) are broad and referred to as the **posterior atlantoaxial membrane**. There are no ligamenta flava between the atlas and the occipital bone; instead, there is a **posterior atlantooccipital membrane** that is relatively thin in order to accommodate flexion of the neck. There are gaps in the posterior atlantooccipital membrane on the left and right that allow the vertebral arteries to pierce the membrane and move into the vertebral foramen to supply blood to the brainstem and spinal cord.

Adjacent spinous processes are connected by **interspinous ligaments** that limit flexion. Similarly, transverse processes are connected by small **intertransverse ligaments** that limit side-bending. These are indistinct in the cervical region, form visible bundles between the thoracic vertebrae, and are present as thin sheets in the lumbar region. The L4 and L5 transverse processes have very strong **iliolumbar ligaments** connecting them to the iliac crest.

Most posteriorly a long **supraspinous ligament** runs along the length of the vertebral column, jumping from the tip of each spinous process from C7 to the coccyx. Fibers of the supraspinous and interspinous ligaments are continuous with each other. Because the supraspinous is the most posterior of the ligaments of the vertebral column, it becomes taut in flexion and limits hyperflexion of the back. The supraspinous ligament terminates as the **superficial posterior sacrococcygeal ligament**, which covers the sacral hiatus. The coccyx is more firmly anchored to the sacrum by the **anterior, lateral, and deep posterior sacrococcygeal ligaments**. In the cervical region, the supraspinous ligament is replaced by the very broad, fan-shaped **nuchal ligament**, which runs from the external occipital protuberance to the posterior tubercle of the atlas and the spinous processes of C2–C7. Like the ligamentum flavum, the nuchal ligament contains elastic fibers. Because of that, the ligament allows cervical flexion but becomes taut as the neck is flexed further and further. Because of its large size, the nuchal ligament also provides a site of attachment for the muscles of the posterior neck.

CLINICAL CORRELATION 9.3   Herniated Nucleus Pulposus—Part 1

If the annulus fibrosus weakens or the nucleus pulposus is compressed too forcefully, it can tunnel through the protective laminae of the annulus fibrosus and protrude outward. This does not tend to occur anteriorly, due to the thick anterior longitudinal ligament, but when the back is flexed, the nucleus pulposus migrates posteriorly and can push through the annulus fibrosus. This is called a herniated nucleus pulposus, or a slipped disc. The thin posterior longitudinal ligament tends to deflect it posterolaterally, where it can compress a nearby spinal nerve.

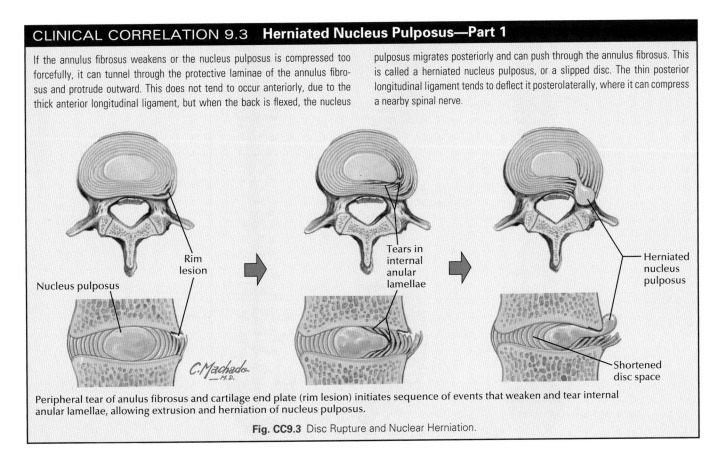

Peripheral tear of anulus fibrosus and cartilage end plate (rim lesion) initiates sequence of events that weaken and tear internal anular lamellae, allowing extrusion and herniation of nucleus pulposus.

Fig. CC9.3 Disc Rupture and Nuclear Herniation.

In the thoracic region there are several ligaments that anchor the vertebrae to the proximal ribs. The **radiate ligament of the head of the rib** forms a continuous circular sheath that connects the head of the rib to the facets or demifacets of the vertebrae. Within the radiate ligament is a small **intraarticular ligament of the head of the rib** that anchors the central part of the rib head to the center of the facet/demifacet. The **costotransverse ligament** extends from the transverse process to the neck of the rib at the same level. A **superior costotransverse ligament** connects the neck of a rib to the transverse process of its superior neighbor (e.g., the superior costotransverse ligament of the 5th rib connects to the transverse process of T4). The **lateral costotransverse ligament** connects the lateral end of the transverse process to the tubercle of the rib, effectively becoming a capsular ligament for the costotransverse joint.

Ligaments of the Vertebral Bodies

Moving on to the vertebral bodies themselves, the broad **anterior longitudinal ligament** travels from the anterior aspect of the axis to the anterior sacrum, connecting the vertebral bodies and their intervertebral discs along its length. This strong ligament becomes taut during extension. In the upper cervical region, the anterior longitudinal ligament is continuous with an **anterior atlantoaxial membrane** and **anterior atlantooccipital membrane**. The anterior atlantooccipital membrane is a stout structure that continues laterally in association with the capsule of the atlantooccipital joint and is continuous with the posterior atlantooccipital membrane, forming a continuous ring of connective tissue running between the atlas and the foramen magnum.

The thinner **posterior longitudinal ligament** connects the posterior aspects of all the vertebral bodies and intervertebral discs from the axis to the sacrum. The **tectorial membrane** continues superiorly from the posterior longitudinal ligament (they are essentially the same ligament but with different names) to cover the dens and its ligaments and the posterior atlas. It runs along the inside of the occipital bone anterior to the foramen magnum.

In general, flexion of the vertebral column is limited by the supraspinous and nuchal ligaments, particularly in the thorax, due to its kyphotic curvature. Extension of the vertebral column is limited by the anterior longitudinal ligament and intervertebral discs. Excessive lordotic curvatures in the cervical and lumbar regions can stretch and eventually weaken the anterior longitudinal ligament (Clinical Correlation 9.4).

Ligaments Related to the Dens (Fig. 9.10)

For such a small structure, the dens of the axis is associated with a bewildering number of ligaments. The small **apical ligament** of the dens extends off its apex to insert on the anterior rim of the foramen magnum. Flanking the apical ligament are two strong **alar ligaments** that extend off the superolateral dens to insert on the anterolateral rim of the foramen magnum. These ligaments allow rotation of the head and atlas using the dens as a pivot point but prevent excessive rotation (e.g., as the head rotates to the right, the right alar ligament will become taut).

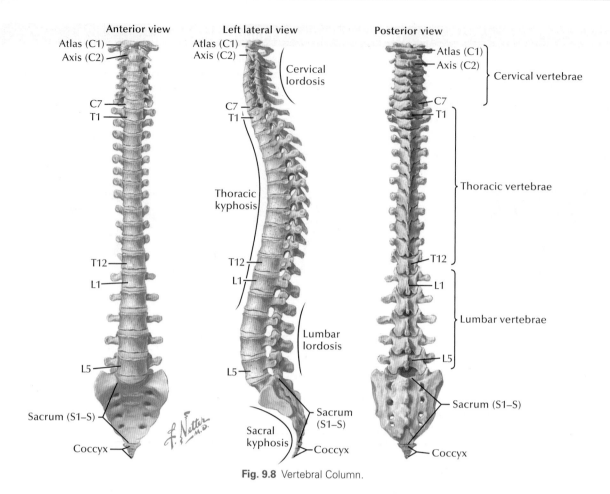

Fig. 9.8 Vertebral Column.

The **cruciate ligament of the atlas** is a composite structure that connects the axis, atlas, and occipital bone. Its horizontal component is the **transverse ligament of the atlas**, which connects the right and left inner sides of the anterior arch, passing posterior to the dens. This ligament actually forms a synovial articulation with the posterior articular facet of the dens. The vertical components of the cruciate ligament of the atlas are the **inferior longitudinal band** (posterior vertebral body of axis to the transverse ligament of atlas) and the **superior longitudinal band** (transverse ligament of atlas to the inner, anterior rim of the foramen magnum), which runs posterior to the apical ligament and anterior to the tectorial membrane (Clinical Correlation 9.5).

MUSCLE GROUPS OF THE BACK (FIG. 9.11A)

The bone, joints, and ligaments of the vertebral column allow the body to balance mobility with stability. However, the large muscles of the back are the structures that actually move and strongly stabilize the vertebral column and the spinal cord within it. The **intrinsic muscles of the back** develop from the epaxial muscles that are derived from the myotome of the somites at that level. These muscles attach to the vertebrae, iliac crest, ribs, and posterior skull. The **extrinsic muscles of the back** are located more superficially and are derived from the hypaxial muscles that migrate to the back. These muscles are attached to the back but primarily act to move the upper limbs,

since they also attach to the scapula, clavicle, and/or humerus. One structure that connects many muscles of the back, both intrinsic and extrinsic, is the thoracolumbar fascia.

Thoracolumbar Fascia (See Fig. 9.11)

The lower back contains a unique multilayered connective tissue structure, the **thoracolumbar fascia**, which connects the ilium, vertebrae, and muscles of the back. The posterior layer is subdivided into two laminae: a superficial lamina that forms a broad, flat tendon of the latissimus dorsi and serratus posterior inferior muscles, and a deep lamina that attaches to the erector spinae muscles. The middle layer of the thoracolumbar fascia marks where the epaxial and hypaxial muscles were separated. It separates the erector spinae muscles from the quadratus lumborum, which connects the iliac crest to the 12th rib. The anterior layer of the thoracolumbar fascia surrounds the anterior aspect of the quadratus lumborum muscle. Anteriorly, the thoracolumbar fascia is continuous with the fascia surrounding the abdominal oblique muscles.

Extrinsic Back Muscles
Latissimus Dorsi Muscle

The **latissimus dorsi muscle** (see Fig. 9.11B) is the most superficial muscle of the inferior back. In English, its name means "widest of the back" and it certainly earns that description. This muscle originates broadly from the iliac crest, sacrum, lumbar and thoracic spinous processes (via thoracolumbar fascia) but

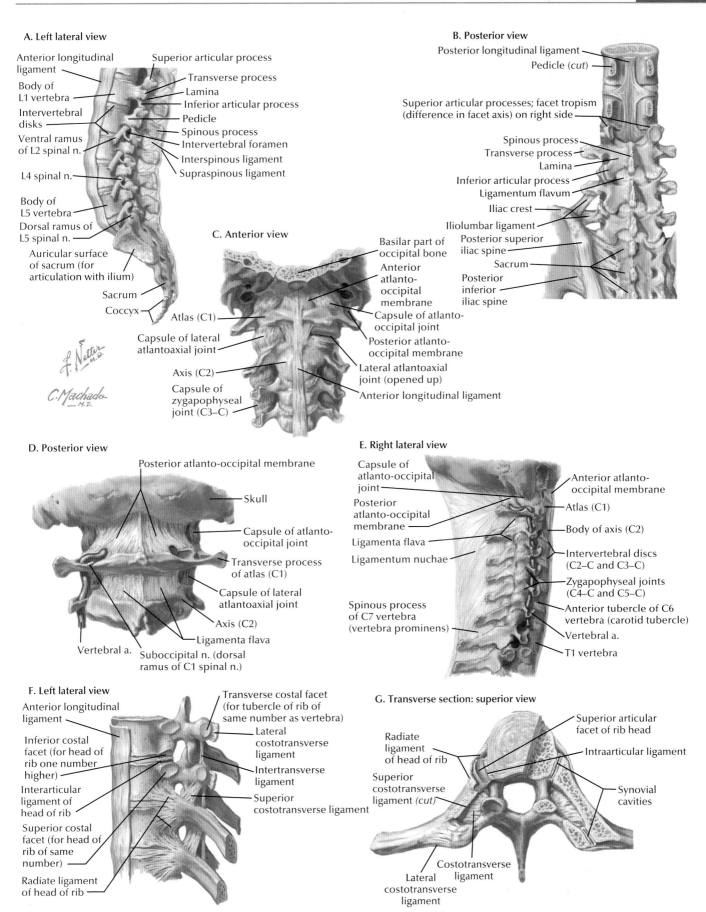

A. Left lateral view

Anterior longitudinal ligament
Body of L1 vertebra
Intervertebral disks
Ventral ramus of L2 spinal n.
L4 spinal n.
Body of L5 vertebra
Dorsal ramus of L5 spinal n.
Auricular surface of sacrum (for articulation with ilium)
Sacrum
Coccyx

Superior articular process
Transverse process
Lamina
Inferior articular process
Pedicle
Spinous process
Intervertebral foramen
Interspinous ligament
Supraspinous ligament

B. Posterior view

Posterior longitudinal ligament
Pedicle (cut)
Superior articular processes; facet tropism (difference in facet axis) on right side
Spinous process
Transverse process
Lamina
Inferior articular process
Ligamentum flavum
Iliac crest
Iliolumbar ligament
Posterior superior iliac spine
Sacrum
Posterior inferior iliac spine

C. Anterior view

Basilar part of occipital bone
Anterior atlanto-occipital membrane
Capsule of atlanto-occipital joint
Posterior atlanto-occipital membrane
Lateral atlantoaxial joint (opened up)
Anterior longitudinal ligament

Atlas (C1)
Capsule of lateral atlantoaxial joint
Axis (C2)
Capsule of zygapophyseal joint (C3–C)

D. Posterior view

Posterior atlanto-occipital membrane
Skull
Capsule of atlanto-occipital joint
Transverse process of atlas (C1)
Capsule of lateral atlantoaxial joint
Axis (C2)
Ligamenta flava
Vertebral a.
Suboccipital n. (dorsal ramus of C1 spinal n.)

E. Right lateral view

Capsule of atlanto-occipital joint
Posterior atlanto-occipital membrane
Ligamenta flava
Ligamentum nuchae
Spinous process of C7 vertebra (vertebra prominens)

Anterior atlanto-occipital membrane
Atlas (C1)
Body of axis (C2)
Intervertebral discs (C2–C and C3–C)
Zygapophyseal joints (C4–C and C5–C)
Anterior tubercle of C6 vertebra (carotid tubercle)
Vertebral a.
T1 vertebra

F. Left lateral view

Anterior longitudinal ligament
Inferior costal facet (for head of rib one number higher)
Interarticular ligament of head of rib
Superior costal facet (for head of rib of same number)
Radiate ligament of head of rib

Transverse costal facet (for tubercle of rib of same number as vertebra)
Lateral costotransverse ligament
Intertransverse ligament
Superior costotransverse ligament

G. Transverse section: superior view

Radiate ligament of head of rib
Superior costotransverse ligament (cut)
Lateral costotransverse ligament
Costotransverse ligament

Superior articular facet of rib head
Intraarticular ligament
Synovial cavities

Fig. 9.9 Vertebral Ligaments: Lumbosacral Region.

CLINICAL CORRELATION 9.4
Hyperflexion and Hyperextension Injuries

When the vertebral column is violently extended or flexed, its muscular tissue, connective tissue, and nervous structures may be torn by the sudden motion. Muscular and ligamentous injuries are very painful but muscular injuries tend to heal more quickly, due to the greater vascularity of skeletal muscle compared to small vessels supplying connective tissue. Injuries of this kind can result in long-term debilitating pain.

Sudden hyperflexion (such as a sudden deceleration in a head-on vehicle collision) will stretch and possibly tear the muscles of the posterior neck as well as the ligaments of the posterior neck (in this order): (1) the nuchal ligament or supraspinous ligament, (2) interspinous ligament, and (3) ligamentum flavum. If the stretching continues it can put traction on the cervical spinal cord and possibly even tear the posterior longitudinal ligament and intervertebral disc. The same process can occur in the lumbar region (such as forced flexion during a sudden deceleration when restrained by a lap belt) and can affect muscles of the lower back and ligaments (in this order): (1) supraspinous, (2) interspinous, and (3) ligamentum flavum. As before, continued stretching may traumatize the cauda equina, posterior longitudinal ligament, and intervertebral disc.

Sudden hyperextension (such as being rear-ended in a vehicle collision without a headrest) will stretch and injure muscles of the anterior neck. If the stretch continues, the anterior longitudinal ligament and intervertebral disc may be torn. These are commonly called "whiplash" injuries and can also cause avulsion of part of the vertebral body as the ligament is torn. Another problem with hyperextension, especially in the cervical region, is the "pinching" of articular facets, pedicles, and spinous processes by their neighbors, possibly fracturing the vertebrae.

narrows to insert onto a small region of the proximal humerus. It will pull the arm closer to the lower back and this makes it a strong extensor of the shoulder, especially when the arm begins in a flexed position. Similarly, it strongly adducts the arm at the shoulder from an abducted position. Since its tendon slightly spirals around the anterior aspect of the humerus, it will also medially (internally) rotate the arm at the shoulder. The thoracodorsal nerve and vessels travel on the anterior surface of the latissimus dorsi and provide innervation and blood to it.

Proximal Attachments	• Iliac crest • Superficial lamina of posterior layer of thoracolumbar fascia (T7 to sacrum)
Distal Attachment	• Intertubercular sulcus of proximal humerus
Functions	• Extension of shoulder from a flexed position • Adduction of shoulder from an abducted position • Medial rotation of arm
Muscle Testing and Signs of Damage	• With the arms abducted at the shoulder, ask the patient to adduct them against resistance, assess any asymmetry in strength. • With the arms flexed at the shoulder, ask the patient to extend them against resistance, assess any asymmetry in strength.
Innervation	• Thoracodorsal nerve
Blood Supply	• Primarily thoracodorsal vessels

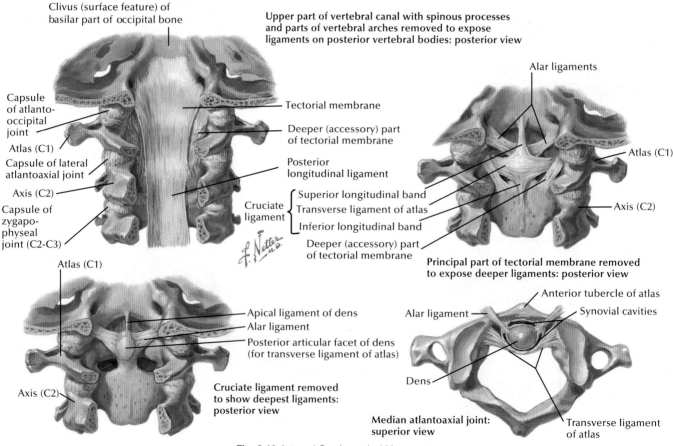

Fig. 9.10 Internal Craniocervical Ligaments.

CLINICAL CORRELATION 9.5 Rupture of the Transverse Ligament of the Atlas and Fracture of the Dens

Sudden compression of the head down onto the neck can put tremendous pressure on the articular facets of the atlas causing it to fracture. The transverse ligament of the atlas is also exposed to rupture when this occurs. Without an intact ligament, the atlas may translocate anteriorly, pinching the spinal cord. A similar problem can occur if the dens is fractured. If the tip of the dens is avulsed by the apical or alar ligaments (type I), there will not be gross instability of the atlas. If the base of the dens (type II) or the anterosuperior body of the axis (type III) is fractured, the dens and atlas are no longer restrained by the transverse ligament of the atlas, allowing anterior translation of the atlas and dens, impinging on the spinal cord.

Trapezius Muscle

The **trapezius** (see Fig. 9.11B) is the most superficial muscle of the superior back. This diamond-shaped muscle originates from the occipital bone, nuchal ligament, and thoracic spinous processes. It focuses this lengthy attachment onto the spine of the scapula, acromion, and distal clavicle. This allows the superior, middle, and inferior parts of the trapezius to elevate, retract, and depress the scapula, respectively. It receives motor innervation from cranial nerve XI (CN XI, spinal accessory nerve) but also has some sensory innervation from cervical spinal nerves. Intriguingly, there are sensory cell bodies (likely proprioceptive

from the trapezius and sternocleidomastoid muscles) associated with CN XI, which is traditionally described as a motor-only nerve. The breadth of this muscle is reflected in its blood supply; it receives blood from branches of the external carotid artery and the thyrocervical trunk in the neck.

Proximal Attachments	• Superior fibers: Medial part of superior nuchal line and external occipital protuberance, nuchal ligament • Middle fibers: nuchal ligament, C7–T5 spinous processes • Inferior fibers: T6–T12 spinous processes
Distal Attachment	• Spine of scapula • Acromion • Distal clavicle
Functions	• Superior fibers: elevate scapula and upper limb • Middle fibers: retract scapula • Inferior fibers: depress scapula
Muscle Testing and Signs of Damage	• Ask patient to elevate shoulders against resistance • Weakness on one side may indicate dysfunction of the trapezius or CN XI.
Innervation	• CN XI—spinal accessory nerve
Blood Supply	• Primarily branches of external carotid artery and thyrocervical trunk (transverse cervical and dorsal scapular vessels)

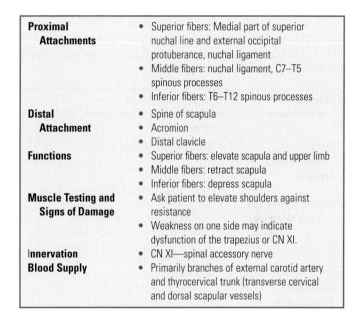

A. Lumbar region of back: cross section transverse section through lumbar region (L2) of back

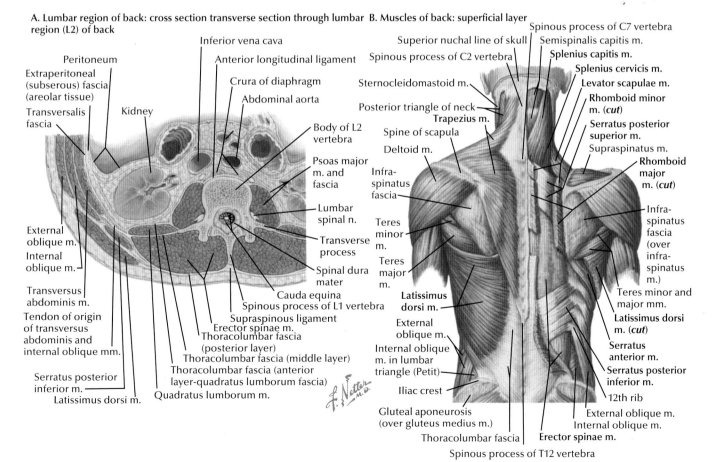

B. Muscles of back: superficial layer

Fig. 9.11 (A) Lumbar region of back: cross-section of transverse section through lumbar region (L2) of back; (B) muscles of back: superficial layer.

Levator Scapulae Muscle

The **levator scapulae muscle** (see Fig. 9.11B) has muscle bellies originating from the transverse processes of the upper cervical vertebrae that fuse and insert onto the superior angle of the scapula. This very steep inferolateral slope makes the levator scapulae good at elevating the scapula (hence its name) but also in rotating the scapula inferiorly, pointing the shoulder "down" and depressing the upper limb. The dorsal scapular nerve passes between the heads of the levator scapulae, innervating it, and is joined by the dorsal scapular artery and vein.

Proximal Attachments	• C1 transverse process • C2–C4 posterior tubercles of the transverse processes
Distal Attachment	• Superior angle of scapula
Functions	• Elevate scapula • Inferior rotation of scapula and glenoid fossa
Muscle Testing and Signs of Damage	• Ask patient to elevate their shoulders bilaterally and watch for asymmetry. • Weakness on one side may indicate weakness of the levator scapulae muscles, but the activity of the superior fibers of the trapezius may mask this weakness.
Innervation	• Dorsal scapular nerve
Blood Supply	• Primarily dorsal scapular vessels

Rhomboid Major and Rhomboid Minor Muscles

The **rhomboid major** and **rhomboid minor muscles** (see Fig. 9.11B) are located deep to the middle and inferior fibers of the trapezius muscle. They travel from the lower cervical and upper thoracic spinous processes to insert on the medial border of the scapula near the scapular spine (minor) and medial to the infraspinatus fossa (major). In the process, both muscles travel in an inferolateral direction. These muscles sometimes fuse, obscuring the exact site of separation between major and minor. Since these muscles travel obliquely, they can retract the scapula but also rotate the scapula inferiorly, which will also shift the entire upper limb inferiorly. These muscles are innervated and perfused by the dorsal scapular nerve and vessels, which continue from the levator scapulae and run along the anterior aspect of the rhomboid muscles.

Proximal Attachments	• Minor: Inferior nuchal ligament, C7 and T1 spinous processes • Major: T2–T5 spinous processes
Distal Attachment	• Minor: Medial border of scapula superior to and at the level of the spine of the scapula • Major: Medial border of scapula from level of the spine of the scapula to near the inferior angle
Functions	• Retraction of scapula. • Inferior rotation of scapula and glenoid fossa.
Muscle Testing and Signs of Damage	• Ask patient to retract their shoulders bilaterally and watch for asymmetry. • Weakness retracting may indicate weakness of the rhomboid muscles, but the activity of the middle fibers of the trapezius may mask this weakness.
Innervation	• Dorsal scapular nerve
Blood Supply	• Primarily dorsal scapular vessels

Serratus Posterior Superior and Inferior Muscles

The **serratus posterior superior and inferior muscles** (Fig. 9.12, see also Fig. 9.11B) are flat, deep muscles that run from spinous processes to the ribs. The serratus posterior superior is located deep to the rhomboid muscles, running in an inferolateral direction. The serratus posterior inferior is deep to the latissimus dorsi muscle, traveling in a superolateral direction. Since the latissimus dorsi and serratus posterior inferior run the same direction and originate from the thoracolumbar fascia, they may fuse to some degree.

Proximal Attachments	• Superior: Inferior aspect of nuchal ligament, C7–T3 spinous processes • Inferior: Superficial lamina of posterior layer of thoracolumbar fascia near T11–L2.
Distal Attachment	• Superior: T2–T5 ribs, at or lateral to the costal angle • Inferior: T9–T12 ribs, lateral to the costal angle
Functions	• Electromyographic studies coupled with their small size suggests that these muscles are primarily proprioceptive in nature. • Superior: may assist in elevating the upper ribs during forced inspiration • Inferior: may assist in depressing the lower ribs during forced expiration
Muscle Testing and Signs of Damage	• These muscles are not typically assessed clinically. • Spasm or irritation of the serratus posterior superior often causes a "trigger point" that does become more painful in forced expiration but is not exacerbated by upper limb movement. This can be treated with manipulation or massage.
Innervation	• Superior: T2–T5 intercostal nerves • Inferior: T9–T11 intercostal nerves, T12 subcostal nerve
Blood Supply	• Superior: T2–T5 intercostal vessels • Inferior: T9–T11 intercostal vessels, subcostal vessels

Intrinsic Back Muscles

The **intrinsic back muscles** are interesting in that many of them do not have distinct origins and insertions. Instead, the erector spinae and transversospinalis groups consist of many small muscles that bundle together, contribute to the body of the muscle, and then leave as their small tendons attach to more superior bones. Other intrinsic back muscles do indeed have well-defined origins and insertions.

Splenius Cervicis and Splenius Capitis Muscles

The **splenius cervicis** and **splenius capitis muscles** (see Figs. 9.11B and 9.12) are located primarily in the cervical region and are immediately superficial to the erector spinae muscles there. They are oriented obliquely in a superolateral direction. These two muscles do not typically have a clear separation between each other and are distinguished by their sites of insertion. One way to distinguish the splenius muscles is that one of the muscle slips of the levator scapulae muscle will travel between the splenius cervicis and capitis to reach the C1 transverse processes.

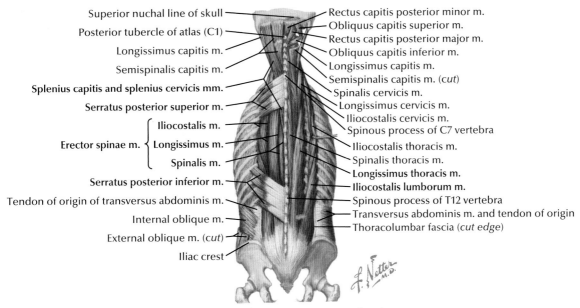

Superior nuchal line of skull
Posterior tubercle of atlas (C1)
Longissimus capitis m.
Semispinalis capitis m.
Splenius capitis and splenius cervicis mm.
Serratus posterior superior m.
Iliocostalis m.
Erector spinae m. { Longissimus m.
Spinalis m.
Serratus posterior inferior m.
Tendon of origin of transversus abdominis m.
Internal oblique m.
External oblique m. (*cut*)
Iliac crest

Rectus capitis posterior minor m.
Obliquus capitis superior m.
Rectus capitis posterior major m.
Obliquus capitis inferior m.
Longissimus capitis m.
Semispinalis capitis m. (*cut*)
Spinalis cervicis m.
Longissimus cervicis m.
Iliocostalis cervicis m.
Spinous process of C7 vertebra
Iliocostalis thoracis m.
Spinalis thoracis m.
Longissimus thoracis m.
Iliocostalis lumborum m.
Spinous process of T12 vertebra
Transversus abdominis m. and tendon of origin
Thoracolumbar fascia (*cut edge*)

Fig. 9.12 Muscles of the Back: Intermediate Layers.

Proximal Attachments	• Cervicis: T3–T6 spinous processes • Capitis: Inferior portion of nuchal ligament, C7–T2 spinous processes • Note: the distinction between splenius cervicis and capitis tends to be indistinct at their proximal attachments.
Distal Attachment	• Cervicis: transverse process of C1, C2–C4 posterior tubercles of the transverse processes • Capitis: Posterior mastoid process of temporal bone, lateral occipital bone between superior and inferior nuchal lines
Functions	• Unilateral contraction: ipsilateral side-bending and rotation of the head (capitis) and neck (cervicis and capitis) • Bilateral contraction: extension of the head (capitis) and neck (cervicis and capitis)
Muscle Testing and Signs of Damage	• With a patient seated upright, palpate the posterior neck and ask the patient to slowly extend and rotate the neck. The splenius muscles may be palpable but they are difficult to isolate since they are deep to the trapezius and superficial to the semispinalis capitis, the most prominent extensor of the head. • If one side is weak, the patient will side-bend and rotate away from the weak side during extension of the neck. Spasm of these muscles will cause the patient to side-bend and rotate toward the affected side.
Innervation	• Posterior rami of cervical spinal nerves near their level of origin
Blood Supply	• Primarily branches of external carotid artery and thyrocervical trunk (transverse cervical vessels)

Erector Spinae

The **erector spinae** (see Fig. 9.12) group of muscles is located deep to the trapezius, latissimus dorsi, rhomboid, and serratus posterior muscles. They run longitudinally along the vertebral column and for this reason they are sometimes referred to as the **paraspinal muscles**. The erector spinae are surrounded posteriorly by the deep lamina of the posterior layer of the thoracolumbar fascia. They have broad origin from the T11 to L5 transverse processes, posterior sacrum, and iliac crest. These muscles ascend (mostly) superolaterally to insert on more lateral and superior structures such as transverse processes, spinous processes, and ribs. Since these muscles travel obliquely, unilateral contraction will side-bend and rotate the body ipsilaterally, bilateral contraction will strongly extend the vertebral column.

The erector spinae are divided into the **iliocostalis**, **longissimus**, and **spinalis muscles**, which will then become further subdivided (buckle up). The iliocostalis has thoracic and cervical sections. The longissimus has lumbar, thoracic, cervical, and capitis sections. The spinalis has thoracic, cervical, and capitis sections.

Proximal Attachments	**Iliocostalis Muscle Group** • Iliocostalis lumborum: L4–L5 transverse processes, posterior sacrum, iliac crest • Iliocostalis thoracis: Ribs 7–12 near costal angle • Iliocostalis cervicis: Ribs 3–6 near costal angle **Longissimus Muscle Group** • Longissimus thoracis: L1–L5 transverse processes, posterior sacrum • Longissimus cervicis: T1–T5 transverse processes • Longissimus capitis: T1–T5 transverse processes, C4–C7 articular processes **Spinalis Muscle Group** • Spinalis thoracis: spinous processes of T10–L2 • Spinalis cervicis: inferior portion of nuchal ligament and T1 spinous process • Spinalis capitis: middle region of the nuchal ligament
Distal Attachment	**Iliocostalis Muscle Group** • Iliocostalis lumborum: Ribs 7–12 at (or lateral) to the costal angle • Iliocostalis thoracis: Ribs 1–6 near the costal angle • Iliocostalis cervicis: C4–C7 transverse processes **Longissimus Muscle Group** • Longissimus thoracis: all thoracic transverse processes and all ribs proximal to the costal angle • Longissimus cervicis: C2–C7 transverse processes • Longissimus capitis: posterior aspect of mastoid process of temporal bone **Spinalis Muscle Group** • Spinalis thoracis: T1–T8 spinous processes • Spinalis cervicis: C7–C2 spinous processes • Spinalis capitis: between superior and inferior nuchal lines of occipital bone, fused with semispinalis capitis
Functions	• Unilateral contraction: ipsilateral side-bending and rotation • Bilateral contraction: extension of vertebral column
Muscle Testing and Signs of Damage	• With a patient seated upright, palpate the paraspinal muscle columns (erector spinae) on the back. Ask the patient to slowly extend the back. Observe any asymmetry or deviation to one side. • If one side is weak, the patient will side-bend and rotate away from the weak side during extension of the back. Spasm of these muscles will cause the patient to side-bend and rotate toward the affected side. • These muscles are commonly strained during heavy lifting. The patient will commonly adopt a position of ease that passively shortens the muscle. He or she will sit or stand, side-bent towards the affected side, letting gravity shorten the affected muscle. Pain typically results from extension of the back, side-bending away from the affected side (stretching the injured muscle), or ACTIVE side-bending toward the affected side or extension (contracting the injured muscle).
Innervation	• Posterior rami of spinal nerves near their level of origin
Blood Supply	• Posterior segmental arteries accompanying the posterior rami

---

BIOMECHANICS BOX 9.2
Transversospinalis Muscles

While the members of the transversospinalis group span many vertebral levels, there are some that are particularly important. The **rotatores thoracis** are the best developed of the rotatores and are particularly prone to strain during jerky rotation of the vertebrae. Because of their proprioceptive and sensory function, they are quite painful when injured. The **multifidus lumborum** is a massive wedge of muscle that stretches between the posterior sacrum, iliac crest, lumbar transverse processes, and lumbar spinous processes. It serves to anchor the vertebral column to the pelvis during flexion and standing. If we think of the spinal column as the extended arm of a crane, the multifidus lumborum is the heavy, stable base of the crane. The **semispinalis cervicis** and **semispinalis capitis** are large, nearly vertical muscles that are major extensors of the head and neck. These can become spastic or hyperactive during muscle-tension headaches.

Transversospinalis Muscle Group

The **transversospinalis muscle group** (Fig. 9.13, see also Fig. 9.12) are the deepest of the intrinsic back muscles and are generally nestled in the groove between transverse and spinous processes of the vertebrae, hence their name. This group runs longitudinally along the vertebral column, but unlike the splenius and erector spinae muscles, they travel in a superomedial direction. With a few exceptions, the transversospinalis muscles will side-bend the back ipsilaterally and rotate the back contralaterally when contracted unilaterally. When contracted bilaterally they will extend the back and head.

The transversospinalis muscles are divided into the **semispinalis**, **multifidus**, and **rotatores muscles**. Since these muscles all originate from transverse processes and insert on spinous processes (or the occipital bone), they are not distinguished by differences in their attachments but by how many vertebral segments they span. Semispinalis muscles span greater than 4 vertebral levels as they ascend, multifidus muscles span 2 to 4 levels, rotatores span 1 to 2 levels. As you might already suspect, they will be further subdivided based on the region of the back in which they reside. The semispinalis muscles have thoracic, cervical, and capitis sections. Due to their vertical orientation, the semispinalis muscles are primarily extensors of the back, with the very large **semispinalis capitis muscle**, which is located deep to the trapezius and splenius muscles, being a powerful extensor of the head and neck. The multifidi have lumbar, thoracic, and cervical sections. Due to their oblique course, they can extend and rotate the vertebrae. The rotatores have lumbar, thoracic, and cervical sections but are best developed in the thoracic region. The rotatores that span two vertebral levels are referred to as **rotatores longus** (a bit hyperbolic for such short muscles), while those spanning one level are **rotatores brevis** (Biomechanics Box 9.2).

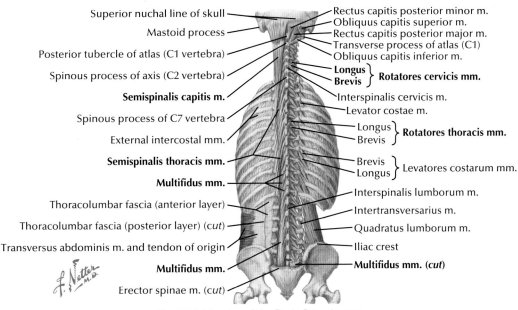

Superior nuchal line of skull
Mastoid process
Posterior tubercle of atlas (C1 vertebra)
Spinous process of axis (C2 vertebra)
Semispinalis capitis m.
Spinous process of C7 vertebra
External intercostal mm.
Semispinalis thoracis mm.
Multifidus mm.
Thoracolumbar fascia (anterior layer)
Thoracolumbar fascia (posterior layer) (*cut*)
Transversus abdominis m. and tendon of origin
Multifidus mm.
Erector spinae m. (*cut*)

Rectus capitis posterior minor m.
Obliquus capitis superior m.
Rectus capitis posterior major m.
Transverse process of atlas (C1)
Obliquus capitis inferior m.
Longus / **Brevis** } **Rotatores cervicis mm.**
Interspinalis cervicis m.
Levator costae m.
Longus / **Brevis** } **Rotatores thoracis mm.**
Brevis / Longus } Levatores costarum mm.
Interspinalis lumborum m.
Intertransversarius m.
Quadratus lumborum m.
Iliac crest
Multifidus mm. (*cut*)

Fig. 9.13 Muscles of the Back: Deep Layers.

Inferior Attachments	• **Semispinalis Muscle Group (spans >4 segments)** • Semispinalis thoracis: T6–T10 transverse processes • Semispinalis cervicis: T1–T5 transverse processes • Semispinalis capitis: C4–T6 transverse processes • **Multifidus Muscle Group (spans 2–4 segments)** • Multifidus lumborum: posterior sacrum, posterior superior iliac spine, lumbar mammillary processes • Multifidus thoracis: thoracic transverse processes • Multifidus cervicis: C4–C7 articular processes • **Rotatores Muscle Group (spans 1–2 segments)** • Rotatores lumborum: L1–L5 transverse processes • Rotatores thoracis: T1–T12 transverse processes • Rotatores cervicis: C3–C7 transverse processes
Superior Attachment	• **Semispinalis Muscle Group (spans >4 segments)** • Semispinalis thoracis: C6–T4 spinous processes • Semispinalis cervicis: C2–C6 spinous processes (C2 insertion is very prominent) • Semispinalis capitis: medial occipital bone between superior and inferior nuchal lines • **Multifidus Muscle Group (spans 2–4 segments)** • Multifidus lumborum: L1–L5 spinous processes • Multifidus thoracis: T1–T12 spinous processes • Multifidus cervicis: C2–C7 spinous processes • **Rotatores Muscle Group (spans 1–2 segments)** • Rotatores lumborum: T12–L4 spinous processes • Rotatores thoracis: C7–T11 spinous processes • Rotatores cervicis: C2–C6 spinous processes
Functions	• **Semispinalis Muscle Group** • Unilateral contraction: ipsilateral side-bending and slight contralateral rotation • Bilateral contraction: extension of the back • The semispinalis capitis strongly extends the head • **Multifidus Muscle Group** • Unilateral contraction: ipsilateral side-bending and contralateral rotation • Bilateral contraction: extension of vertebral column • The multifidus lumborum anchors the lumbar vertebrae to the sacrum and ilium. • **Rotatores Muscle Group** • Unilateral contraction: weak ipsilateral side-bending and contralateral rotation • Bilateral contraction: very weak extension of vertebral column • These muscles are too small to move the vertebrae notably. They may stabilize the vertebral column somewhat but are primarily proprioceptive.
Muscle Testing and Signs of Damage	• These muscles are rarely tested clinically but they are a possible source of back pain due to injury, strain, or atrophy. • If a patient has back pain caused by spasm or injury to one of these muscles, it can be localized by asking the patient to extend his or her back. Thereafter, side-bending away from the affected muscle will stretch it and cause pain. If the pain is localized to the deep back and becomes even worse with ipsilateral rotation, it is probably originating from a transversospinalis muscle.
Innervation	• Posterior rami of spinal nerves near their level of origin
Blood Supply	• Lumbar and thoracic divisions: posterior segmental arteries accompanying the posterior rami • Cervical and capitis divisions: branches of external carotid artery and thyrocervical trunk (transverse cervical and dorsal scapular vessels)

Suboccipital Muscles

The **suboccipital muscles** (Fig. 9.14, see also Figs. 9.12 and 9.13) are a collection of four short muscles clustered between the spinous process of the axis and the posterior occipital bone. The **suboccipital triangle** is formed by **rectus capitis posterior major** (medial border), **obliquus capitis inferior** (inferior), and **obliquus capitis superior** (superior). The **rectus capitis posterior minor** is medial to the triangle. This triangle contains the vertebral artery as it passes across the posterior arch of the atlas to pierce the posterior atlantooccipital membrane. It also contains the posterior ramus of C1, called the **suboccipital nerve**, which innervates the suboccipital muscles. The **greater occipital nerve** (C2 posterior ramus) is a large sensory nerve that passes immediately inferior to the obliquus capitis inferior muscle to reach the posterior scalp (Clinical Correlation 9.6).

Proximal Attachments	• Rectus capitis posterior minor: posterior tubercle of C1 • Rectus capitis posterior major: spinous process of C2 • Obliquus capitis inferior: spinous process of C2 • Obliquus capitis superior: transverse process of C1
Distal Attachment	• Rectus capitis posterior minor: medial aspect of inferior nuchal line • Rectus capitis posterior major: lateral aspect of inferior nuchal line • Obliquus capitis inferior: transverse process of C1 • Obliquus capitis superior: lateral aspect of occipital bone between superior and inferior nuchal lines
Functions	• Unilateral contraction: ipsilateral side-bending • Bilateral contraction: extension of the atlantoaxial and atlantooccipital joints
Muscle Testing and Signs of Damage	• The suboccipital muscles may become spastic or hyperactive during muscle-tension headaches. Patients may complain of their head feeling "locked down." • Manipulation or massage at the base of the skull can help to temporarily relieve this pain.
Innervation	• Suboccipital nerve (C1 posterior ramus)
Blood Supply	• Branches of external carotid artery and vertebral vessels.

Minor Deep Back Muscles (See Fig. 9.13)

There are several very small, mostly proprioceptive muscles in the back. They are not able to move the back appreciably but act to stabilize the vertebrae and ribs and provide proprioceptive feedback based on the tension and stretch they experience. Left and right **interspinales muscles** connect adjacent spinous processes and are separated by the midline interspinous ligament. **Intertransversarii muscles** connect adjacent transverse processes on each side of the vertebrae. The **levatores costarum muscles** extend inferiorly from the transverse processes to the proximal ribs. Those that extend inferiorly by one rib are the **levatores costarum brevis**; those that reach two ribs lower are the **levatores costrum longus**.

Superior Attachments	• Interspinales: inferior aspect of spinous processes (indistinct in thoracic region) • Intertransversarii: inferior aspect of transverse processes (indistinct in thoracic region) • Levatores costarum brevis: transverse processes from C7 to T11 • Levatores costarum longus: transverse processes from C7 to T10
Inferior Attachment	• Interspinales: superior aspect of spinous processes of the neighboring inferior vertebra • Intertransversarii: superior aspect of transverse processes of the neighboring inferior vertebra • Levatores costarum: area near costal tubercle of rib (brevis—1 rib lower; longus—2 ribs lower)
Functions	• Stabilize adjacent vertebrae and proximal ribs. • Proprioceptive feedback regarding tension and position of vertebrae and ribs.
Muscle Testing and Signs of Damage	• Spasm of these muscles may produce focal deep back pain that is exacerbated by flexion (interspinales), contralateral side-bending (contralateral intertransversarii), and deep exhalation (levatores costarum). • Manipulation or massage at the tender area may temporarily relieve this pain.
Innervation	• Interspinales: Posterior rami of C2–L5 • Intertransversarii: anterior (cervical) and posterior (lumbar) rami. Thoracic levels may be indistinct due to possible absence of intertransversarii. • Levatores costarum: Posterior rami of C8–T11
Blood Supply	• Superficial and deep transverse cervical vessels • Posterior divisions of intercostal and lumbar segmental vessels

Other Muscles

There are other muscles that are seen in the back but have their greatest effect elsewhere. The **external abdominal oblique muscle** originates from the ribs and iliac crest before wrapping around the abdomen. Deep to the latissimus dorsi, serratus posterior inferior, and erector spinae muscles is the quadratus lumborum muscle, which is part of the posterior abdominal wall. It originates from the posteromedial iliac crest and inserts on the lumbar transverse processes and inferior aspect of rib 12. It may be a source of tension and deep back pain that is exacerbated by side-bending away from the affected side. These muscles will be discussed in more detail in the section on the abdomen (Clinical Correlation 9.7).

THE VERTEBRAL CANAL

Within the vertebral canal are the three **meninges** that surround the spinal cord and the spinal nerves. The dura mater is the outermost protective layer, but it does not take up all the space within the canal. A great deal of **epidural fat** (adipose tissue) and an extensive **internal vertebral venous plexus** surround the dura mater in the **epidural space** (Fig. 9.15).

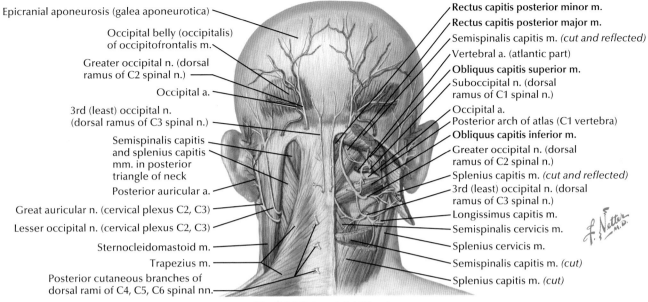

Epicranial aponeurosis (galea aponeurotica)

Occipital belly (occipitalis) of occipitofrontalis m.

Greater occipital n. (dorsal ramus of C2 spinal n.)

Occipital a.

3rd (least) occipital n. (dorsal ramus of C3 spinal n.)

Semispinalis capitis and splenius capitis mm. in posterior triangle of neck

Posterior auricular a.

Great auricular n. (cervical plexus C2, C3)

Lesser occipital n. (cervical plexus C2, C3)

Sternocleidomastoid m.

Trapezius m.

Posterior cutaneous branches of dorsal rami of C4, C5, C6 spinal nn.

Rectus capitis posterior minor m.

Rectus capitis posterior major m.

Semispinalis capitis m. (cut and reflected)

Vertebral a. (atlantic part)

Obliquus capitis superior m.

Suboccipital n. (dorsal ramus of C1 spinal n.)

Occipital a.

Posterior arch of atlas (C1 vertebra)

Obliquus capitis inferior m.

Greater occipital n. (dorsal ramus of C2 spinal n.)

Splenius capitis m. (cut and reflected)

3rd (least) occipital n. (dorsal ramus of C3 spinal n.)

Longissimus capitis m.

Semispinalis cervicis m.

Splenius cervicis m.

Semispinalis capitis m. (cut)

Splenius capitis m. (cut)

Fig. 9.14 Suboccipital Triangle.

CLINICAL CORRELATION 9.6 Myodural Bridges

The dura mater is exquisitely sensitive to pain and is frequently the source of severe headaches. One intriguing aspect of the suboccipital muscles are the myodural bridges running between the suboccipital muscles and cervical dura mater. Distinct bands of connective tissue extend from the anterior surface of the rectus capitis posterior minor, rectus capitis posterior major, and obliquus capitis inferior to pierce the posterior atlantoaxial and atlantooccipital membranes and fuse with the underlying dura mater. This direct connection may explain how suboccipital muscle spasm or dysfunction can cause headaches that are too severe to be explained by tension of these small muscles alone. The function of the myodural bridges is still being debated. Since the posterior atlantoaxial and atlantooccipital membranes are not as elastic as the ligamentum flavum present at other levels, the myodural bridges may allow the suboccipital muscles to pull the dura mater posteriorly during extension of the neck and prevent it from folding forward to push on the spinal cord.

CLINICAL CORRELATION 9.7 Lumbar Triangle and Lumbar Hernia

The **lumbar triangle** is formed by the latissimus dorsi muscle (medial border), external abdominal oblique (lateral border), and iliac crest (inferior border) (see Fig. 9.11B). The floor of this triangle is made by two other abdominal muscles, the internal oblique and transversus abdominis muscles. The lumbar triangle constitutes a weak spot in the abdominal wall since it is covered by only two muscles instead of three. When intraabdominal pressure rises, portions of the small or large intestines can push through this weak spot, creating a lumbar hernia. The herniated gut may slide in and out of the defect or it may become stuck and strangulated in the narrow opening.

Meninges (See Fig. 9.15)

The **dura mater** sits within the vertebral canal, surrounded by the epidural space and surrounding the spinal cord and spinal nerve roots. The dura mater is a tough and relatively inelastic connective tissue structure made primarily from type I collagen that truly does protect the spinal cord (it is not hyperbole that *dura mater* translates into English as "tough mother"). The entire open space inside the dura mater is referred to as the **dural sac**. The epidural space surrounds the dura mater along the entirety of the vertebral canal. Superiorly, the spinal dura mater becomes the cranial dura mater as it enters the foramen magnum. As this happens the **meningeal dura mater** fuses with the internal periosteum of the skull's calvarium, which is sometimes called the **periosteal dura mater**. As each spinal nerve exits the intervertebral foramen, a sleeve of dura mater surrounds it (and the spinal roots that create it). These **dural root sheaths** fuse with the periosteum of the vertebrae, forming the intervertebral foramen. Inferiorly, the dural sac ends approximately at the S2 vertebral level. However,

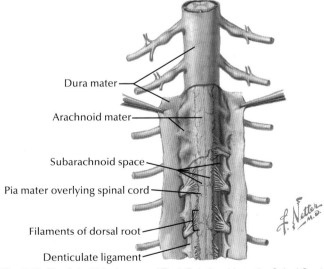

Dura mater

Arachnoid mater

Subarachnoid space

Pia mater overlying spinal cord

Filaments of dorsal root

Denticulate ligament

Fig. 9.15 The Spinal Meninges and Their Relationship to the Spinal Cord.

multiple dural root sheaths continue around the S3–Co1 spinal nerve roots until they each meet their foramina. A single long midline extension of dura mater, the **filum terminale externum**, fuses to the posterior coccyx and anchors the dural sac inferiorly.

Deep to the dura mater is the next layer of the meninges, the **arachnoid mater**. This structure gets its name ("spidery mother") from the diffuse, cobweb-like nature of its fibers. In the gross anatomy laboratory, this layer is typically seen plastered to the outside of the spinal cord. But in life it is pushed outward by **cerebrospinal fluid (CSF)** in the **subarachnoid space** and into contact with the dura mater. Between the dura and arachnoid mater is a potential space that is only seen when blood or some other mass pushes the two layers apart, the **subdural space**. The arachnoid mater consists of wispy type I collagen fibers alongside elastic fibers. It is avascular and derives nutrition from the CSF, yet it helps support blood vessels as they approach and depart from the spinal cord. **Arachnoid trabeculae** extend from the arachnoid mater and fuse to the next layer, the pia mater.

The **pia mater** is the final, and deepest, layer of the meninges. It is intimately bound to all surfaces of the central nervous system, including the spinal cord, spinal roots, and spinal nerves. The very end of the spinal cord, the conus medullaris, narrows to leave only the outer layer of pia mater, which extends all the way down to the posterior coccyx as the **filum terminale internus** within the filum terminale externum. However, this is not the only way the pia mater stabilizes the spinal cord. Denticulate ligaments are pial extensions that leave the spinal cord on the left and right (≈20 to 22 pairs) to pierce the arachnoid mater and insert onto the dura mater. They are present along the length of the cord and can be identified as they separate into anterior and posterior roots.

My favorite metaphor for appreciating the arrangement of the meninges is to liken them to sleeping in a sleeping bag. The tough sleeping bag surrounds everything in a big sac like the dura mater. The pajamas a person wears are much lighter, much like the arachnoid mater. Finally, the skin beneath the pajamas is just like the pia mater. It cannot be removed without damaging the underlying body/spinal cord.

The subarachnoid space contains the CSF that keeps the spinal cord and spinal nerve roots buoyant. The CSF leaves the ventricular system of the cerebral hemispheres and fills the subarachnoid space around the brain, brainstem, and spinal cord. CSF leaves the subarachnoid space by draining through arachnoid granulations into a huge dural venous sinus (the superior sagittal sinus) in the head. It was long believed that the dural sac was a blind pouch for CSF. But small arachnoid granulations of the dural root sheaths also remove CSF from the spinal subarachnoid space and deposit it into nearby radicular veins (Clinical Correlation 9.8).

INNERVATION OF THE BACK

The neuroanatomy of the spinal cord has been described already. For the rest of this chapter we will discuss how the spinal cord innervates the muscles of the back and the overlying skin with reference to the anatomy, histology, and physiology of the area.

Spinal Levels and the Cauda Equina

The spinal cord gives off a spinal nerve for each vertebral level. In the back, each of these nerves will supply a strip of skin that extends from the midline of the back to the anterior midline (Fig. 9.16).

CLINCAL CORRELATION 9.8   Lumbar Puncture

It is sometimes useful to get a sample of the CSF to diagnose infections of the meninges or to administer anesthetics. To perform a lumbar puncture (spinal tap) the needle is directed through the skin, subcutaneous fat, thoracolumbar fascia (if the needle is inserted off the midline), supraspinous ligament (if the needle is inserted on the midline), interspinous ligament, nuchal ligament, epidural space, dura mater, arachnoid mater, and (finally) the subarachnoid space and CSF. This is done in the lower lumbar region so that the needle cannot accidentally contact the spinal cord but passes between the spinal nerve roots, which are mobile enough to not get stuck by the needle tip. To aid in the process of needle insertion, the patient is asked to flex forward to spread the lumbar laminae away from each other to make it less likely that the needle will impact them. Anesthesia can also be administered into the subarachnoid space using this route.

To numb the sacral nerves during childbirth, anesthetic can be injected into the epidural space around the spinal nerve roots, spinal nerves, and their dural sleeves. Caudal epidural anesthesia is administered by directing a needle through the sacral hiatus using the sacral cornua as palpatory landmarks. Alternatively, the needle can be inserted through a posterior sacral foramen to bathe the nerves via a transsacral epidural anesthesia.

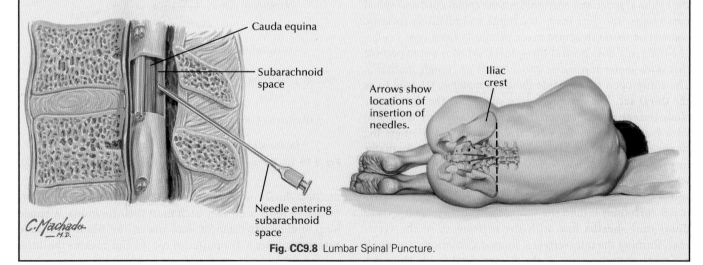

Fig. CC9.8 Lumbar Spinal Puncture.

Cauda equina

Subarachnoid space

Iliac crest

Arrows show locations of insertion of needles.

Needle entering subarachnoid space

C.Machado —M.D.

- 8 cervical spinal nerves exit superior to the corresponding vertebra (e.g., C4 spinal nerve exits between C3 and C4 vertebrae). The one exception is that the C8 spinal nerve exits between C7 and T1 vertebrae.
- 12 thoracic spinal nerves exit inferior to corresponding vertebra (e.g., T4 spinal nerve exits between T4 and T5 vertebrae).
- 5 lumbar spinal nerves exit inferior to the corresponding vertebra (e.g., L4 spinal nerve exits between L4 and L5 vertebrae).
- 5 sacral spinal nerves exit through the intervertebral foramen and anterior and posterior sacral foramina inferior to the corresponding vertebra (e.g., S4 spinal nerve exits between fused S4 and S5 vertebrae).
- 1 to 2 coccygeal spinal nerves exit in the vicinity of the proximal coccyx.

The Spinal Cord in Detail (Fig. 9.17A and B)

The interior of the spinal cord has a core of butterfly-shaped gray matter (nerve cells) with the central canal of the ventricular system at the center.

The internal structures of interest for each spinal nerve are:

- **Posterior horn**: contains neuron cell bodies associated with sensory tracts as well as interneurons that connect to other regions of the spinal gray matter.

- **Anterior horn**: contains lower motor neurons that project their axons out through the anterior spinal roots to innervate skeletal muscle.
- **Intermediate zone**: contains:
  - **Interneurons**: present at all levels, communicate with other regions of the spinal cord.
  - **Spinal accessory nucleus (CN XI)**: present in upper cervical region only, provides motor innervation to the trapezius and sternocleidomastoid muscles.
  - **Intermediolateral cell column**: present from T1 to L2, supplies preganglionic sympathetic axons to innervate visceral structures of the body.

The large white-matter regions on the outside of the spinal cord are called **columns** or **lemnisci** and consist of sensory (afferent) axons ascending toward the cortex as well as motor (efferent) axons descending to the gray matter of the cord.

- **Dorsal columns**: contain ascending sensory tracts conveying proprioceptive, vibration, and fine touch stimuli (dorsal column-medial lemniscal system) that synapse with nuclei in the medulla.
- **Lateral columns**: contain descending motor tracts to control willful motion (lateral corticospinal and rubrospinal tracts) that synapse with nerves in the anterior horn. The lateral column also contains ascending sensory tracts (dorsal and ventral spinocerebellar tracts) to the cerebellum.

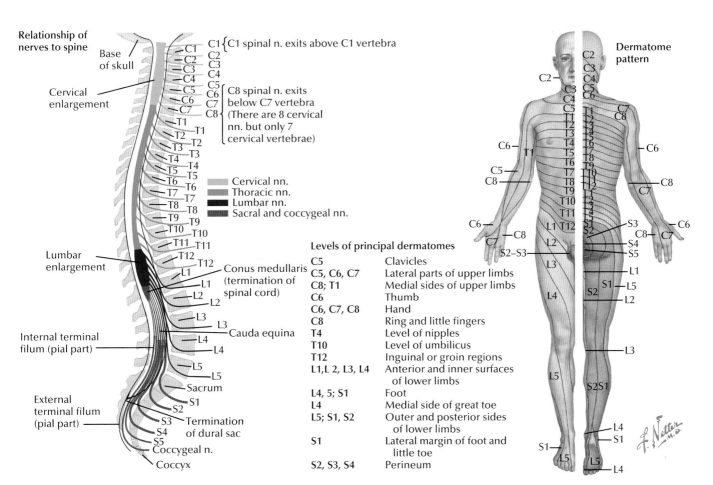

Fig. 9.16 Spinal Nerves and Sensory Dermatomes.

- **Anterior columns**: the most medial portions contain descending motor tracts (anterior corticospinal, medial and lateral vestibulospinal, reticulospinal, and tectospinal tracts) that synapse with nerve cells in the anterior horn. More laterally, where the anterior column overlaps with the lateral column, is the anterolateral system, an ascending sensory tract that conveys pain, temperature, and crude touch stimuli to nuclei in several regions of the brainstem.

Upper motor neurons (see Figs. 8.12, 8.14, and 8.17-8.20) from several parts of the central nervous system descend to reach the gray matter of the spinal cord. Within the spinal cord, these axons are protected by **oligodendrocytes** that send processes outward to surround segments of several nearby axons with **myelin sheaths**.

- **Precentral gyrus of cortex**: projects axons through the lateral corticospinal tracts in the lateral columns, as well as the anterior corticospinal tracts in the anterior columns
- **Red nucleus of midbrain**: sends axons through the rubrospinal tracts in the lateral columns
- **Tectal nuclei in midbrain**: axons descend through the tectospinal tracts of the anterior columns
- **Reticular formation**: projects axons through the reticulospinal tracts in the anterior columns
- **Vestibular nuclei of the medulla**: send axons through the medial and lateral vestibular tracts in the anterior columns

Upper motor neurons that innervate proximal trunk muscles (including intrinsic muscles of the back) leave their tracts and synapse with **lower motor neurons** (see Fig. 8.14) in the medial aspect of the anterior horn. Synapses between upper and lower motor neurons are mediated by interneurons and the neurotransmitter **glutamate**. After being released into the synaptic cleft, glutamate binds to **glutamatergic receptors** that have both ionotropic and metabotropic properties. Ionotropic receptors allow Na^+ and Ca^{2+} to enter the lower motor neuron, causing a net depolarization and making generation of an action potential more likely. Glutamate is cleared from the synaptic cleft by Na+-dependent **glutamate transporters** of the nearby astrocytes.

Lower motor neurons at each level of the spinal cord project their axons out through the anterolateral side of the column through multiple rootlets. At each vertebral level these rootlets combine to form a single **anterior spinal root** that contains somatic lower motor neurons as well as visceral motor preganglionic sympathetic axons. Anterior spinal roots travel laterally from the spinal cord to reach muscles. As they travel, they meet the posterior spinal roots (see below) that convey sensory information from that level and fuse to form a **spinal nerve**.

Just as the anterior spinal roots carry motor axons from neurons in the anterior horn, posterior roots convey sensory axons from the **posterior root ganglia**. These ganglia sit alongside the posterolateral aspect of the spinal cord. The sensory neurons in the ganglia are derived from neural crest cells. These pseudounipolar nerve cells are characterized by the large size of their cell body, central nucleus (making the cell look like an over-easy fried egg), and many small satellite cells located around the body. They also have a single axon that departs from the cell body before splitting into a medial and lateral branch. Together, the medial and lateral branches from the posterior root ganglion are collectively called a **posterior spinal root**.

- **Medial branch**: extends from the posterior root ganglion to the spinal cord. It will ascend briefly before synapsing in the posterior horn or traveling superiorly in the posterior columns.
- **Lateral branch**: extends from the posterior root ganglion through the intervertebral foramen (joining the anterior root in the process and forming the spinal nerve) to reach sensory receptors in the muscles, skin, and organs.

Spinal nerves are formed by the convergence of anterior roots and posterior roots. They leave the vertebral column by traveling through the intervertebral foramen at each level. After a spinal nerve exits an intervertebral foramen it divides to form posterior and anterior rami, which each contain both motor and sensory axons. The dura mater in the vicinity of the intervertebral foramen fuses with the periosteum of the vertebrae that form the foramen. Since the CSF and pia mater are no longer present around the rami, the **epineurium** covers and protects the spinal nerves and all peripheral nerves that are derived from them. Prior to forming anterior and posterior rami, the spinal nerve gives off several **meningeal branches** (also called recurrent meningeal nerves) that convey pain sensations from the nearby vertebral ligaments, intervertebral discs, and dura mater. These meningeal branches also carry postganglionic sympathetic axons to the blood vessels that supply those structures.

Anterior rami also leave the spinal nerves at each level and project anteriorly. They innervate muscles derived from the hypomere of each myotome, the muscles of the body wall and limbs. Unlike the posterior rami, they do not innervate muscles in a segmental manner. They frequently form interconnected plexi before forming terminal nerves that reach their target muscles.

Posterior rami (see Fig. 9.17C) leave the spinal nerves at each level of the spinal cord and project posteriorly. They provide motor innervation to all the intrinsic back muscles as well as cutaneous sensation from the overlying skin. After leaving the spinal nerve, each posterior ramus will divide into lateral, medial, and (sometimes) intermediate branches. Articular branches from the medial branch of each posterior ramus will innervate vertebral facet joints on both sides of the intervertebral foramen (Clinical Correlation 9.9).

Autonomic Innervation and the Spinal Nerve (See Fig. 9.17A and B)

In addition to controlling blood flow to the organs, the sympathetic nervous system innervates sweat glands in the skin as well as the smooth muscle sphincters that regulate blood flow to skeletal muscles, including those in the back. **Preganglionic sympathetic axons** from the **intermediolateral cell columns** (present at the T1–L2 levels) project their axons through the anterior roots, spinal nerve, and anterior rami. These axons exit the anterior ramus as **white rami communicans** (*white* because these axons are lightly myelinated B fibers) to reach the **paravertebral ganglia** associated with each spinal level within the **sympathetic chain**. Since they come from the intermediolateral cell column, there are only white rami communicans present from T1 to L2. These

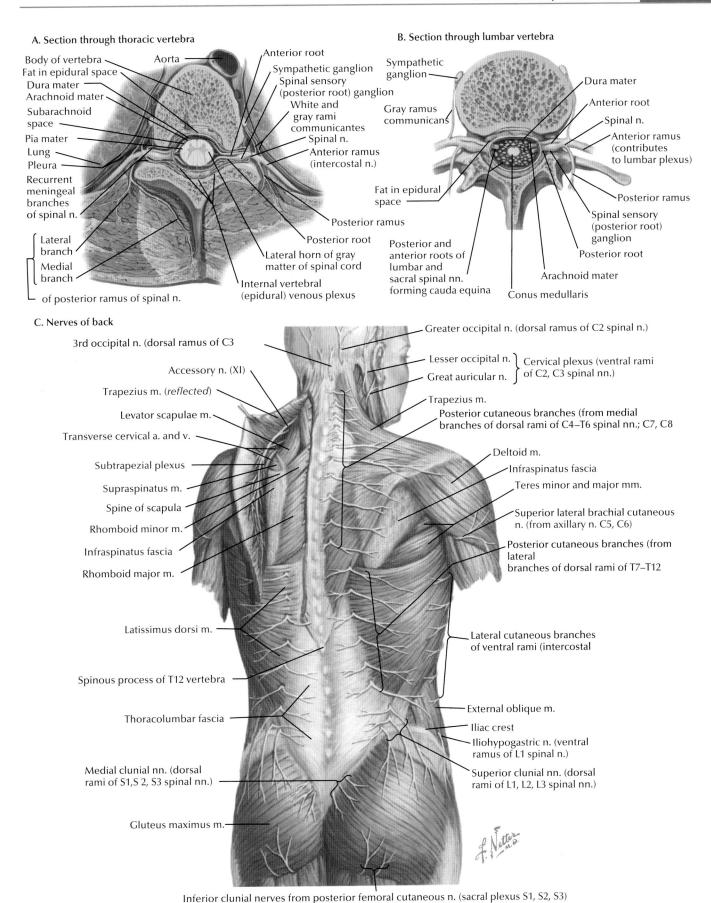

A. Section through thoracic vertebra

Body of vertebra
Fat in epidural space
Dura mater
Arachnoid mater
Subarachnoid space
Pia mater
Lung
Pleura
Recurrent meningeal branches of spinal n.
{ Lateral branch
Medial branch }
of posterior ramus of spinal n.

Aorta
Anterior root
Sympathetic ganglion
Spinal sensory (posterior root) ganglion
White and gray rami communicantes
Spinal n.
Anterior ramus (intercostal n.)
Posterior ramus
Posterior root
Lateral horn of gray matter of spinal cord
Internal vertebral (epidural) venous plexus

B. Section through lumbar vertebra

Sympathetic ganglion
Gray ramus communicans
Fat in epidural space
Posterior and anterior roots of lumbar and sacral spinal nn. forming cauda equina

Dura mater
Anterior root
Spinal n.
Anterior ramus (contributes to lumbar plexus)
Posterior ramus
Spinal sensory (posterior root) ganglion
Posterior root
Arachnoid mater
Conus medullaris

C. Nerves of back

3rd occipital n. (dorsal ramus of C3
Accessory n. (XI)
Trapezius m. (*reflected*)
Levator scapulae m.
Transverse cervical a. and v.
Subtrapezial plexus
Supraspinatus m.
Spine of scapula
Rhomboid minor m.
Infraspinatus fascia
Rhomboid major m.
Latissimus dorsi m.
Spinous process of T12 vertebra
Thoracolumbar fascia
Medial clunial nn. (dorsal rami of S1,S 2, S3 spinal nn.)
Gluteus maximus m.

Greater occipital n. (dorsal ramus of C2 spinal n.)
Lesser occipital n. } Cervical plexus (ventral rami
Great auricular n. } of C2, C3 spinal nn.)
Trapezius m.
Posterior cutaneous branches (from medial branches of dorsal rami of C4–T6 spinal nn.; C7, C8
Deltoid m.
Infraspinatus fascia
Teres minor and major mm.
Superior lateral brachial cutaneous n. (from axillary n. C5, C6)
Posterior cutaneous branches (from lateral branches of dorsal rami of T7–T12
Lateral cutaneous branches of ventral rami (intercostal
External oblique m.
Iliac crest
Iliohypogastric n. (ventral ramus of L1 spinal n.)
Superior clunial nn. (dorsal rami of L1, L2, L3 spinal nn.)

Inferior clunial nerves from posterior femoral cutaneous n. (sacral plexus S1, S2, S3)

Fig. 9.17 Spinal Nerve Cross Section.

axons may ascend or descend within the sympathetic chain before synapsing or they may synapse at the level at which they entered.

For somatic targets, including the skin and muscles of the back, the preganglionic axons synapse with postganglionic nerve cells in the paravertebral ganglia. The **postganglionic sympathetic axons** leave the chain via **gray rami communicans** (*gray* because these axons are unmyelinated C fibers) that carry them to the spinal nerve at the level of departure. Since the sympathetic chain stretches to all levels of the vertebral column, there are gray rami present at all spinal levels. Once in the spinal nerve, these postganglionic sympathetic axons will follow posterior rami, anterior rami, and the resultant peripheral nerves to reach sweat glands, arrector pili muscles, and precapillary sphincters in the skin, as well as precapillary sphincters and smooth muscles in the vessels to the skeletal muscles of the back.

THE BLOOD SUPPLY TO THE BACK

The vertebrae and spinal cord have an extensive and complex blood supply. In the cervical region, the ascending cervical, deep cervical, and vertebral arteries provide the majority of the arterial blood to the vertebrae. The thoracic and lumbar vertebrae receive blood from the intercostal, subcostal, lumbar segmental, and iliolumbar arteries. The sacrum receives blood from the median sacral, lateral sacral, and iliolumbar arteries (Fig. 9.18).

The large vessels near each vertebra give off **equatorial branches** that pierce the perimeter of the vertebral body to supply it. **Posterior branches** continue from the large vessels and supply the transverse, articular, and spinous processes as well as **muscular branches** to the overlying back muscles. These posterior branches are often found running alongside the posterior rami. **Spinal branches** enter the intervertebral foramina and split into:

- **postcentral (anterior vertebral canal) branch**: located posterior to the vertebral body. It supplies a large **nutrient artery** to the vertebral body through the basivertebral foramen.
- **prelaminar (posterior vertebral canal) branch**: located within the vertebral canal near pedicles and laminae.

These vessels also have small contributions to the longitudinal arteries of the spinal cord itself, the two **posterior spinal arteries** and one **anterior spinal artery**. These arteries originate at the base of the skull from the large left and right **vertebral arteries**. While the vertebral arteries are very large, they are not able to supply enough blood to perfuse the entire spinal cord. Thankfully, each spinal branch (at each level) gives off **radicular**

CLINICAL CORRELATION 9.9   Herniated Nucleus Pulposus—Part 2

When a herniated nucleus pulposus (HNP) pushes its way out of the annulus fibrosus, it projects posteriorly. Due to the narrow intervertebral foramen in the cervical and upper thoracic levels, it will tend to impinge on the spinal nerve exiting at that level. However, in the lumbar (and lowest thoracic) levels, the intervertebral foramina are elongated from top to bottom. Spinal nerves exit in the superior region of the foramen and the intervertebral disc is in the inferior region of the intervertebral foramen.

Because of this, a cervical HNP will affect the nerve exiting at that level. Since a named cervical spinal nerve exits superior to its named vertebrae (e.g., the C5 spinal nerve exits at the C4–C5 intervertebral level), the nerve affected by an HNP is the one exiting at that level. In contrast, a lumbar HNP will push into

the lowest part of an intervertebral foramen and miss the nerve exiting at that level. The nerve exiting at the level immediately inferior is nearby and is likely to be impinged. So, if the L4–L5 disc is herniated, it will miss the L4 spinal nerve (exiting at that level) but impinge on the next nerve, L5.

You will notice that despite the differences in how spinal nerves exit relative to their named vertebrae, it typically works out if you list an intervertebral disc (e.g., C4–C5, L2–L3, or L5–S1), the lowest level will correspond to the spinal nerve that is impinged (C5, L3, and S1, respectively). HNP in the thoracic region are relatively rare due to the stability afforded by the ribcage. HNP cannot occur in the sacrum for (what I hope is) an obvious reason.

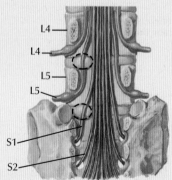

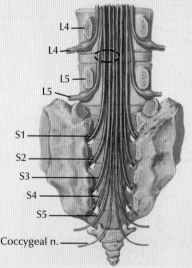

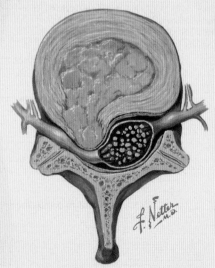

A. Lumbar disk protrusion. Does not usually affect nerve exiting above disk. Lateral protrusion at disk level L4–L5 affects L5 spinal n., not L4 spinal n. Protrusion at disk level L5–S1 affects S1 spinal n., not L5 spinal n.

B. Medial protrusion at disk level L4–L5. Rarely affects L4 spinal n. but may affect L5 spinal n. and sometimes S1–S4 spinal nn.

C. Schematic cross section showing compression of nerve root

Fig. CC9.10 Lumbar Disc Herniation.

or **segmental medullary arteries** that travel along the spinal nerve and roots. Radicular arteries only supply the roots and spinal nerve. **Segmental medullary arteries** (either anterior or posterior) are larger and feed into the anterior or posterior spinal arteries perfusing the cord at that level. They are most prominent near the cervical and lumbosacral enlargements. In the lower thoracic or upper lumbar region, there is typically a **great anterior segmental medullary artery (of Adamkiewicz)** that supplies a massive boost to the blood volume in the spinal vessels. It is typically located on the left and must be preserved during operations on the posterior thorax or abdomen, since loss of this vessel will cause ischemia of the inferior spinal cord and possible hemiplegia.

Within the cord, the anterior spinal artery sends a **sulcal branch** through the anterior median fissure of the spinal cord. It provides the majority of blood to the gray matter, anterior columns, and part of the lateral columns. The posterior spinal arteries supply the posterior columns, a small area of the posterior gray matter, and some of the lateral columns.

Multiple **spinal veins** (Fig. 9.19) run parallel to spinal arteries and interconnect as they pass along the length of the cord. Blood in these veins drains to **anterior medullary, posterior medullary, and radicular veins** that empty into an extensive series of veins sitting in the adipose tissue of the epidural space, the **internal vertebral venous plexus**. The posterior and anterior portions of the internal vertebral venous plexus are quite extensive. The large **basivertebral veins** drain the red marrow (an important source of new blood cells) of the vertebral bodies into the anterior portion of the internal vertebral venous plexus. Superiorly, this plexus can drain to cerebral veins or dural venous sinuses. In the rest of the spinal cord, they drain to **intervertebral veins** that carry blood to the **external vertebral venous plexus** that surrounds the vertebrae. From there, the venous blood will drain to any large nearby vein such as deep cervical, vertebral, intercostal, subcostal, or lumbar veins (Clinical Correlation 9.10).

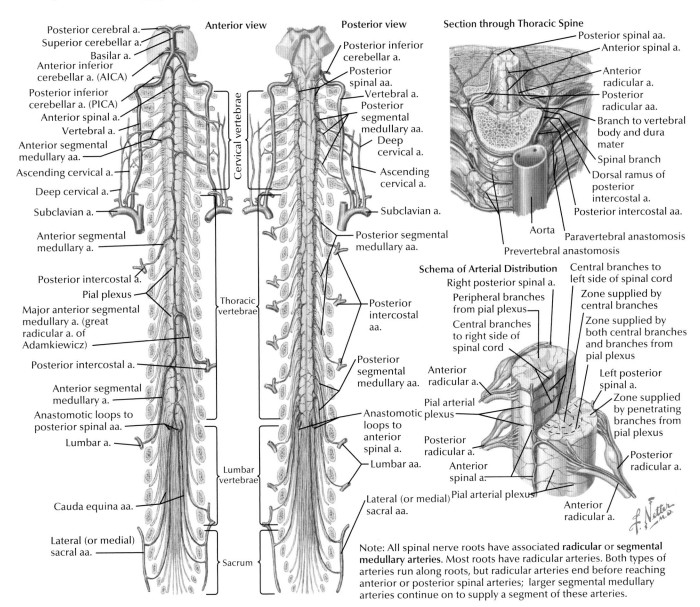

Fig. 9.18 Arteries of the Spinal Cord.

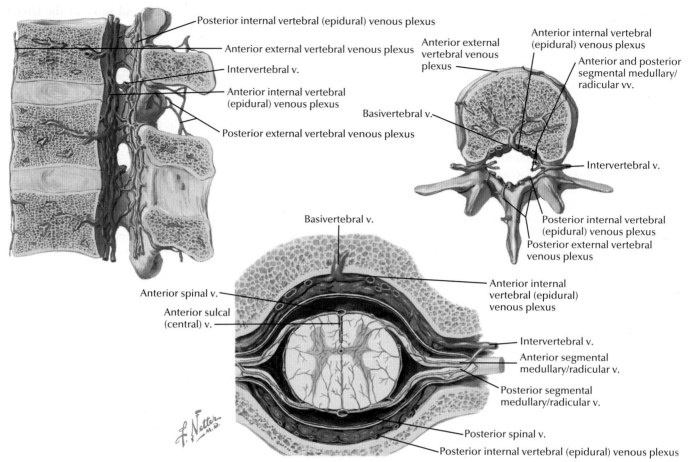

Fig. 9.19 Veins of the Spinal Cord and Vertebrae.

CLINICAL CORRELATION 9.10   Vertebral Venous Plexi and Tumor Metastasis

The internal and external vertebral venous plexi form an extensive and interconnected network of veins that stretch from the coccyx to the base of the skull. These veins are interconnected to many of the large veins near the midline of the body and have no valves in their walls. Metastatic tumors that have invaded veins can send tumor cells into the bloodstream. Prostate, breast, and lung cancers frequently spread to the spine, carried by the valveless veins of the external and internal vertebral venous plexus. This entire system is sometimes referred to as the Batson venous plexus.

Clinical Anatomy of the Upper Limb

INTRODUCTION

The upper limb is connected to the back by its extrinsic muscles (latissimus dorsi, trapezius, rhomboid major and minor, levator scapulae) and to the chest by large muscles of the thoracic wall (pectoralis major and minor, serratus anterior). In addition, the clavicle connects the sternum to the scapula, bridging the two regions.

BONES, LIGAMENTS, AND JOINTS OF THE UPPER LIMB

The **pectoral (shoulder) girdle** is formed by the clavicle and scapula on each side of the body and it anchors the upper limbs to the torso. The manubrium of the sternum is not technically a part of the girdle, but it does interact with both clavicles. The **shoulder** is a collection of structures where the humerus interacts with the pectoral girdle.

Clavicle and the Sternoclavicular Joint (Fig. 10.1, See Also Fig. 2.23)

The **clavicle** is an elongated bone that appears mostly flat when viewed anteriorly but has a pronounced double curvature when viewed from a superior vantage point. The **sternal end** of the clavicle is a medial expansion of the bone that articulates with the manubrium of the sternum at a sternal facet. If you examine this articulation on dry bone, it does not look remotely comfortable and the two surfaces do not interface easily. This is because in life there is typically an **articular disc** made from fibrocartilage between the two bones that allows them to move across each other smoothly at the **sternoclavicular joint**. This allows the distal clavicle to move anteriorly, posteriorly, superiorly, or inferiorly along with a little bit of rotation. The **anterior sternoclavicular and posterior sternoclavicular ligaments** are capsular ligaments that are thickenings of the sternoclavicular joint capsule. Continuous with the sternoclavicular ligaments is the **interclavicular ligament**, which connects the medial sides of the left and right clavicles and crosses the jugular notch of

the manubrium. The sternocleidomastoid muscle inserts on the superior aspect of the manubrium and proximal clavicle. Immediately lateral to the sternal facet on the inferior side of the clavicle is the **impression for the costoclavicular ligament**, which links the clavicle to the first rib.

The only feature of note along the elongated clavicular **shaft** is the **groove for the subclavius muscle**, which also connects the inferior aspect of the clavicle to the first rib. The clavicular head of the pectoralis major muscle originates from the anterior aspect of the shaft. The lateral clavicle has an expanded **acromial end** that ends in an articular facet that interacts with the acromial process of the scapula. The distal clavicle is an attachment site for the trapezius muscle and the anterior belly of the deltoid muscle (Clinical Correlation 10.1).

Acromioclavicular Joint (Fig. 10.2, See Also Fig. 10.1)

The **acromioclavicular joint** is enclosed by a strong capsule that features a strong **acromioclavicular ligament** on the superior aspect. There is often fibrocartilage between the acromion and clavicle, but it does not always form a complete disc. The inferior aspect of the lateral clavicle hosts the **conoid tubercle** and the **trapezoid line**, where the **coracoclavicular ligaments** (**conoid** and **trapezoid ligaments**) attach to stabilize the distal clavicle. While the two ligaments are distinct, they are located very close together, have similar functions, and tend to be damaged simultaneously (see Clinical Correlation 2.1).

Scapula (See Fig. 10.1)

We noted in Chapter 9 that many of the extrinsic back muscles attach to the scapula to move the upper limb. The scapula is the most proximal bone of the upper limb and is only connected to the torso through the clavicle. This gives the scapula a wide range of possible motions that are constrained and stabilized by the many muscles that attach it to the back, thorax, and upper limb. The triangular **body of the scapula** has an oblique **lateral border** that meets the vertical **medial border** at the scapula's **inferior angle**. The medial border extends

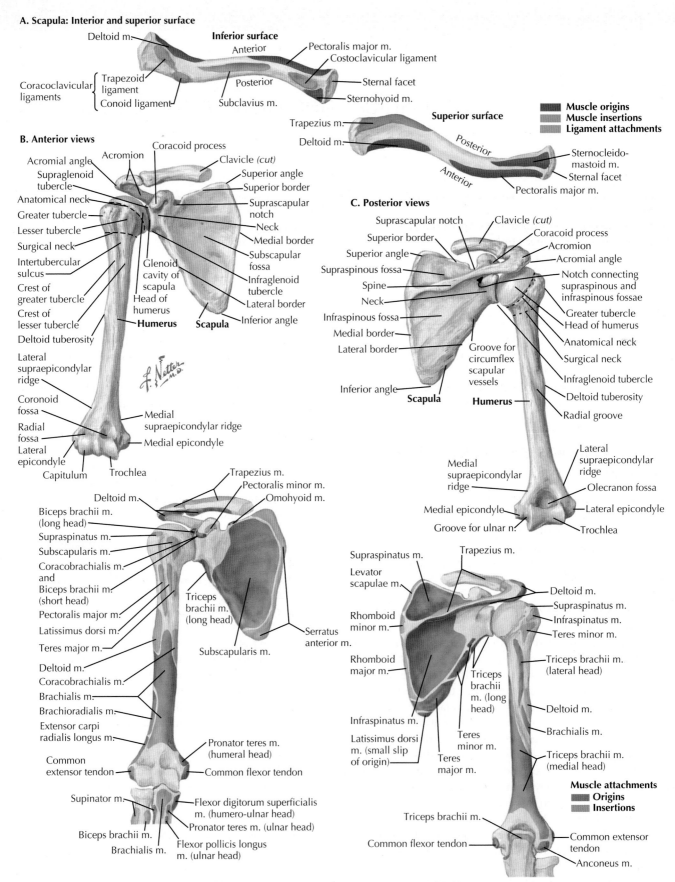

A. Scapula: Interior and superior surface

Deltoid m.

Inferior surface

Anterior

Pectoralis major m.

Costoclavicular ligament

Coracoclavicular ligaments

Trapezoid ligament

Conoid ligament

Posterior

Subclavius m.

Sternal facet

Sternohyoid m.

Trapezius m.

Deltoid m.

Superior surface

Posterior

Anterior

Sternocleido-mastoid m.

Sternal facet

Pectoralis major m.

■ Muscle origins
■ Muscle insertions
■ Ligament attachments

B. Anterior views

Coracoid process

Acromial angle

Acromion

Clavicle *(cut)*

Supraglenoid tubercle

Superior angle

Superior border

Anatomical neck

Suprascapular notch

Greater tubercle

Neck

Lesser tubercle

Medial border

Surgical neck

Subscapular fossa

Intertubercular sulcus

Glenoid cavity of scapula

Infraglenoid tubercle

Crest of greater tubercle

Lateral border

Crest of lesser tubercle

Head of humerus

Inferior angle

Deltoid tuberosity

Humerus

Scapula

Lateral supraepicondylar ridge

Coronoid fossa

Medial supraepicondylar ridge

Radial fossa

Medial epicondyle

Lateral epicondyle

Capitulum

Trochlea

C. Posterior views

Suprascapular notch

Clavicle *(cut)*

Superior border

Coracoid process

Superior angle

Acromion

Supraspinous fossa

Acromial angle

Spine

Notch connecting supraspinous and infraspinous fossae

Neck

Infraspinous fossa

Greater tubercle

Medial border

Head of humerus

Lateral border

Anatomical neck

Groove for circumflex scapular vessels

Surgical neck

Infraglenoid tubercle

Inferior angle

Deltoid tuberosity

Scapula

Humerus

Radial groove

Medial supraepicondylar ridge

Lateral supraepicondylar ridge

Olecranon fossa

Medial epicondyle

Lateral epicondyle

Groove for ulnar n.

Trochlea

Trapezius m.

Pectoralis minor m.

Deltoid m.

Omohyoid m.

Biceps brachii m. (long head)

Supraspinatus m.

Subscapularis m.

Coracobrachialis m. and Biceps brachii m. (short head)

Triceps brachii m. (long head)

Pectoralis major m.

Latissimus dorsi m.

Teres major m.

Serratus anterior m.

Deltoid m.

Subscapularis m.

Coracobrachialis m.

Brachialis m.

Brachioradialis m.

Extensor carpi radialis longus m.

Pronator teres m. (humeral head)

Common extensor tendon

Common flexor tendon

Supinator m.

Flexor digitorum superficialis m. (humero-ulnar head)

Biceps brachii m.

Pronator teres m. (ulnar head)

Brachialis m.

Flexor pollicis longus m. (ulnar head)

Supraspinatus m.

Trapezius m.

Levator scapulae m.

Deltoid m.

Rhomboid minor m.

Supraspinatus m.

Infraspinatus m.

Teres minor m.

Rhomboid major m.

Triceps brachii m. (lateral head)

Triceps brachii m. (long head)

Deltoid m.

Infraspinatus m.

Brachialis m.

Latissimus dorsi m. (small slip of origin)

Teres minor m.

Teres major m.

Triceps brachii m. (medial head)

Muscle attachments
■ Origins
■ Insertions

Triceps brachii m.

Common flexor tendon

Common extensor tendon

Anconeus m.

Fig. 10.1 Humerus and Scapula: Insertions and Origins.

CLINICAL CORRELATION 10.1 Bone Fractures and Fracture of the Clavicle

There are several types of fractures that can affect bones, particularly the long bones of the limbs (Fig. CC10.1A). Other specialized fractures may affect certain bones (e.g., burst fracture of the vertebral bodies), but here are the common types of fractures. Note that these are not mutually exclusive, and fractures can be described by using one or more of these terms simultaneously.

- **Closed fractures** do not rupture the skin.
- **Compound (open) fractures** have broken through the skin and are open to the external environment, making infection a concern.
- **Transverse fractures** run perpendicular (90 degrees) to the long axis of the bone.
- **Linear fractures** run along the long axis of a bone.
- **Oblique fractures** pass diagonally along the long axis of a bone.
- **Spiral fractures** also pass diagonally along the long axis of a bone but in a twisting fashion.
- **Stable fractures** have their fractured ends in their original position despite the fracture.
- **Displaced fractures** have separation between the fractured ends of the bone.
- **Comminuted fractures** are broken into several pieces, some of which may be small.
- **Segmental fractures** occur when two fractures create a "loose" piece between the other two.
- **Stress fractures** are commonly caused by overuse and impact causing small, painful, hairline fractures.
- **Compression fractures** occur when the bone cannot hold the loads it is exposed to and collapses on itself.

- **Torus fractures** result from bending and collapse of the bone on one side without fracture on the opposite side.
- **Greenstick fractures** are common in children and occur when a fracture affects one side of the bone and the other side does not break but bends.
- **Avulsion fractures** occur when a tendon or ligament pulls so strongly on a bone that it tears away a portion of that bone.
- **Pathologic fractures** occur when the bone has been weakened by another disease process (such as a tumor in the bone) and fractures since the bone cannot support the normal forces that the bone encounters.
- **Salter-Harris fractures** are fractures that include cartilage growth plates. These were discussed in Chapter 7.

The clavicle is a very frequently fractured bone, especially in children (see Fig. CC10.1B). It can be fractured by direct trauma or by falling onto an outstretched arm and having the force of the fall transmitted up along the upper limb where it snaps the clavicle. It typically fractures just proximal to the coracoclavicular ligaments or in the middle third of the bone. When this happens, the sternocleidomastoid muscle elevates the end of the proximal fragment and the weight of the upper limb pulls the distal segment (and the rest of the limb) inferiorly. Tension of the pectoral muscles, latissimus dorsi, and other adducting muscles can shorten the fragments, causing the distal end to migrate more medially. Surgical repair can be done in the case of comminuted fractures but the injury is frequently reduced (the ends of the bone are brought together), splinted, and allowed to heal without surgical intervention.

A. Types of fracture

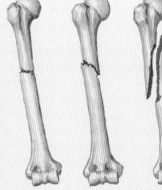

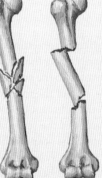
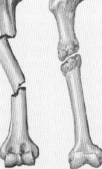
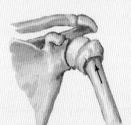
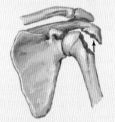
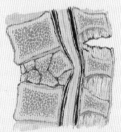
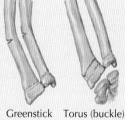

Transverse fracture

Oblique fracture

Spiral fracture

Comminuted fracture

Segmental fracture

Pathologic fracture (tumor or bone disease)

Avulsion (greater tuberosity of humerus avulsed by supraspinatus)

Impacted fracture

Greenstick fracture   Torus (buckle) fracture

In children

Compression fracture

B. Fracture of the clavicle

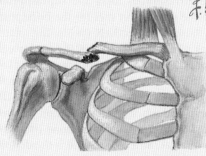
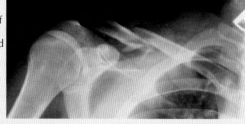

f. Netter M.D.

Fracture of middle third of clavicle (most common). Medial fragment displaced upward by pull of sternocleidomastoid m.; lateral fragment displaced downward by weight of shoulder. Fractures occur most often in children.

Anteroposterior radiograph. Fracture of middle third of clavicle.

Fig. CC10.1 Types of Fracture.

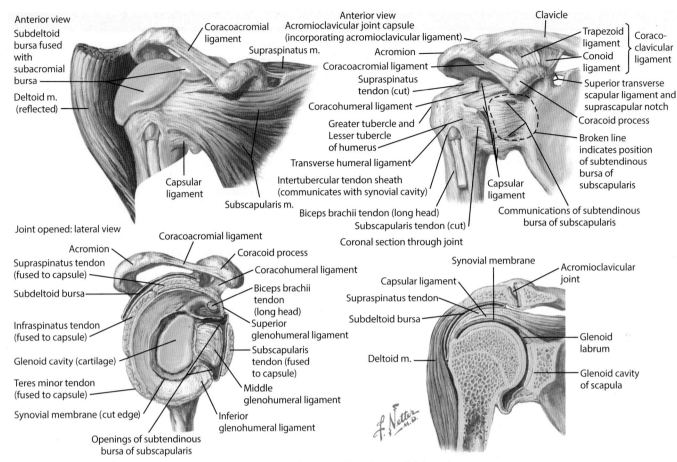

Fig. 10.2 Shoulder: Glenohumeral Joint.

from the T7 to T2 vertebral level to the **superior angle** where it meets the **superior border** of the scapula. The rhomboid major and minor muscles attach to the medial border and the levator scapulae muscles attach along the scapula's superior angle. The superior border has a small but distinct impression along its distal third, the **suprascapular notch**, which is covered by a small but strong **superior transverse scapular ligament**. Occasionally this ligament will ossify, enclosing a **suprascapular foramen**. The small omohyoid muscle attaches to the superior border near the suprascapular notch. Immediately lateral to the suprascapular notch is a massive, thumb-shaped strut of bone that extends anteriorly, the **coracoid process**. In addition to the two coracoclavicular ligaments, the pectoralis minor, coracobrachialis, and short head of the biceps brachii muscles also insert on the coracoid process. The superior border of the scapula meets the lateral border at the **lateral angle** of the scapula. This complex area forms a narrowed, ovoid extension of bone, the **neck of the scapula**, before expanding into the large, circular **head of the scapula** that articulates with the head of the humerus through the **glenoid cavity**. Immediately superior and inferior to the glenoid cavity are the **supraglenoid tubercle** and **infraglenoid tubercle**, origination sites for the long head of the biceps brachii and long head of the triceps muscles, respectively.

The scapula has a concave **costal surface** on its anterior side where it glides across the ribs. The smooth appearance of this surface is sometimes interrupted by lateral lines that extend primarily along the axial plane. The majority of the costal surface is devoted to the **subscapular fossa**, where the subscapularis muscle, one of the four rotator cuff muscles, originates. Just medial to the subscapular fossa is a rougher area parallel to the medial border of the scapula where the serratus anterior muscle originates. The **scapulothoracic joint** is a very unusual articulation. It is not a synovial joint and has no capsule. The loose connective tissue between the anterior scapula and the lateral ribcage is rich in proteoglycans that cushion and lubricate the scapula as it elevates, depresses, protracts, retracts, and rotates across the thorax.

The **posterior surface** of the scapula is convex and hosts two smooth areas, the **infraspinous fossa** and **supraspinous fossa**. These fossae are the origination sites for the infraspinatus and supraspinatus muscles, respectively (two of the rotator cuff muscles). The teres minor muscle (last of the rotator cuff muscles) originates from the lateral border of the scapula. Just inferior to it is the origin of the teres major muscle, the attachment point of which almost reaches the inferior angle of the scapula. The infraspinatus and supraspinatus fossae on the posterior surface are divided by an elevated strut of bone, the **spine of the scapula**. On the medial third of the spine is the **deltoid tubercle** for the posterior belly of the deltoid muscle. The spine of the scapula continues laterally and loses its connection to the rest of the bone, creating the **scapular notch** where it connects to the neck of the scapula. The scapular notch allows vessels and nerves to travel between the supraspinous and infraspinous fossae. The lateral extension of the spine creates the **acromion**. It turns anteriorly, creating a variably sized **acromial angle** before terminating at the **clavicular facet**, where it meets the distal clavicle. A broad and surprisingly strong **coracoacromial ligament** connects the acromion to the lateral aspect of the coracoid process. Since both the acromion and coracoid process are part of the scapula, damage to this ligament is infrequent. The trapezius muscle inserts along the superior aspect of the distal clavicle, acromion, and spine of the scapula. The deltoid muscle originates from the same three bony landmarks but extends inferiorly to insert on the humerus.

Proximal Humerus (See Fig. 10.1)

The bone at the core of the arm is the humerus. The most prominent aspect of the proximal humerus is its smooth and rounded **head** that articulates with the glenoid cavity of the scapula. More laterally are two sites for muscle attachment, the **lesser tubercle** and the very large **greater tubercle**, which continue inferiorly as the **crest of the lesser tubercle** and **crest of the greater tubercle**. Between the two tubercles is the deep **intertubercular sulcus**, also known as the bicipital groove. The **transverse humeral ligament** stretches across the greater tubercle and lesser tubercle, keeping the tendon of the long head of the biceps brachii tethered in place.

The humeral head and tubercles are separated from each other by the **anatomical neck** of the humerus, a shallow depression marking where ossification centers fused to create a continuous bone. The tubercles and their crests narrow as they extend inferiorly onto the **shaft** of the humerus. The narrowed area just below the tubercles marks the **surgical neck** of the humerus, which is a common site for both fractures and orthopedic operations. Travelling along the greater tubercle from inferior to superior, we encounter the attachment sites for the teres minor, infraspinatus, and supraspinatus muscles. The lesser tubercle marks the insertion site of the subscapularis muscle. The pectoralis major muscle tendon inserts along the crest of the greater tubercle while the crest of the lesser tubercle is the site where the latissimus dorsi and teres major muscles insert.

Glenohumeral Joint (See Fig. 10.2)

The head of the humerus articulates with the shallow glenoid cavity at the **glenohumeral joint**. To deepen the articulation, there is a fibrocartilage ring around the outside of the glenoid fossa named the **glenoid labrum**. The **superior glenohumeral**, **middle glenohumeral**, and **inferior glenohumeral ligaments** are intracapsular ligaments that are most visible from within the joint itself. They limit adduction, external rotation, and abduction, respectively. The **coracohumeral ligament** extends from the lateral base of the coracoid process to the medial aspect of the greater tubercle to cover and reinforce the capsule. The glenohumeral joint allows a wide range of motions: flexion/extension, abduction/adduction, internal/external rotation. It can also circumduct, moving through several motions simultaneously. As the glenohumeral joint approaches its limits in abduction, flexion, and extension, the scapula will rotate to

shift the angle of the glenohumeral joint (Clinical Correlations 10.2–10.4).

Humeral Shaft and Distal Humerus (Fig. 10.3, See Also Fig. 10.1)

The shaft does not have a completely circular cross-section but is more of a rounded triangle with anteromedial, anterolateral, and posterior surfaces. The **deltoid tuberosity** is a notable elevation on the lateral aspect of the shaft where all three bellies of the deltoid muscle insert. The radial groove runs in an inferolateral direction along the posterior surface and marks where the radial nerve and deep brachial artery are found. The posterior surface is also where the lateral and medial heads of the triceps brachii originate. The coracobrachialis muscle inserts midway down the shaft on the anterolateral surface of the humerus. The brachialis muscle originates from a very broad region on the anterolateral and anteromedial surfaces of the distal humerus. The posterior surface of the humerus flattens considerably near its inferior end, creating a prominent medial border and lateral border ending in a prominent **medial supraepicondylar ridge** and a **lateral supraepicondylar ridge**. The brachioradialis and extensor carpi radialis longus muscles originate from the lateral supraepicondylar ridge.

The distal end of the humerus, the **humeral condyle** (sometimes subdivided into medial and lateral condyles although there is no clear division between the two), articulates with the radius and the ulna. The lateral side of the condyle ends in an articular surface for the radial head, the **capitulum**. Immediately superior to the capitulum on the anterior humerus is a depression, the **radial fossa**, where the rounded perimeter of the radial head can sit during full flexion of the elbow. The medial side of the condyle ends in the **trochlea**, where the ulna will articulate. Just superior to the trochlea on the anterior side is the **coronoid fossa** and on the posterior aspect is the **olecranon fossa**, where the coronoid process and olecranon process will reside during full flexion or extension of the elbow, respectively. Immediately lateral to the capitulum is a raised and palpable prominence called the **lateral epicondyle**, which is an attachment site for the common extensor tendon and is continuous with the lateral supraepicondylar ridge. Medial to the trochlea is an even larger **medial epicondyle** where part of the pronator teres muscle and the common flexor tendon originate. Superiorly it fuses with the medial supraepicondylar ridge and on its posterior aspect is a very deep depression running from superior to inferior, the **groove for the ulnar nerve** (Clinical Correlation 10.5).

Proximal Ulna and Radius (Fig. 10.4, See Also Fig. 10.3)

The most prominent part of the proximal ulna is the massive **olecranon process**, the single insertion point for all three heads of the triceps brachii muscle. The anconeus muscle attaches to a broad expanse of the proximal, posterolateral aspect of the ulna, including part of the olecranon. On the ulna's anterior, proximal side is a C-shaped depression, the **trochlear notch**, which has a slightly elevated guiding ridge that helps keep it aligned with the trochlea of the humerus. Opposite the olecranon, the guiding ridge terminates anteriorly at the prominent

CLINICAL CORRELATION 10.2   Shoulder (Glenohumeral) Dislocation

The rotator cuff muscles, coracoacromial ligament, glenoid labrum, and glenohumeral joint capsule all keep the humeral head in place. However, excessive abduction, extension, and rotation of the humerus cause displacement of the head of the humerus from the glenoid cavity, a **shoulder dislocation**. Excessive abduction can force the humeral head inferiorly, after which it may be pulled anterior (most common) or posterior to the glenoid fossa by muscles attaching to the proximal humerus. A humeral head that has been displaced anteriorly can come to rest in a **subcoracoid** (most common), **subglenoid**, or **subclavicular** position. Simultaneously, the head of the humerus may be pressed against the rim of the glenoid cavity, creating a wedge-shaped region of compressed bone on the head of the humerus, which is called a **Hill-Sachs lesion.** This is often accompanied by ruptures of the glenohumeral joint capsule and traction on the axillary or musculocutaneous nerves.

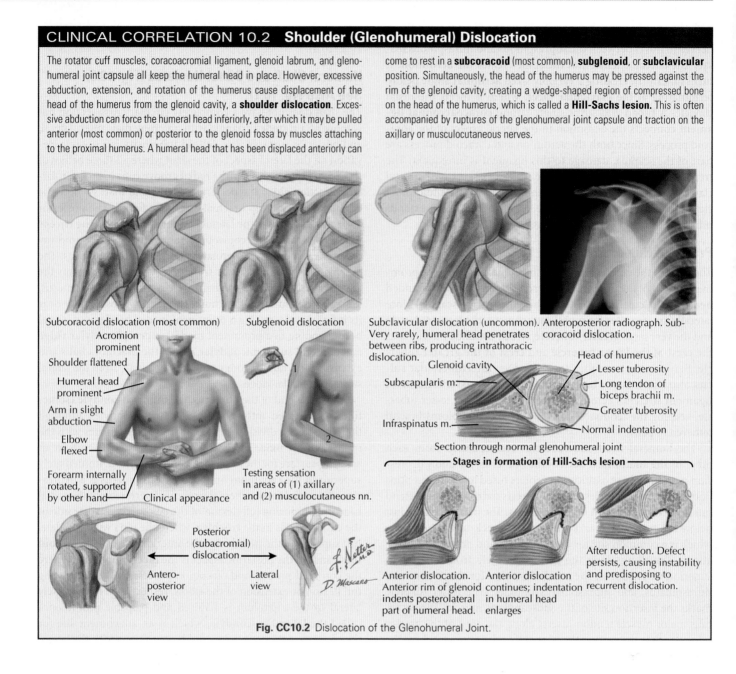

Fig. CC10.2 Dislocation of the Glenohumeral Joint.

coronoid process. Just distal to the coronoid process on the anterior aspect is the **ulnar tuberosity** where the brachialis muscle inserts. The ulnar head of the pronator teres and part of the flexor digitorum superficialis muscles originate just medial to this area. The lateral side of the trochlear notch is continuous with another articular surface, the **radial notch**, where the head of the radius articulates with the ulna. Immediately distal to the radial notch on the lateral side of the proximal ulna is the **supinator crest**, the origin of the supinator muscle, which wraps around the posterior side of the head of the radius before inserting on it.

The **head of the radius** is the expanded proximal part of the bone that contributes to the elbow joint complex. More specifically, the articular facet of the head of the radius, a slightly depressed region at the superior end of the bone is what articulates with the capitulum of the humerus. The smooth **articular circumference** of the head of the radius slides across the radial notch of the ulna, kept in place by the **anular ligament**. The radius narrows considerably at the **neck** before expanding again as the **shaft** of the radius. The proximal shaft has a notable process, the **radial tuberosity,** where the tendon for the biceps brachii muscle attaches.

Elbow Joint (Fig. 10.5)

The **elbow joint** is a combination of three distinct articulations: the humeroulnar, humeroradial, and proximal radioulnar joints that are collected within the capsule of the elbow joint. The **humeroulnar joint** between the trochlea of the humerus and trochlear notch of the ulna allows a great deal of flexion and extension. Flexion is limited by the coronoid process reaching the coronoid fossa of the distal humerus; likewise, extension is limited by the olecranon process reaching the olecranon fossa

CLINICAL CORRELATION 10.3   Glenoid Labrum Tear

Repetitive motion at the shoulder or extremely forceful movements of the proximal humerus can cause tears to develop in the glenoid labrum. During an anterior dislocation of the humerus, it is common for the anteroinferior glenoid labrum to become ruptured; this is called a **Bankart lesion**. Extreme tension conveyed through the long head of the biceps tendon can cause tears in the superior glenoid labrum. These **SLAP lesions** (superior labral tear from anterior to posterior) commonly occur in athletes who have to violently whip their arms downward, such as when spiking a volleyball or pitching in baseball or cricket.

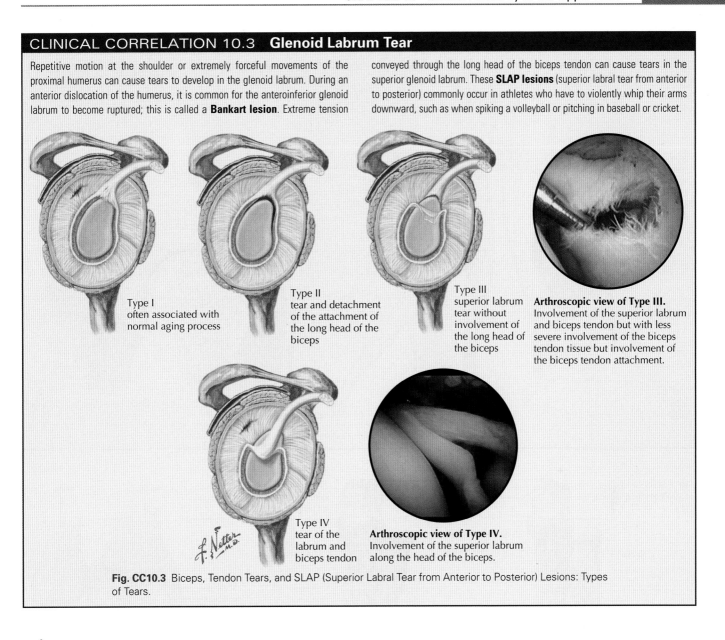

Type I
often associated with normal aging process

Type II
tear and detachment of the attachment of the long head of the biceps

Type III
superior labrum tear without involvement of the long head of the biceps

Arthroscopic view of Type III.
Involvement of the superior labrum and biceps tendon but with less severe involvement of the biceps tendon tissue but involvement of the biceps tendon attachment.

Type IV
tear of the labrum and biceps tendon

Arthroscopic view of Type IV.
Involvement of the superior labrum along the head of the biceps.

Fig. CC10.3 Biceps, Tendon Tears, and SLAP (Superior Labral Tear from Anterior to Posterior) Lesions: Types of Tears.

of the humerus. The medial side of the ulna is connected to the medial side of the distal humerus by a strong, fan-shaped **ulnar collateral ligament** (also known as the medial collateral ligament of the elbow). The **humeroradial joint** between the capitulum of the humerus and the articular facet of the head of the radius allows the radial head to rotate around the capitulum during supination and pronation. The **anular ligament** wraps around the head and neck of the radius and keeps the radial head in place during pronation and supination. The stability of the radial head is ensured by the small **quadrate ligament**, which extends from the radial notch of the ulna to the radial neck. It prevents excessive supination and pronation at the elbow. The **radial collateral ligament** (lateral collateral ligament of the elbow) connects the anular ligament to the distal, lateral aspect of the humerus. Medially the anular ligament attaches to either side of the ulna's radial notch and on the lateral side it is connected to the radial collateral ligament. This keeps the head of the radius in close contact with the radial notch of the ulna, forming the **proximal radioulnar joint**, which allows for pronation and supination. A small pouch of the elbow's synovial lining, the sacciform recess, extends inferiorly out of the anular ligament (Clinical Correlation 10.6).

Distal Ulna and Radius (See Figs. 10.3 and 10.4)

The **shaft/body** of the ulna extends distally and has three flattened areas; the medial surface is separated from the anterior surface by the anterior border, and from the posterior surface by the posterior border. The anterior and posterior surfaces are separated by the **interosseous border** of the ulna, marking where the interosseous membrane attaches to the ulna. The shaft becomes narrower as it approaches the **head** of the ulna at its distal end. A smooth **articular circumference** can be distinguished around its periphery. The posteromedial side of the head ends with a small but prominent **ulnar styloid process**.

Regarding the radius, the lateral surface of the shaft is separated from the anterior surface and posterior surface by the

CLINICAL CORRELATION 10.4   Frozen Shoulder/Adhesive Capsulitis

Inflammation around the shoulder due to dislocation, rupture of the labrum, tendonitis of the long head of the biceps brachii, rotator cuff injury, or bursitis can cause the connective tissue of the glenohumeral joint to become scarred. This will result in adhesive capsulitis, which limits the mobility of the joint, preventing abduction past 45 degrees. Treatment often involves placing the patient under anesthesia and aggressively manipulating the humerus, tearing through the adhesions, and then keeping subsequent inflammation from re-freezing the shoulder.

Markedly limited range of motion on right side compared with that on left side. Slight abduction capability largely due to elevation and rotation of scapula.

Posterior view reveals atrophy of scapular and deltoid mm. Broken lines, indicating position of spine of scapula and axis of humerus on each side, show little or no motion in right shoulder

Adhesions of peripheral capsule to distal articular cartilage

Adhesions obliterating axillary fold of capsule

Coronal section of shoulder shows adhesions between capsule and periphery of humeral head

Fig. CC10.4 Adhesive Capsulitis of the Shoulder (Frozen Shoulder).

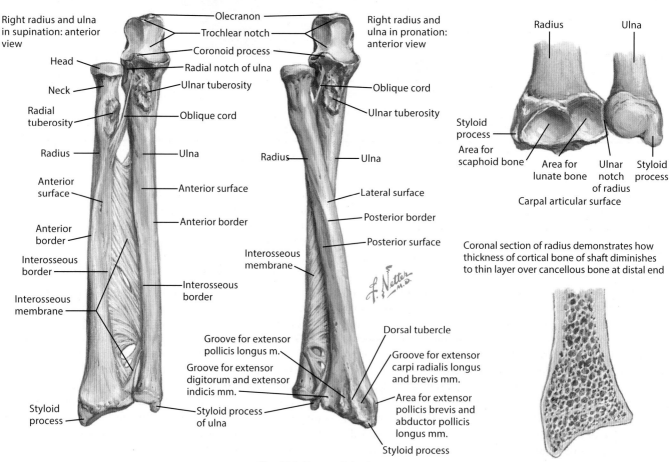

Right radius and ulna in supination: anterior view

- Head
- Neck
- Radial tuberosity
- Radius
- Anterior surface
- Anterior border
- Interosseous border
- Interosseous membrane
- Styloid process

- Olecranon
- Trochlear notch
- Coronoid process
- Radial notch of ulna
- Ulnar tuberosity
- Oblique cord
- Ulna
- Anterior surface
- Anterior border
- Interosseous border
- Groove for extensor pollicis longus m.
- Groove for extensor digitorum and extensor indicis mm.
- Styloid process of ulna

Right radius and ulna in pronation: anterior view

- Radius
- Oblique cord
- Ulnar tuberosity
- Ulna
- Lateral surface
- Posterior border
- Posterior surface
- Interosseous membrane
- Dorsal tubercle
- Groove for extensor carpi radialis longus and brevis mm.
- Area for extensor pollicis brevis and abductor pollicis longus mm.
- Styloid process

Radius   Ulna

- Styloid process
- Area for scaphoid bone
- Area for lunate bone
- Ulnar notch of radius
- Styloid process
- Carpal articular surface

Coronal section of radius demonstrates how thickness of cortical bone of shaft diminishes to thin layer over cancellous bone at distal end

Fig. 10.3 Bones of the Forearm.

The humerus is a stout bone, but there are a few sites where it is more prone to fracture than others. A **fracture of the surgical neck of the humerus** can occur when torsional force is exerted on the proximal humerus, particularly if the bone is weakened by osteoporosis or lack of activity. This leaves the humeral head present within the capsule of the glenohumeral joint. The strong tendons inserting on the greater and lesser tubercles can pull those bony prominences off the rest of the bone, causing **avulsion fractures**. The shaft of the humerus can undergo a **transverse** or **spiral fracture**. Depending on exactly where the fracture occurs, the proximal fragment may be directed laterally by the pull of the deltoid muscle or the distal fragment may be pulled superiorly, overriding the proximal fragment. The **intercondylar region of the distal humerus** can be fractured by forced hyperextension of the olecranon into the olecranon fossa, separating the medial and lateral condyles from the rest of the humerus.

lateral end. Just proximal to it is a **suprastyloid crest** where part of the brachioradialis muscle attaches. The posterior side of the distal radius has several **grooves for extensor tendons** that are separated by bony ridges. From lateral to medial, they are: the groove for the extensor carpi radialis tendons, the **dorsal (Lister) tubercle**, the groove for the extensor pollicis longus tendon, and the groove for the extensor digitorum and extensor indicis tendons. The medial side of the distal radius hosts an **ulnar notch** that articulates with the head of the ulna.

The **interosseous membrane** is not a joint per se but is a collection of connective tissue fibers that tether the shaft of the ulna to the shaft of the radius. The collagen fibers of the membrane run primarily in an inferomedial direction. It allows pronation and supination but keeps the two bones connected even when one or both are fractured. A related **oblique cord** runs inferolaterally from the base of the ulnar coronoid process to the radial tuberosity.

Several muscles share attachment sites across the humerus, radius, ulna, and the intervening interosseous membrane. On the anterior side: flexor digitorum superficialis, flexor digitorum profundus, flexor pollicis longus, and most distally, the pronator quadratus. Posteriorly are the: flexor carpi ulnaris, extensor carpi ulnaris, abductor pollicis longus, extensor pollicis longus, extensor pollicis brevis, and the extensor indicis (Clinical Correlation 10.7).

anterior border and posterior border, respectively. The supinator muscle inserts along the proximal anterior border and the pronator teres inserts just a bit more inferiorly, sometimes leaving a distinct **pronator tuberosity**. Like the ulna, the anterior and posterior surfaces are separated by the **interosseous border** of the radius. The distal end of the radius expands notably near its articulation with the proximal row of carpal bones, terminating with a **radial styloid process** at its most

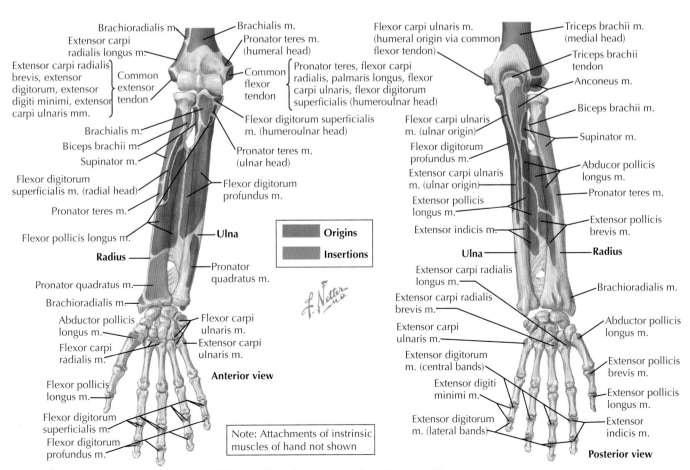

Fig. 10.4 Bony Attachments of the Muscles of Forearm.

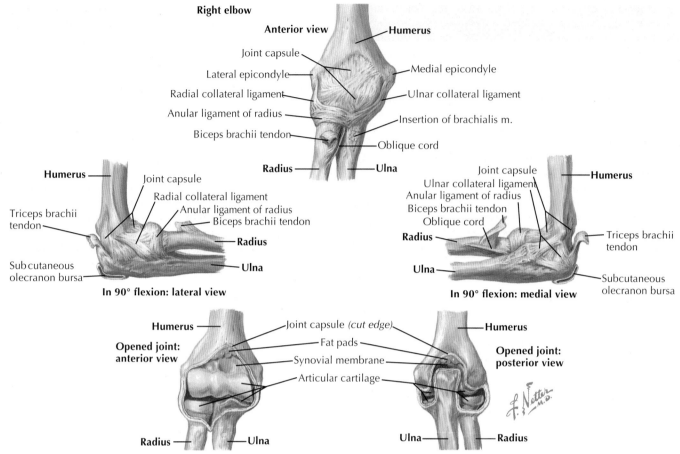

Fig. 10.5 Ligaments of the Elbow.

Carpal Bones (Fig. 10.6)

The **proximal row** of carpal bones from lateral to medial are the scaphoid, lunate, triquetrum, and pisiform bones.

- **Scaphoid**: this boat-shaped bone has a laterally directed scaphoid **tubercle** that is separated from the rest of the bone by a narrow **waist**. The scaphoid has large articular surfaces for the radius and capitate and smaller articular surfaces for the trapezium, trapezoid, and lunate (Clinical Correlation 10.8).
- **Lunate**: half-moon (crescent) shaped; it articulates with the radius, scaphoid, triquetrum, capitate, and hamate.
- **Triquetrum**: has three articular surfaces for the lunate, hamate, and pisiform.

- **Pisiform**: the smallest carpal bone, it articulates exclusively with the triquetrum. The pisiform is a distinct attachment point for the flexor carpi ulnaris and some hypothenar muscles. It has a small **groove for the ulnar artery** on its lateral aspect.

The **distal row** of carpal bones is formed by the trapezium, trapezoid, capitate, and hamate bones.

- **Trapezium**: has a **tubercle** on its medial palmar aspect and a nearby groove for the tendon of the flexor carpi radialis tendon. It has articular surfaces for the scaphoid and trapezoid, as well as a large saddle-shaped articular surface for the 1st metacarpal, while the 2nd metacarpal has a very small articulation medially.
- **Trapezoid**: a wedge-shaped bone with large articular surfaces for the trapezium, capitate, and 2nd metacarpal and a tiny surface for the scaphoid.
- **Capitate**: the largest carpal bone is centrally located in the wrist. Its large convex articular surface faces proximally and articulates with the scaphoid and lunate. Its lateral and medial aspects articulate with the trapezoid and hamate. The flattened, distal end articulates with the 2nd, 3rd, and (inconstantly) 4th metacarpals.
- **Hamate**: distinguished by the elongated **hook (hamulus) of the hamate** on its palmar side. It articulates with the capitate, triquetrum, and with the 4th and 5th metacarpals via an expansive distal end.

CLINICAL CORRELATION 10.7 Fracture of the Forearm

Because of their connection with the interosseous membrane, the radius and ulna often fracture together when they are traumatized. When a person falls and stops their descent by reaching out the arm, the distal radius can break, causing a **Colles fracture**. This is characterized by a "dinner fork deformity" as the distal fragment displaces posteriorly.

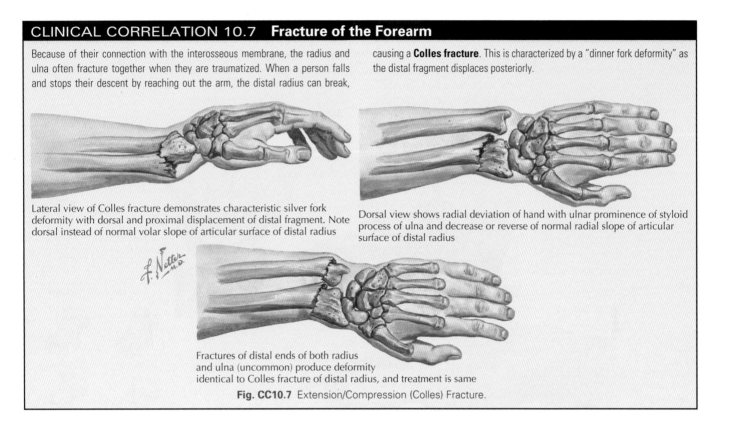

Lateral view of Colles fracture demonstrates characteristic silver fork deformity with dorsal and proximal displacement of distal fragment. Note dorsal instead of normal volar slope of articular surface of distal radius

Dorsal view shows radial deviation of hand with ulnar prominence of styloid process of ulna and decrease or reverse of normal radial slope of articular surface of distal radius

Fractures of distal ends of both radius and ulna (uncommon) produce deformity identical to Colles fracture of distal radius, and treatment is same

Fig. CC10.7 Extension/Compression (Colles) Fracture.

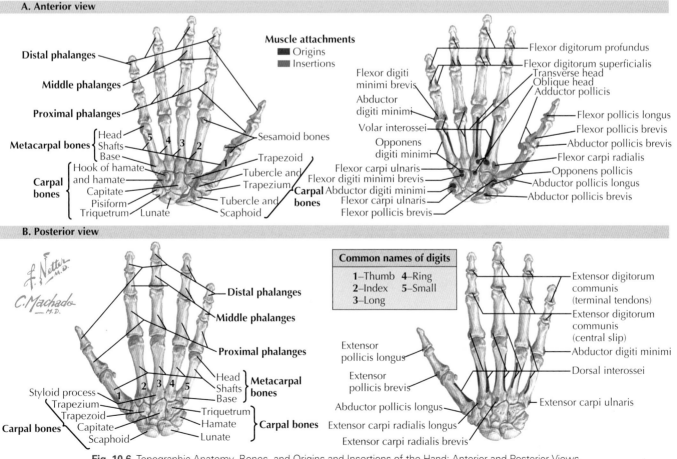

A. Anterior view

Distal phalanges

Middle phalanges

Proximal phalanges

Metacarpal bones { Head, Shafts, Base }

Carpal bones { Hook of hamate and hamate, Capitate, Pisiform, Triquetrum }

Lunate

Muscle attachments
■ Origins
▨ Insertions

Sesamoid bones

Trapezoid

Tubercle and Trapezium

Tubercle and Scaphoid

Flexor digitorum profundus
Flexor digitorum superficialis
Transverse head
Oblique head — Adductor pollicis
Flexor digiti minimi brevis
Abductor digiti minimi
Volar interossei
Opponens digiti minimi
Flexor carpi ulnaris
Flexor digiti minimi brevis
Abductor digiti minimi
Flexor carpi ulnaris
Flexor pollicis brevis

Flexor pollicis longus
Flexor pollicis brevis
Abductor pollicis brevis
Flexor carpi radialis
Opponens pollicis
Abductor pollicis longus
Abductor pollicis brevis

Carpal bones

B. Posterior view

Distal phalanges

Middle phalanges

Proximal phalanges

{ Head, Shafts, Base } **Metacarpal bones**

Styloid process
Trapezium
Trapezoid
Capitate
Scaphoid

Carpal bones

Triquetrum
Hamate
Lunate

Carpal bones

Common names of digits	
1–Thumb	4–Ring
2–Index	5–Small
3–Long	

Extensor digitorum communis (terminal tendons)
Extensor digitorum communis (central slip)
Abductor digiti minimi
Dorsal interossei
Extensor carpi ulnaris

Extensor pollicis longus
Extensor pollicis brevis
Abductor pollicis longus
Extensor carpi radialis longus
Extensor carpi radialis brevis

Fig. 10.6 Topographic Anatomy, Bones, and Origins and Insertions of the Hand: Anterior and Posterior Views.

CLINICAL CORRELATION 10.8   *Avascular Necrosis of the Scaphoid*

The scaphoid can be injured when a person falls and reaches their hand outward to stop their descent. Sudden pressure on the wrist can cause a fracture of the scaphoid, most commonly at the narrow waist. Since the blood supply to the scaphoid enters the bone distally from a branch of the radial artery, the proximal segment of the fractured bone may become deprived of blood, causing

avascular necrosis and wrist pain. As we have seen, falling onto an outstretched limb puts a great deal of stress on the bones of the upper limb and can cause a fracture in a variety of places: the scaphoid, distal radius, or clavicle, or wherever the "weak link" happens to be.

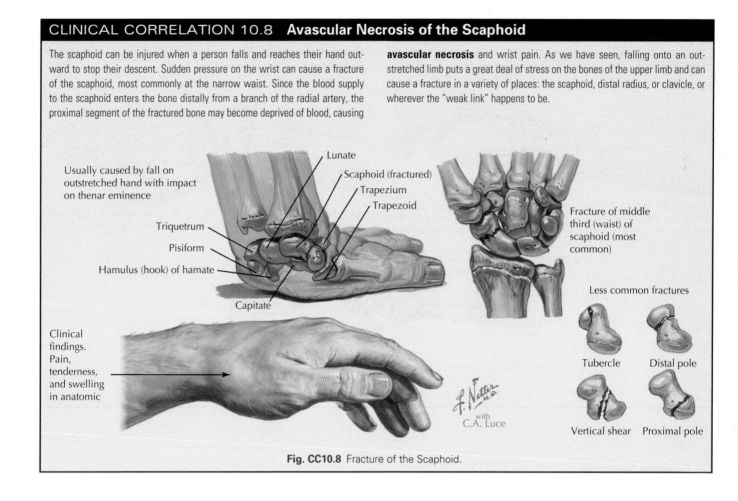

Fig. CC10.8 Fracture of the Scaphoid.

Metacarpal Bones (See Fig. 10.6)

The hand itself has five long **metacarpal bones** at its core. The **base** of each metacarpal bone associates with one or more distal carpal bones and projects forward as a long **body/shaft**. At the end of the body, the **head** of each metacarpal has a bulbous convexity that articulates with their corresponding phalanges. The **interosseous metacarpal spaces** between adjacent metacarpals is where the dorsal and palmar interosseous muscles originate. The head of the 1st metacarpal is associated with two small **sesamoid bones** that sit within the adductor pollicis and flexor pollicis brevis muscles near the metacarpophalangeal (MCP) joint. Another sesamoid bone may be found near the 2nd MCP joint.

- **1st metacarpal**: has a saddle-shaped articulation with the trapezium.
- **2nd metacarpal**: has a very deep concavity at its base where it articulates with the trapezium, trapezoid, capitate, and the base of the 3rd metacarpal.
- **3rd metacarpal**: has a **styloid process** projecting laterally from the dorsal base of the bone. It articulates with the capitate as well as the bases of the neighboring metacarpals.
- **4th metacarpal**: articulates with the hamate as well as the bases of the neighboring metacarpals.
- **5th metacarpal**: articulates with the hamate as well as the base of the 4th metacarpal.

Wrist Joint (Figs. 10.7 and 10.8)

Like the elbow, the **wrist** is a joint that is formed from multiple articulations. Many, many articulations. The distal radius and ulna interact with the proximal row of carpal bones and every carpal bone has an articulation with each of its neighbors.

The **distal radioulnar joint** is formed by the head of the ulna, the ulnar notch of the radius, and the **articular disc** of the wrist; it allows pronation and supination to occur. This articulation is stabilized by **dorsal and palmar radioulnar ligaments**. The radius rotates around the head of the ulna, with the styloid process of the ulna serving as the axis of rotation. The articular disc forms a fibrocartilage cap over the head of the ulna and creates an articular surface that is continuous with the carpal articular surface of the radius; this continuous articular surface is concave and forms the proximal side of the **radiocarpal joint**. The scaphoid, lunate, and triquetrum form the joint's distal, convex surface. The pisiform does not contribute to the radiocarpal joint but articulates with the triquetrum and is anchored in place by the **pisohamate** and **pisometacarpal ligaments**. The radiocarpal joint has a great degree of freedom since the bones that form it are concave/convex in two planes, allowing the wrist to flex and extend (better at flexion) as well as to abduct and adduct, which is referred to as radial deviation and ulnar deviation (better at ulnar deviation).

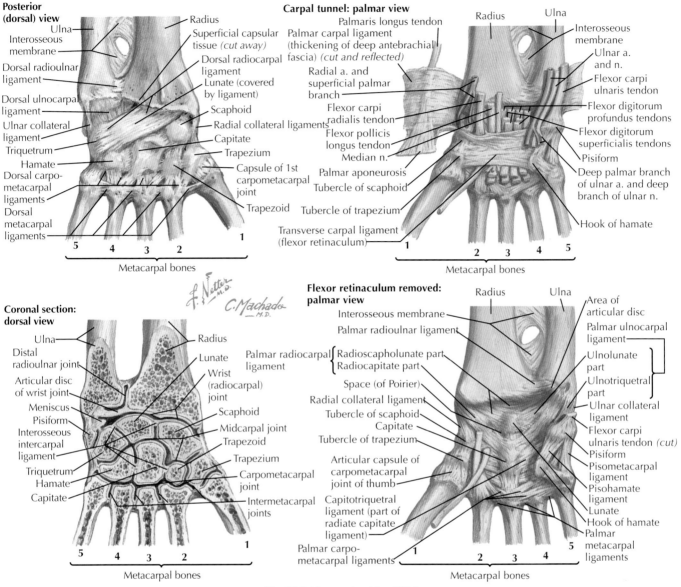

Posterior (dorsal) view

Ulna
Interosseous membrane
Dorsal radioulnar ligament
Dorsal ulnocarpal ligament
Ulnar collateral ligament
Triquetrum
Hamate
Dorsal carpo-metacarpal ligaments
Dorsal metacarpal ligaments

Radius
Superficial capsular tissue *(cut away)*
Dorsal radiocarpal ligament
Lunate (covered by ligament)
Scaphoid
Radial collateral ligaments
Capitate
Trapezium
Capsule of 1st carpometacarpal joint
Trapezoid

5 4 3 2 1
Metacarpal bones

Carpal tunnel: palmar view

Palmaris longus tendon
Palmar carpal ligament (thickening of deep antebrachial fascia) *(cut and reflected)*
Radial a. and superficial palmar branch
Flexor carpi radialis tendon
Flexor pollicis longus tendon
Median n.
Palmar aponeurosis
Tubercle of scaphoid
Tubercle of trapezium
Transverse carpal ligament (flexor retinaculum)

Radius
Ulna
Interosseous membrane
Ulnar a. and n.
Flexor carpi ulnaris tendon
Flexor digitorum profundus tendons
Flexor digitorum superficialis tendons
Pisiform
Deep palmar branch of ulnar a. and deep branch of ulnar n.
Hook of hamate

1 2 3 4 5
Metacarpal bones

Coronal section: dorsal view

Ulna
Distal radioulnar joint
Articular disc of wrist joint
Meniscus
Pisiform
Interosseous intercarpal ligament
Triquetrum
Hamate
Capitate

Radius
Lunate
Wrist (radiocarpal) joint
Scaphoid
Midcarpal joint
Trapezoid
Trapezium
Carpometacarpal joint
Intermetacarpal joints

5 4 3 2 1
Metacarpal bones

Flexor retinaculum removed: palmar view

Interosseous membrane
Palmar radioulnar ligament
Palmar radiocarpal ligament { Radioscapholunate part
Radiocapitate part
Space (of Poirier)
Radial collateral ligament
Tubercle of scaphoid
Capitate
Tubercle of trapezium
Articular capsule of carpometacarpal joint of thumb
Capitotriquetral ligament (part of radiate capitate ligament)
Palmar carpo-metacarpal ligaments

Radius
Ulna
Area of articular disc
Palmar ulnocarpal ligament
Ulnolunate part
Ulnotriquetral part
Ulnar collateral ligament
Flexor carpi ulnaris tendon *(cut)*
Pisiform
Pisometacarpal ligament
Pisohamate ligament
Lunate
Hook of hamate
Palmar metacarpal ligaments

1 2 3 4 5
Metacarpal bones

Fig. 10.7 Ligaments of the Wrist.

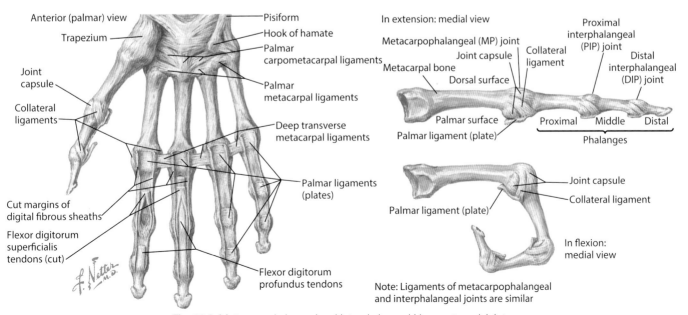

Anterior (palmar) view

Trapezium
Joint capsule
Collateral ligaments
Cut margins of digital fibrous sheaths
Flexor digitorum superficialis tendons (cut)

Pisiform
Hook of hamate
Palmar carpometacarpal ligaments
Palmar metacarpal ligaments
Deep transverse metacarpal ligaments
Palmar ligaments (plates)
Flexor digitorum profundus tendons

In extension: medial view

Metacarpophalangeal (MP) joint
Joint capsule
Metacarpal bone
Dorsal surface
Palmar surface
Palmar ligament (plate)

Collateral ligament
Proximal interphalangeal (PIP) joint
Distal interphalangeal (DIP) joint
Proximal   Middle   Distal
Phalanges

Joint capsule
Collateral ligament
Palmar ligament (plate)

In flexion: medial view

Note: Ligaments of metacarpophalangeal and interphalangeal joints are similar

Fig. 10.8 Metacarpophalangeal and Interphalangeal Ligaments and Joints.

The **midcarpal joint** is the collection of articulations of the proximal carpal row with the distal row of carpal bones. Its complex articular surface allows a slight degree of flexion/extension (better at extension) and ulnar/radial deviation (better at radial deviation).

For both the radiocarpal and midcarpal joint, flexion/extension is limited by muscle tension as well as ligaments on both sides of the wrist, the **dorsal radiocarpal, dorsal ulnocarpal, palmar radiocarpal, palmar ulnocarpal, dorsal intercarpal, and palmar intercarpal ligaments**. These can be subdivided by listing the exact carpal bone to which each ligament attaches. The intercarpal ligaments also define the synovial joint capsule for each articulation. Just in case this was not complex enough already, there are also **interosseous intercarpal ligaments** within the synovial joint capsules. Radial/ulnar deviation is significantly limited by collateral ligaments on each side. The **radial collateral ligament of the wrist** connects the radial styloid process to the scaphoid, trapezium, and first metacarpal while the **ulnar collateral ligament of the wrist** connects the ulnar styloid process to the triquetrum and pisiform.

The **carpometacarpal joints** are the articulations that exist between the distal row of carpal bones and the bases of metacarpals 1 to 5. There are also **intermetacarpal joints** between the bases of metacarpals 2 to 5. These articulations are stabilized by **dorsal carpometacarpal, palmar carpometacarpal, dorsal metacarpal, palmar metacarpal, and interosseous metacarpal ligaments**. The carpometacarpal joint of the thumb (1st digit) is often treated separately since it has several unique features. The 1st metacarpal only articulates with the trapezium via a saddle-shaped surface that allows flexion/extension and adduction/abduction. A combination of thumb abduction, flexion, and adduction at this joint creates a movement that brings the thumb in contact with the other digits, called opposition.

The bases of metacarpals 2 to 5 each articulate with the distal row of carpal bones and neighboring metacarpals. The carpometacarpal joints allow a small degree of flexion/extension (biased toward flexion) so that objects can be "cupped" in the palm. As a whole, the carpal and metacarpal bones are concave on the palmar side. This concavity is reinforced by the **flexor retinaculum**, a very strong band of connective tissue that connects the trapezium to the pisiform and hamate bones. This forms a "roof" over a space on the palmar wrist called the **carpal tunnel**. The floor of the carpal tunnel is a collection of palmar intercarpal ligaments fanning out from the capitate bone that are referred to as the **radiate carpal ligament**. Abduction of the heads of metacarpals 2 to 5 is prevented by the **deep transverse metacarpal ligament**, which connects the head of each metacarpal to its neighbor.

Phalanges (See Figs. 10.6 and 10.7)

The thumb or **pollux** (1st digit) has two segments, formed by a **proximal phalanx** and **distal phalanx**. The fingers (2nd to 5th digits) have three segments, a **proximal**, **middle**, and **distal phalanx**. Each phalanx appears like a shrunken metacarpal, with a proximal **base**, **shaft/body**, and distal **head**. The distal phalanges have flared-out **tuberosities** just proximal to their heads.

On the palmar side, the flexor pollicis brevis and flexor pollicis longus tendons insert on the base of the proximal and distal phalanx of the 1st digit. Similarly, the flexor digitorum superficialis and profundus tendons insert on the bases of the middle and distal phalanges of the 2nd to 5th digits. On the dorsal side, the extensor pollicis brevis and extensor pollicis longus tendons insert on the base of the proximal and distal phalanx of the 1st digit. The extensor digitorum muscle has tendinous bands that insert on the bases of the middle and distal phalanges of digits 2 to 5; the extensor indicis tendon inserts on the bases of the middle and distal phalanges of digit 2, the index finger.

Joints of the Digits (See Fig. 10.8)

Digits 2 to 5 each have metacarpophalangeal (MCP) proximal interphalangeal (PIP), and distal interphalangeal (DIP) joints that allow the fingers to move. The 1st digit (thumb/pollux) has an MCP joint but only one interphalangeal joint since it has no middle phalanx. At the **MCP joints**, the head of each metacarpal is rounded and fits into a concave (sometimes saddle-shaped) depression at the base of each proximal phalanx that allow the digits to flex/extend and abduct/adduct. There are stout **medial collateral** and **lateral collateral ligaments** on each side of the MCP that are tense in flexion and loose in extension. This makes adduction/abduction of the digits possible when the MCP is extended but not when flexed. Lastly, there are **palmar ligaments** (palmar plates) that stabilize the palmar side of the MCP. They limit extension of the MCP and also connect to the deep transverse metacarpal ligament.

The PIP and DIP **joints** are very similar to the MCP, with **medial collateral**, **lateral collateral**, and **palmar ligaments** limiting abduction, adduction, and extension. The heads of the proximal and middle phalanges are convex but with a central depression that forms a track that allows the interphalangeal joints to flex/extend but prevents abduction/adduction. To further stabilize the digits, the collateral ligaments of the PIP and DIP are tight in both flexion and extension, so no abduction or adduction is possible at those joints unless the result of trauma.

MUSCLE GROUPS OF THE UPPER LIMB

It might be useful to review the section on the upper limb in Chapter 3 or Table 10.1 before moving into the detailed anatomy of the muscles in the upper limbs.

Upper Limb Muscles Originating from the Back

The extrinsic muscles of the back are located in the back but have their major effect on the upper limb. The **latissimus dorsi, trapezius, rhomboid major, rhomboid minor, levator scapulae muscles** were discussed in Chapter 9, so we will only revisit them in these tables.

TABLE 10.1   Muscle Groups of the Upper Limb

Muscle Region	Major Function(s)	Source of Innervation
Inferior back	Adduction and extension of arm at shoulder	Thoracodorsal nerve
Superior back	Elevation, retraction, depression of scapula	Spinal accessory nerve (CN XI)
Lateral chest wall	Protraction of scapula	Long thoracic nerve
Anterior chest wall	Flexion and adduction of arm at shoulder	Medial and lateral pectoral nerves
Shoulder	Abduction, adduction, flexion, extension, rotation of arm at shoulder	Axillary, subscapular, suprascapular nerves
Anterior arm	Flexion of forearm at elbow	Musculoskeletal nerve
Posterior arm	Extension of forearm at elbow	Radial nerve
Posterior forearm	Extension of wrist, extension of digits, supination	Radial nerve
Anterior forearm	Flexion of wrist, flexion of digits, pronation	Median and ulnar nerves
Palm of hand	Flexion, adduction of digits, extension of phalanges	Median and ulnar nerves
Dorsum of hand	Abduction of digits	Ulnar nerve

Latissimus Dorsi

Proximal attachments	• Iliac crest
	• Superficial lamina of posterior layer of thoracolumbar facia (T7 to sacrum)
Distal attachment	• Intertubercular sulcus of proximal humerus
Functions	• Extension of shoulder from a flexed position
	• Adduction of shoulder from an abducted position
	• Medial rotation of arm
Muscle testing and signs of damage	• With the arms abducted at the shoulder, ask the patient to adduct them against resistance, assess any asymmetry in strength.
	• With the arms flexed at the shoulder, ask the patient to extend them against resistance, assess any asymmetry in strength.
Innervation	• Thoracodorsal nerve (C6–C8)
Blood supply	• Primarily thoracodorsal vessels

Trapezius

Proximal attachments	• Superior fibers: Medial part of superior nuchal line and external occipital protuberance, nuchal ligament
	• Middle fibers: nuchal ligament, C7–T5 spinous processes
	• Inferior fibers: T6–T12 spinous processes
Distal attachment	• Spine of scapula
	• Acromion
	• Distal clavicle
Functions	• Superior fibers: elevate scapula and upper limb
	• Middle fibers: retract scapula
	• Inferior fibers: depress scapula
Muscle testing and signs of damage	• Ask patient to elevate shoulders against resistance.
	• Weakness on one side may indicate dysfunction of the trapezius or Cranial Nerve XI
Innervation	• CN XI—Spinal accessory nerve
Blood supply	• Primarily branches of external carotid artery and thyrocervical trunk (transverse cervical and dorsal scapular vessels)

CLINICAL CORRELATION 10.9   Triangle of Auscultation

On the superior back is an area that is covered by less musculature than the surroundings. This triangle of auscultation is formed by the lateral border of the trapezius, superior border of the latissimus dorsi, and medial border of the scapula. The space can be expanded by having the patient adduct their arms across the front of the body (i.e., "Give yourself a hug.") while flexing the torso. This triangle has been considered a desirable place to listen to (auscultate) the lungs but modern stethoscopes have made it less relevant; this anatomical landmark lives on primarily in exam questions.

Levator Scapulae

See Clinical Correlation 10.9.

Proximal attachments	• C1 transverse process
	• C2–C4 posterior tubercles of the transverse processes
Distal attachment	• Superior angle of scapula
Functions	• Elevate scapula
	• Inferior rotation of scapula and glenoid fossa
Muscle testing and signs of damage	• Ask patient to elevate their shoulders bilaterally and watch for asymmetry
	• Weakness on one side may indicate weakness of the levator scapulae muscles, but the activity of the superior fibers of the trapezius may mask this weakness
Innervation	• Dorsal scapular nerve
Blood supply	• Primarily dorsal scapular vessels

Rhomboid Minor and Major

Proximal attachments	• Minor: Inferior nuchal ligament, C7 and T1 spinous processes • Major: T2–T5 spinous processes
Distal attachment	• Minor: Medial border of scapula superior to and at the level of the spine of the scapula • Major: Medial border of scapula from level of the spine of the scapula near the inferior angle
Functions	• Retraction of scapula • Inferior rotation of scapula and glenoid fossa
Muscle testing and signs of damage	• Ask patient to retract their shoulders bilaterally and watch for asymmetry • Weakness on one side may indicate weakness of the rhomboid muscles, but the activity of the middle fibers of the trapezius may mask this weakness
Innervation	• Dorsal scapular nerve
Blood supply	• Primarily dorsal scapular vessels

Upper Limb Muscles Originating From the Lateral Chest Wall

The **serratus anterior muscle** (Fig. 10.9) originates from the lateral thorax as distinct muscular slips that fuse as they travel posteriorly, wrapping around the body wall and inserting on the medial scapula. In slender, muscular individuals this muscle has a saw-tooth (serrated) appearance just inferior and lateral to the pectoralis major. Uniform contraction of the multiple slips of this muscle cause protraction of the scapula, which brings it closer to the thorax so that movements of the torso are translated to the arm and vice-versa. If this did not occur, every time a person would push something away with their arm, the scapula would bulge posteriorly. Contraction of the lower slips of the serratus anterior will rotate the glenoid fossa superiorly so that the arm can be raised past 90 degrees of abduction. It is innervated by the long thoracic nerve, which descends along the lateral surface of the muscle alongside its major source of blood, the lateral thoracic artery. Other nearby vessels like the thoracodorsal and intercostal arteries also supply some blood to the serratus anterior muscle.

Serratus Anterior

Proximal attachments	• Lateral aspects of ribs 1–8
Distal attachment	• Anterior aspect of medial border of the scapula, immediately medial to the subscapularis muscle
Functions	• Protraction of the scapula, fixing it to the thorax • Contraction of the lower slips will rotate the glenoid fossa superiorly so that the arm can be raised past 90 degrees of abduction
Muscle testing and signs of damage	• Weakness of serratus anterior results in a "winged scapula" that does not protract toward the body wall but gets pushed posteriorly as force is applied along the arm. Have a patient lean forward with palms against a wall. As he or she pushes away, a winged scapula will bulge outward away from the thorax. Fit patients can be asked to do a push up while the observer watches for a winged scapula. There will also be weakness abducting the upper limb superior to the horizontal plane
Innervation	• Long thoracic nerve (C5–C7)
Blood supply	• Lateral thoracic artery, thoracodorsal artery, and/or intercostal arteries

Upper Limb Muscles Originating From the Anterior Chest Wall (See Fig. 10.9)

The broad **pectoralis major muscle** originates from the inferior clavicle, sternum, costal cartilages, and ribs before focusing its contraction onto the intertubercular sulcus of the humerus. It is covered on its anterior and posterior surfaces by a distinct **pectoral fascia**. This fascia allows it to be separated from the underlying **pectoralis minor muscle** that stretches from the anterior ribs 3 to 5 to the coracoid process. The pectoralis minor is contained within **clavipectoral fascia** that stretches from the clavicle and subclavius muscle, around the pectoralis minor, and fuses with the fascia of the axilla. The pectoralis major is a very strong adductor and flexor of the arm at the shoulder. The popular bench press exercise is directed at this muscle. Since its tendon wraps around the anterior shaft of the humerus, it also medially/internally rotates the arm. The pectoralis minor helps to fix the scapula to the body wall by pulling anteriorly and inferiorly on the coracoid process. These muscles are innervated by the medial and lateral pectoral nerves and receive blood from many nearby arteries.

In contrast to the massive pectoralis major is the small subclavius muscle. In humans this muscle has minimal functional importance since it cannot maneuver the clavicle through much of a range of motion but acts as a stabilizer. It is very useful during fractures of the clavicle since it prevents displacement of the fragments due to its insertion along the inferior shaft of the bone.

One anomalous muscle that can sometimes be found in the anterior chest is the **sternalis muscle**. This odd muscle is unusual (~3% to 5%) and extends along the lateral border of the sternum between the xiphoid process and the medial clavicle and sternocleidomastoid muscle.

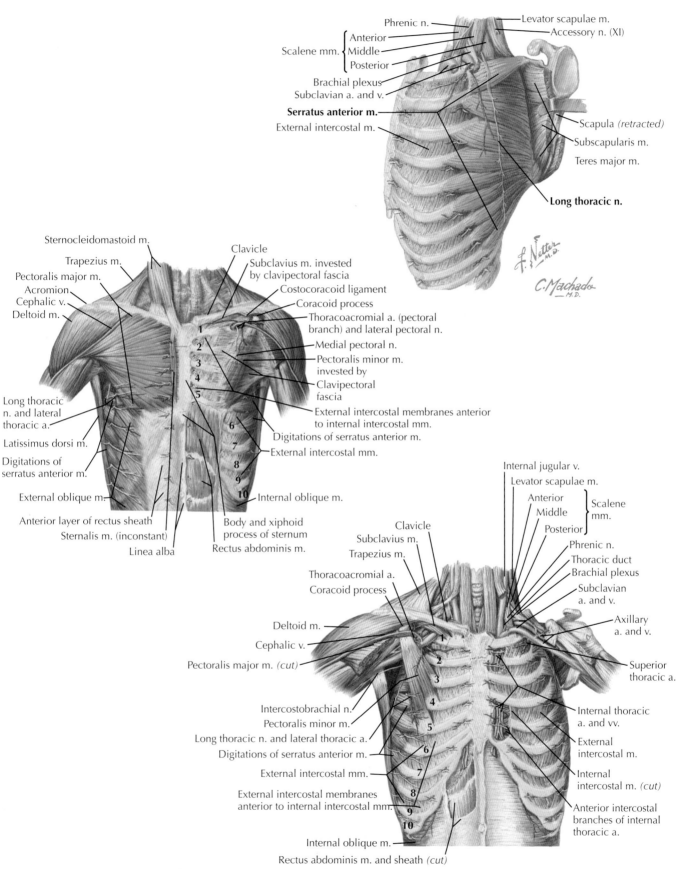

Fig. 10.9 Upper Limb Muscles Originating from the Lateral Chest Wall.

Pectoralis Major and Minor

Proximal attachments	• Major:
	  • Clavicular head: medial aspect of the anterior clavicle
	  • Sternocostal head: anterior sternum and costal cartilages 1–6
	  • Abdominal head: a small area shared with the aponeurosis of the external abdominal oblique muscle
	  • Minor: anterior aspects of ribs 3–5

Distal attachment	• Major: lateral aspect of intertubercular sulcus and crest of the greater tubercle • Minor: medial aspect of the coracoid process of scapula
Functions	• Major: flexes and adducts the humerus at the shoulder. Also medially rotates the humerus • Minor: pulls the coracoid process and scapula anteriorly and inferiorly across the superior aspect of the thorax
Muscle testing and signs of damage	• Weakness of one pectoralis major muscle will result in asymmetric weakness in adduction and flexion of the arm at the shoulder. This may be masked by the activity of other muscles (latissimus dorsi and deltoid) that also effect these motions. Weakness of the clavicular head (lateral pectoral nerve) will primarily affect shoulder flexion while weakness of the sternocostal and abdominal heads (medial pectoral nerve) will affect adduction • Isolated weakness of the pectoralis minor is difficult to diagnose due to the deep location of the muscle and its narrow range of motion
Innervation	• Major: clavicular head is innervated by the lateral pectoral nerve (C5–C7) while the sternocostal and abdominal heads are innervated by the medial pectoral nerve (C8–T1) • Minor: medial pectoral nerve (C8–T1)
Blood supply	• Pectoral branch of thoracoacromial trunk, lateral thoracic, internal thoracic, anterior intercostal arteries

Subclavius

Proximal attachments	• Superior aspect of the first costal cartilage and adjacent first rib
Distal attachment	• Inferior aspect of the middle portion of the shaft of the clavicle
Functions	• Slight depression of clavicle • Stabilization of the sternoclavicular joint • The subclavius may prevent jagged ends of a recently fractured clavicle from displacing and lacerating subclavian vessels and the brachial plexus.
Muscle testing and signs of damage	• Spasm of the subclavius may depress the clavicle and compress the subclavian vessels and brachial plexus • Venous catheters may be pinched by the muscle if they are inserted through its tissues during a lateral approach to the subclavian vein
Innervation	• Nerve to subclavius (C5–C6)
Blood supply	• Branches of thoracoacromial trunk, possibly superior thoracic artery

Muscles of the Shoulder

The most prominent muscle of the shoulder is the **deltoid** (see Fig. 10.8), which is covered by investing **deltoid fascia** and innervated by the axillary nerve. This muscle has anterior, middle, and posterior heads that flex, abduct, and extend the shoulder, respectively. Since other muscles complement those motions, loss of deltoid activity does not obliterate movements of the arm at the shoulder but weakens them. Friction caused by the deltoid crossing the greater tubercle of the humerus is minimized by a **subdeltoid** or **subacromial bursa**, a connective tissue sac filled with synovial fluid that is present between the muscle and bone.

Deltoid

Proximal attachments	• Anterior head: distal clavicle • Middle head: acromion • Posterior head: spine of scapula
Distal attachment	• Deltoid tuberosity
Functions	• Anterior head: flex and medially rotate the arm at the shoulder • Middle head: abduct the arm at the shoulder from 15 to 90 degrees. Further abduction requires superior rotation of glenoid fossa by serratus anterior or trapezius muscles • Posterior head: extend and externally rotate the arm at the shoulder
Muscle testing and signs of damage	• Anterior head: weakness flexing the shoulder against resistance. Note that the pectoralis major and coracobrachialis also flex the arm at the shoulder and may mask deltoid weakness • Middle head: inability to maintain an arm at a 90-degree angle (sticking straight out to the side of the body) against resistance or gravity is indicative of dysfunction of the middle head of the deltoid • Posterior head: asymmetric weakness extending the shoulder against resistance. Note that latissimus dorsi muscle also extends the arm and may mask deltoid weakness • In cases of de-innervation, atrophy of the deltoid is often visually apparent due to the muscle's prominence on the shoulder
Innervation	• Anterior head: lateral pectoral nerve (C5–C7) and axillary nerve (C5–C6) • Middle and posterior heads: axillary nerve (C5–C6)
Blood supply	• Deltoid branch of thoracoacromial trunk, anterior circumflex humeral, posterior circumflex humeral, and deep brachial arteries

Deep to the deltoid are muscles of the **rotator cuff: supraspinatus, infraspinatus, teres minor**, and **subscapularis** (Fig. 10.10, see also Fig. 10.9). These muscles originate from the scapula and form a cuff around the head of the humerus that keeps it in place. Individually they rotate or abduct the arm at the shoulder. The subdeltoid/subacromial bursa also minimizes friction between the supraspinatus and overlying acromion. A separate **subtendinous bursa of the subscapularis muscle**

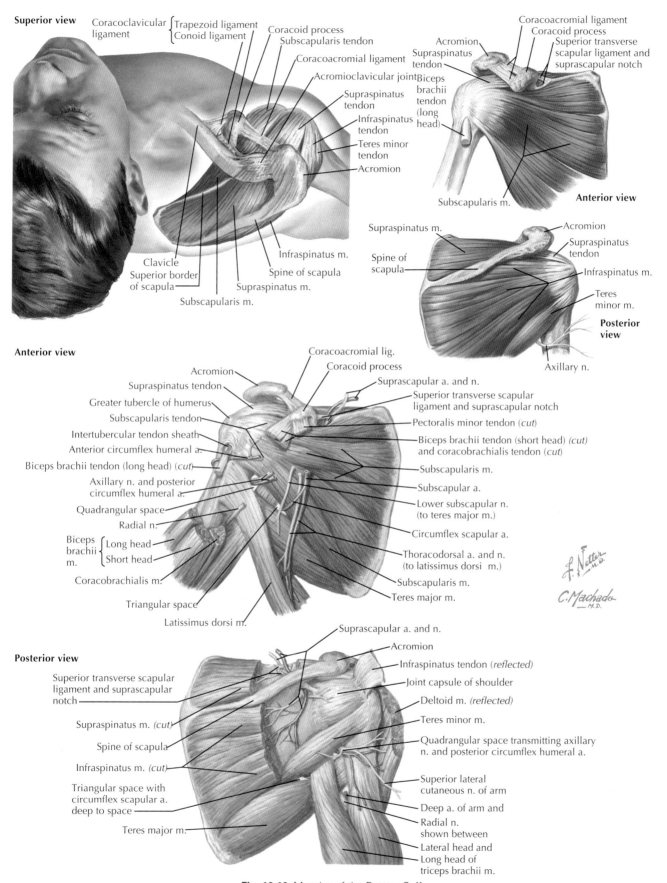

Fig. 10.10 Muscles of the Rotator Cuff.

minimizes friction between the muscle and the neck of the scapula and typically communicates directly with the glenohumeral joint space. The supraspinatus muscle has a distinct investing **supraspinous fascia**, but it is minimal when compared to the incredibly stout **infraspinous fascia**, which serves to stabilize the spine of the scapula and also provides an additional origin surface for the infraspinatus muscle. This infraspinous fascia often covers part of the teres minor muscle. The nearby **teres major** (see Fig. 10.10) is not part of the rotator cuff but acts in a similar way to the latissimus dorsi.

Rotator Cuff

Proximal attachments	• Anterior and posterior surfaces of the scapula
Distal attachment	• Greater and lesser tubercles of the humerus
Group functions	• Forms a muscular cuff around the head of the humerus that maintains its position in the glenoid fossa

Supraspinatus

See Clinical Correlation 10.10.

Proximal attachments	• Supraspinous fossa of scapula
Distal attachment	• Anterosuperior aspect of greater tubercle of the humerus
Functions	• Initiates abduction of the arm at the shoulder from 0 to 15 degrees. The deltoid continues abduction beyond that point
Muscle testing and signs of damage	• The supraspinatus muscle is the most frequently injured member of the rotator cuff. Weakness or paralysis of this muscle will result in an inability to initiate abduction of the arm from the side of the body or pain when carrying out the abduction. Be sure your patients do not sway sideways to get an assist from momentum
	• Since this muscle is so frequently injured, a wide array of special tests exists to assess its function
Innervation	• Suprascapular nerve (C5–C6)
Blood supply	• Suprascapular artery

CLINICAL CORRELATION 10.10 Calcific Tendonitis of the Shoulder

Overuse and inflammation of the supraspinatus tendon can result in deposition of calcium within it as it inserts on the greater tubercle of the humerus. This causes pain as the arm is abducted between 50 and 130 degrees since it places the inflamed tendon against the underside of the acromion. This can cascade into additional inflammation of the subacromial/subdeltoid bursa, tendon rupture, and adhesive capsulitis.

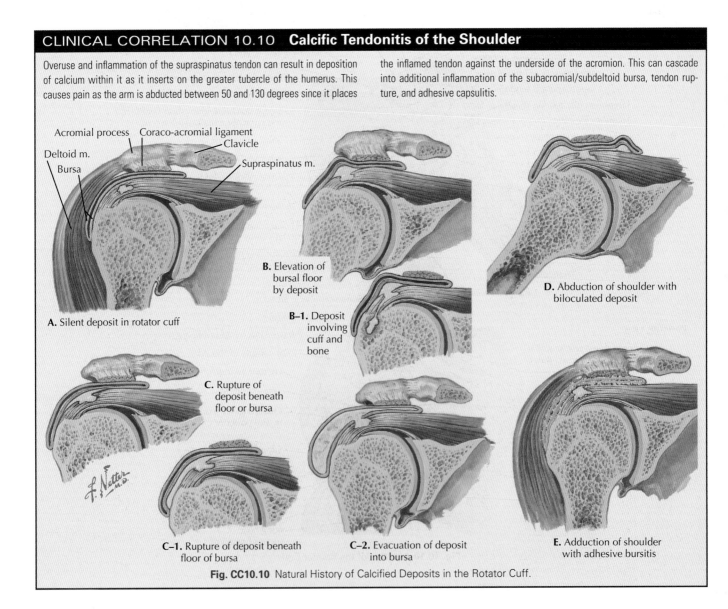

A. Silent deposit in rotator cuff

B. Elevation of bursal floor by deposit

B–1. Deposit involving cuff and bone

C. Rupture of deposit beneath floor or bursa

D. Abduction of shoulder with biloculated deposit

C–1. Rupture of deposit beneath floor of bursa

C–2. Evacuation of deposit into bursa

E. Adduction of shoulder with adhesive bursitis

Acromial process — Coraco-acromial ligament — Clavicle — Supraspinatus m.
Deltoid m. — Bursa

Fig. CC10.10 Natural History of Calcified Deposits in the Rotator Cuff.

Infraspinatus

Proximal attachments	• Infraspinous fossa of scapula
Distal attachment	• Posterosuperior aspect of greater tubercle of the humerus
Functions	• Externally rotates arm at the shoulder
Muscle testing and signs of damage	• Injury or de-innervation of the infraspinatus will manifest as an inability to externally rotate the humerus against resistance and/or as a persistently internally rotated humerus due to the unopposed action of the subscapularis.
Innervation	• Suprascapular nerve (C5–C6)
Blood supply	• Suprascapular, circumflex scapular, dorsal scapular arteries

Teres Minor

Proximal attachments	• Medial border of scapula immediately superior to teres major muscle
Distal attachment	• Posterior aspect of greater tubercle of the humerus
Functions	• Externally rotates arm at the shoulder
Muscle testing and signs of damage	• Injury or de-innervation of the teres minor muscle will manifest in the same ways as the infraspinatus muscle
Innervation	• Axillary nerve (C5–C6)
Blood supply	• Suprascapular and circumflex scapular arteries

Subscapularis

Proximal attachments	• Subscapular fossa on the anterior, costal surface of the scapula
Distal attachment	• Lesser tubercle of the humerus
Functions	• Internally rotates arm at the shoulder
Muscle testing and signs of damage	• Injury or de-innervation of the subscapularis will manifest as an inability to internally rotate the humerus against resistance and/or as a persistently externally rotated humerus due to the unopposed action of the infraspinatus and teres minor
Innervation	• Upper subscapular nerve (C5) • Lower subscapular nerve (C6)
Blood supply	• Subscapular, thoracodorsal, circumflex scapular arteries

Teres Major

See Clinical Correlations 10.11 and 10.12.

Proximal attachments	• Inferior angle and lateral border of scapula inferior to teres minor
Distal attachment	• Medial aspect of intertubercular sulcus and crest of the lesser tubercle
Functions	• Adduction of shoulder from an abducted position • Medial rotation of arm
Muscle testing and signs of damage	• With the arms abducted at the shoulder, ask the patient to adduct them against resistance, assess any asymmetry in strength
Innervation	• Lower subscapular nerve (C6)
Blood supply	• Suprascapular, circumflex scapular, dorsal scapular arteries

CLINICAL CORRELATION 10.11 **Injury of the Rotator Cuff Muscles**

The supraspinatus muscle is the most frequently damaged of the rotator cuff muscles since it is the smallest and it passes through a tight tunnel of bone formed by the spine of the scapula, acromion, and distal clavicle. Repetitive motions, sudden stretching, and degenerative tendonitis can cause weakness and pain in any of the rotator cuff muscles. This is the basis for many of the clinical tests of rotator cuff motion.

Muscles of the Anterior Arm (Fig. 10.11)

The three muscles of the **anterior compartment of the arm** have investing fascia around each individual muscle but are also contained in a stout sleeve of **brachial fascia** that defines the compartment. This fascia fuses to the humerus on each side, forming the **lateral and medial intermuscular septae**, which separates the anterior arm from the posterior arm. The individual muscles in this region, the **coracobrachialis**, **biceps brachii**, and **brachialis** each have unique features but as a group they flex the forearm at the elbow and are innervated by the musculocutaneous nerve. The coracobrachialis and short head of the biceps brachii both originate from the tip of the coracoid process of the scapula and may be fused in that region before separating to attach to the humerus or joining the long head of the biceps. The musculocutaneous nerve typically pierces the medial aspect of the coracobrachialis before running in a plane between the biceps brachii and brachialis before proceeding laterally to become the lateral cutaneous nerve of the forearm.

The long head of the biceps brachii originates within the glenohumeral joint just above the glenoid cavity. The tendon travels through the synovial space, exits the anterior aspect of the capsule, runs deep to the transverse humeral ligament within the intertubercular sulcus, and finally joins the short head of the biceps brachii. Distally it has two insertions, a well-defined tendinous insertion on the radial tuberosity and a flimsier (but still functional) insertion into the fascia of the anterior forearm. A **bicipitoradial bursa** is present between the distal biceps tendon and the radial tuberosity, preventing irritation as the muscle approaches its attachment site.

The brachialis is the deepest of the muscles and runs immediately anterior to the capsule of the elbow joint. Some of its fibers insert onto the fibrous layer of the capsule so that it does not get pinched and compressed during flexion of the elbow. It is always involved in elbow flexion, but this action is supplemented by other muscles like the biceps brachii and brachioradialis.

CLINICAL CORRELATION 10.12　Special Tests for the Rotator Cuff Muscles

There are many specialized tests for muscle function and stability. Here are a few of the more common physical examination techniques related to the rotator cuff. Note that the arm is considered to be at 0 degrees when it is laying alongside the body with the fingers pointing to the ground.

Supraspinatus Muscle

- **Drop Arm Test:** start with the arm abducted to 180 degrees overhead. The patient is asked to slowly lower her/his arm to the side. Pain or uncontrolled dropping of the arm is considered to be a positive test. If the arm suddenly drops between 180 and 90 degrees, the serratus anterior and trapezius muscles may be damaged. If it drops between 90 and 15 degrees, the deltoid may be dysfunctional. If it descends in a controlled way to ~15 degrees and then drops, the supraspinatus muscle is likely damaged or painful.
- **Hawkins Kennedy Test:** the arm is flexed at 90 degrees at the shoulder with the elbow bent at 90 degrees. The arm is slowly internally rotated, pain is considered a positive test. This can be due to supraspinatus dysfunction, labral tears, or acromioclavicular damage.
- **Empty Can (Jobe's) Test:** the patient begins the exam with arms flexed anteriorly at the shoulder with the forearms over-pronated (thumbs down). The evaluator places gentle pressure on the distal forearms to push them inferiorly. Pain or an inability to push symmetrically against resistance is a positive test.
- **Full Can (Jobe's) Test:** the patient begins the exam with arms flexed anteriorly at the shoulder with the forearms in the thumbs up position. The evaluator places gentle pressure on the distal forearms to push them inferiorly. Pain or an inability to push symmetrically against resistance is a positive test.
- **Neer's Test:** the examiner will stabilize the scapula with one arm and internally rotate the arm with support at the elbow. The arm is elevated into flexion and lifted over the head, compressing the structures in the subacromial space. Pain anteriorly is associated with subacromial/subdeltoid bursitis while deeper pain is associated with supraspinatus dysfunction.

Infraspinatus and Teres Minor Muscles

- **External rotation lag sign in neutral:** the patient starts with the arm slightly abducted at roughly 20 degrees and the elbow flexed at 90 degrees. The examiner gently externally rotates the arm to its non-painful limit and helps to maintain it in that position with support at the elbow and wrist. The examiner asks the patient to maintain that externally rotated position as the support at the wrist is withdrawn. If the arm recoils into internal rotation and drops, damage to the infraspinatus or supraspinatus is likely.
- **External rotation lag sign in abduction:** the patient has her/his arm abducted to 90 degrees with the elbow flexed at 90 degrees and the palm forward (i.e., "High Five!") while the examiner supports the elbow and wrist in external rotation. The examiner asks the patient to maintain that position as the support is withdrawn from the wrist. If the arm rotates internally (palm downward) then the infraspinatus or teres minor muscles are likely to be damaged.
- **Hornblower sign:** the patient begins with the arms abducted and the elbows flexed (i.e., elbows sticking out to the side) and the hands together at the mouth with the examiner supporting the elbows. The patient is asked to maintain this position as the support is withdrawn. If the infraspinatus and/or teres minor are damaged, the patient will be unable to stop the affected elbow from dropping down, as though he or she is blowing a horn.

Subscapularis Muscle

- **Lift-off test:** the patient places (with or without assistance) the dorsum of the hand against the lower back. The patient is asked to lift the hand away from the back, testing internal rotation and the subscapularis muscle. The test is positive if the motion cannot be performed or is painful.
- **Bear hug test:** the patient is positioned with the palm of the hand resting on the opposite shoulder with the fingers extended or in a fist. The examiner attempts to lift the hand off the shoulder (upward) and the patient is told to resist. The test is positive if there is pain, the patient cannot resist the elevation of the hand, or there is gross asymmetry on one side compared to the other.

Coracobrachialis

Proximal attachments	• Anterior tip of coracoid process of scapula
Distal attachment	• Medial aspect of the middle shaft of the humerus
Functions	• Flex arm at the shoulder • Adduct arm at the shoulder • Prevents inferior displacement of the head of the humerus
Muscle testing and signs of damage	• Weakness in flexing and adduction of the shoulder might result from selective damage to the coracobrachialis muscle, but since other, larger muscles also contribute to these motions it may not be discernable.
Innervation	• Musculocutaneous nerve (C5–C7)
Blood supply	• Branches of axillary and brachial arteries

Biceps Brachii

See Clinical Correlation 10.13.

Proximal attachments	• Short head: anterior tip of coracoid process of scapula • Long head: supraglenoid tubercle of scapula
Distal attachment	• The strong biceps tendon inserts on the radial tuberosity • The bicipital aponeurosis fans out to fuse with the anteromedial aspect of the antebrachial fascia
Functions	• Strongly supinates a flexed forearm • Once the forearm is flexed, the biceps brachii supinates the forearm at the elbow • Like the coracobrachialis, the short head also prevents inferior displacement of the head of the humerus
Muscle testing and signs of damage	• Weakness in flexing a supinated forearm against resistance is a sign of biceps weakness.
Innervation	• Musculocutaneous nerve (C5–C7)
Blood supply	• Branches of axillary and brachial arteries

Superficial layer

Coracoacromial ligament
Subdeltoid bursa
Greater tubercle,
Lesser tubercle
of humerus
Intertubercular
tendon sheath
Deltoid m.
(reflected)
Pectoralis major
m. (reflected)
Anterior circumflex
humeral a.
Biceps {Long head
brachii m. Short head
Brachial a. (cut)
Median n. (cut)
Brachialis m.
Lateral antebrachial
cutaneous n.
Bicipital aponeurosis
Biceps brachii tendon
Brachioradialis m.
Pronator teres m.
Flexor carpi radialis m.

Acromion
Coracoid process
Pectoralis minor tendon (cut)
Subscapularis m.
Musculocutaneous n. (cut)
Coracobrachialis m.
Circumflex scapular a. (cut)
Teres major m.
Latissimus dorsi m.

Deep layer

Biceps brachii
tendons (cut)
Short head
Long head

Coracobrachialis m.
Musculocutaneous n.
Branch to biceps brachii (cut)
Deltoid m. (cut)

Brachialis m.
Medial
intermuscular
septum
Medial
epicondyle
of humerus

Lateral intermuscular septum
Lateral epicondyle of humerus
Lateral antebrachial cutaneous n.
Head of radius
Biceps brachii tendon
Radial tuberosity
Tuberosity of ulna

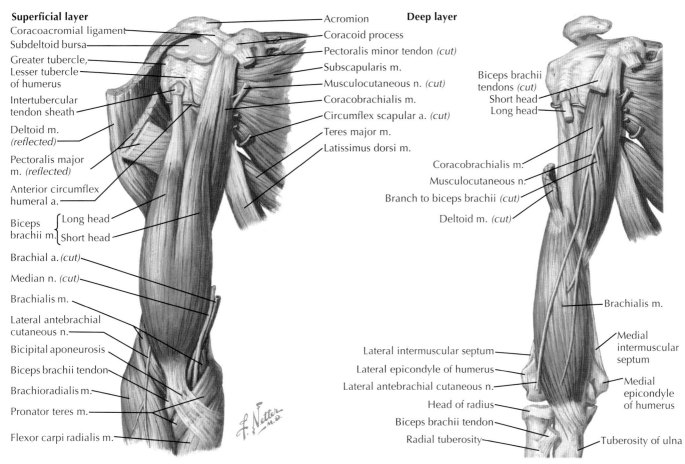

Fig. 10.11 Arm Muscles with Portions of Arteries and Nerves: Anterior Views.

CLINICAL CORRELATION 10.13 Biceps Tendonitis, Dislocation, Rupture

The tendon of the long head of the biceps brachii has an extended course from the supraglenoid tubercle through the glenohumeral joint, before it takes a sharp turn inferiorly within a synovial tendon sheath, descending in the intertubercular sulcus before finally entering the anterior arm and fusing with the short head. This long pathway, along with frequent use, can cause painful **biceps tendonitis** as microtrauma occurs to the dense regular connective tissue of the tendon. Another issue related to this tendon occurs when it displaces itself from the intertubercular sulcus, rolling out from under a weakened transverse humeral ligament. This **biceps tendon dislocation** often occurs during rotation of the arm and is noted for the painful "strumming" of the tendon as it rolls across the greater or lesser tubercle of

the humerus. The tendon may require treatment to be re-positioned properly. Prolonged inflammation of the tendon of the long head of the biceps brachii weakens it and may result in **rupture**. This can also occur if too much force is exerted by the biceps brachii and the tendon tears in half. If it ruptures, the long head of the biceps will "bunch up" with the short head in the anterior arm creating a visible lump in the middle of the anterior arm. It is also possible to have a distal biceps tendon rupture. In this case the long and short heads will retract into the upper part of the anterior arm, causing a large lump. In both cases, the bunched-up biceps muscle is often referred to as "Popeye" sign despite the fact that the cartoon character Popeye the Sailor Man has ludicrously oversized forearms, not biceps.

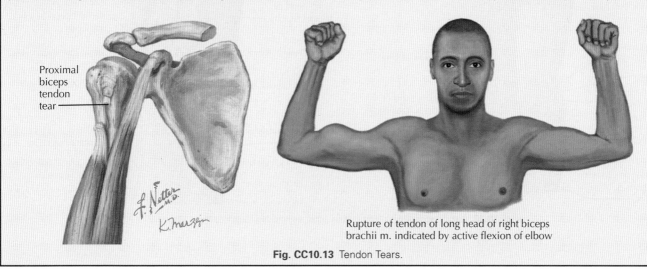

Proximal
biceps
tendon
tear

Rupture of tendon of long head of right biceps
brachii m. indicated by active flexion of elbow

Fig. CC10.13 Tendon Tears.

Brachialis

Proximal attachments	• Anterior aspect of the distal humerus
Distal attachment	• Ulnar tuberosity and coronoid process of ulna
Functions	• Flex forearm at the elbow
Muscle testing and signs of damage	• With the elbow midway between pronation and supination, check for weakness in flexing the forearm against resistance.
Innervation	• Musculocutaneous nerve (C5–C7)
Blood supply	• Branches of brachial, radial, radial recurrent, ulnar, and ulnar recurrent arteries

Muscles of the Posterior Arm (Fig. 10.12)

The two muscles of the **posterior compartment of the arm** are also contained in a stout sleeve of brachial fascia that fuses to the humerus at the **lateral** and **medial intermuscular septae**. The individual muscles in this compartment are the **triceps brachii and anconeus**, they are innervated by the radial nerve and extend the forearm at the elbow.

The three heads of the triceps brachii all converge on the olecranon to focus their contraction onto that single point. The **long head of the triceps brachii** originates from the infraglenoid tubercle of the scapula while the **lateral head** and **medial head** originate from the posterior humerus, lateral and medial to the radial groove, respectively. The medial head is typically deep to the long head and difficult to see from a superficial view. The **anconeus** is a smaller muscle that originates from the lateral epicondyle and fans out across the lateral aspect of the olecranon and posterior ulna. There are a variety of bursae associated with the olecranon and tendon of the triceps brachii. A **subtendinous olecranon bursa** sits between the distal end of the triceps brachii tendon and olecranon. A **subcutaneous olecranon bursa** rests between the skin and the olecranon. It is prone to becoming inflamed if it gets repeatedly irritated resulting in **subcutaneous olecranon bursitis**. Other subcutaneous bursae around the medial epicondyle, lateral epicondyle, and anconeus may become inflamed and mimic olecranon bursitis.

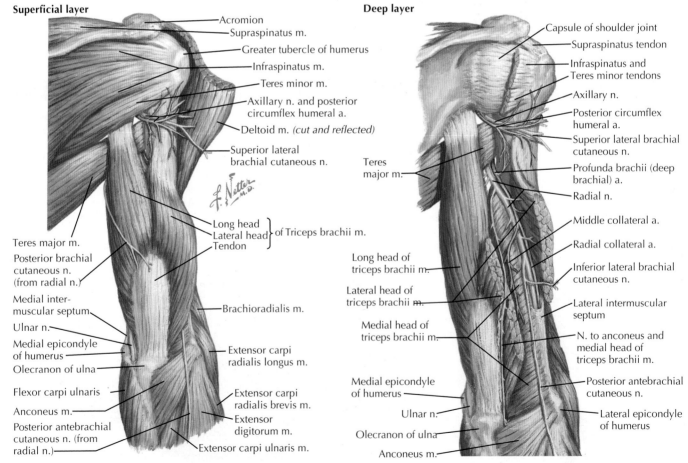

Superficial layer

- Acromion
- Supraspinatus m.
- Greater tubercle of humerus
- Infraspinatus m.
- Teres minor m.
- Axillary n. and posterior circumflex humeral a.
- Deltoid m. *(cut and reflected)*
- Superior lateral brachial cutaneous n.
- Long head
- Lateral head } of Triceps brachii m.
- Tendon
- Brachioradialis m.
- Extensor carpi radialis longus m.
- Extensor carpi radialis brevis m.
- Extensor digitorum m.
- Extensor carpi ulnaris m.

- Teres major m.
- Posterior brachial cutaneous n. (from radial n.)
- Medial intermuscular septum
- Ulnar n.
- Medial epicondyle of humerus
- Olecranon of ulna
- Flexor carpi ulnaris
- Anconeus m.
- Posterior antebrachial cutaneous n. (from radial n.)

Deep layer

- Capsule of shoulder joint
- Supraspinatus tendon
- Infraspinatus and Teres minor tendons
- Axillary n.
- Posterior circumflex humeral a.
- Superior lateral brachial cutaneous n.
- Profunda brachii (deep brachial) a.
- Radial n.
- Middle collateral a.
- Radial collateral a.
- Inferior lateral brachial cutaneous n.
- Lateral intermuscular septum
- N. to anconeus and medial head of triceps brachii m.
- Posterior antebrachial cutaneous n.
- Lateral epicondyle of humerus

- Teres major m.
- Long head of triceps brachii m.
- Lateral head of triceps brachii m.
- Medial head of triceps brachii m.
- Medial epicondyle of humerus
- Ulnar n.
- Olecranon of ulna
- Anconeus m.

Fig. 10.12 Arm Muscles with Portions of Arteries and Nerves: Posterior Views.

Triceps Brachii

Proximal attachments	• Long head: infraglenoid tubercle of the scapula • Lateral head: superolateral shaft of the humerus, lateral to the radial groove • Medial head: posterior aspect of the humerus, medial to the radial groove and deep to the long head
Distal attachment	• Posterosuperior aspect of the olecranon
Functions	• All heads of the triceps extend the forearm at the elbow • The long head of the triceps brachii can adduct and extend the arm, particularly when it is initially positioned over the head. It also prevents inferior displacement of the head of the humerus
Muscle testing and signs of damage	• Weakness or de-innervation of the triceps brachii would manifest as pronounced weakness extending the forearm at the elbow. Testing should look for asymmetric weakness.
Innervation	• Radial nerve (C5–T1)
Blood supply	• Anterior and posterior circumflex humeral, circumflex scapular, scapular, deep brachial, ulnar collateral, radial recurrent, and branches of the brachial artery

Anconeus

See Clinical Correlation 10.14.

Proximal attachments	• Posterior aspect of the lateral epicondyle of the humerus
Distal attachment	• Posterior aspect of the fibrous capsule of the elbow joint • Lateral aspect of the olecranon and posterior ulna
Functions	• Assists in extension of the forearm at the elbow • Stabilizes the olecranon to resist abduction of the forearm • Puts traction on the joint capsule to prevent pinching during full extension
Muscle testing and signs of damage	• Weakness of this muscle would be very difficult to detect
Innervation	• Radial nerve (C5–T1)
Blood supply	• Branches of deep brachial and radial recurrent arteries

Muscles of the Posterior Forearm (Fig. 10.13)

As we move from the arm to the forearm, the fascial support remains similar. Each muscle is surrounded by an investing fascia and the forearm as a whole is covered by **antebrachial fascia** that, along with the interosseous membrane, separates the anterior and posterior compartments of the forearm from each other. The muscles of the posterior forearm are varied but (mercifully) share several traits that help us to understand them. They are all innervated by branches of the radial nerve, many of them originate from a common tendon of the lateral humeral epicondyle, most of them are extensors of the wrist or digits, and their names describe their location or major function.

Superficial Layer of the Posterior Forearm

The **brachioradialis** is a bit of an anomaly since it originates near the other extensors and is innervated by the radial nerve but mainly acts to flex the elbow. It seems to blend characteristics of the anterior and posterior compartments of the arm since it originates from the lateral supraepicondylar area of the humerus and inserts on the distal, lateral radius.

A bit further inferiorly on the lateral humerus are the **extensor carpi radialis longus** (long head) and **extensor carpi radialis brevis** (short head). They insert on the base of the 2nd and 3rd metacarpals, respectively. The extensor carpi radialis longus is immediately posterior to the brachioradialis and the brevis is posterior and a bit inferior to the longus. These muscles will strongly extend the wrist when contracted in coordination with the extensor carpi ulnaris, but when they contract in coordination with the flexor carpi radialis, they will cause abduction/radial deviation of the wrist. While these and the other extensor muscles extend the wrist, they have an under-appreciated function in that they contract during strong flexion of the wrist to stabilize it and allow the digital flexors to work efficiently.

The **extensor digitorum** is located immediately medial to the extensor carpi radialis brevis and both originate from the common extensor origin of the lateral epicondyle of the humerus. This broad muscle passes across the carpus and dorsum of the hand to reach the posterior side of digits 2 to 5. On the dorsum of the hand, proximal to the MCP joints, the four tendons are usually connected by three **intertendinous connections** that reinforce the tendons and make isolated extension of digits 3 and 4 very difficult. The slender **extensor digiti minimi muscle** also originates from the common extensor origin and travels alongside the medial aspect of the extensor digitorum to also insert on the posterior side of the 5th digit. These muscles insert on the dorsal aspect of the digits via an **extensor expansion** that will be described in more detail after the other muscles that insert into it from the palmar side of the hand have been described.

The **extensor carpi ulnaris** muscle is the final extensor muscle in this layer. It originates from the lateral epicondyle and the proximal ulna. It attaches to the base of the 5th metacarpal. In conjunction with the extensor carpi radialis it can extend and stabilize the wrist. Working with the flexor carpi ulnaris it causes adduction/ulnar deviation of the wrist.

Brachioradialis

Proximal attachments	• Lateral supraepicondylar ridge of humerus
Distal attachment	• Lateral aspect of the distal radius, proximal to radial styloid process
Functions	• Flexion of the forearm at the elbow joint, particularly when the forearm is neither pronated nor supinated
Muscle testing and signs of damage	• Ask the patient to put their hand in the "thumbs up" position (in-between pronation and supination) and to flex the elbow against resistance. This muscle tends to bulge outward visibly when tested. Asymmetric weakness may be a sign of brachioradialis dysfunction
Innervation	• Radial nerve (C5–T1)
Blood supply	• Branches of deep brachial, radial recurrent, radial arteries

CLINICAL CORRELATION 10.14   Olecranon Fracture or Avulsion

Because of the exposed location of the olecranon, it can be fractured in a fall when the point of the elbow contacts the ground or other solid surface. Once fractured, the triceps brachii will often displace the fragment superiorly into the posterior arm. While uncommon, the triceps brachii can sometime contract so forcefully that it avulses an otherwise healthy olecranon from the ulna.

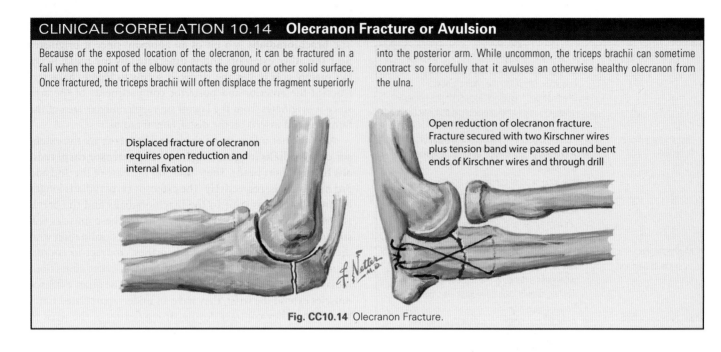

Displaced fracture of olecranon requires open reduction and internal fixation

Open reduction of olecranon fracture. Fracture secured with two Kirschner wires plus tension band wire passed around bent ends of Kirschner wires and through drill

Fig. CC10.14 Olecranon Fracture.

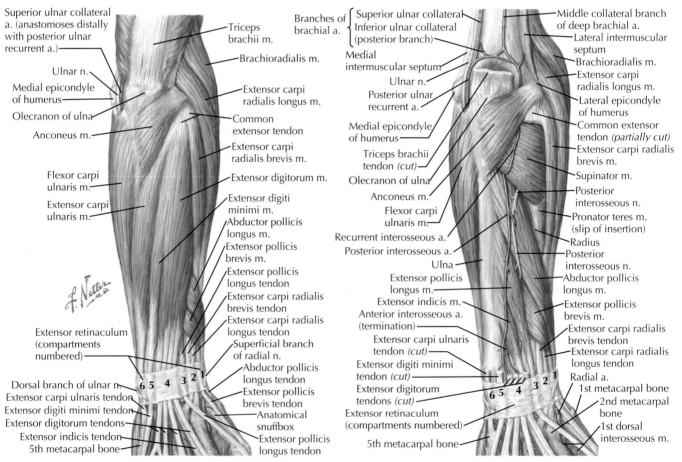

Fig. 10.13 Muscles of the Forearm with Arteries and Nerves (Posterior View).

Extensor Carpi Radialis Longus and Brevis

Proximal attachments	• Longus (long head): lateral supraepicondylar ridge of humerus, just superior to lateral epicondyle • Brevis (short head): common extensor origin from lateral epicondyle of the humerus
Distal attachment	• Longus: base of 2nd metacarpal on the dorsal aspect of the hand • Brevis: base of 3rd metacarpal on the dorsal aspect of the hand
Functions	• Both muscles will contract in conjunction with extensor carpi ulnaris to extend the hand at the wrist • Both muscles will contract in conjunction with flexor carpi radialis to cause radial deviation/lateral deviation/abduction of the hand at the wrist • Both muscles, but particularly the long head, contract to stabilize the hand and wrist during flexion of the digits or to form a tight fist
Muscle testing and signs of damage	• Weakness or de-innervation of the extensor carpi radialis muscles will result in a weak grip, weak extension of the wrist, and weak abduction of the wrist. Since other muscles also contribute to these motions, they may be asymmetrically weak but not completely lost. The examiner may attempt to have the patient simultaneously abduct and extend the wrist against resistance to isolate the extensor carpi radialis muscles
Innervation	• Longus: Radial nerve (C5–T1) • Brevis: Deep branch of radial nerve (C7–C8)
Blood supply	• Branches of deep brachial, radial recurrent, radial arteries

Extensor Digitorum

Proximal attachments	• Common extensor origin from lateral epicondyle of the humerus
Distal attachment	• Extensor expansions of digits 2–5
Functions	• Strongly extends the MCP joints of digits 2–5 • Tethered to each other by intertendinous connections
Muscle testing and signs of damage	• With the forearm resting on a table or other flat surface, have the patient extend the metacarpophalangeal joint against light resistance
Innervation	• Deep branch of radial nerve (C7–C8)
Blood supply	• Branches of deep brachial, radial recurrent, radial arteries

Extensor Digiti Minimi

Proximal attachments	• Common extensor origin from lateral epicondyle of the humerus
Distal attachment	• Extensor expansions of digit 5
Functions	• Strongly extends the MCP joint of digit 5 in conjunction with the final tendon of the extensor digitorum muscle
Muscle testing and signs of damage	• The examiner flexes digits 2–5 and asks the patient to extend the 5th digit against light resistance
Innervation	• Deep branch of radial nerve (C7–C8)
Blood supply	• Branches of deep brachial, radial recurrent, radial arteries

Extensor Carpi Ulnaris

See Clinical Correlation 10.15.

Proximal attachments	• Common extensor origin from lateral epicondyle of the humerus and the proximal, lateral ulna
Distal attachment	• Base of 5th metacarpal on the dorsal aspect of the hand
Functions	• The extensor carpi ulnaris contracts in conjunction with long and short heads of the extensor carpi radialis to extend the hand at the wrist • It also contracts in conjunction with flexor carpi ulnaris to cause ulnar deviation/medial deviation/adduction of the hand at the wrist
Muscle testing and signs of damage	• Weakness of the extensor carpi ulnaris muscles will result in a weak grip, weak extension of the wrist, and weak adduction of the wrist. Since other muscles also contribute to these motions, they may be asymmetrically weak but not completely lost. The examiner may attempt to have the patient simultaneously adduct and extend the wrist against resistance to isolate the extensor carpi ulnaris muscles
Innervation	• Deep branch of radial nerve (C7–C8)
Blood supply	• Branches of deep brachial, radial recurrent arteries

CLINICAL CORRELATION 10.15 Lateral Epicondylitis

Repeated forceful contractions of the carpal and digital extensors can cause inflammation and pain at the attachment of the common extensor origin into the lateral epicondyle of the humerus. This condition is also known as tennis elbow because it can be aggravated by the backswing of a tennis racket and it is difficult to treat since any strong extension or radial deviation of the wrist can further inflammation. One mode of treatment is to apply pressure to the affected muscles a few centimeters distal to the lateral epicondyle. This functionally moves the site of contraction from the bone to the compressed part of the muscle, giving the bone time to heal without additional aggravation.

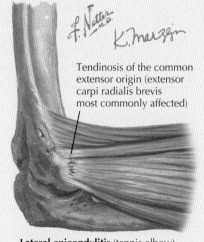

Tendinosis of the common extensor origin (extensor carpi radialis brevis most commonly affected)

Lateral epicondylitis (tennis elbow)

Fig. CC10.15 Lateral Epicondylitis (Tennis Elbow).

Deep Layer of the Posterior Forearm

Deep to the flexor carpi radialis, extensor digitorum, extensor digiti minimi, and extensor carpi ulnaris are additional muscles. The **supinator** takes an oblique course from the lateral epicondyle of the humerus and the supinator crest of the ulna around the proximal ulna, before inserting on the proximal anterior border of the radius. The deep branch of the radial nerve passes through the supinator muscle and continues distally as the posterior interosseous nerve, which innervates the muscles in this region.

Further distally, the **abductor pollicis longus** originates broadly from the posterior middle portion of the ulna, interosseous membrane, and radius. A bit more distally, the **extensor pollicis brevis** muscle originates from the distal third of the radius and interosseous membrane. The tendons of these two muscles travel together superficial to the tendons of the extensor carpi radialis brevis and longus. They insert onto the base of the 1st metacarpal and dorsal aspect of the base of the proximal phalanx of the 1st digit, respectively.

The **extensor pollicis longus** muscle originates from the middle third of the posterior ulna and interosseous membrane. Its tendon crosses the posterior side of the distal radius before inserting on the dorsal aspect of the base of the distal phalanx of the 1st digit. The nearby **extensor indicis** muscle originates just distal to the extensor pollicis longus muscle from the distal third of the ulna and interosseous membrane on their posterior side. Distally, its tendon joins the extensor expansion of the 2nd digit along with one of the tendons from the extensor digitorum.

Supinator

Proximal attachments	• Humerus: lateral epicondyle • Ulna: supinator crest
Distal attachment	• Proximal anterior border of the radius
Functions	• Supinates the forearm when the elbow is extended
Muscle testing and signs of damage	• Weakness of the supinator can be detected by having the patient resist pronation of the forearm with the elbow extended. The biceps brachii supinates the forearm when the elbow is flexed, so flexion of the elbow must be minimized
Innervation	• Deep branch of radial nerve (C7–C8)
Blood supply	• Radial recurrent and recurrent interosseous arteries

Abductor Pollicis Longus (APL), Extensor Pollicis Brevis (EPB), Extensor Pollicis Longus (EPL)

Proximal attachments	• APL: Middle third of the posterior ulna, radius, and interosseous membrane • EPB: Distal third of the posterior radius and adjacent interosseous membrane • EPL: Middle third of posterior ulna and adjacent interosseous membrane
Distal attachment	• APL: Lateral aspect of the base of the 1st metacarpal • EPB: Dorsal base of the proximal phalange of the 1st digit • EPL: Dorsal base of the distal phalanx of the 1st digit
Functions	• APL: Abduct the 1st metacarpal and digit. Slight extension of the 1st digit • EPB: Extension of 1st digit at the carpometacarpal and metacarpophalangeal joints • EPL: Extension of 1st digit at the carpometacarpal, metacarpophalangeal, and interphalangeal joints
Muscle testing and signs of damage	• Starting with the thumb adducted (pressed close to the rest of the hand), have the patient attempt to abduct the thumb (give a "thumbs up") against resistance and slowly shift between abduction and extension. The tendons of these muscles will protrude from the lateral side of the wrist if they are intact
Innervation	• Posterior interosseous nerve (C7–C8)
Blood supply	• Posterior interosseous artery

Extensor Indicis

Proximal attachments	• Distal third of posterior ulna and adjacent interosseous membrane
Distal attachment	• Extensor expansion of the 2nd digit (index finger)
Functions	• Strongly extends the MCP joint of digit 2 in conjunction with the first tendon of the extensor digitorum muscle
Muscle testing and signs of damage	• The examiner flexes digits 2–5 and asks the patient to extend the 2nd digit against light resistance
Innervation	• Posterior interosseous nerve (C7–C8)
Blood supply	• Posterior interosseous artery

Muscles of the Anterior Forearm (Fig. 10.14)

In many ways, the muscles of the anterior compartment of the forearm correspond to those in the posterior compartment: they are also covered by antebrachial fascia; instead of extensors, they tend to be flexors; the common flexor tendon is from the medial epicondyle of the humerus, rather than the lateral epicondyle; instead of the radial nerve, they are innervated by the median and ulnar nerves; and their names describe their location or major function.

A. Superficial layer: anterior view

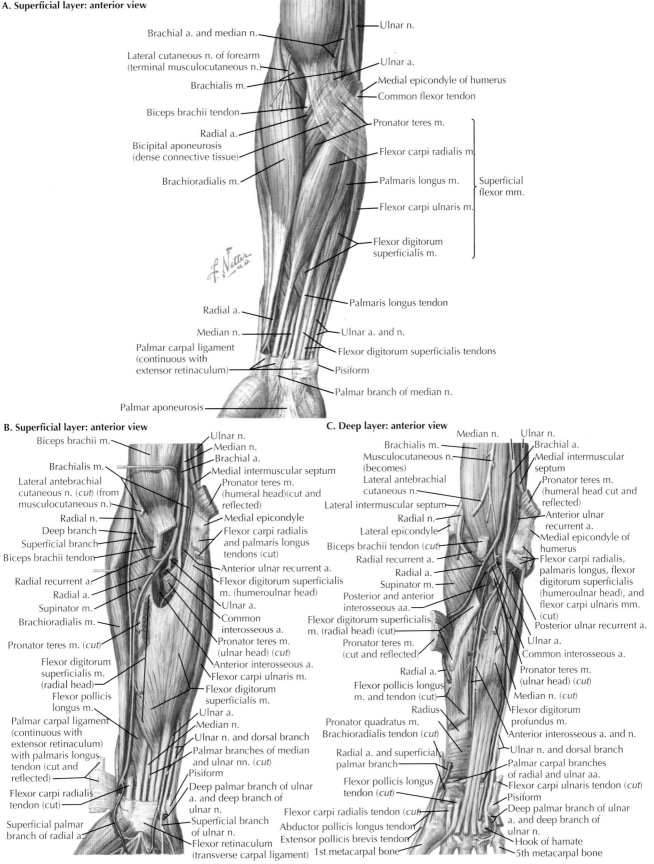

Ulnar n.

Brachial a. and median n.

Lateral cutaneous n. of forearm
(terminal musculocutaneous n.)

Brachialis m.

Ulnar a.

Medial epicondyle of humerus

Common flexor tendon

Biceps brachii tendon

Radial a.

Bicipital aponeurosis
(dense connective tissue)

Brachioradialis m.

Pronator teres m.

Flexor carpi radialis m.

Palmaris longus m.

Flexor carpi ulnaris m.

Superficial
flexor mm.

Flexor digitorum
superficialis m.

Radial a.

Palmaris longus tendon

Median n.

Ulnar a. and n.

Palmar carpal ligament
(continuous with
extensor retinaculum)

Flexor digitorum superficialis tendons

Pisiform

Palmar branch of median n.

Palmar aponeurosis

B. Superficial layer: anterior view

Biceps brachii m.

Ulnar n.

Median n.

Brachial a.

Brachialis m.

Medial intermuscular septum

Lateral antebrachial
cutaneous n. (cut) (from
musculocutaneous n.)

Pronator teres m.
(humeral head)(cut and
reflected)

Radial n.

Deep branch

Superficial branch

Biceps brachii tendon

Medial epicondyle

Flexor carpi radialis
and palmaris longus
tendons (cut)

Anterior ulnar recurrent a.

Radial recurrent a.

Radial a.

Flexor digitorum superficialis
m. (humeroulnar head)

Supinator m.

Ulnar a.

Brachioradialis m.

Common
interosseous a.

Pronator teres m. (cut)

Pronator teres m.
(ulnar head) (cut)

Flexor digitorum
superficialis m.
(radial head)

Anterior interosseous a.

Flexor carpi ulnaris m.

Flexor pollicis
longus m.

Flexor digitorum
superficialis m.

Palmar carpal ligament
(continuous with
extensor retinaculum)
with palmaris longus
tendon (cut and
reflected)

Ulnar a.

Median n.

Ulnar n. and dorsal branch

Palmar branches of median
and ulnar nn. (cut)

Pisiform

Flexor carpi radialis
tendon (cut)

Deep palmar branch of ulnar
a. and deep branch of
ulnar n.

Superficial branch
of ulnar n.

Superficial palmar
branch of radial a.

Flexor retinaculum
(transverse carpal ligament)

C. Deep layer: anterior view

Median n.

Ulnar n.

Brachialis m.

Brachial a.

Musculocutaneous n.
(becomes)

Lateral antebrachial
cutaneous n.

Medial intermuscular
septum

Pronator teres m.
(humeral head cut and
reflected)

Lateral intermuscular septum

Anterior ulnar
recurrent a.

Radial n.

Lateral epicondyle

Biceps brachii tendon (cut)

Radial recurrent a.

Radial a.

Supinator m.

Posterior and anterior
interosseous aa.

Medial epicondyle of
humerus

Flexor carpi radialis,
palmaris longus, flexor
digitorum superficialis
(humeroulnar head), and
flexor carpi ulnaris mm.
(cut)

Posterior ulnar recurrent a.

Ulnar a.

Common interosseous a.

Flexor digitorum superficialis
m. (radial head) (cut)

Pronator teres m.
(cut and reflected)

Radial a.

Flexor pollicis longus
m. and tendon (cut)

Radius

Pronator quadratus m.

Brachioradialis tendon (cut)

Radial a. and superficial
palmar branch

Flexor pollicis longus
tendon (cut)

Flexor carpi radialis tendon (cut)

Abductor pollicis longus tendon

Extensor pollicis brevis tendon

1st metacarpal bone

Pronator teres m.
(ulnar head) (cut)

Median n. (cut)

Flexor digitorum
profundus m.

Anterior interosseous a. and n.

Ulnar n. and dorsal branch

Palmar carpal branches
of radial and ulnar aa.

Flexor carpi ulnaris tendon (cut)

Pisiform

Deep palmar branch of ulnar
a. and deep branch of
ulnar n.

Hook of hamate

5th metacarpal bone

Fig. 10.14 Muscles of the Forearm.

Superficial Layer of the Anterior Forearm

The **pronator teres** muscle counters the supinator; it strongly pronates the arm whether the elbow is flexed or extended. Its humeral head originates from the common flexor origin on the medial epicondyle of the humerus, while the ulnar head arises from the coronoid process of the ulna. The median nerve travels between the two heads and may become entrapped by them as they descend obliquely to insert on the anterolateral radius, approximately midway along its shaft.

Also originating off the common flexor origin is the **flexor carpi radialis** muscle, which crosses from medial to lateral as it descends to insert on the palmar side of the base of the 2nd metatarsal. It causes strong flexion of the wrist when it contracts in conjunction with the flexor carpi ulnaris, and it causes radial deviation/lateral deviation/abduction of the wrist and hand when it contracts with the two heads of the extensor carpi radialis.

The **palmaris longus** originates from the common flexor origin, quickly gives off a long, thin tendon that crosses the wrist and fans out into a triangular sheet of tough connective tissue that covers and protects the structures of the palm, the **palmar aponeurosis**. It weakly helps to flex the wrist. This muscle often has a short belly and long, thin tendon but it can sometimes have a longer muscle belly or may be entirely absent in ~14% of people. The palmaris longus can be demonstrated (if present) by strongly pinching the thumb and 5th digit together in opposition while flexing the wrist; its tendon will tend to "bowstring" fairly dramatically. Since it is not a major mover of the wrist, the tendon of the palmaris longus is clinically important as a source of tendon autografts.

The large **flexor carpi ulnaris** originates from the common flexor origin of the humeral medial epicondyle and the nearby posterior border of the ulna from the medial olecranon to approximately mid-shaft of the bone. It descends along the medial aspect of the forearm before inserting on the pisiform bone, hook of the hamate, and base of the 5th metacarpal. Contracting with the flexor carpi radialis, it strongly flexes the wrist, and contracting with the extensor carpi ulnaris it will cause ulnar deviation/medial deviation/adduction.

Pronator Teres

Proximal attachments	• Humerus: common flexor origin from the medial epicondyle of the humerus • Ulna: medial aspect of coronoid process
Distal attachment	• Lateral surface of radius, approximately mid-shaft
Functions	• Pronates the forearm
Muscle testing and signs of damage	• Weakness of the pronator teres can be detected by having the patient resist supination. The examiner will palpate the area of the medial epicondyle to feel for contraction of the muscle and note any asymmetric weakness
Innervation	• Median nerve (C6–T1)
Blood supply	• Ulnar collateral, ulnar recurrent, ulnar, and radial arteries

Flexor Carpi Radialis

Proximal attachments	• Common flexor origin from medial epicondyle of humerus
Distal attachment	• Base of 2nd metacarpal on the palmar aspect of the hand
Functions	• The flexor carpi radialis contracts in conjunction with the flexor carpi ulnaris to flex the hand at the wrist • It contributes to radial deviation/lateral deviation/abduction of the hand at the wrist in conjunction with the two heads of the extensor carpi radialis
Muscle testing and signs of damage	• Dysfunction of the flexor carpi radialis muscle will result in weak flexion of the wrist. These motions may be asymmetrically weak but not completely lost since other muscles also contribute • The tendon can be palpated when flexion and abduction of the wrist are combined, as if trying to touch the anterior forearm with the thumb
Innervation	• Median nerve (C6–T1)
Blood supply	• Ulnar collateral, ulnar recurrent, ulnar, and radial arteries

Palmaris Longus

Proximal attachments	• Common flexor origin from medial epicondyle of humerus
Distal attachment	• Flexor retinaculum and palmar aponeurosis
Functions	• Weakly flexes the hand at the wrist
Muscle testing and signs of damage	• Isolated weakness of the palmaris longus is unlikely to be detectable. The presence of the muscle and tendon can be established by having the patient oppose the thumb and fifth digit while flexing the wrist
Innervation	• Median nerve (C6–T1)
Blood supply	• Ulnar collateral, ulnar recurrent, and ulnar arteries

Flexor Carpi Ulnaris

Proximal Attachments	• Humerus: common flexor origin from the medial epicondyle of the humerus • Ulna: posterior border of ulna from the medial olecranon to mid-shaft
Distal attachment	• Pisiform bone, hook of hamate, base of 5th metacarpal on palmar side
Functions	• The flexor carpi ulnaris contracts in conjunction with the flexor carpi radialis to flex the hand at the wrist • It also contributes to ulnar deviation/medial deviation/adduction of the hand at the wrist in conjunction with the extensor carpi ulnaris
Muscle testing and signs of damage	• Weakness of the flexor carpi ulnaris muscle will result in profoundly weak flexion and adduction of the wrist as it is a major contributor to both motions. To test for it specifically, its tendon can be palpated when flexion and adduction of the wrist are combined, as if trying to touch the anterior forearm with the little finger
Innervation	• Median nerve (C6–T1)
Blood supply	• Ulnar collateral, ulnar recurrent, and ulnar arteries

Intermediate Layer of the Anterior Forearm

The single muscle occupying this layer is the **flexor digitorum superficialis**. This muscle has an oblique origin that crosses all the bones in the area but not the interosseous membrane, which begins just inferior to the muscle's sites of origin. The humeroulnar head originates from an oblique line crossing from the common flexor origin on the medial epicondyle across the superomedial aspect of the coronoid process. The radial head originates from the anterior border of the radius beginning below the radial tuberosity and ending mid-shaft on the bone. The two heads fuse and then re-separate to form four elongated tendons that pass through the **carpal tunnel** before one of each of the tendons travels to digits 2 to 5. As the tendons pass into the digits, they split into medial and lateral bands that insert on the medial and lateral sides of the palmar bases and shafts of the middle phalanges. Contraction will flex the MCP and PIP joints but not the DIP joints, which is accomplished by the flexor digitorum profundus in the deep layer of the anterior forearm.

Flexor Digitorum Superficialis

See Clinical Correlation 10.16.

Proximal attachments	• Humeroulnar: common flexor origin on medial epicondyle of humerus and the superomedial coronoid process of ulna • Radial: anterior border of radius between radial tuberosity and mid-shaft
Distal attachment	• The medial and lateral aspects of the bases and shafts of the middle phalanges on their palmar aspect
Functions	• Strongly flexes the PIP and MCP joints of digits 2–5. • Thereafter it will flex the wrist
Muscle testing and signs of damage	• Weakness of this muscle as a whole will result in a reduction in grip strength, but this will be masked if the flexor digitorum profundus is functional • Since these tendons travel independently to each of the digits 2–5, they can be tested individually in case of tendon rupture. Each digit is flexed at the PIP joint (while the MCP and DIP joints are kept in an extended position) and the patient resists gentle extension
Innervation	• Median nerve (C6–T1)
Blood supply	• Ulnar recurrent, ulnar, and radial arteries

Deep Layer of the Anterior Forearm

The median nerve and ulnar artery pass between the humeroulnar and radial heads of the flexor digitorum superficialis to reach the space between the intermediate and deep layer of the anterior forearm. Within the deep layer are three muscles. The **flexor digitorum profundus** originates from the proximal

CLINICAL CORRELATION 10.16   Medial Epicondylitis

Repeated forceful contractions of the carpal and digital flexors can cause inflammation and pain at the attachment of the common flexor origin onto the medial epicondyle of the humerus. This condition is also known as golfer's elbow because it can be aggravated by the strong stroke of a golf club when teeing off. Like lateral epicondylitis, it is challenging to treat since any strong flexion or ulnar deviation of the wrist can create further inflammation. One mode of treatment is to apply pressure to the affected muscles a few centimeters distal to the medial epicondyle. This functionally moves the site of contraction from the bone to the compressed part of the muscle, giving the bone time to heal without additional aggravation.

Tendinosis of the origin of the flexor-pronator mass (pronator teres and flexor carpi radialis most commonly affected)

Medial epicondylitis (golfer's elbow)

Fig. CC10.16 Medial Epicondylitis (Golfer's Elbow).

two-thirds of the ulna's anterior surface starting just inferior to the coronoid process and the adjacent interosseous membrane. The muscle will give off four tendons that pass through the carpal tunnel and then to digits 2 to 5. As the tendons pass into the digits, they split into medial and lateral bands that insert on the medial and lateral sides of the bases of the distal phalanges. It is the only muscle that can flex the DIP, but continued contraction will also flex the PIP, MCP, and wrist joints.

The **flexor pollicis longus** originates broadly from the anterior surface of the radius just inferior to the origin of the flexor digitorum superficialis and the adjacent interosseous membrane. This large muscle gives off a single tendon that passes through the carpal tunnel and then inserts on the palmar base of the distal phalanx of the 1st digit. It is the only muscle that flexes the interphalangeal joint of the thumb.

The deepest muscle in the anterior forearm is the **pronator quadratus**, which tethers the distal ulna to the distal radius. Its contraction will initiate pronation of the forearm and when stretched it will prevent excessive supination of the distal radius from the ulna. It also keeps the distal ends of both bones connected and prevents distraction of them from each other. The anterior interosseous nerve and artery pass deep (posterior) to it as they travel distally.

Flexor Digitorum Profundus

Proximal attachments	• Superior 2/3rd of the anterior surface of the ulna and the adjacent interosseous membrane
Distal attachment	• The palmar bases of the distal phalanges of digits 2–5.
Functions	• Strongly flexes the DIP joints of digits 2–5
	• Thereafter it will flex the PIP, MCP joints and the wrist
Muscle testing and signs of damage	• Weakness of this muscle as a whole will result in weakness in grip strength but this will be masked if the flexor digitorum superficialis is functional
	• Since these tendons travel independently to each of the digits 2–5, they can be tested individually in case of tendon rupture. The MCP and PIP of each digit is extended and the patient is asked to flex the DIP joint against gentle resistance
Innervation	• Medial aspect: ulnar nerve (C8–T1)
	• Lateral aspect: anterior interosseous nerve (C8–T1)
Blood supply	• Ulnar and anterior interosseous arteries

Flexor Pollicis Longus

Proximal attachments	• Middle region of anterior surface of the radius and nearby interosseous membrane
Distal attachment	• The palmar base of the distal phalanx of the 1st digit
Functions	• Strongly flexes the interphalangeal joint of the 1st digit
	• Thereafter it will flex the MCP joint
Muscle testing and signs of damage	• The MCP joint of the thumb is kept in an extended position and the interphalangeal joint is flexed against gentle extension
Innervation	• Anterior interosseous nerve (C8–T1)
Blood supply	• Radial and anterior interosseous arteries

Pronator Quadratus

Medial attachment	• Distal ¼ of the anterior surface of the ulna just superior to the ulnar head
Lateral attachment	• Distal ¼ of the anterior surface of the radius, just superior to brachioradialis insertion
Functions	• Pronates forearm and resists excessive supination
	• Resists distraction of radius from the ulna
Muscle testing and signs of damage	• Dysfunction of the pronator quadratus will manifest as weakness in pronation but this can be masked by arm positioning and activity of the pronator teres
Innervation	• Anterior interosseous nerve (C8–T1)
Blood supply	• Anterior interosseous arteries

Fascial Structures of the Wrist and Hand (Figs. 10.14 and 10.15, See Also Fig. 10.13)

The **dorsal** and **palmar fascia** are continuous with the posterior and anterior antebrachial fasciae and cover their respective regions of the hand. There is very little to say about the dorsal fascia apart from its connection to the **extensor retinaculum** of the wrist, a tough connective tissue sheet that tethers the extensor and abductor pollicis tendons to the bones so they do not lose their mechanical advantage or bowstring outward as the hand moves through a variety of positions. As the tendons cross deep to the extensor retinaculum they pass through **synovial tendon sheaths**. These are structures that surround tendons to lubricate their movements and allow them to glide smoothly across the wrist. Crossing the posterior aspect of the head of the ulna within its own synovial sheath is the extensor carpi ulnaris. Moving laterally, there is a single sheath along the gap between the ulna and radius for the tendon of the extensor digiti minimi. Continuing laterally along the posterior side of the radius, the next sheath contains all the tendons of the extensor digitorum and extensor indicis and then another, single sheath for the extensor pollicis longus. The dorsal tubercle of the radius separates it from the next sheath, which contains the extensor carpi radialis longus and brevis tendons. The final synovial tendon sheath lies on the lateral side of the radius and contains the extensor pollicis brevis and abductor pollicis longus tendons.

On the opposite side, the anterior antebrachial fascia thickens to form the **palmar carpal ligament**. The tendons of the flexor carpi ulnaris and palmaris longus travel superficially across it while the other long flexor tendons travel deep to it as well as the much thicker **flexor retinaculum**, which forms the roof of the **carpal tunnel**. The carpal tunnel is a single large space that contains several synovial tendon sheaths (see Fig. 10.15). Laterally, the flexor carpi radialis tendon occupies its own sheath and is immediately lateral to the **tendon sheath of the tendon of the flexor pollicis longus**. More medially, the tendons of the flexor digitorum profundus and superficialis occupy a single, large **common flexor sheath** that conveys them across the wrist and into the palmar hand.

More superficially on the palmar hand, the palmar fascia creates many distinct structures, spaces, and compartments. Centrally it forms a tough **palmar aponeurosis** (previously discussed along with the palmaris longus muscle) that protects the palm (see Fig. 10.15). Distally, the palmar aponeurosis fans outward from the wrist toward each finger (digits 2 to 5), creating distinct **digital bands** that cover the tendons going to those digits. Before reaching each digit, over the heads of the metacarpals, there is a **superficial transverse metacarpal ligament** that connects the fascia at the base of each finger to its neighbor. Each digital band of the palmar aponeurosis also extends deeply toward the underlying metacarpal to form a **fibrous digital sheath** that surrounds a **synovial tendon sheath of the finger**, which (in turn) surrounds and lubricates the tendons of the flexor digitorum superficialis and profundus as they travel to the middle and distal phalanges. While the tendon sheathes of digits 1 to 4 are separate from each other, the tendon sheath of the 5th digit connects with the common flexor sheath. The collagen fibers of the fibrous digital sheaths have **anular parts** oriented in a circular direction as well as **cruciform parts** oriented in a crisscross manner. This helps stabilize the tendons and prevents bowstringing during flexion. As the tendons cross the MCP, PIP, and DIP joints, they are supported by thickenings of the joint capsule, the palmar plates/ligaments. The extensor expansion of each digit fuses laterally and medially with the palmar plate of

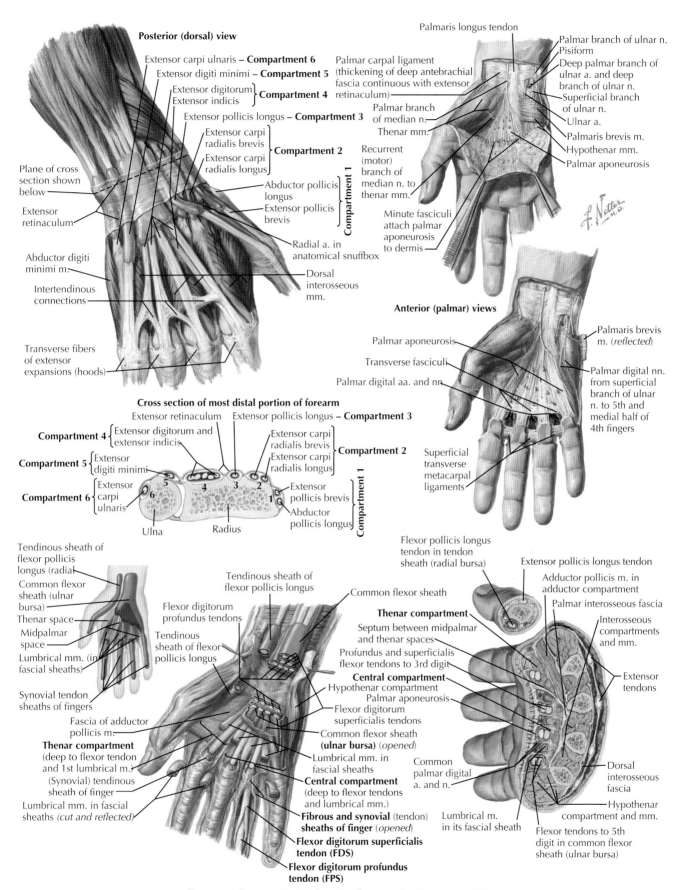

Posterior (dorsal) view

Extensor carpi ulnaris – **Compartment 6**
Extensor digiti minimi – **Compartment 5**
Extensor digitorum
Extensor indicis } **Compartment 4**
Extensor pollicis longus – **Compartment 3**
Extensor carpi radialis brevis
Extensor carpi radialis longus } **Compartment 2**
Abductor pollicis longus
Extensor pollicis brevis } **Compartment 1**
Radial a. in anatomical snuffbox

Plane of cross section shown below
Extensor retinaculum

Abductor digiti minimi m.
Intertendinous connections
Transverse fibers of extensor expansions (hoods)

Dorsal interosseous mm.

Palmaris longus tendon
Palmar carpal ligament (thickening of deep antebrachial fascia continuous with extensor retinaculum)
Palmar branch of median n.
Thenar mm.
Recurrent (motor) branch of median n. to thenar mm.
Minute fasciculi attach palmar aponeurosis to dermis

Palmar branch of ulnar n.
Pisiform
Deep palmar branch of ulnar a. and deep branch of ulnar n.
Superficial branch of ulnar n.
Ulnar a.
Palmaris brevis m.
Hypothenar mm.
Palmar aponeurosis

Cross section of most distal portion of forearm

Extensor retinaculum   Extensor pollicis longus – **Compartment 3**

Compartment 4 { Extensor digitorum and extensor indicis
Compartment 5 { Extensor digiti minimi
Compartment 6 { Extensor carpi ulnaris

Extensor carpi radialis brevis
Extensor carpi radialis longus } **Compartment 2**
Extensor pollicis brevis
Abductor pollicis longus } **Compartment 1**

Ulna   Radius

Anterior (palmar) views

Palmar aponeurosis
Transverse fasciculi
Palmar digital aa. and nn.

Palmaris brevis m. (*reflected*)
Palmar digital nn. from superficial branch of ulnar n. to 5th and medial half of 4th fingers

Superficial transverse metacarpal ligaments

Tendinous sheath of flexor pollicis longus (radial)
Common flexor sheath (ulnar bursa)
Thenar space
Midpalmar space
Lumbrical mm. (in fascial sheaths)
Synovial tendon sheaths of fingers
Fascia of adductor pollicis m.
Thenar compartment (deep to flexor tendon and 1st lumbrical m.)
(Synovial) tendinous sheath of finger
Lumbrical mm. in fascial sheaths (cut and reflected)

Tendinous sheath of flexor pollicis longus
Tendinous sheath of flexor pollicis longus
Flexor digitorum profundus tendons

Common flexor sheath
Profundus and superficialis flexor tendons to 3rd digit
Hypothenar compartment
Palmar aponeurosis
Flexor digitorum superficialis tendons
Common flexor sheath (ulnar bursa) (opened)
Lumbrical mm. in fascial sheaths
Central compartment (deep to flexor tendons and lumbrical mm.)
Fibrous and synovial (tendon) **sheaths of finger** (opened)
Flexor digitorum superficialis tendon (FDS)
Flexor digitorum profundus tendon (FPS)

Flexor pollicis longus tendon in tendon sheath (radial bursa)
Thenar compartment
Septum between midpalmar and thenar spaces
Central compartment

Common palmar digital a. and n.
Lumbrical m. in its fascial sheath
Flexor tendons to 5th digit in common flexor sheath (ulnar bursa)

Extensor pollicis longus tendon
Adductor pollicis m. in adductor compartment
Palmar interosseous fascia
Interosseous compartments and mm.
Extensor tendons
Dorsal interosseous fascia
Hypothenar compartment and mm.

Fig. 10.15 Extensor Indicis Proprius Extensor Tendons at the Wrist.

the MCP joint. Also, the palmar plates at the MCP joint of digits 2 to 5 are interconnected by the **deep transverse metacarpal ligament**, which prevents them from distracting too far from each other (Clinical Correlations 10.17 and 10.18).

Returning to the base of the hand, the palmar aponeurosis lies superficial to the large **central compartment** of the palm. A **medial fibrous septum** connects the medial side of the palmar aponeurosis to the 5th metacarpal, creating the **hypothenar**

CLINICAL CORRELATION 10.17   Ganglion (Synovial) Cysts of the Wrist

Excessive synovial fluid or weakness of a tendon sheath can cause a firm nodule to appear on the dorsal side of the wrist that is associated with one of the extensor tendon sheaths. These ganglion or synovial cysts may or may not be painful.

They sometimes resolve spontaneously but may require aspiration or lancing. Despite being called "ganglion" cysts, they have nothing to do with neuron cell bodies. These can also arise from the palmar synovial tendon sheaths.

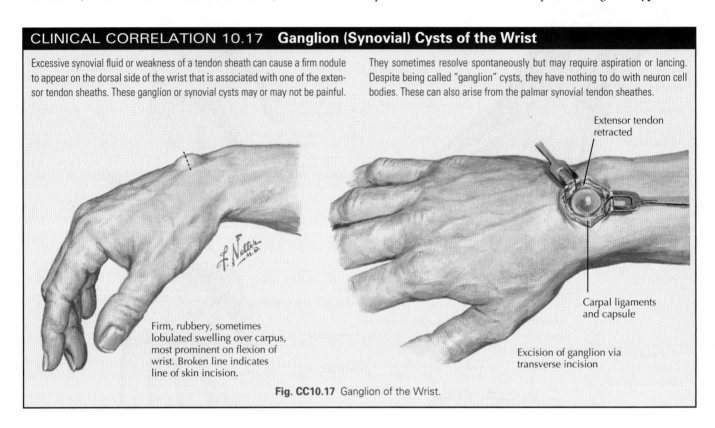

Firm, rubbery, sometimes lobulated swelling over carpus, most prominent on flexion of wrist. Broken line indicates line of skin incision.

Extensor tendon retracted

Carpal ligaments and capsule

Excision of ganglion via transverse incision

Fig. CC10.17 Ganglion of the Wrist.

CLINICAL CORRELATION 10.18   Trigger Finger

Nodules can sometimes develop in the long tendons of the flexor digitorum superficialis or profundus that make it difficult for that region of the tendon to enter the digital sheathes of the fingers. If the nodule is stuck proximal to the sheath, the finger will be persistently flexed. Patients can often use their other hand to forcibly extend the digit, pulling the nodule into the sheath. These **trigger fingers** will frequently produce an audible snap as the nodule enters the sheath during extension and leaves it during flexion.

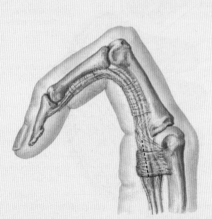
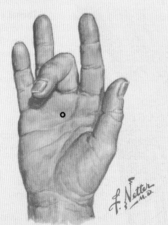
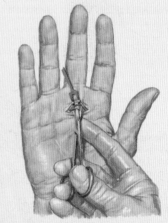

Inflammatory thickening of fibrous sheath (pulley) of flexor tendons with fusiform nodular enlargement of both tendons. Broken line indicates line for incision of lateral aspect of pulley.

Patient unable to extend affected finger. It can be extended passively, and extension occurs with distinct and painful snapping action. Circle indicates point of tenderness where nodular enlargement of tendons and sheath is usually palpable.

Incision of thickened pulley via small transverse skin incision just distal to distal flexion crease releases constriction, permitting flexor tendons to glide freely and inflammation to subside.

Fig. CC10.18 Trigger Finger.

CLINICAL CORRELATION 10.19 Dupuytren Contracture

The palmar aponeurosis can undergo progressive fibrosis of its digital bands, particularly those projecting to digits 4–5. This will begin with firm nodules in the palmar fascia and aponeurosis that form fibrous contractures that persistently flex and form raised "spokes" leading to the affected digits. No single cause for this condition has been found but it tends to affect people after the age of 50 and is likely hereditary. Treatment involves surgically detaching the fibrous bands.

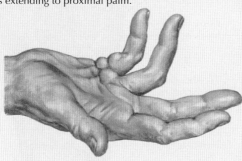

Flexion contracture of 4th and 5th fingers (most common). Dimpling and puckering of skin. Palpable fascial nodules near flexion crease of palm at base of involved fingers with cordlike formations extending to proximal palm.

Partial excision of palmar fascia. Proximal portion of fascia divided and freed via thenar incision, then drawn up into palmar incision, where it is further dissected with care to avoid neurovascular bundles. Dissection is then continued into fingers. Buttonholing of skin must be avoided. Nodules and cordlike fascial thickening are apparent.

Fig. CC10.19 Dupuytren Disease.

compartment, covered by thin **hypothenar fascia**. Likewise, the **lateral fibrous septum** connects the lateral aspect of the palmar aponeurosis to the 3rd metacarpal, creating the **thenar compartment**, covered by thenar fascia. Deep to the central compartment is the **adductor compartment** and deep/dorsal to all of the previously named compartments are the four **interosseous compartments** between the metacarpals. Note that some sources list additional compartments within these, formed by subdivisions of the palmar fascia. Superficial to the hypothenar compartment and inserting onto the proximal medial border of the palmar aponeurosis is the **palmaris brevis muscle**, which inserts onto the skin overlying the base of the hypothenar eminence. This muscle creates a crease in the skin and is not seen in all persons (Clinical Correlation 10.19).

Muscles of the Palm of the Hand (Fig. 10.16, See Also Fig. 10.15)

In the **hypothenar compartment** there are three muscles, all of which are associated with the 5th digit, or digiti minimi, and all are innervated by the deep branch of the ulnar nerve. The **abductor digiti minimi** is the most medial, stretching from the pisiform bone to the medial aspect of the base of the 5th digit's proximal phalanx. When it contracts, it will abduct the 5th digit, moving it medial and away from the centerline of the hand. The **flexor digiti minimi brevis** originates from the flexor retinaculum and the hook of the hamate and inserts onto the same location as the abductor digiti minimi. Because of its more anterior origin, it flexes the MCP joint instead of abducting it. The **opponens digiti minimi** shares the same site of origin as the flexor digiti minimi brevis but inserts on the medial aspect

of the body of the 5th metacarpal. Contraction of this muscle will cause opposition of the 5th digit and its metacarpal toward the center of the palm.

Abductor Digiti Minimi (ADM), Flexor Digiti Minimi Brevis (FDMB), Opponens Digiti Minimi (ODM)

Proximal attachments	• ADM: Pisiform bone • FDMB and ODM: Hook of hamate and flexor retinaculum
Distal attachment	• ADM and FDMB: Medial side of base of proximal phalanx of 5th digit • ODM: Medial side of the shaft/body of the 5th metacarpal
Functions	• ADM: Abducts (moves medially) the 5th digit • FDMB: Flex the MCP joint of the 5th digit • ODM: Opposes the hypothenar eminence, pulling it toward the center of palm
Muscle testing and signs of damage	• Atrophy of the hypothenar eminence is one sign of de-innervation of the muscles in this compartment. Abduction of the 5th digit away from the rest of the hand is a unique function of the ADM and loss of this action points to an issue in the hypothenar compartment. Opposition of the hypothenar eminence is a bit subtle and other muscles flex the MCP joint of the 5th digit
Innervation	• Deep branch of the ulnar nerve (C8–T1)
Blood supply	• Superficial palmar arch, deep palmar arch, common palmar digital, palmar metacarpal arteries

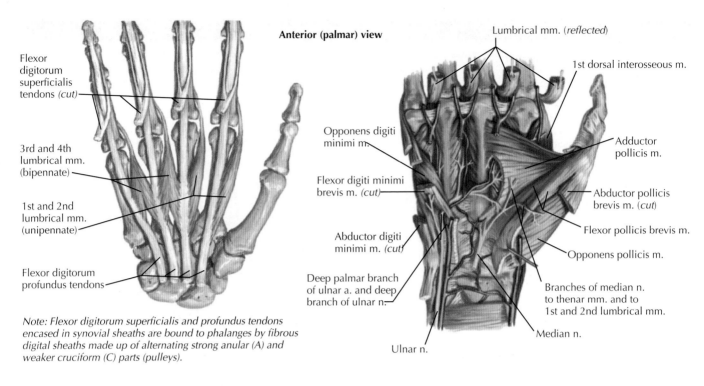

Anterior (palmar) view

Flexor digitorum superficialis tendons (cut)

3rd and 4th lumbrical mm. (bipennate)

1st and 2nd lumbrical mm. (unipennate)

Flexor digitorum profundus tendons

Lumbrical mm. (reflected)

1st dorsal interosseous m.

Opponens digiti minimi m.

Flexor digiti minimi brevis m. (cut)

Abductor digiti minimi m. (cut)

Deep palmar branch of ulnar a. and deep branch of ulnar n.

Ulnar n.

Adductor pollicis m.

Abductor pollicis brevis m. (cut)

Flexor pollicis brevis m.

Opponens pollicis m.

Branches of median n. to thenar mm. and to 1st and 2nd lumbrical mm.

Median n.

Note: Flexor digitorum superficialis and profundus tendons encased in synovial sheaths are bound to phalanges by fibrous digital sheaths made up of alternating strong anular (A) and weaker cruciform (C) parts (pulleys).

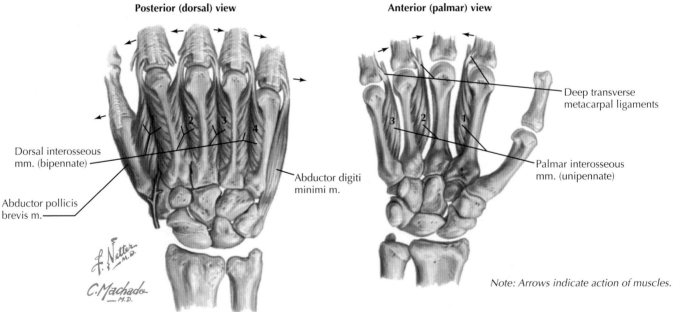

Posterior (dorsal) view

Dorsal interosseous mm. (bipennate)

Abductor pollicis brevis m.

Abductor digiti minimi m.

Anterior (palmar) view

Deep transverse metacarpal ligaments

Palmar interosseous mm. (unipennate)

Note: Arrows indicate action of muscles.

Finger in extension: lateral (radial) view

Insertion of extensor tendon to base of middle phalanx

Insertion of extensor tendon to base of distal phalanx

Extensor expansion (hood)

Long extensor tendon

Interosseous mm.

Lumbrical m.

Flexor digitorum profundus tendon

Flexor digitorum superficialis tendon

Note: Black arrows indicate pull of long extensor tendon; red arrows indicate pull of interosseous and lumbrical mm.

Fig. 10.16 Muscles of the Hand.

In the **thenar compartment** there are three muscles, all of which are associated with the 1st digit, thumb, or pollicis. Two of these muscles, the **abductor pollicis brevis** and **flexor pollicis brevis**, originate from the flexor retinaculum, scaphoid, and trapezium and both insert close together on the lateral/palmar aspect of the base of the proximal phalanx of the 1st digit. The abductor pollicis brevis is more lateral, making its motion abduction of the 1st MCP joint than its neighbor, which originates more medially and therefore tends to flex the same joint. The flexor pollicis brevis has two heads, the superficial head is innervated by the recurrent branch of the median nerve and the deep head by the deep branch of the ulnar nerve. Deep to both of these muscles is the **opponens pollicis**. It shares nearly the same site of origin as the other muscles in this compartment and it inserts on the lateral, palmar side of the body of the 1st metacarpal. When it contracts it will roll the entire thenar eminence, 1st metacarpal and the digits, toward the center of the palm, causing opposition.

Abductor Pollicis Brevis (APB), Flexor Pollicis Brevis (FPB), Opponens Pollicis (OP)

Proximal attachments	• APB, FPB (superficial and deep head), OP: Flexor retinaculum, scaphoid, trapezium
Distal attachment	• APB and FPB: palmar/lateral aspect of base of proximal phalanx of 1st digit • OP: palmar/lateral aspect of 1st metacarpal
Functions	• APB: Abducts (moves laterally) the 1st digit away from the rest of the hand • FPB: Flexes the MCP joint of the 1st digit • OP: Causes opposition of the thenar eminence, moving the 1st metacarpal and digits toward the center of palm
Muscle testing and signs of damage	• Atrophy of the thenar eminence points to de-innervation of the compartment • Opposition of the thenar eminence by the opponens pollicis is a very important motion that is unique to this compartment. It is tested with the palm facing upward so that gravity cannot assist in opposition • Flexion and abduction of the thumb are complemented by other muscles and isolated loss of the FPB and APB muscles may not be easy to diagnose
Innervation	• APB, FPB (superficial head), OP: recurrent branch of median nerve (C8–T1) • FPB (deep head): Deep branch of the ulnar nerve (C8–T1)
Blood supply	• Superficial and deep palmar arches, princeps pollicis arteries

The **adductor compartment** is located deep to the thenar muscles and contains the adductor pollicis muscle, which is innervated by the deep branch of the ulnar nerve. This muscle has oblique and transverse heads that originate broadly from the 2nd and 3rd metacarpals, capitate, and trapezoid to insert on the medial aspect of the base of the proximal phalanx of the 1st digit. This allows it to adduct the thumb toward the rest of the hand, which is different from opposition in that the 1st metacarpal remains in the same plane as the other metacarpals. It is located just anterior to the 1st interosseous muscle. The adductor pollicis typically contains two, small sesamoid bones near the 1st MCP joint and may contain a single sesamoid bone near the 2nd MCP joint.

Adductor Pollicis

Proximal attachments	• Transverse head: shaft of the 3rd metacarpal • Oblique head: trapezoid, capitate, and bases of the 2nd and 3rd metacarpals
Distal attachment	• Medial aspect of base of proximal phalanx of 1st digit
Functions	• Adducts the thumb toward the rest of the hand
Muscle testing and signs of damage	• In the event of a deep ulnar nerve lesion, isolated dysfunction of this muscle would leave the patient unable to adduct the thumb against resistance. It is important to isolate adduction from opposition and flexion of the thumb
Innervation	• Deep branch of the ulnar nerve (C8–T1)
Blood supply	• Superficial and deep palmar arches, dorsal metacarpal, princeps pollicis arteries

The major structures in the **central compartment** of the palmar hand are the tendons of the flexor pollicis longus, flexor digitorum superficialis, and flexor digitorum profundus as well as vessels and nerves that will be discussed shortly. The central compartment is where some unusual muscles, the **lumbricals**, originate. The four lumbrical muscles are strange in that instead of bone, they originate from the tendons of the flexor digitorum profundus. The **1st and 2nd lumbrical muscles** are unipennate (single bellied) muscles that extend off the lateral aspect of the flexor digitorum profundus tendons to digits 2 and 3. They are innervated by the median nerve. The **3rd and 4th lumbrical muscles** are bipennate and arise from the tendons going to digits 3 and 4 (3rd lumbrical), and 4 and 5 (4th lumbrical), respectively. They are innervated by the deep branch of the ulnar nerve. Another bizarre aspect of the lumbricals is their insertion. They each cross the palmar aspect of their corresponding MCP joint (1st lumbrical = 2nd digit, 2nd lumbrical = 3rd digit, 3rd lumbrical = 4th digit, 4th lumbrical = 5th digit) before inserting onto the dorsolateral aspect of the extensor expansion of that digit. Because they are travelling along the palmar side of the metacarpal head, they flex the MCP when they contract. However, since they insert into the extensor expansion proximal to the middle phalanx, they are strong extensors of the PIP and DIP.

Lumbrical Muscles

Proximal attachments	• All lumbricals originate from the tendons of the flexor digitorum profundus
	  • 1st lumbrical: lateral aspect of tendon to digit 2
	  • 2nd lumbrical: lateral aspect of tendon to digit 3
	  • 3rd lumbrical: medial aspect of tendon to digit 3 and lateral aspect of tendon to digit 4
	  • 4th lumbrical: medial aspect of tendon to digit 4 and lateral aspect of tendon to digit 5

Distal attachment	• Extensor expansion between MCP and PIP joints on the lateral side of digits 2–5
Functions	• Each lumbrical will flex the MCP joint, but this can be countered by the digital extensor muscles to keep the joints extended • Each lumbrical can also strongly extend its associated PIP and DIP joint. No other muscles are able to do this effectively
Muscle testing and signs of damage	• In the case of lumbrical dysfunction, when the patient is asked to extend the fingers strongly, the MCP joints will extend strongly but the PIP and DIP joints will extend weakly. Flexion of MCP, PIP, and DIP joints will be unaffected since other muscles contribute to flexion of the digits • Damage to the median nerve will cause dysfunction related to the 1st and 2nd lumbrical, affecting digits 2 and 3 • Damage to the ulnar nerve or deep ulnar nerve will cause dysfunction related to the 3rd and 4th lumbricals, affecting digits 4 and 5
Innervation	• 1st and 2nd: median nerve • 3rd and 4th: deep branch of ulnar nerve
Blood supply	• Superficial palmar arch, common palmar digital arteries

There are two distinct sets of muscles within the interosseous compartments between the metacarpal bones. These interosseous muscles have some characteristics in common with the lumbricals in that their tendons cross the MCP joints before inserting onto the extensor expansions of digits 2 to 5. Because of this they can flex the MCP and (weakly) extend the PIP and DIP joints. However, since their insertions are close to the medial and lateral side of the extensor expansion, they adduct and abduct the digits. The reference point for abduction and adduction of the digits is the midline of the 3rd digit. If a digit moves away from that line, it is abduction, moving toward it is adduction.

There are three unipennate **palmar interossei** that adduct digits 2, 4, 5 toward the 3rd digit (mnemonic: **PAD** = **P**almar **AD**duct). The 3rd digit cannot adduct since it cannot move closer to its own midline. The first palmar interosseous muscle originates from the medial side of the 2nd metacarpal and inserts on the medial aspect of the 2nd digit's extensor expansion. The other two palmar interosseous muscles originate from the lateral aspect of the 4th and 5th metacarpals and insert on the lateral aspect of the corresponding extensor expansions. The separate adductor pollicis muscle is responsible for moving the 1st digit toward the hand's midline.

There are four **dorsal interossei** and they abduct digits 2, 3, and 4 away from the midline of the 3rd digit (mnemonic: **DAB** = **D**orsal **AB**duct). Both medial and lateral motions of the 3rd digit are called abduction since both motions shift it away from its neutral midline. Unlike the palmar interossei, the dorsal interossei are bipennate and originate from two neighboring metacarpals. The very large first dorsal interosseous muscle originates from the 1st and 2nd metacarpals and inserts on the lateral aspect of the 2nd digit's extensor expansion. The second, from 2nd and 3rd metacarpals inserts on the lateral side of the 3rd digit's extensor expansion, while the third dorsal interosseous muscle originates from the 3rd and 4th metacarpals and inserts on the medial side of the 3rd digit's extensor expansion. The fourth dorsal interosseous originates between the 4th and 5th metacarpals and inserts on the medial aspect of the 4th digit's extensor expansion. Recall that a separate muscle, the abductor digiti minimi, abducts the 5th digit.

Palmar and Dorsal Interosseous Muscles

See Clinical Correlation 10.20.

Proximal attachments	• Palmar: (1st) medial aspect of metacarpal 2; (2nd and 3rd) lateral aspect of metacarpals 4 and 5 • Dorsal: (1st) between metacarpals 1 and 2; (2nd) between metacarpals 2 and 3; (3rd) between metacarpals 3 and 4; (4th) between metacarpals 4 and 5
Distal attachment	• Palmar: (1st) medial extensor expansion of digit 2 and (2nd and 3rd) lateral extensor expansion of digits 4–5 • Dorsal: (1st and 2nd) lateral side of extensor expansion of digits 2–3, and medial extensor expansion of digits 3–4
Functions	• Both palmar and dorsal interossei can flex MCP and extend PIP and DIP joints although not very strongly • Palmar: Adduct digits 2, 4, and 5 toward the 3rd digit • Dorsal: Abduct digits 2, 3, and 4 away from the 3rd digit's neutral midline
Muscle testing and signs of damage	• Damage to an interosseous muscle tendon can result in isolated loss of function • Palmar interossei are tested by seeing if the patient can maintain active adduction of the digits against gentle pressure. They can also be assessed by having a patient hold a sheet of paper between the digits as the examiner pulls on it • Dorsal interossei can be tested by having the patient actively abduct the digits against gentle pressure • Since the palmar and dorsal interossei share the same innervation, both groups are affected by damage to the deep branch of the ulnar nerve
Innervation	• Deep branch of the ulnar nerve (C8–T1)
Blood supply	• Deep palmar arches, palmar metacarpal, radialis indicis arteries

CLINICAL CORRELATION 10.20 Injuries to the Hand and Digits

Because we use our hands to interact with our environment, they are often exposed to injury. The metacarpals and phalanges can be fractured by direct trauma or crushing injury. A common injury of the 4th and 5th metacarpals is a **boxer's fracture**, which occurs when a punch is too powerful for the hand (often due to a loosely held fist) and the impact breaks the metacarpals. These typically leave a bump that grows less pronounced with age.

When an extended finger is suddenly flexed, the distal insertion of the extensor expansion can be torn, often causing an avulsion at its attachment onto the dorsal base of the distal phalanx. In this state, the pull of the flexor digitorum profundus will cause the distal interphalangeal (DIP) to be permanently flexed. Someone thought this looked like a hammer and named it **mallet finger**. This often occurs when the fingers are jammed by a ball or when sliding finger-first into a base during a game of baseball. For this reason, it is also sometimes called baseball finger.

On the opposite side of the digit, **jersey finger** results from sudden, forceful extension of the DIP joint (as if trying to grab a football or rugby jersey with a fingertip), which can rupture the tendon of the flexor digitorum profundus or avulse its attachment to the palmar side of the base of the distal phalanx.

Skier's thumb results from forceful abduction of the thumb away from the head of the 1st metacarpal. This injury ruptures the medial collateral ligament at the metacarpophalangeal joint of the pollux. This occurs when the thumb is forced back while the rest of the hand continues forward, as when a skier falls and their hand pushes into powdery snow but the thumb is pushed upward by a ski pole. This condition was formerly called **game-keeper's thumb** due to the strain caused by repeated shooting of firearms with grips that recoiled into the medial aspect of the thumb, forcing it posteriorly. The adductor pollicis may also be strained in this injury.

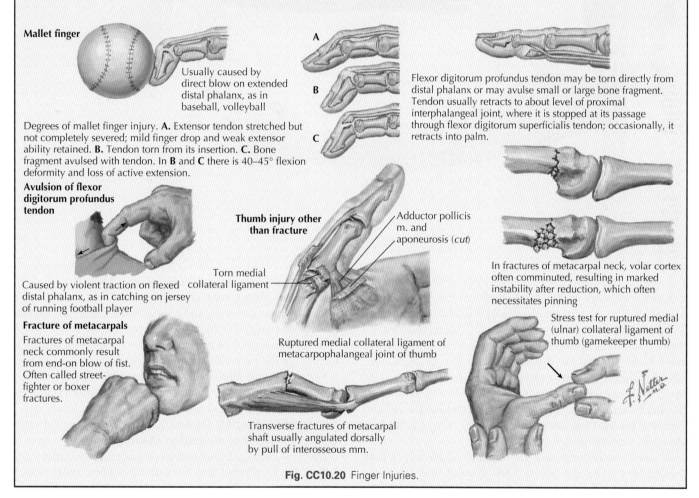

Mallet finger

Usually caused by direct blow on extended distal phalanx, as in baseball, volleyball

Degrees of mallet finger injury. **A.** Extensor tendon stretched but not completely severed; mild finger drop and weak extensor ability retained. **B.** Tendon torn from its insertion. **C.** Bone fragment avulsed with tendon. In **B** and **C** there is 40–45° flexion deformity and loss of active extension.

Avulsion of flexor digitorum profundus tendon

Caused by violent traction on flexed distal phalanx, as in catching on jersey of running football player

Fracture of metacarpals

Fractures of metacarpal neck commonly result from end-on blow of fist. Often called street-fighter or boxer fractures.

Thumb injury other than fracture

Torn medial collateral ligament

Adductor pollicis m. and aponeurosis (cut)

Ruptured medial collateral ligament of metacarpophalangeal joint of thumb

Transverse fractures of metacarpal shaft usually angulated dorsally by pull of interosseous mm.

Flexor digitorum profundus tendon may be torn directly from distal phalanx or may avulse small or large bone fragment. Tendon usually retracts to about level of proximal interphalangeal joint, where it is stopped at its passage through flexor digitorum superficialis tendon; occasionally, it retracts into palm.

In fractures of metacarpal neck, volar cortex often comminuted, resulting in marked instability after reduction, which often necessitates pinning.

Stress test for ruptured medial (ulnar) collateral ligament of thumb (gamekeeper thumb)

Fig. CC10.20 Finger Injuries.

INNERVATION OF THE UPPER LIMBS

The Spinal Nerves to the Upper Limb and Dermatomes (Fig. 10.17)

The neuroanatomy of the spinal cord, spinal nerve, posterior and anterior rami have been described in Chapters 4 and 9. Since we have already discussed the long motor and sensory tracts affecting muscles of the upper limb, we will not be discussing them separately. In this chapter we will discuss how the C4 to T2 anterior rami innervate the muscles of the upper limb and convey sensation from it. These rami interconnect and then

separate to form all the nerves associated with the upper limb. The dermatomes associated with each spinal nerve remain as distinct strips of skin along the upper limb, even if the axons conveying sensation from a dermatome return along several different peripheral nerves.

The dermatomes on the dorsal side of the upper and lower limbs appear neatly segmented; however, on the other side the dermatomes converge on a ventral axial line that separates C5 from T1. The C4 dermatome extends only as far as the top of the shoulder, the C5 dermatome stretches from the anterior chest onto the ventral side of the arm and forearm, following

Note: Schematic demarcation of dermatomes (according to Keegan and Garrett) shown as distinct segments. There is actually considerable overlap between adjacent dermatomes.

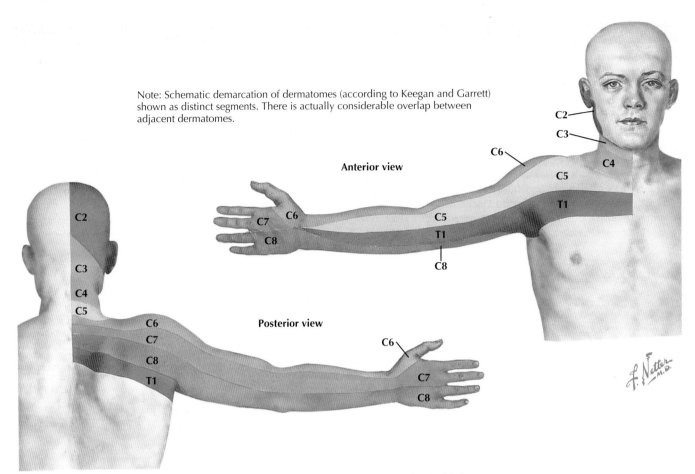

Fig. 10.17 Dermal Segmentation of the Upper Limb.

the ventral axial line. C6 progresses along both the anterior and posterior sides of the lateral shoulder, arm, forearm, and 1st digit. C7 is seen along the posterior shoulder, arm, forearm, and on the posterior and anterior sides of the hand and 2nd-3rd digits. The C8 dermatome lies along the anterior and posterior sides of the 4th and 5th digits and hand. The T1 dermatome stretches along the anterior and posterior inferior aspects of the upper limb, inferior to the ventral axial line. The T2 dermatome has been variably described as being present on the inferior aspect of the proximal arm and axilla or as being absent from the upper limb altogether.

It would be convenient if the muscles of the upper limb formed strips like the dermatomes. Instead, the myotomal mesenchymal cells fuse with others as they migrate down the limb and insert onto the developing bones. They drag their nerve supply behind them, creating the brachial plexus as they do so.

Brachial Plexus and the Axilla (Fig. 10.18)

C4 and T2 have small contributions to the skin of the superior shoulder and medial arm, respectively. It is the anterior rami of C5 to T1 that provide the majority of the axons that create the **brachial plexus**, which will innervate the skin and muscles of the upper limb. As C5 to T1 anterior rami exit each intervertebral foramen they travel laterally, passing between the anterior and middle scalene muscles to enter the axilla. The

axilla (armpit) is a large, pyramid-shaped space that contains the brachial plexus, subclavian artery and vein, many lymph nodes, lymphatic vessels, and a sometimes-staggering amount of adipose tissue. The medial border of the axilla is the thoracic wall and serratus anterior muscle, the anterior border is formed by the pectoralis minor and major muscles, the posterior wall is the subscapularis and latissimus dorsi muscles, the lateral wall is the medial aspect of the humerus, and the inferior wall is just the skin of the axilla. The subclavian artery and vein run alongside the brachial plexus for a considerable distance, wrapped in the **axillary sheath**, a protective layer of connective tissue. As the brachial plexus progresses more distally, it can be divided into five distinct regions: **roots** (which are really just anterior rami), **trunks, divisions, cords,** and **terminal nerves**.

Roots and Trunks of the Brachial Plexus

The C5 and C6 roots fuse to create the **superior trunk** of the brachial plexus; a small number of axons from C4 may join the C5 root and reach the superior trunk. The C7 root continues laterally and becomes the **middle trunk**. C8 and T1 roots fuse to create the **inferior trunk**.

The C5 root contributes to the **phrenic nerve (C3–C5)**, which descends along the anterior aspect of the anterior scalene muscle to enter the thorax and innervate the thoracic diaphragm. The **dorsal scapular nerve (C4–C5)** (Fig. 10.19) arises primarily

A. Brachial plexus: schema

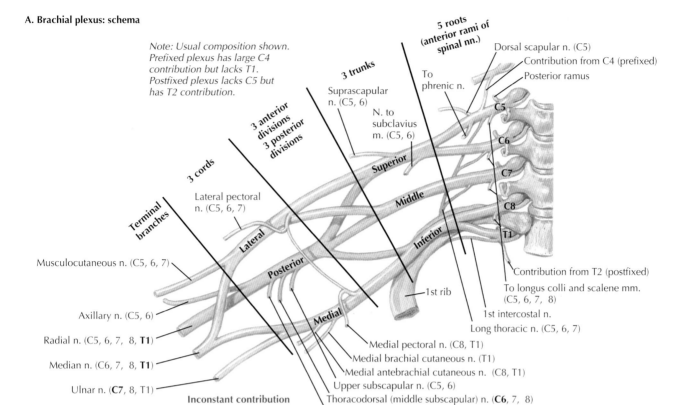

Note: Usual composition shown. Prefixed plexus has large C4 contribution but lacks T1. Postfixed plexus lacks C5 but has T2 contribution.

5 roots (anterior rami of spinal nn.)

3 trunks

3 anterior divisions / 3 posterior divisions

3 cords

Terminal branches

Suprascapular n. (C5, 6)

N. to subclavius m. (C5, 6)

To phrenic n.

Dorsal scapular n. (C5)

Contribution from C4 (prefixed)

Posterior ramus

C5

C6

C7

C8

T1

Superior

Middle

Inferior

Lateral

Posterior

Medial

1st rib

Lateral pectoral n. (C5, 6, 7)

Musculocutaneous n. (C5, 6, 7)

Axillary n. (C5, 6)

Radial n. (C5, 6, 7, 8, **T1**)

Median n. (C6, 7, 8, **T1**)

Ulnar n. (**C7**, 8, T1)

Inconstant contribution

Medial pectoral n. (C8, T1)

Medial brachial cutaneous n. (T1)

Medial antebrachial cutaneous n. (C8, T1)

Upper subscapular n. (C5, 6)

Thoracodorsal (middle subscapular) n. (**C6**, 7, 8)

Lower subscapular n. (C5, 6)

Contribution from T2 (postfixed)

To longus colli and scalene mm. (C5, 6, 7, 8)

1st intercostal n.

Long thoracic n. (C5, 6, 7)

B. Axilla (dissection): anterior view

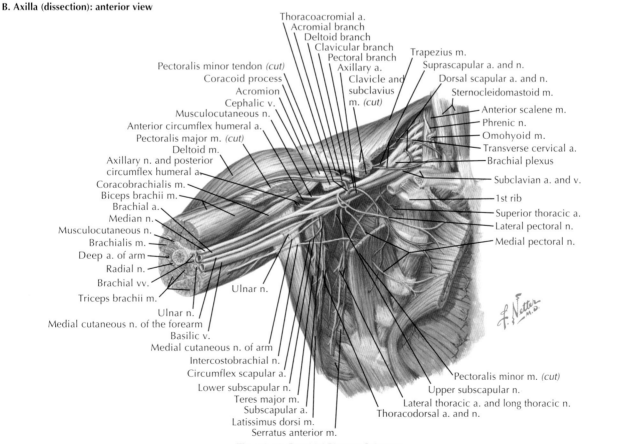

Thoracoacromial a.
Acromial branch
Deltoid branch
Clavicular branch
Pectoral branch
Axillary a.
Clavicle and subclavius m. (cut)

Pectoralis minor tendon (cut)
Coracoid process
Acromion
Cephalic v.
Musculocutaneous n.
Anterior circumflex humeral a.
Pectoralis major m. (cut)
Deltoid m.
Axillary n. and posterior circumflex humeral a.
Coracobrachialis m.
Biceps brachii m.
Brachial a.
Median n.
Musculocutaneous n.
Brachialis m.
Deep a. of arm
Radial n.
Brachial vv.
Triceps brachii m.
Ulnar n.

Ulnar n.
Medial cutaneous n. of the forearm
Basilic v.
Medial cutaneous n. of arm
Intercostobrachial n.
Circumflex scapular a.
Lower subscapular n.
Teres major m.
Subscapular a.
Latissimus dorsi m.
Serratus anterior m.

Trapezius m.
Suprascapular a. and n.
Dorsal scapular a. and n.
Sternocleidomastoid m.
Anterior scalene m.
Phrenic n.
Omohyoid m.
Transverse cervical a.
Brachial plexus
Subclavian a. and v.
1st rib
Superior thoracic a.
Lateral pectoral n.
Medial pectoral n.

Pectoralis minor m. (cut)
Upper subscapular n.
Lateral thoracic a. and long thoracic n.
Thoracodorsal a. and n.

Fig. 10.18 Brachial Plexus: Schema.

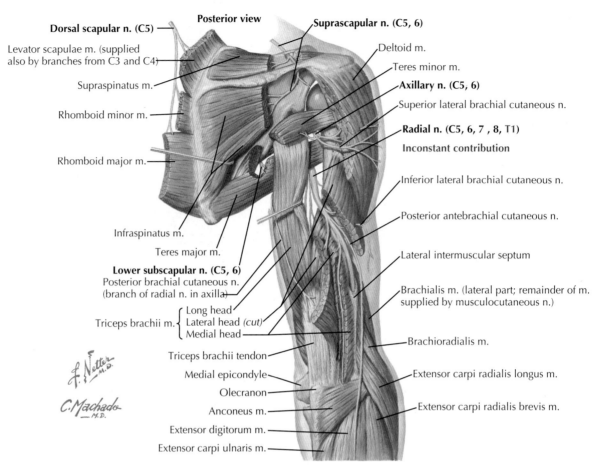

Posterior view

Dorsal scapular n. (C5)

Levator scapulae m. (supplied also by branches from C3 and C4)

Suprascapular n. (C5, 6)

Deltoid m.

Teres minor m.

Supraspinatus m.

Axillary n. (C5, 6)

Superior lateral brachial cutaneous n.

Rhomboid minor m.

Radial n. (C5, 6, 7 , 8, T1)

Inconstant contribution

Rhomboid major m.

Inferior lateral brachial cutaneous n.

Posterior antebrachial cutaneous n.

Lateral intermuscular septum

Infraspinatus m.

Teres major m.

Brachialis m. (lateral part; remainder of m. supplied by musculocutaneous n.)

Lower subscapular n. (C5, 6)
Posterior brachial cutaneous n. (branch of radial n. in axilla)

Triceps brachii m. { Long head / Lateral head *(cut)* / Medial head }

Brachioradialis m.

Triceps brachii tendon

Medial epicondyle

Extensor carpi radialis longus m.

Olecranon

Extensor carpi radialis brevis m.

Anconeus m.

Extensor digitorum m.

Extensor carpi ulnaris m.

Fig. 10.19 Scapular, Axillary, and Radial Nerves.

from C5 and descends along the posterior thorax to innervate the levator scapulae, rhomboid major and minor muscles. The C5 to C7 roots give off branches that form the **long thoracic nerve (C5–C7)** (see Fig. 10.9) that travels inferiorly along the thoracic wall to innervate the serratus anterior muscle. Short individual branches from the C5, C6, C7, and C8 roots extend anteromedially to innervate the longus coli and longus capitis muscles in the anterior neck.

The **subclavius nerve** (C5–C6) originates from the superior trunk and travels to the inferior aspect of the clavicle to reach the subclavius muscle. It frequently contributes an accessory root that joins the phrenic nerve. The superior trunk also gives off the much larger **suprascapular nerve (C5–C6)** (see Fig. 10.19) that moves laterally and posteriorly to pass deep to the superior transverse scapular ligament, through the scapular notch, to innervate the supraspinatus muscle. It continues inferiorly, crossing lateral to the scapular notch to innervate the infraspinatus muscle. No nerves typically leave the middle or inferior trunks.

Divisions of the Brachial Plexus

Each trunk splits into a posterior division and an anterior division. These divisions mark the dorsal and ventral muscle masses during development of the upper limb and their migration to their respective sides of the upper limb. The **posterior cord** is formed by the fusion of all three of the

posterior divisions and it will innervate the extensor muscles of the upper limb. The anterior divisions of the superior and middle trunks fuse to form the **lateral cord** while the anterior division of the inferior cord continues alone to form the **medial cord**. The nerves derived from the anterior divisions, and thereafter the lateral and medial cords, innervate flexor muscles.

Branches and Terminal Nerves from the Posterior Cord of the Brachial Plexus

The posterior cord gives off three small but important nerves before terminating: the **upper subscapular (C5), thoracodorsal (C6–C8)**, and **lower subscapular (C6) nerves** (see Fig. 10.18). The upper and lower subscapular nerves extend posteriorly to innervate the subscapularis muscle, the lower subscapular nerve also innervates the teres major muscle. The **thoracodorsal nerve** stretches inferiorly across the subscapularis muscle to reach the latissimus dorsi muscle, which it innervates. The posterior cord ends when it bifurcates into its two terminal branches, the **axillary** and **radial nerves**.

The **axillary nerve (C5–C6)** (Fig. 10.20, see also Fig. 10.19) wraps around the posterior aspect of the surgical neck of the humerus to pass through the quadrangular space (bounded laterally by the humerus, medially by the long head of the triceps brachii, superiorly by the teres minor muscle, and inferiorly by the teres major muscle) to innervate the teres minor and deltoid

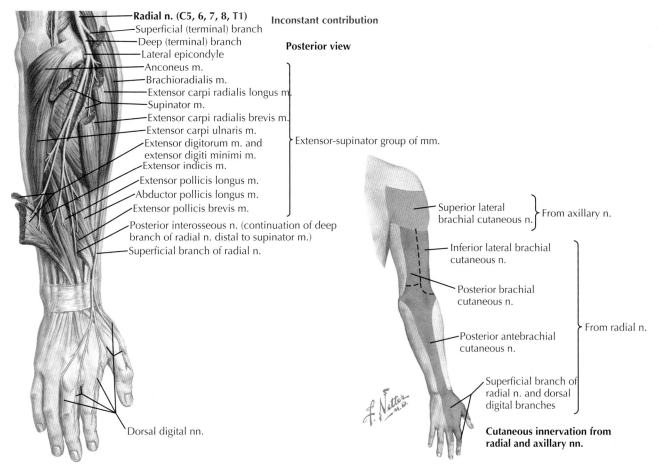

Fig. 10.20 Radial Nerve in the Forearm.

muscles. A cutaneous branch of the axillary nerve, the **superior lateral brachial cutaneous nerve**, conveys sensations from the lateral shoulder (Clinical Correlation 10.21).

The massive **radial nerve (C5–T1)** (see Figs. 10.19 and 10.20) passes posteriorly through the triangular interval (bounded medially by the long head of the triceps brachii, laterally by the lateral head of the triceps brachii, and superiorly by the teres major muscle) to wrap around the posterior aspect of the humeral shaft within the radial groove,

innervating all three heads of the triceps brachii and the anconeus muscle along the way. In the arm the radial nerve gives off three large sensory branches that convey sensations from the regions indicated by their names. They are the **inferior lateral brachial cutaneous nerve**, the **posterior brachial cutaneous nerve**, and the long **posterior antebrachial cutaneous nerve**. The posterior antebrachial cutaneous nerve pierces the lateral head of the triceps brachii muscle and then descends along the posterolateral aspect of the forearm. The rest of the radial nerve continues inferiorly within the lateral intermuscular septum, passing across the lateral aspect of the elbow, and innervating the brachioradialis and long head of the extensor carpi radialis muscles. Some branches from the radial nerve may innervate parts of the brachialis muscle. As the radial nerve continues across the lateral epicondyle of the humerus it splits into a superficial and deep branch. The **superficial branch of the radial nerve** travels along the extensor carpi radialis tendons and conveys sensations from the posterolateral wrist and lateral dorsum of the hand before it splits into **dorsal digital nerves** that convey sensations from the dorsal aspect of digits 1 to 3, excluding area around the fingernails. The **deep branch of the radial nerve (C7–C8)** continues distally through the posterior forearm, innervating the short head of the extensor carpi radialis and the supinator, which it passes through to reach the extensor digitorum, extensor digiti minimi, and

CLINICAL CORRELATION 10.22   Damage to the Radial Nerve

Damage to the Radial Nerve Near the Shoulder

If the radial nerve is damaged shortly after it leaves the posterior cord, all of the muscles it innervates in the posterior arm and forearm will be paralyzed, with the exception of the brachioradialis, which often receives additional axons from the musculocutaneous nerve. This will manifest with weakness: extending the forearm at the elbow, supinating the forearm when the elbow is extended, and extending the wrist and all digits at the metacarpophalangeal (MCP) joints. Due to this, **wrist drop** is a common sign of radial nerve injury. Grip strength will also be compromised since contraction of the digital and carpal flexors must be counter-balanced by the extensors to maintain an optimal grip. Sensory losses will be noted across the posterior and lateral arm, posterior forearm, and dorsum of the hand, including the dorsal aspects of the digits 1, 2, and the lateral side of digit 3. The radial nerve is especially vulnerable during a spiral fracture of the humerus as it crosses the posterior side of the bone along the radial groove. However, the function of the triceps brachii is often spared in this instance since many of those motor axons leave the radial nerve before it reaches the radial groove.

Damage to the Radial Nerve Near the Elbow

Lacerations of the radial nerve's branches in the forearm produce very distinct clinical signs. Injury to the superficial radial nerve will generally produce only sensory losses on the dorsal aspect of the hand and digits 1–3. The exact area involved can vary considerably. The deep radial nerve contains only motor neurons. Injury to it will cause flaccid paralysis to any "downstream" muscles that receive axons from it or the posterior interosseous nerve. The exact muscles involved will depend on precisely where the nerve was damaged. Weakness extending digits 2–5 at the MCP or making the tendons of the "anatomical snuff box" stand out are indicative of damage to the deep branch of the radial nerve or posterior interosseous nerve.

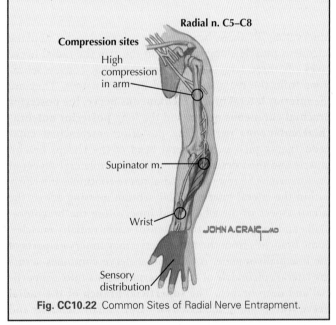

Fig. CC10.22 Common Sites of Radial Nerve Entrapment.

Branches and Terminal Nerves from the Lateral Cord of the Brachial Plexus

The lateral cord gives off a **lateral pectoral nerve (C5–C7)** (see Fig. 10.18) that innervates the clavicular head of the pectoralis major muscle as well as the anterior belly of the deltoid muscle (may be shared with axillary nerve). The lateral cord bifurcates to form the musculocutaneous nerve and a lateral contribution to the median nerve. The **musculocutaneous nerve (C5–C7)** (Fig. 10.21) dives into the anterior compartment of the arm, piercing the coracobrachialis muscle before moving into the short and long heads of the biceps brachii muscle. It descends on the anterior surface of the brachialis muscle, which it also innervates. It also travels across the anterior aspect of the lateral epicondyle and frequently innervates part of the brachioradialis muscle before giving off the cutaneous **lateral cutaneous nerve of the forearm**. This nerve splits into an anterior branch and posterior branch that convey sensation from the lateral forearm from the elbow to the wrist (Clinical Correlation 10.23).

Branches and Terminal Nerves from the Medial Cord of the Brachial Plexus

The medial cord gives off the **medial pectoral nerve (C8–T1)** (see Fig. 10.18), which passes posterior to the axillary artery before innervating the pectoralis minor muscle. It continues through the pectoralis minor to reach and innervate the sterno-costal and abdominal portions of the pectoralis major muscle. Like the lateral pectoral nerve, it gets its name from the cord from which it originates. In fact, on the chest it is usually seen more laterally than the lateral pectoral nerve. Interestingly, a small branch of the lateral pectoral nerve passes anterior to the axillary artery to join the medial pectoral nerve. Two cutaneous nerves, the **medial antebrachial cutaneous nerve (C8–T1)** and **medial brachial cutaneous nerve (C8–T1)** arise from the medial cord distal to the medial pectoral nerve. They descend on the medial aspect of the arm and forearm, providing cutaneous sensation along their courses. The medial cord terminates as the ulnar nerve and a medial contribution to the median nerve.

The **ulnar nerve (C8–T1)** (Fig. 10.22) continues inferiorly on the medial side of the arm, passing posterior to the medial epicondyle of the humerus, in the **cubital tunnel**, before entering the anterior compartment of the forearm, where it innervates two muscles, the flexor carpi ulnaris and the medial (ulnar) side of the flexor digitorum profundus, which sends flexor tendons to digits 4 and 5. Before crossing the wrist, the ulnar nerve gives off a **dorsal branch** that travels posteriorly to convey sensory innervation from the medial dorsal side of the hand, as well as the 5th digit and the medial half of the 4th digit via **dorsal digital nerves**. The ulnar nerve also branches to create the **palmar branch** that innervates the medial side of the wrist and base of the hypothenar eminence. The rest of the nerve passes deep to the palmar carpal ligament to pass between the pisiform bone and the hook of the hamate, making the **ulnar canal** (of Guyon). After exiting the canal and entering the palmar hand, the ulnar nerve splits into a deep branch and superficial branch. The **superficial branch of the ulnar nerve** is cutaneous and innervates the skin of the hypothenar eminence and the medial side of the 5th digit via a **proper palmar digital nerve**. It

extensor carpi ulnaris in the posterior forearm. The final motor branch of the radial nerve is the **posterior interosseous nerve (C7–C8)**, which runs along the posterior aspect of the interosseous membrane, innervating the abductor pollicis longus, extensor pollicis brevis, extensor pollicis longus, and extensor indicis muscles (Clinical Correlation 10.22).

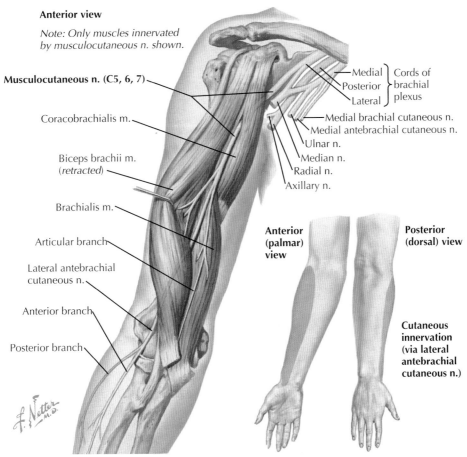

Anterior view

*Note: Only muscles innervated
by musculocutaneous n. shown.*

Musculocutaneous n. (C5, 6, 7)

Coracobrachialis m.

Biceps brachii m.
(*retracted*)

Brachialis m.

Articular branch

Lateral antebrachial
cutaneous n.

Anterior branch

Posterior branch

Medial ⎤
Posterior ⎬ Cords of
Lateral ⎦ brachial plexus

Medial brachial cutaneous n.
Medial antebrachial cutaneous n.
Ulnar n.
Median n.
Radial n.
Axillary n.

Anterior
(palmar)
view

Posterior
(dorsal) view

Cutaneous
innervation
(via lateral
antebrachial
cutaneous n.)

Fig. 10.21 Musculocutaneous Nerve.

CLINICAL CORRELATION 10.23 Damage to the Musculocutaneous Nerve

The musculocutaneous nerve enters the anterior compartment of the arm shortly after leaving the lateral cord. Therefore it does not frequently get injured in isolation. When this does occur, it would result in flaccid paralysis of the coracobrachialis, biceps brachii, and brachialis muscles. This would result in profound weakness flexing the forearm at the elbow (the brachioradialis is often dually innervated by the musculocutaneous and radial nerves and would still allow some flexion to occur) and supinating the forearm in a flexed position. There will be altered or absent sensation along an elongated patch of skin on the lateral forearm.

also gives off a **common palmar digital nerve** that splits to become the **proper palmar digital nerves** for the lateral side of the 5th digit and the medial side of the 4th digit. The exclusively motor **deep branch of the ulnar nerve** arches laterally across the deep palm to innervate the muscles of the hypothenar eminence, palmar and dorsal interossei, lumbricals 3 and 4 (to digits 4 and 5), and the adductor pollicis. Rarely, the 1st dorsal interosseous and adductor pollicis muscles can be innervated by axons from the superficial radial nerve (Clinical Correlation 10.24).

The **lateral (C6–C7)** and **medial roots (C8–T1)** of the median nerve converge from their respective cords to create the **median nerve (C6–T1)** (Fig. 10.23). The median nerve travels inferiorly along the medial aspect of the humerus and then along the anterior

midline of the forearm. Aside from the two forearm muscles innervated by the ulnar nerve, the median nerve innervates all the muscles of the forearm: pronator teres, flexor carpi radialis, palmaris longus, flexor carpi ulnaris, and the flexor digitorum superficialis. The median nerve gives off a deep branch, the **anterior interosseous nerve** that travels along the anterior aspect of the interosseous membrane between the radius and ulna. It innervates the lateral (radial) side of the flexor digitorum profundus, the flexor pollicis longus, and pronator quadratus muscles. Before leaving the forearm, the median nerve gives off a **palmar branch** that innervates the skin over the flexor retinaculum. The rest of the median nerve then travels through the carpal tunnel alongside the tendons of the flexor digitorum superficialis, flexor digitorum profundus, and flexor pollicis longus. After it passes through the carpal tunnel, the median nerve gives off the **recurrent branch of the median nerve**, which innervates the muscles of the thenar eminence. In the hand, it innervates the 1st and 2nd lumbricals (to digits 2 and 3) and branches into three cutaneous **common palmar digital nerves** that continue branching into **proper palmar digital nerves** for digits 1, 2, 3, and the lateral half of digit 4 (Clinical Correlations 10.25 and 10.26).

Autonomic Innervation of the Upper Limb (Fig. 10.24)

In the upper and lower limbs, the sympathetic nervous system innervates sweat glands in the skin as well as the smooth muscle sphincters that regulate blood flow to skeletal muscles. For the

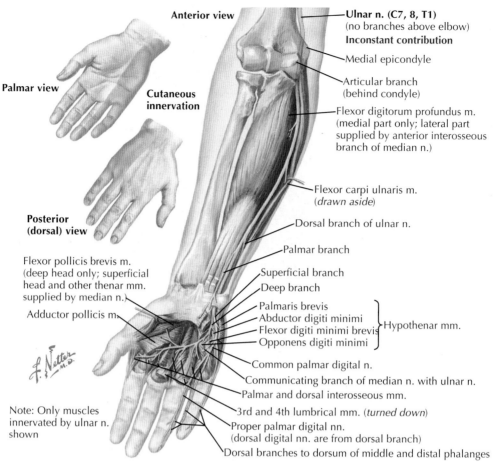

Anterior view

Ulnar n. (C7, 8, T1)
(no branches above elbow)
Inconstant contribution

Medial epicondyle

Articular branch
(behind condyle)

Flexor digitorum profundus m.
(medial part only; lateral part
supplied by anterior interosseous
branch of median n.)

Flexor carpi ulnaris m.
(*drawn aside*)

Dorsal branch of ulnar n.

Palmar branch

Superficial branch

Deep branch

Palmaris brevis
Abductor digiti minimi
Flexor digiti minimi brevis
Opponens digiti minimi
Hypothenar mm.

Common palmar digital n.

Communicating branch of median n. with ulnar n.

Palmar and dorsal interosseous mm.

3rd and 4th lumbrical mm. (*turned down*)

Proper palmar digital nn.
(dorsal digital nn. are from dorsal branch)

Dorsal branches to dorsum of middle and distal phalanges

Palmar view

Cutaneous innervation

Posterior (dorsal) view

Flexor pollicis brevis m.
(deep head only; superficial
head and other thenar mm.
supplied by median n.)

Adductor pollicis m.

Note: Only muscles
innervated by ulnar n.
shown

Fig. 10.22 Ulnar Nerve.

upper limbs specifically, pre-ganglionic sympathetic axons from the intermediolateral cell columns from T1 to T5 project their axons through their respective anterior roots, spinal nerves, and anterior rami. These axons leave the anterior rami as white rami communicans to reach the sympathetic chain, specifically the middle cervical, inferior cervical, and 1st thoracic ganglia. A stellate ganglion is frequently seen in this area and is simply a fusion of the inferior cervical and first thoracic ganglia. Within these ganglia are the post-ganglionic sympathetic nerve cells that project their axons back to the spinal nerve along gray rami communicans. Once in the spinal nerve, the post-ganglionic axons can travel to the back via posterior rami or to the upper limb via the anterior rami and brachial plexus. These axons travel along all the peripheral nerves, leaving along the way to innervate the smooth muscle sphincters within skeletal muscle as well as sweat glands, arrector pili muscles, and pre-capillary sphincters in the skin (Clinical Correlation 10.27).

THE BLOOD SUPPLY TO THE UPPER LIMBS

Proximal Arteries of the Upper Limb and Subclavian Artery (Fig. 10.25)

In addition to the arteries that supply the thoracic organs, the thoracic aorta gives off **posterior intercostal arteries** that supply blood to intercostal spaces 3 to 11. While these supply blood to the intercostal muscles and overlying skin,

they also contribute blood to the serratus anterior and pectoralis major muscles (as anterior intercostal arteries) near the sternum.

The **subclavian artery** arises from the brachiocephalic trunk on the right and directly from the arch of the aorta on the left side. It has several important branches that characteristically arise from it, but one must always remember that variation around this pattern is very common.

- **Internal thoracic artery:** supplies the anterior thoracic wall, sternum, and medial aspect of the pectoralis major muscles, meeting the anterior intercostal arteries as mentioned above.
- **Vertebral artery**: ascends through the transverse foramina of C6 up to C1 to supply blood to the brainstem and cerebrum.
- **Thyrocervical trunk:** this single trunk splits into several arteries, which may branch directly from the subclavian artery in some cases. Some branches like the inferior thyroid, ascending cervical, deep cervical, and supreme intercostal arteries do not supply blood to the upper limb; however, other branches do supply proximal limb structures.
- **Suprascapular artery:** passes posteriorly to run alongside the suprascapular nerve. It runs lateral to the inferior belly of the omohyoid muscle and superior to the transverse scapular ligament to provide branches to the supraspinatus muscle. It follows the suprascapular nerve laterally around the scapular notch and gives off branches to the infraspinatus muscle. Within the muscle it forms

CLINICAL CORRELATION 10.24 Damage to the Ulnar Nerve

Damage to the Ulnar Nerve Superior to the Forearm

The ulnar nerve has a long course down the medial aspect of the arm, forearm, and wrist and it can be injured at several points along its descent. The first motor axons do not leave the nerve until it reaches the medial forearm, so injuries between the proximal forearm and its origin from the medial cord can cause total loss of function related to the ulnar nerve. This can occur due to penetrating trauma and may also be caused by a fracture of the distal humerus that displaces the medial epicondyle and stretches or lacerates the ulnar nerve within the cubital tunnel. Avulsion of the medial epicondyle by the common flexor tendon or ulnar collateral ligaments also frequently cause ulnar nerve signs. The ulnar nerve can also be compressed by the humeral and ulnar heads of the flexor carpi ulnaris muscle in the same region. Damage in this area will result in weakness flexing the wrist (flexor carpi ulnaris) and the DIP joints of digits 4–5 (ulnar side of the flexor digitorum profundus). The unbalanced pull from the intact flexor carpi radialis and extensor carpi radialis muscle will cause persistent radial deviation of the wrist.

Past the wrist, this injury will manifest with weakness in the muscles of the hypothenar eminence, lumbricals 3–4 (to digits 4 and 5), the adductor pollicis, a portion of the flexor pollicis brevis, and the palmar and dorsal interosseous muscles. Sensory loss along the medial aspect of the hand (5th digit and the medial aspect of the 4th digit) on the dorsum and palmar sides will also typically occur. Damage to the ulnar nerve in the arm or proximal elbow will result in weakness flexing the distal interphalangeal (DIP) joints of digits 4–5. This is useful clinically since the patient will be unable to make a tight fist when asked to do so, with digits 4 and 5 remaining somewhat extended. This clinical sign is known as the **claw hand** and is accompanied by atrophy of the interosseous muscles. Slightly paradoxically, since the lumbrical muscles to digits 4 and 5 are affected, the patient will also be unable to strongly extend the proximal interphalangeal and DIP joints of those digits.

Damage to the Ulnar Nerve at the Wrist and Hand

The ulnar nerve is prone to becoming compressed as it passes through the ulnar canal covered by the pisohamate ligament. This compression can occur when prolonged pressure is applied to the pisiform or hamate bones by the handlebars of bicycles or motorcycles (**cyclist's palsy/neuropathy**) and will cause sensory loss along the medial aspect of the hand and the muscles in the hand that are listed above. Since the forearm muscles are not affected by a lesion in this location, the claw hand sign will not be seen.

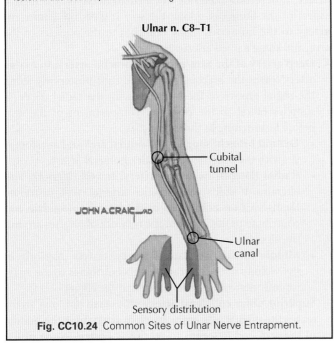

Fig. CC10.24 Common Sites of Ulnar Nerve Entrapment.

significant anastomoses with the dorsal scapular and circumflex scapular arteries.

- The **transverse cervical artery** (also called the **cervicodorsal trunk**) gives rise to two branches that supply structures related to the upper limb.
  - **Superficial cervical artery**: runs parallel to the spinal accessory nerve on the anterior aspect of the trapezius.
  - **Dorsal scapular artery**: passes posteriorly to weave between the heads of the levator scapulae muscle (which it perfuses), descending along the medial border of the scapula and supplying blood to the rhomboid minor and major muscles. The dorsal scapular artery may also arise directly from the subclavian artery.

Axillary Artery (See Fig. 10.25)

Once the subclavian artery crosses the lateral border of the first rib, the vessel changes its name to become the **axillary artery**, denoting its location in the axilla. The axillary artery passes posterior to the pectoralis minor muscle, which is a handy spatial reference for keeping track of the most common branching pattern of the vessels that originate from it.

The first section of the axillary artery is located proximal to the pectoralis minor muscle and has one branch.

- **Superior thoracic artery**: supplies blood to intercostal spaces 1 and 2, which are too far superior to receive posterior intercostal arteries from the aorta. It also typically provides blood to the subclavius and pectoralis major muscles.

The second section of the axillary artery is located posterior to the pectoralis minor muscle and has two branches that further subdivide.

- **Thoracoacromial artery/trunk**: this arterial trunk splits into four daughter arteries very quickly after leaving the axillary artery and passing medial to the pectoralis minor muscle. Note that these daughter arteries can sometimes leave the axillary artery directly.
  - **Clavicular branch**: travels superiorly toward the subclavius muscle.
  - **Pectoral branch**: travels inferiorly toward the pectoral muscles.
  - **Acromial branch**: travels superior to the coracoid process to reach the anterior aspect of the acromion and contributes to the **acromial anastomosis** along with the suprascapular and anterior circumflex humeral arteries.
  - **Deltoid branch**: travels laterally in the deltopectoral groove alongside the cephalic vein and a branch of the lateral pectoral nerve to supply the anterior belly of the deltoid and pectoralis major.
- **Lateral thoracic artery**: descends along the lateral wall of the thorax alongside the long thoracic nerve to supply the serratus anterior muscle, pectoralis major, nearby intercostal muscles, and the lateral breast. It sometimes originates as a branch of the thoracoacromial artery or from the third section of the axillary artery.

The third section of the axillary artery is located distal to the pectoralis minor muscle and has three branches that continue branching thereafter.

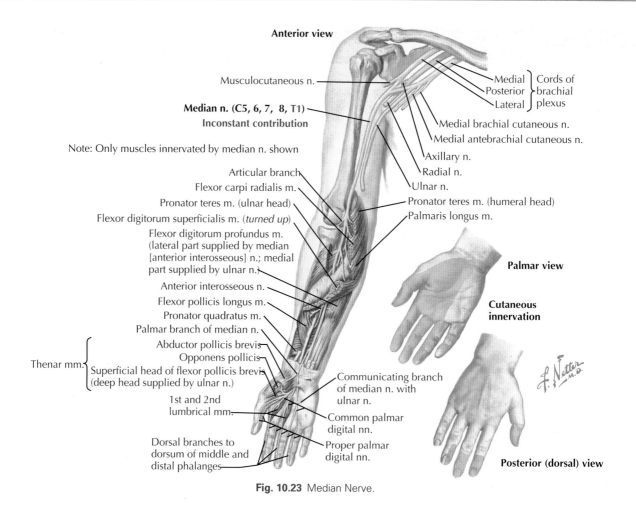

Anterior view

Musculocutaneous n.

Median n. (C5, 6, 7, 8, T1)
Inconstant contribution

Note: Only muscles innervated by median n. shown

Articular branch
Flexor carpi radialis m.
Pronator teres m. (ulnar head)
Flexor digitorum superficialis m. (*turned up*)
Flexor digitorum profundus m.
(lateral part supplied by median
[anterior interosseous] n.; medial
part supplied by ulnar n.)
Anterior interosseous n.
Flexor pollicis longus m.
Pronator quadratus m.
Palmar branch of median n.
Abductor pollicis brevis
Opponens pollicis
Superficial head of flexor pollicis brevis
(deep head supplied by ulnar n.)
Thenar mm.
1st and 2nd
lumbrical mm.
Dorsal branches to
dorsum of middle and
distal phalanges

Medial ⎱ Cords of
Posterior ⎬ brachial
Lateral ⎰ plexus
Medial brachial cutaneous n.
Medial antebrachial cutaneous n.
Axillary n.
Radial n.
Ulnar n.
Pronator teres m. (humeral head)
Palmaris longus m.

Palmar view

**Cutaneous
innervation**

Communicating branch
of median n. with
ulnar n.
Common palmar
digital nn.
Proper palmar
digital nn.

Posterior (dorsal) view

Fig. 10.23 Median Nerve.

- **Subscapular artery**: briefly descends along the lateral aspect of the subscapularis muscle before splitting into two large branches.
  - **Circumflex scapular artery**: passes superior to the teres major muscle as it travels posteriorly to reach the teres minor and infraspinatus muscles. It is a major contributor to the anastomoses in the infraspinous fossa along with the suprascapular and dorsal scapular arteries.
  - **Thoracodorsal artery**: continues inferiorly alongside the thoracodorsal nerve on the anterior side of the latissimus dorsi muscle, to which it is the major blood supply.
- **Anterior circumflex humeral artery**: this small artery crosses into the anterior compartment of the arm, moving along the surgical neck of the humerus while providing blood to the overlying muscles. It forms a significant anastomosis with the posterior circumflex humeral artery and also contributes to the acromial anastomosis.
- **Posterior circumflex humeral artery**: a large vessel that passes posteriorly along the surgical neck of the humerus, running parallel to the axillary nerve. It supplies all nearby muscles (posterior and middle bellies of deltoid, long and lateral heads of triceps brachii, teres minor and major) and anastomoses with the anterior circumflex humeral artery and deep brachial artery (Clinical Correlation 10.28).

Brachial Artery (Fig. 10.26)

As the axillary artery crosses the inferior border of the teres major muscle, it again changes its name to become the **brachial artery**. It descends alongside the median nerve on the medial aspect of the humerus. Along the way it gives off a **nutrient artery to the humerus**, many branches to the muscles of the arm, and some named arteries.

- **Deep artery of the arm/profunda brachii artery**: this large artery leaves the brachial artery and runs posteriorly along the radial groove of the humerus with the radial nerve. It supplies blood to the posterior compartment of the arm before terminating as three branches.
  - **Deltoid branch**: supplies the deltoid area and anastomoses with the posterior circumflex humeral artery.
  - **Radial (lateral) collateral artery**: travels inferiorly and laterally. It splits into smaller arteries that distribute themselves on both sides of the lateral epicondyle and contribute to the anastomotic network of arteries around the elbow.
  - **Middle (medial) collateral artery**: travels inferiorly in the vicinity of the olecranon and contributes to the anastomotic network of arteries around the elbow.
- **Superior ulnar collateral artery**: this small but long artery leaves the medial side of the brachial artery near the middle of the arm and descends to reach the posterior side of the

CLINICAL CORRELATION 10.25 Damage to the Median Nerve

Damage to the Median Nerve at or Superior to the Elbow

If the median nerve is damaged shortly after it forms from the lateral and medial cords, all of the muscles it innervates will be paralyzed, manifesting as loss of grip strength, pronation, and clumsiness of the thumb due to de-innervation of the flexor pollicis longus and thenar muscles (aside from part of the flexor pollicis brevis muscle). Sensory losses on the palmar side of digits 1–3 and the lateral ½ of the 4th digit will also occur. Damage to the median nerve in this area will affect the flexor digitorum superficialis, flexor pollicis longus, and part of the flexor digitorum profundus (specifically the tendons to digits 2 and 3). This is useful in clinical testing since the affected patients will have weakness flexing the interphalangeal joint of digit 1, the proximal interphalangeal joints of digits 2–5, and will be specifically unable to flex the distal interphalangeal joints of digits 2–3. When asked to make a tight fist, the affected patient will be unable to do so, with digits 2 and 3 remaining somewhat extended. This clinical sign is known as the **hand of benediction**. Occasionally a strut of bone, the supracondylar process, extends from the medial humeral shaft and projects a ligament (of Struthers) to the medial epicondyle. If that is the case, the median nerve passes deep to the ligament and can be compressed at that site. The median nerve can also be compressed by the bicipital aponeurosis or entrapped by the two heads of the pronator teres as it passes through the muscle. This may spare the flexor carpi radialis, palmaris longus, and flexor digitorum superficialis, which are innervated before the median nerve enters the pronator teres. This can be assessed by testing muscles innervated by the anterior interosseous nerve, which branches distal to the pronator teres. The affected patient will also be unable to strongly contract the flexor pollicis longus and the radial side of the flexor digitorum profundus to digits 2 and 3. The patient is asked to make a circle by pushing the tips of digits 1 and 2 (or 3) together strongly. The examiner may try to separate the fingers to find if strength is symmetric or weak on one side. This is a positive **weak pinch sign**. Another assessment involves gripping the patient's hand in a handshake grip and telling the patient to pronate the forearm against resistance. If the median nerve is entrapped in the pronator teres, this maneuver will exacerbate symptoms. The median nerve passes posteriorly between the humeroulnar and radial heads of the flexor digitorum superficialis and can be compressed there as well.

Damage to the Median Nerve Near the Wrist

Inflammation of the tendons of the flexor digitorum superficialis, flexor digitorum profundus, and flexor pollicis longus can compress the median nerve as they all pass through the carpal tunnel. **Carpal tunnel syndrome** typically manifests first as altered sensation along the skin innervated by the median nerve in the hand, the palmar aspects of digits 1–3 and the lateral palmar side of digit 4 along with the nail bed region of those same digits on the dorsal side. Later there will be motor losses associated with lumbricals 1 and 2 (to digits 2 and 3) and the thenar eminence via the recurrent branch of the median nerve. Atrophy of the thenar eminence may become visibly pronounced as this condition progresses. The muscles in the forearm that are innervated by the median nerve will not be affected. It is worth noting that a synovial cyst of the common digital tendon sheath can also compress the area and cause carpal tunnel syndrome. The irritated median nerve can be assessed by the **Tinel test** at the wrist, wherein the wrist is extended and the flexor retinaculum is percussed. The test is positive if the tapping results in radicular (shooting) pain along the sensory distribution of the median nerve in the hand; however, aggressive percussion can result in a positive test in those without carpal tunnel syndrome. The **Phalen test/maneuver** is another, more sensitive, test for carpal tunnel syndrome. In this test the dorsal aspects of both hands are pushed together for 45–60 s. A positive test results in the same sort of radicular pain as was described above.

One final note about the median nerve in the hand: because the median and ulnar nerves both innervate muscles and skin in the hand and because the C8–T1 roots contribute to both nerves, it is not uncommon to have some of the axons that would typically travel on one nerve arrive at their destination by following the other. This should be remembered when clinical signs do not fall neatly into median or ulnar neuropathies; there may be compression affecting one nerve that mimics the signs you would associate with the other. A Martin-Gruber anastomosis occurs when there is a direct connection between the distal branches of the median and ulnar nerves.

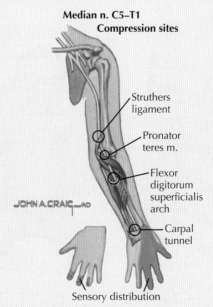

Median n. C5–T1
Compression sites

Struthers ligament

Pronator teres m.

Flexor digitorum superficialis arch

Carpal tunnel

JOHN A. CRAIG AD

Sensory distribution

Fig. CC10.25 Common Sites of Median Nerve Entrapment.

CLINICAL CORRELATION 10.26 Brachial Plexopathy

It is easier to understand damage to the rest of the brachial plexus (**brachial plexopathy**) after learning how injuries to the terminal nerves will manifest clinically. We can now interpret how more proximal injuries will manifest.

Damage to the Posterior Cord
Damage to the posterior cord will affect the axillary and radial nerves. This will cause a loss of sensation from the lateral shoulder (axillary), posterolateral arm, posterior forearm, dorsum of the hand, and dorsal aspects of digits 1–3 (radial). Motor dysfunctions will include the deltoid muscle (axillary), and extensor muscles of the arm, forearm, carpus, and digits (radial). In addition to the two terminal nerves, the subscapular and thoracodorsal nerves can also be affected, compromising the latissimus dorsi, subscapularis, and teres major muscles.

Damage to the Lateral Cord
Damage to the lateral cord will profoundly affect the musculocutaneous nerve and partially lesion the median nerve. This will cause a loss of sensation along the lateral forearm (musculocutaneous) as well as the palm and palmar aspect (and dorsal nail beds) of digits 1–3 and the lateral aspect of digit 4 (median). Motor losses will include all muscles of the anterior arm, which will make elbow flexion profoundly weak or absent (musculocutaneous). In the forearm, there will likely be weakness in pronation due to de-innervation of the pronator teres as some diffuse weakness in wrist and digit flexion because of partial de-innervation of the flexor carpi radialis, palmaris longus, flexor carpi ulnaris, and flexor digitorum superficialis muscles. These muscles will be weak rather than flaccid because some axons to these muscles come into the median nerve from the medial cord and they would not be affected. The lateral pectoral nerve may be affected, which would weaken the clavicular head of the pectoralis major muscle.

Damage to the Medial Cord
Damage to the medial cord will cause sensory losses including the palmar aspect of digit 3, as well as both palmar and dorsal sides of digits 4–5. Since the medial antebrachial cutaneous nerve and medial brachial cutaneous nerves both arise from the medial cord, sensory loss will include the C8–T1 dermatomes from the medial hand, forearm, and arm. Damage to the medial cord will also affect the median nerve but the more proximal muscles innervated by the lateral root of the

median nerve will likely be spared. However, the deep forearm muscles innervated by the medial root of the median nerve and all muscles innervated by the ulnar nerve will be weakened. This will cause an inability to flex the wrist and digits, as well as weakness pronating the forearm. The medial pectoral nerve may be affected, affecting the pectoralis major and minor muscles.

Damage to the Superior Trunk
Damage to the C5 root, C6 root, or superior trunk of the brachial plexus results from forceful traction of the head away from the shoulder, which can occur during a fall onto the neck or during a difficult birth when the head is side-bent excessively, putting traction on the upper brachial plexus. This causes **Erb-Duchenne palsy** and primarily affects proximal muscles of the upper limb, manifesting as difficulty abducting and externally rotating the arm along with flexion the elbow since C5–C6 are major contributors to suprascapular, axillary, and musculocutaneous nerves. This will cause a persistently internally rotated arm that is extended at the elbow. This is called **waiter's tip sign** since it used to be common practice for a waiter or maître-d to turn away from a customer with an internally rotated and extended arm so that the patron could discretely slip a tip into his hand to get a better table in a restaurant. The dorsal scapular, subclavian, and long thoracic nerves would also likely be affected but do not contribute to the waiter's tip appearance. Erb-Duchenne palsy can also develop gradually as a result of wearing a heavy backpack that compresses the superior trunk.

Damage to the Inferior Trunk
Damage to the C8 root, T1 root, or inferior trunk of the brachial plexus occurs less frequently but can result from sudden, forceful abduction of the arm, putting traction on the inferior axilla and nerves of the inferior brachial plexus. Since the inferior trunk contributes almost all the axons to the medial cord, clinical signs will be very similar to damage to the medial cord. There may be additional deficits affecting the distal extensor muscles of the posterior forearm because the deep branch of the radial nerve receives some axons from the inferior trunk. This is known as Klumpke paralysis and can happen when a person falls and grasps something that arrests their fall but jerks their arm superiorly. Forceful traction on a newborn's arm during the birthing process can also cause this condition since the muscles are not developed and cannot resist the excessive abduction.

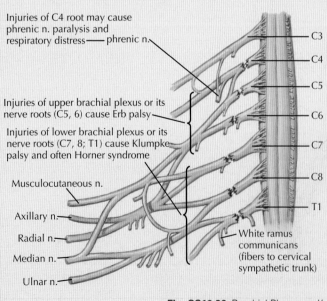

Injuries of C4 root may cause phrenic n. paralysis and respiratory distress —— phrenic n.

Injuries of upper brachial plexus or its nerve roots (C5, 6) cause Erb palsy

Injuries of lower brachial plexus or its nerve roots (C7, 8; T1) cause Klumpke palsy and often Horner syndrome

Musculocutaneous n.

Axillary n.

Radial n.

Median n.

Ulnar n.

C3
C4
C5
C6
C7
C8
T1

White ramus communicans (fibers to cervical sympathetic trunk)

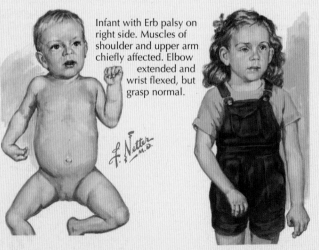

Infant with Erb palsy on right side. Muscles of shoulder and upper arm chiefly affected. Elbow extended and wrist flexed, but grasp normal.

Young girl with Klumpke palsy on right side. Muscles of forearm and hand chiefly affected. Grasp weak and affected limb small. Horner syndrome present, due to interruption of fibers to cervical sympathetic trunk.

Fig. CC10.26 Brachial Plexus and/or Cervical Nerve Root Injuries at Birth.

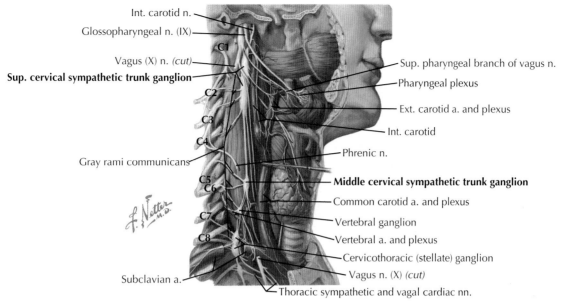

Int. carotid n.
Glossopharyngeal n. (IX)
Vagus (X) n. *(cut)*
Sup. cervical sympathetic trunk ganglion
C1
C2
C3
C4
Gray rami communicans
C5
C6
C7
C8
Subclavian a.

Sup. pharyngeal branch of vagus n.
Pharyngeal plexus
Ext. carotid a. and plexus
Int. carotid
Phrenic n.
Middle cervical sympathetic trunk ganglion
Common carotid a. and plexus
Vertebral ganglion
Vertebral a. and plexus
Cervicothoracic (stellate) ganglion
Vagus n. (X) *(cut)*
Thoracic sympathetic and vagal cardiac nn.

Fig. 10.24 Autonomic Nerves in the Neck.

CLINICAL CORRELATION 10.27
Autonomic Dysfunction of the Upper Limb

Raynaud syndrome is characterized by pronounced contraction of the pre-capillary sphincters that lead to fingers. This causes the fingers to become pale, cyanotic, and ache painfully. The cause is not always known but this ischemia of the digits can occur when stress or intense emotions result in increased sympathetic activity, constricting these blood vessels. **Hyperhidrosis** occurs when the sympathetic nervous system is overactive and causes frequent (or constant) sweating from the axilla, palms, or elsewhere. Such conditions can be treated by selectively cutting the gray rami communicans leaving the sympathetic chain to join the brachial plexus or by lesioning pre-ganglionic sympathetic nerves within the sympathetic chain itself.

medial epicondyle. In that region it joins the anastomotic network of the elbow.
- **Inferior ulnar collateral artery**: this smaller artery leaves the brachial artery near the elbow and briefly travels inferiorly before contributing to the anastomotic network of arteries around the elbow.

Arteries of the Forearm (See Fig. 10.26)

In the cubital fossa, the brachial artery crosses deep and lateral to the median nerve before passing deep to the bicipital aponeurosis. Typically, it will divide just distal to the elbow joint to form the ulnar and radial arteries, which supply blood to the structures of the anterior and posterior compartments of the forearm as well as the palm and dorsum of the hand. Note that the radial and ulnar arteries sometimes separate in the arm and will descend on either side of the median nerve.

In the forearm the **ulnar artery** travels on the medial side of the forearm deep to the superficial layer of flexor muscles to reach the medial side of the anterior forearm. In some people (~3%) the ulnar artery is located superficial to the flexor muscles on the medial side of the arm, making it vulnerable to shallow

trauma. Shortly after branching off the brachial artery, the ulnar artery gives off several proximal branches, including a **nutrient artery of the ulna**. Thereafter, it falls alongside the ulnar nerve just lateral to the flexor carpi ulnaris muscle and tendon as it descends toward the wrist.
- **Anterior ulnar recurrent artery**: travels medially and proximally along the anterior side of the medial epicondyle of the humerus to anastomose primarily with the inferior ulnar collateral artery.
- **Posterior ulnar recurrent artery**: travels medially and proximally along the posterior side of the medial epicondyle to anastomose with the superior ulnar collateral artery.
- **Common interosseous artery**: branches off the lateral side of the ulnar artery and quickly divides into branches on both sides of the interosseous membrane.
  - **Anterior interosseous artery**: travels alongside the anterior interosseous nerve to supply the deep flexor muscles of the anterior forearm. It passes deep to the pronator quadratus muscle before piercing the interosseous membrane to reach the dorsal side of the hand and the dorsal carpal arch, which comes from the radial artery.
    - **Median artery**: during early development of the limb, this artery runs along the anterior side of the interosseous membrane and through the carpal tunnel to reach the palm. It typically dwindles to leave behind the anterior interosseous artery as the radial and ulnar arteries enlarge; however, it may persist in some people.
  - **Posterior interosseous artery**: leaves the anterior compartment of the forearm by passing between the oblique cord and the interosseous membrane. Unsurprisingly, it then runs alongside the posterior interosseous nerve on the posterior side of the interosseous membrane. It supplies blood to the deep structures of the posterior forearm and disappears near the wrist but it may sometimes contribute to the dorsal carpal arch.

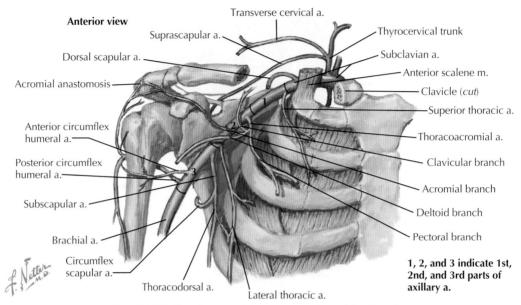

Anterior view

Transverse cervical a.

Suprascapular a.

Dorsal scapular a.

Acromial anastomosis

Anterior circumflex humeral a.

Posterior circumflex humeral a.

Subscapular a.

Brachial a.

Circumflex scapular a.

Thoracodorsal a.

Lateral thoracic a.

Thyrocervical trunk

Subclavian a.

Anterior scalene m.

Clavicle (*cut*)

Superior thoracic a.

Thoracoacromial a.

Clavicular branch

Acromial branch

Deltoid branch

Pectoral branch

1, 2, and 3 indicate 1st, 2nd, and 3rd parts of axillary a.

Fig. 10.25 Axillary Artery and Anastomoses Around the Scapula.

- **Recurrent interosseous artery** leaves the posterior interosseous artery shortly after it enters the posterior compartment of the forearm and travels proximally along the surface of the supinator muscle to anastomose with the middle collateral artery from the deep brachial artery.

The **radial artery** travels along the lateral aspect of the anterior forearm deep to the brachioradialis muscle but distally it crosses laterally around the distal radius to reach the dorsal side of the lateral carpal bones and hand. In the proximal forearm, the radial artery gives off several muscular branches, a **nutrient artery of the radius**, and one named branch.

- **Radial recurrent artery**: leaves the lateral side of the radial artery and travels proximally along the anterior aspect of the lateral epicondyle to the humerus. It will meet the most lateral branch of the deep brachial artery, the radial collateral artery (Clinical Correlations 10.29 and 10.30).

Arteries of the Wrist and Hand (See Fig. 10.26)

The ulnar and radial arteries both cross the wrist to supply the carpal bones and structures of the hand. They will form several complex anastomoses during this process. The ulnar artery travels lateral to the tendon of the flexor carpi ulnaris and pisiform bone as it enters the ulnar canal, deep to the palmar carpal ligament. Before entering the canal it gives off two vessels to the wrist.

- **Dorsal carpal branch**: this artery travels medially around the distal ulna to feed into the small (but important) dorsal carpal arch, which receives most of its blood from the radial artery.
- **Palmar carpal branch**: this artery exits the lateral side of the ulnar artery to supply the distal forearm and proximal carpus. It anastomoses with a similar branch from the radial artery.

Once it has passed through the ulnar canal, the ulnar artery gives off two branches to the palm.

- **Superficial palmar arch**: the majority of the blood in the distal ulnar artery travels into the superficial palmar arch,

which is typically found just deep to the palmar aponeurosis. It is joined by the superficial palmar branch of the radial artery.

- **Common palmar digital arteries**: three of these arteries leave the superficial palmar arch, running between the metacarpals 2 and 3, 3 and 4, and 4 and 5.
  - **Proper palmar digital arteries**: these vessels branch off each common palmar digital artery to supply the digits themselves.
    - The 1st common palmar digital artery branches into the proper palmar digital arteries for the medial side of digit 2 and the lateral side of digit 3.
    - The 2nd common palmar digital artery branches into the proper palmar digital arteries for the medial side of digit 3 and the lateral side of digit 4.
    - The 3rd common palmar digital artery branches into the proper palmar digital arteries for the medial side of digit 4 and the lateral side of digit 5.
    - A separate proper palmar digital artery for the medial side of digit 5 branches directly off the superficial palmar arch.
    - The proper palmar digital arteries to the lateral side of the 2nd digit and both sides of the 1st digit come from the radial artery. More on that shortly.
- **Deep palmar branch**: a smaller vessel that exits the lateral side of the ulnar artery that runs anterior to the interosseous muscles and anastomoses with the deep palmar arch, which arises primarily from the radial artery.

The **radial artery** travels along the lateral aspect of the distal radius but shifts dorsally in the vicinity of the scaphoid bone. While still in the distal forearm it has two important branches.

- **Palmar carpal branch**: this artery leaves the medial side of the radial artery and crosses the distal forearm to anastomose with the equivalent branch from the ulnar artery, forming the **palmar carpal arch.**

The upper limb receives the entirety of its blood supply from the subclavian artery and its tributaries, particularly the axillary and brachial arteries. The dorsal scapular and suprascapular arteries arise from the subclavian artery and supply blood to the medial, superior, and posterior aspects of the scapula. The circumflex scapular artery is a tributary of the third portion of the axillary artery and it supplies the lateral and posterior sides of the scapula. If a blockage (such as arteriosclerosis) occurs in the distal subclavian or proximal axillary artery, an anastomotic channel may enlarge using these vessels to bypass the blockage. The dorsal scapular and suprascapular arteries will convey blood across the infraspinous fossa to the circumflex scapular artery. Flow through this artery will reverse its typical direction, moving blood into the subscapular and axillary artery before supplying the brachial artery and backfilling the proximal axillary artery. Sudden ligation of the proximal axillary artery (such as repairing a rupture to the axillary artery) will deprive the upper limb of blood and there may not be enough time for a significant anastomotic re-routing to preserve tissues of the upper limb.

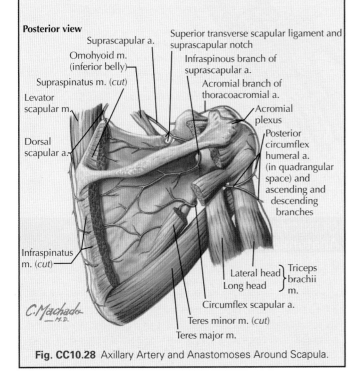

Posterior view

Suprascapular a.
Omohyoid m. (inferior belly)
Supraspinatus m. (cut)
Levator scapular m.
Dorsal scapular a.
Superior transverse scapular ligament and suprascapular notch
Infraspinous branch of suprascapular a.
Acromial branch of thoracoacromial a.
Acromial plexus
Posterior circumflex humeral a. (in quadrangular space) and ascending and descending branches
Infraspinatus m. (cut)
Lateral head
Long head
Triceps brachii m.
Circumflex scapular a.
Teres minor m. (cut)
Teres major m.
C. Machado M.D.

Fig. CC10.28 Axillary Artery and Anastomoses Around Scapula.

- **Superficial palmar branch**: this branch leaves the anterior side of the radial artery to travel across the palm deep to the abductor pollicis brevis muscle and palmar aponeurosis. It contributes to the superficial palmar arch, which typically receives most of its blood from the ulnar artery.

After it has crossed to the dorsal side of the wrist, the radial artery gives off several branches.

- **Dorsal carpal branch**: this artery leaves the medial side of the radial artery and crosses anterior to the tendons of the extensor carpi radialis muscles to anastomose with the dorsal carpal branch of the ulnar artery. This anastomosis forms the **dorsal carpal arch.**
  - **Dorsal metacarpal arteries**: these arteries extend distally off the dorsal carpal arch (and the radial artery) alongside the metacarpal bones.

- **Dorsal digital arteries**: these arteries branch off the dorsal metacarpal arteries to provide blood to each side of the digits.
  - The 1st dorsal metacarpal artery (from the radial artery) branches into dorsal digital arteries on the medial side of digit 1 and the lateral side of digit 2.
  - The 2nd dorsal metacarpal artery (from the dorsal carpal arch) branches into dorsal digital arteries on the medial side of digit 2 and lateral side of digit 3.
  - The 3rd dorsal metacarpal artery (off the dorsal digital arch) branches into dorsal digital arteries on the medial side of digit 3 and the lateral side of digit 4.
  - The 4th dorsal metacarpal artery (off the dorsal digital arch) branches into dorsal digital arteries on the medial side of digit 4 and the lateral side of digit 5.
  - The dorsal digital artery to the medial side of digit 5 branches directly off the dorsal carpal arch or the dorsal carpal branch of the ulnar artery.

Thereafter, the radial artery pierces the two heads of the 1st dorsal interosseous muscle and enters the palmar side of the hand to give off its final three branches.

- **Princeps pollicis artery**: this large vessel travels along the medial side of the 1st metacarpal before branching into the two proper palmar digital arteries of the 1st digit.
- **Radialis indicis artery**: this artery runs along the lateral aspect of the 2nd metacarpal before transitioning into the proper palmar digital artery on the lateral aspect of the 2nd digit.
- **Deep palmar arch**: the radial artery provides the majority of the blood to this arch but is supplemented by blood from the deep palmar branch of the ulnar artery. It is found anterior to the interosseous muscles and gives off branches that will fuse with the overlying common palmar digital arteries.
  - **Palmar metacarpal arteries**: three of these vessels branch off the deep palmar arch and fuse with the three common palmar digital arteries, providing another route for blood to reach the digits (Clinical Correlations 10.31 and 10.32).

Veins of the Upper Limbs (Fig. 10.27)

In general, each named artery has a vein running anti-parallel to it, draining blood from the regions supplied by the artery. However, venous pathways are far more variable than arterial pathways and there are frequently multiple veins running along a large artery. When these veins form an interconnected network along the surface of the artery, they are known as **venae comitantes**, accompanying veins. Veins of the upper limb tend to have valves in their lumen to prevent the retrograde flow of venous blood, which is particularly important when venous drainage needs to operate against gravity. The pulsation of large arteries may help propel venous blood proximally as the expansion of the artery will compress the veins and push blood superiorly past another valve. Another major driver of venous drainage against gravity is muscle contraction within the compartments of the limbs. Since the fascia surrounding each compartment does not allow tremendous expansion, the increased pressure will compress veins in the compartment, propelling blood proximally with valves preventing the blood from returning distally.

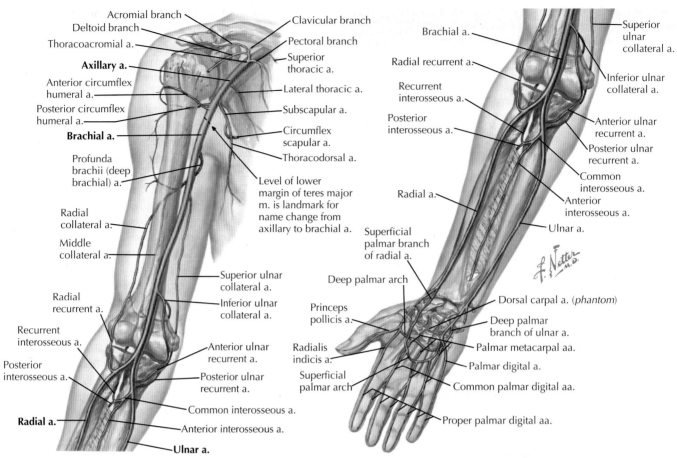

Fig. 10.26 Arteries of the Arm and Forearm.

CLINICAL CORRELATION 10.29
Anastomoses Around the Elbow (See Fig. 10.26)

Aside from the brachial artery, there are several arterial connections that also cross the elbow.
- Superior ulnar collateral and posterior ulnar recurrent arteries
- Inferior ulnar collateral and anterior ulnar recurrent arteries
- Radial collateral branch of the deep brachial and radial recurrent arteries
- Middle collateral branch of the deep brachial and the recurrent interosseous artery.

If the brachial artery is damaged, ligated, or compressed for a prolonged period of time, one or more of these channels may enlarge to carry blood past the blockage to perfuse the forearm and hand.

CLINICAL CORRELATION 10.31 The Anatomical Snuff Box (See CC10.32)

If a patent is asked to strongly stick her or his thumb "up," abducting and extending it, two tendinous ridges will bulge from the lateral wrist. The more lateral of the two ridges is formed by the abductor pollicis longus and extensor pollicis brevis tendons, while the more medial ridge is created by the extensor pollicis longus tendon. The small depression in between is known as the anatomical snuff box. People used to (and some still do) snort snuff, finely ground tobacco, from this space. Within this space is the radial artery, which can be palpated in the snuff box, along with the scaphoid bone. When there is a fracture or avascular necrosis of the scaphoid bone, palpation of this space will often elicit pain.

CLINICAL CORRELATION 10.30
Branching of the Brachial Artery

The radial artery frequently (~9%) originates high in the arm from the brachial, or less frequently, the axillary artery as the **brachioradial artery**. This variation should be considered when the radial artery is considered for an autograft or during trauma of the arm. Another common (~10%) variation is the **median artery**, which originates from the brachial artery and travels between the radial and ulnar arteries through the carpal tunnel to the palmar arches.

In the upper limb, there are some subcutaneous veins of special significance. They do not have an arterial partner and can often be found just below the skin or protruding from the skin in people with low body fat. Venous blood from the palmar and medial side of the hand and forearm tends to drain into tributaries of the **basilic vein of the forearm**, which travels along the medial side of the forearm toward the medial epicondyle of the humerus. It will continue superiorly on the medial aspect of the arm as the **basilic vein** for several centimeters before it dives into the **brachial vein** in the anterior compartment of the arm. The brachial vein crosses the teres major to become the **axillary**

There are a few typical sites at which the pulse rate can be checked in the upper limb. While ultrasound is being used more frequently, palpating these arteries by hand is still very common.

- Brachial artery: the pulse can be felt as the artery is compressed against the medial aspect of the humeral shaft. It may also be palpable in the cubital fossa just medial to the biceps tendon. This is often where the pulse will be assessed by stethoscope during a blood pressure exam with a cuff.
- Radial artery: somewhat palpable within the anatomical snuff box but more readily felt between the tendons of the flexor carpi radialis and abductor pollicis longus muscles.
- Ulnar artery: palpable just lateral to the pisiform bone and tendon of the flexor carpi ulnaris muscle. It is deep and the examiner may need to push into the skin to find the pulse.

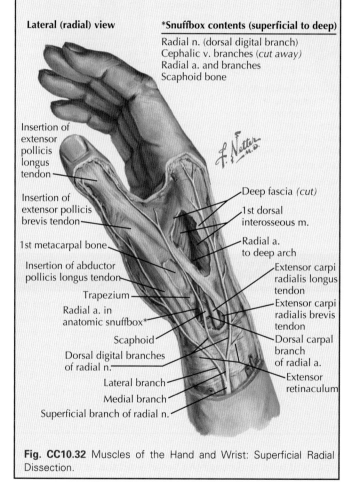

Lateral (radial) view

*Snuffbox contents (superficial to deep)
Radial n. (dorsal digital branch)
Cephalic v. branches (cut away)
Radial a. and branches
Scaphoid bone

Insertion of extensor pollicis longus tendon

Insertion of extensor pollicis brevis tendon

1st metacarpal bone

Insertion of abductor pollicis longus tendon

Trapezium

Radial a. in anatomic snuffbox*

Scaphoid

Dorsal digital branches of radial n.

Lateral branch

Medial branch

Superficial branch of radial n.

Deep fascia (cut)

1st dorsal interosseous m.

Radial a. to deep arch

Extensor carpi radialis longus tendon

Extensor carpi radialis brevis tendon

Dorsal carpal branch of radial a.

Extensor retinaculum

Fig. CC10.32 Muscles of the Hand and Wrist: Superficial Radial Dissection.

vein, which receives venous blood from other tributaries in the area until it crosses the first rib and changes its name to the **subclavian vein**. The subclavian vein will then enter the thorax as it fuses with the internal jugular vein (Clinical Correlation 10.33).

Blood from the dorsum of the hand moves from the digital veins and **intercapitular veins** (between adjacent digits) into **dorsal metacarpal veins** into the **dorsal venous network of the hand**. Some of this blood may drain to the basilic vein of the forearm but the majority of the dorsal blood, along with blood from the lateral side of the forearm, drains toward the elbow in

the **cephalic vein of the forearm**. This vessel continues superiorly on the lateral arm as the **cephalic vein**, which will run along the deltopectoral groove before going deep to join the subclavian vein. A nearby **thoracoacromial vein** draining the area around the anterior shoulder may join the cephalic vein before it terminates.

Returning to the cubital fossa, there is typically a **median cubital vein** that connects the cephalic and basilic veins as they cross from the forearm into the arm. This vessel is variable and may be very large, duplicated, or absent altogether. When present, there is typically a midline **median antebrachial vein** draining blood directly to it from the anterior forearm. All of these superficial veins have small perforating veins that dive through the underlying brachial or antebrachial fascia to reach deeper veins that run alongside the arteries of the upper limb (Clinical Correlation 10.34).

LYMPHATIC DRAINAGE OF THE UPPER LIMB (FIG. 10.28)

There are deep lymphatic vessels that more or less parallel the arteries and veins of the hand, forearm, arm, and axilla. Superficial lymphatic vessels of the palm dive deep to meet the deep lymphatic vessels around the palmar arches. Lymphatic fluid from the digits drains through small superficial lymphatic vessels toward the dorsum of the hand. These small vessels enlarge as they travel proximally and fuse with one another. As the vessels get larger they tend to run parallel to the superficial veins like the cephalic and basilic veins. Lymphatic vessels from the dorsum of the hand, lateral forearm, and lateral arm tend to run alongside the cephalic vein. These afferent vessels carry lymphatic fluid to **deltopectoral lymph nodes** that sit next to the cephalic vein just before it reaches the axillary or subclavian vein. Lymphatic vessels from the palmar hand and anteromedial forearm converge on the cubital fossa and the **cubital lymph nodes** located there. Lymphatic fluid from the cubital nodes passes proximally along the basilic vein to reach deep lymphatic vessels along the brachial vessels. These vessels will continue proximally until they reach the **lateral (humeral) axillary lymph nodes**.

The **axillary lymph nodes** are an important group of lymph nodes with several members whose positions are indicated by their names. The lateral (humeral) axillary lymph nodes run along the medial aspect of the proximal humerus and carry the majority of the lymphatic fluid from the upper limb. The **posterior (subscapular) axillary lymph nodes** are found anterior to the subscapularis muscle. The **anterior (pectoral) axillary lymph nodes** are found on the posterior surfaces of the pectoralis major and minor muscles and drain the anterolateral chest and lateral breast. There are also **interpectoral lymph nodes** between the two muscles. At the core of the axilla are the **central axillary lymph nodes** that receive lymphatic vessels from the posterior, lateral, and anterior axillary nodes. Lymphatic fluid from the central nodes, along with collateral lymph vessels from the other axillary lymph nodes, passes proximally to the **apical axillary lymph nodes**, which are located at the upper limit of

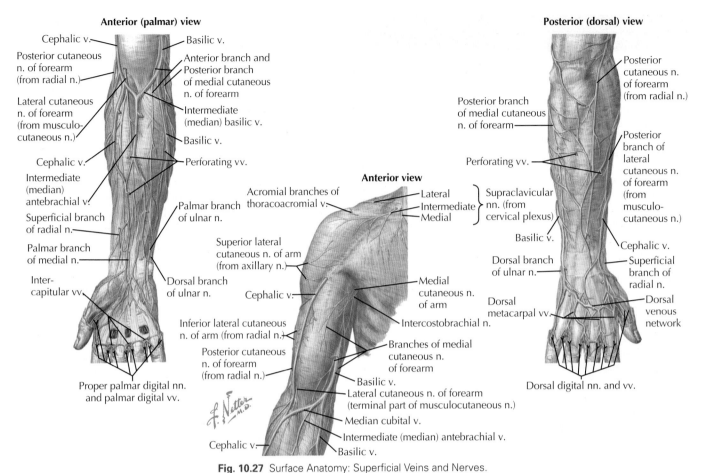

Fig. 10.27 Surface Anatomy: Superficial Veins and Nerves.

CLINICAL CORRELATION 10.33
Neurovascular Relationships in the Neck (See Fig. 10.18)

The subclavian vessels and brachial plexus are located very close to each other in the base of the neck and injuries to this area can result in significant hemorrhage and de-innervation related to the upper limb. The subclavian vein crosses superior to the first rib and inferior to the clavicle before passing anterior to the anterior scalene muscle and phrenic nerve as it drains blood from the upper limb and neck. The axillary artery and brachial plexus are a bit better protected as they leave the neck and pass between the anterior and middle scalene muscles. Further distally they will pass inferior to the clavicle and superior to the first rib. These relationships are important to consider when placing a central line into the subclavian vein. Also, sudden deceleration injuries, such as during a motor vehicle accident, can fracture the first rib and potentially lacerate the subclavian/axillary vessels.

CLINICAL CORRELATION 10.34 The Cubital Fossa (See Fig. 10.27)

The anterior aspect of the elbow is an area called the cubital fossa and it is a common site for accessing venous blood from the median cubital vein. It has a triangular shape with one of the points directed distally. Its borders are the forearm flexors (medially), the forearm extensors (laterally), and a line between the medial and lateral epicondyles (superiorly). The floor of this space is the brachialis and supinator muscles. While it is a relatively safe place to draw blood, there are some important structures in the cubital fossa: brachial, radial, and ulnar arteries and veins as well as the median nerve, and the tendon of the biceps brachii.

---

the axilla. From there, lymphatic fluid goes to **supraclavicular lymph nodes**. Thereafter, the lymphatic fluid travels in a **subclavian lymph trunk** that drains into the right or left subclavian vein. On the left side, it may join the thoracic duct before reaching the subclavian vein (Clinical Correlation 10.35).

NEUROVASCULAR BUNDLES

There are several locations in the upper limb where large vessels and nerves travel alongside each other. Injuries in these areas will tend to damage the vessels and the nerves, causing hemorrhage and de-innervation injuries. Hemorrhage from veins will tend to seep out, although the volume of blood in these veins can be very impressive. Hemorrhage involving arteries will have a pulsatile nature, spurting in time with the pulse.

Shoulder and Axillary Region

- **Cords of the brachial plexus/axillary vessels**: the cords of the brachial plexus (posterior, lateral, and medial) are found on their respective sides of the axillary artery. These are held together by connective tissue that surrounds the bundle, the **axillary sheath.** Deep penetrating trauma to the axilla can

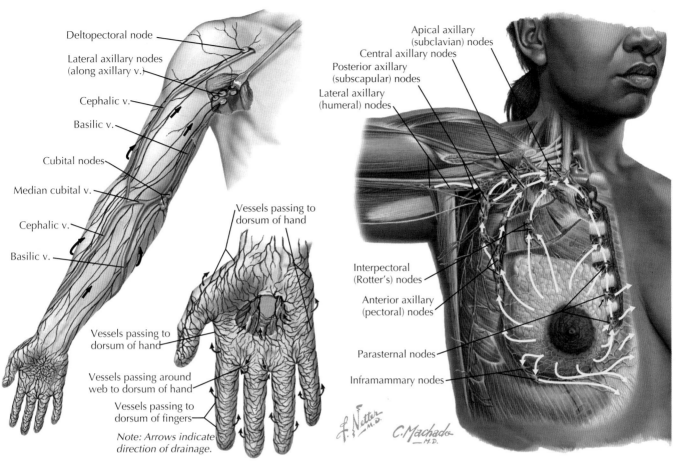

Fig. 10.28 Lymphatic Drainage.

cause damage to one or more of the cords, massive hemorrhage from the axillary artery, and possibly the nearby axillary vein.

- **Long thoracic nerve and lateral thoracic vessels**: the long thoracic nerve leaves the roots of the brachial plexus and falls in line with the lateral thoracic artery, a branch of the 2nd part of the axillary artery. Damage to this bundle will result in hemorrhage along the lateral thoracic wall and paralysis of some or all of the serratus anterior muscle.
- **Suprascapular nerve and vessels**: the suprascapular nerve branches off the superior trunk of the brachial plexus and travels alongside the suprascapular artery after it leaves the thyrocervical trunk or other branch of the subclavian artery.

Penetrating trauma to the area superior and anterior to the scapula may damage this bundle causing hemorrhage and paralysis to the supraspinatus and infraspinatus muscles.

- **Thoracodorsal nerve and vessels**: the thoracodorsal nerve arises from the posterior cord of the brachial plexus and runs along the anterior surface of the latissimus dorsi muscle with the thoracodorsal artery, a branch of the subscapular artery and 3rd part of the axillary artery. Damage to this bundle can occur due to trauma along the posterior axillary fold and would cause hemorrhage and loss of function to the latissimus dorsi muscle.

Arm

- **Axillary nerve and posterior circumflex humeral vessels**: the axillary nerve is a branch of the posterior cord of the brachial plexus. It falls alongside the posterior circumflex humeral artery, a branch of the 3rd portion of the axillary artery and both travel through the quadrangular space of the shoulder across the posterior side of the surgical neck of the humerus. A fracture in this area can result in hemorrhage, paralysis of the deltoid and teres minor muscles, and absent sensation on a patch of skin on the lateral shoulder.
- **Radial nerve and deep brachial vessels**: the radial nerve is a branch of the posterior cord of the brachial plexus that travels anterior to the long head of the triceps brachii muscle

with the deep brachial artery, a branch of the brachial artery in the proximal arm. The bundle travels inferolaterally along the radial groove of the posterior humerus between the lateral and medial heads of the triceps brachii. A fracture (such as a spiral fracture) of the humerus can damage this bundle and cause hemorrhage, paralysis of the muscles that supinate, extend the forearm, carpal bones, and digits, as well as absent/altered sensation on the posterior forearm and dorsum of the hand. Since motor and sensory branches to the muscles (triceps brachii) and skin of the posterolateral arm may have left the radial nerve proximal to the site of injury, they may remain unaffected.

- **Median nerve and brachial vessels**: the median nerve runs alongside the brachial artery and vein medial to the humerus. In the upper arm the nerve is found anterior to the vessels, but it shifts to a more medial position as it approaches the elbow. Since this bundle is not in direct contact with the humerus, it is not frequently injured by a fracture. However, trauma to the anteromedial arm can affect it, resulting in hemorrhage and weakness flexing the wrist, digits, and moving the thumb.

Forearm

- **Superficial radial nerve and radial vessels**: after the radial nerve divides into deep and superficial branches, the superficial branch of the radial nerve briefly travels along the radial artery in the lateral aspect of the anterior forearm. This bundle is protected by the brachioradialis muscles. In the event this bundle was damaged, there would be hemorrhage in the area and a loss of sensation along the distal posterior forearm and dorsum of the hand.
- **Ulnar nerve and vessels**: the ulnar nerve crosses posterior to the medial epicondyle and descends along the medial side of the anterior forearm, lateral to the flexor carpi ulnaris muscle. Roughly mid-way down the forearm it is joined by the ulnar artery (and accompanying vein) after it branches from the brachial artery in the cubital fossa. This bundle is frequently damaged by lacerations of the wrist that penetrate the tendon of the flexor carpi ulnaris. This will result in hemorrhage, loss of sensation of the medial hand, and paralysis of the muscles of the hand innervated by the deep ulnar nerve.

- **Anterior interosseous nerve and vessels**: the anterior interosseous nerve and artery are branches of the median nerve and ulnar artery respectively. Due to their deep location in the forearm, it is unusual for them to be damaged in isolation. They could be affected by forearm fractures with significant displacement, which would result in hemorrhage deep in the anterior forearm and paralysis of the deep flexor muscles of digits 1 to 3.
- **Posterior interosseous nerve and vessels**: the posterior interosseous nerve and artery are deep branches of the radial nerve and ulnar artery respectively. Like the anterior interosseous bundle, they are difficult to damage in isolation but could be affected by trauma to the posterior forearm or displaced fractures. Damage to this bundle would result in hemorrhage in the posterior forearm and paralysis of extensor and abductor muscles of the thumb and the extensor indicis.
- **Cephalic vein and lateral antebrachial cutaneous nerve**: the cephalic vein in the forearm is in close proximity to branches of the lateral antebrachial cutaneous nerve. Trauma to the superficial, lateral forearm could result in venous hemorrhage and loss of sensation on the lateral forearm.
- **Basilic vein and medial antebrachial cutaneous nerve**: the basilic vein of the forearm and the arm is found in the same area as the medial antebrachial cutaneous nerve. Superficial trauma to the medial forearm can result in venous hemorrhage and loss of sensation over the medial forearm.

Hand

- **Common palmar digital nerves and vessels**: Trauma to the hand and digits is a frequent occurrence. Since the common palmar digital arteries (from the superficial palmar arch) and the common palmar digital nerves (from median and ulnar nerves) are located deep in the palm, penetrating trauma to this area may cause hemorrhage and sensory loss along the digits that are innervated by the common palmar digital nerve.
- **Proper palmar digital arteries and nerves**: The proper palmar digital nerves and arteries are located on the lateral and medial palmar sides of the digits. They are frequently injured together by lacerations, which result in hemorrhage and loss of sensation distal to the injury on the affected side of the digit.

Clinical Anatomy of the Lower Limb

INTRODUCTION

The lower limbs resemble the upper limbs in many ways. Instead of shoulder, arm, forearm, wrist, and hand segments, there are hip, thigh, leg, ankle, and foot. The muscles are grouped into flexor and extensor compartments with distinctive patterns of innervation, large vessels travel deeply within the limb, and large superficial veins drain blood from the subcutaneous tissues. However, the lower limbs differ significantly from the upper limbs because they must bear the body's weight, often on one limb. For this reason, the bones and muscles of the lower limb tend to be larger, the joints tend to be less mobile (and therefore more stable), and the foot is not optimized for grasping like the hand but for bearing weight and walking. The lower limb is connected to the back by the articulation of the ilium with the sacrum. Other ligamentous and tendinous connections keep the lower limb strongly connected to the vertebral column.

BONES, LIGAMENTS, AND JOINTS OF THE UPPER LIMB

The **pelvic girdle** is a bony ring formed by the sacrum as well as the right and left os coxae, which are also called the hip, pelvic, or innominate bones. Whichever term is used, this apparently single bone is formed by the fusion of three separate bones during early life: the ilium, ischium, and pubis. The three bones come together at the acetabulum and provide a stable articular site for the head of the femur.

Ilium and Sacroiliac Joint (Figs. 11.1 and 11.2)

The ilium is the largest of the three os coxae, and it meets the auricular (ear-shaped) surface of the sacrum at its own **auricular surface** to form the synovial portion of the **sacroiliac joint**. Immediately superior to it is the **iliac tuberosity**, which gives off a great mass of fibrous connective tissue, the **interosseous sacroiliac ligament**, to anchor the ilium to the sacrum. Just posterior to this, the **posterior sacroiliac ligament** extends in a superior-to-inferior direction, further reinforcing the joint. Likewise, the **anterior sacroiliac ligament** connects the iliac crest to the ala of the sacrum and forms the anterior border of

the synovial sacroiliac joint. It is supplemented by ligaments extending from the transverse processes of L4 and L5 to the iliac crest, the **iliolumbar ligaments**.

Extending anteriorly from the auricular surface is a ridge, the **arcuate line**, which is immediately superior to the **body of the ilium**. Extending superiorly and laterally from the arcuate line is the **ala/wing** of the ilium. The smooth, medial surface of the ala is the **iliac fossa**, where the iliacus muscle originates. The lateral surface of the ala is the **gluteal surface**. In many specimens it will appear nearly as smooth as the iliac surface, but several nested ridges of bone, the **posterior gluteal line, anterior gluteal line**, and **inferior gluteal line**, can sometimes be seen. The gluteus medius originates between the posterior and anterior gluteal lines, while the gluteus minimus originates between the anterior and inferior gluteal lines. At the summit between the medial and lateral sides of the ala is a massive **iliac crest** that extends from posterior to anterior and anchors many of the abdominal muscles. The iliac crest meets the iliac fossa at its **inner lip** and meets the gluteal surface at the **outer (external) lip**, with a roughened **intermediate zone** between the two lips. At its most superior limit, the iliac crest has an enlarged region, the **tuberculum**. The iliac crest terminates anteriorly as the **anterior superior iliac spine** and a slightly lower **anterior inferior iliac spine**. Similarly, the iliac crest terminates posteriorly as the **posterior superior iliac spine** with a smaller **posterior inferior iliac spine** just inferior to it. Inferior to the posterior inferior iliac spine is a large indentation, the **greater sciatic notch**, marking where the ilium fuses with the ischium.

Ischium

At the inferior end of the greater sciatic notch is the pointed **ischial spine**, with another indentation, the **lesser sciatic notch**, just inferior to it. The **body of the ischium** is located immediately anterior to the ischial spine. Inferior to the lesser sciatic notch is the massive **ischial tuberosity**, where the long members of the hamstring muscle group attach. Continuing anteriorly from the ischial tuberosity is a strut of bone that connects the ischium and pubis, the **ischial ramus**. The sacrum is tethered to the ischium by two strong ligaments that pass between it and the ischium. The **sacrotuberous ligament** continues inferiorly

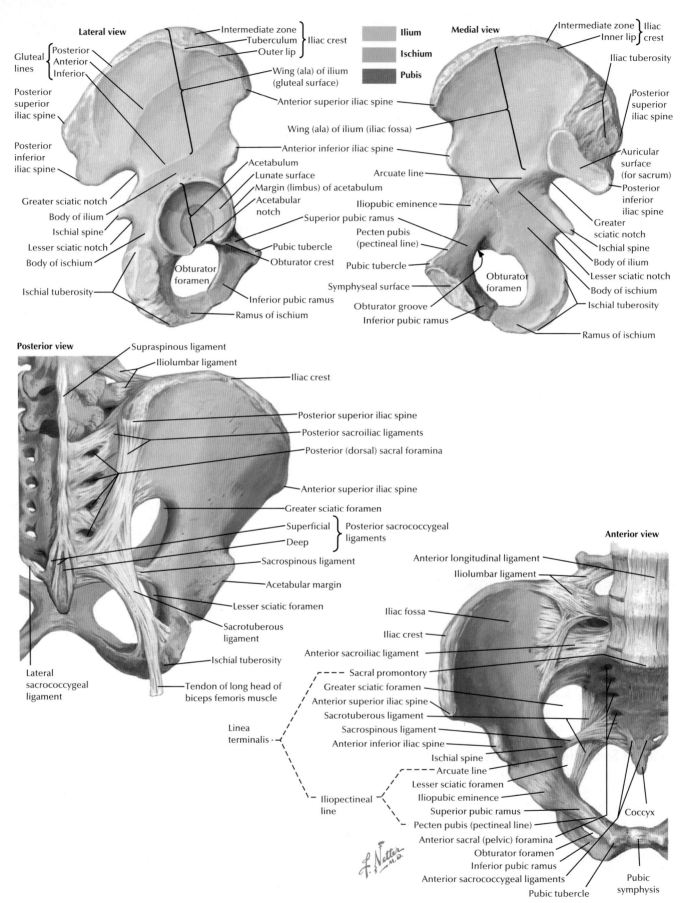

Fig. 11.1 Bones and Ligaments of the Pelvis.

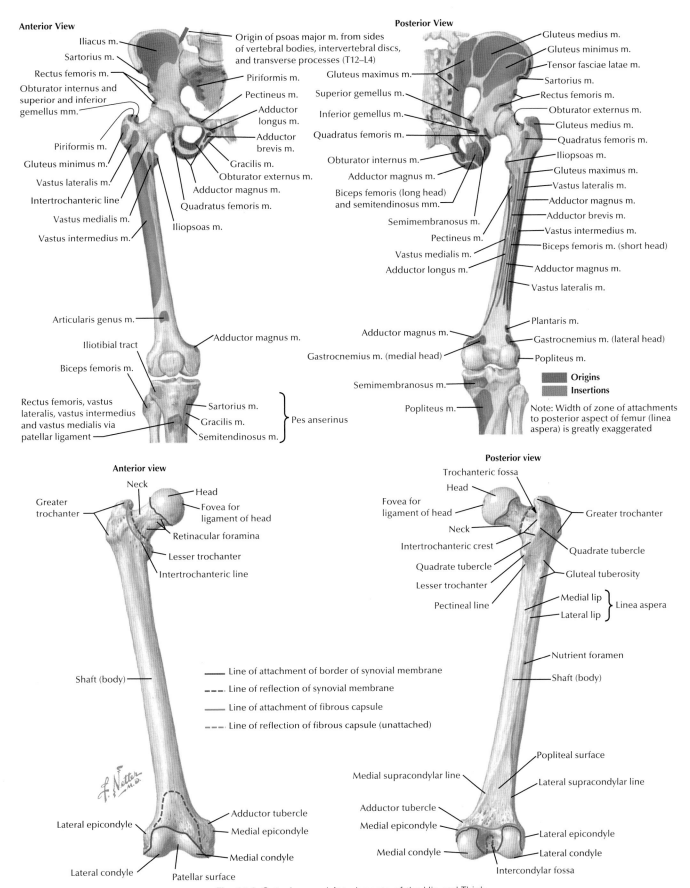

Anterior View

Iliacus m.
Sartorius m.
Rectus femoris m.
Obturator internus and superior and inferior gemellus mm.
Piriformis m.
Gluteus minimus m.
Vastus lateralis m.
Intertrochanteric line
Vastus medialis m.
Vastus intermedius m.

Origin of psoas major m. from sides of vertebral bodies, intervertebral discs, and transverse processes (T12–L4)
Piriformis m.
Pectineus m.
Adductor longus m.
Adductor brevis m.
Gracilis m.
Obturator externus m.
Adductor magnus m.
Quadratus femoris m.
Iliopsoas m.

Articularis genus m.
Iliotibial tract
Biceps femoris m.
Rectus femoris, vastus lateralis, vastus intermedius and vastus medialis via patellar ligament

Adductor magnus m.

Sartorius m.
Gracilis m.
Semitendinosus m.
} Pes anserinus

Posterior View

Gluteus maximus m.
Superior gemellus m.
Inferior gemellus m.
Quadratus femoris m.
Obturator internus m.
Adductor magnus m.
Biceps femoris (long head) and semitendinosus mm.
Semimembranosus m.
Pectineus m.
Vastus medialis m.
Adductor longus m.

Gluteus medius m.
Gluteus minimus m.
Tensor fasciae latae m.
Sartorius m.
Rectus femoris m.
Obturator externus m.
Gluteus medius m.
Quadratus femoris m.
Iliopsoas m.
Gluteus maximus m.
Vastus lateralis m.
Adductor magnus m.
Adductor brevis m.
Vastus intermedius m.
Biceps femoris m. (short head)
Adductor magnus m.
Vastus lateralis m.

Adductor magnus m.
Gastrocnemius m. (medial head)
Semimembranosus m.
Popliteus m.

Plantaris m.
Gastrocnemius m. (lateral head)
Popliteus m.

■ **Origins**
■ **Insertions**

Note: Width of zone of attachments to posterior aspect of femur (linea aspera) is greatly exaggerated

Anterior view

Neck
Greater trochanter
Head
Fovea for ligament of head
Retinacular foramina
Lesser trochanter
Intertrochanteric line

Shaft (body)

_____ Line of attachment of border of synovial membrane
- - - - Line of reflection of synovial membrane
_____ Line of attachment of fibrous capsule
- - - - Line of reflection of fibrous capsule (unattached)

Lateral epicondyle
Lateral condyle
Adductor tubercle
Medial epicondyle
Medial condyle
Patellar surface

Posterior view

Trochanteric fossa
Head
Fovea for ligament of head
Neck
Intertrochanteric crest
Quadrate tubercle
Lesser trochanter
Pectineal line

Greater trochanter
Quadrate tubercle
Gluteal tuberosity
Medial lip
Lateral lip
} Linea aspera

Nutrient foramen
Shaft (body)

Popliteal surface
Medial supracondylar line
Adductor tubercle
Medial epicondyle
Medial condyle

Lateral supracondylar line
Lateral epicondyle
Lateral condyle
Intercondylar fossa

Fig. 11.2 Osteology and Attachments of the Hip and Thigh.

from the posterior sacroiliac ligament to the ischial tuberosity. The nearby **sacrospinous ligament** connects the anterolateral sacrum and ischial spine. In addition to stabilization, these ligaments form two foramina that are not visible when examining dry bones. They enclose the greater and lesser sciatic notches to create the **greater sciatic foramen** and **lesser sciatic foramen**, which allow muscles, nerves, and vessels to leave the pelvis and reach the lower limb and pelvis.

Pubis

The pubis is a V-shaped bone with one leg of the V formed by the **inferior pubic ramus** (which connects it to the ischial ramus) and the other leg formed by the **superior pubic ramus**. Between the two rami and the ischium is the large, round **obturator foramen**. In life, the **obturator membrane** covers the majority of the foramen, leaving a small gap, the **obturator canal**, at its anterior end. The overlying superior pubic ramus hosts an **obturator groove** for the nerve and vessels of the same name near the superior rim of the obturator foramen. The **body of the pubis** is located where the two rami converge. On the superior aspect of the pubic body is a bump, the **pubic tubercle**. The left and right pubic bodies meet each other at their **symphyseal surfaces** and are typically connected by a fibrocartilage disc at the **pubic symphysis**. The **pubic crest** connects the right and left pubic tubercles along their superior surfaces with **superior** and **inferior pubic ligaments** reinforcing the pubic symphysis. The **obturator crest** stretches laterally from the pubic tubercle toward the acetabulum, just superior to the obturator foramen. The superior pubic ramus meets the ilium at the **iliopubic eminence**, just superior to the acetabulum. On the medial side of the superior pubic ramus and iliopubic ramus is the raised **pectineal line**, which is continuous with the arcuate line of the ilium.

Acetabulum

The acetabulum is not a separate bone but is a massive depression in the lateral os coxae at the point where all three bones converge. The depression itself is properly called the **acetabular fossa** and has a surrounding rim of bone that allows it to form a massive ball-in-socket joint with the femoral head. The rim is the **acetabular margin**, while the smooth, horseshoe-shaped medial aspect of the fossa that actually contacts the femoral head is the **lunate surface** of the acetabulum. There is a discontinuity in the acetabular fossa, margin, and lunate surface on its anteroinferior aspect, the **acetabular notch**.

Proximal Femur and Shaft (See Fig. 11.2)

The spherical **head of the femur** articulates with the acetabulum. A narrower **neck** connects the head of the femur to a large knot of bone at its superolateral end, the massive **greater trochanter**, where the gluteus medius and minimus muscles attach. The medial side of the greater trochanter has a depression, the **trochanteric fossa**, where the lateral rotators of the thigh insert. Just inferior to the femoral neck on the medial side of the proximal femur is the **lesser trochanter**, where the iliopsoas muscle inserts. Extending inferiorly from the lesser trochanter is a small raised patch, the **pectineal (spiral) line** where

the pectineus muscle inserts. Anteriorly, the two trochanters are connected by a roughened **intertrochanteric line**. Posteriorly the trochanters are connected by a larger **intertrochanteric crest**. Midway along the intertrochanteric crest is the attachment site for the quadratus femoris muscle, which may form a distinct **quadrate tubercle**. Inferior to the quadrate tubercle is the **gluteal tuberosity**, a major insertion site for the gluteus maximus. It extends inferiorly down the posterior **shaft** of the femur as the **linea aspera**, which has a **medial and lateral lip** where the medial and lateral intermuscular septae of the thigh and adductor muscles insert. The lateral, anterior, and medial sides of the femoral shaft are very smooth with no obvious surface features.

Coxofemoral Joint (Fig. 11.3)

The coxofemoral (hip) joint is formed by the articulation of the round head of the femur with the acetabulum. A stout **acetabular labrum** made of fibrocartilage deepens the cavity in which the head of the femur sits, allowing this ball-and-socket joint to flex/extend, abduct/adduct, and internally/externally rotate without dislocating. The acetabular labrum is discontinuous along the acetabular notch, but this area is bridged by the **transverse acetabular ligament**. A small **ligament of the head of the femur** connects a shallow fovea for the ligament of the head of the femur to the acetabular notch. Along with the labrum, the capsule surrounding the joint is one of the major factors in limiting its motion. As the fibrous layer of the coxofemoral joint capsule travels distally to insert on the femur, it spirals so that extension of the hip will tighten the fibers and pull the femoral head into the acetabulum. The capsule becomes more lax in flexion. The capsule also thickens in the vicinity of the femoral neck, creating the **zona orbicularis**, a region that helps to prevent the femoral head from leaving the acetabulum. Three strong intracapsular ligaments also contribute to the coxofemoral joint (Clinical Correlations 11.1 and 11.2).

- **Iliofemoral ligament:** Stretches across the anterior aspect of the joint capsule from the anterior inferior iliac spine and anterior ilium. It splits into transverse and descending parts that travel toward the greater and lesser trochanters, respectively. It helps to limit extension of the hip.
- **Ischiofemoral ligament:** Spirals superiorly across the posterior side of the capsule from the inferior aspect of the ischium toward the greater trochanter.
- **Pubofemoral ligament:** Extends from the underside of the superior pubic ramus toward the descending part of the iliofemoral ligament and intertrochanteric line. It tightens in extension but also during abduction of the hip.

Distal Femur and Patella (See Figs. 11.2, 2.14, and 2.15)

As the linea aspera continues inferiorly down the posterior side of the femoral shaft, it fans outward to create the **medial supracondylar line** and **lateral supracondylar line**. The smooth space between the two lines is the smooth **popliteal surface**. The distal end of the femur terminates in two large, smooth articular surfaces for the tibia, the **medial condyle** and **lateral condyle**. The medial and lateral femoral condyles curve posteriorly and

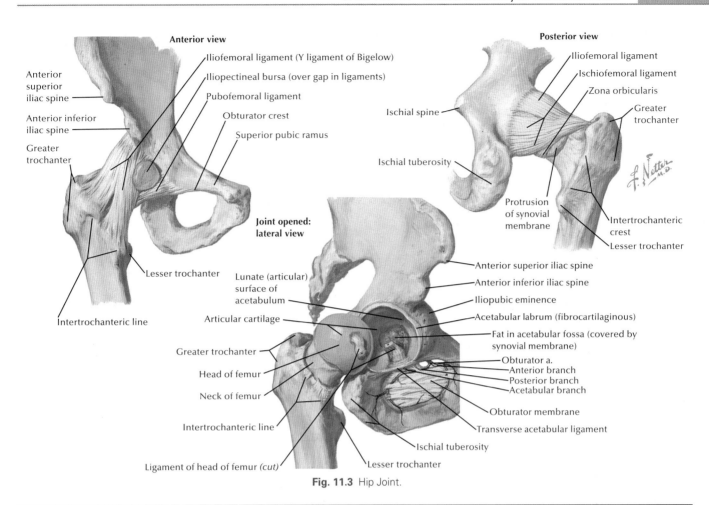

Fig. 11.3 Hip Joint.

CLINICAL CORRELATION 11.1 Hip Dislocation

Traumatic dislocation of the femoral head from the acetabulum requires significant force because the coxofemoral joint is deep and stabilized by strong muscles and ligaments. If the femur is driven posteriorly with the hip in a flexed position (e.g., in a head-on vehicle collision when the knee is pushed backward) a **posterior dislocation of the hip** can occur. In such an instance the femoral head can rupture the joint capsule in the weak spot between the iliofemoral and ischiofemoral ligaments or just burst through the weak ischiofemoral ligament. This will often compress or damage the sciatic nerve, which can compromise muscles of the posterior thigh, leg, and foot. Less frequently, hyperextension or external rotation (or both simultaneously) can cause an **anterior dislocation of the hip**, with the femoral head sitting inferior to the acetabulum or obturator foramen. Note that because so much force is required to dislocate the hip joint, accompanying fractures of the acetabulum are not uncommon.

Posterior dislocation of the hip

Dislocated femoral head lies posterior and superior to acetabulum. Femur adducted and internally rotated; hip flexed. Sciatic nerve may be stretched.

AP radiograph shows superior position of femoral head and no apparent fracture of the acetabulum.

Anterior dislocation of the hip

Anterior view. Femoral head in obturator foramen of pelvis; hip flexed and femur widely abducted and externally rotated

Anteroposterior radiograph shows obturator-type dislocation

Fig. CC11.1 Dislocation of the Hip.

CLINICAL CORRELATION 11.2   Fracture of the Proximal Femur

The neck of the femur is a frequent site of fracture for several reasons. It is the narrowest part of the bone, and it extends medially at an angle from the shaft of the femur. This makes it prone to fracture because it must bear a great deal of the body's weight and redirect it toward the head of the femur in the acetabulum. Femoral neck fractures tend to be contained within the coxofemoral joint capsule. To repair such intracapsular fractures, internal fixation (hardware to repair the femoral neck is within the bone) is used so that movement can occur thereafter. Intertrochanteric fractures take place between the greater and lesser trochanters and tend to be extracapsular, which allows the use of external hardware to align the bones. In both cases the lower limbs will be externally rotated due to the pull of the gluteus maximus on the detached distal fragment.

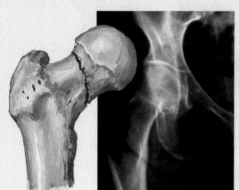

Nondisplaced femoral neck fracture

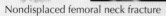

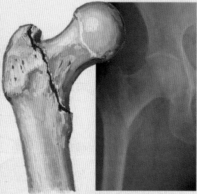

Two-part, minimally displaced intertrochanteric femur fracture

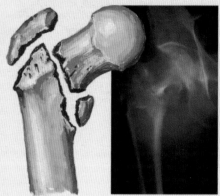

Comminuted four-part intertrochanteric femur fracture

Fig. CC11.2 Fracture of Femoral Neck and Intertrochanteric Fracture of Femur.

---

are separated by a depression, the **intercondylar fossa**, with the **intercondylar line** at its superior limit. Extending from the lateral femoral condyle is a large mound of bone, the **lateral epicondyle**. There is a palpable **groove for the popliteus tendon** on the lateral epicondyle just superior to the lateral condyle. The **medial epicondyle** extends along the shaft from the medial condyle with a prominent **adductor tubercle** projecting superiorly. Anteriorly, the two condyles come together at the smooth **patellar surface**.

The patella (kneecap) has a posterior **articular surface** that glides along the patellar surface of the femur, using a lateral and medial facet to stay in place. It has a rounded **base** along its superior aspect and a roughened **anterior surface** where the quadriceps muscles insert onto the bone. The patellar ligament extends inferiorly off the **apex** of the patella to reach the tibial tuberosity.

Proximal Tibia and Fibula (Figs. 11.2 and 11.4)

The **tibia** has a broad flat **superior articular surface** that sits atop a **medial condyle** and **lateral condyle** to articulate with the medial and lateral femoral condyles. The tibial condyles are separated from each other by an **intercondylar eminence** that hosts the raised **medial intercondylar tubercle** and **lateral intercondylar tubercle**. On either side of the intercondylar tubercles are two intercondylar areas: the anterior cruciate ligament and anterior ends of the menisci attach in the **anterior intercondylar area**, while the posterior cruciate ligament and posterior ends of the menisci attach in the **posterior intercondylar area**.

On the proximal tibia, the **anterolateral (Gerdy) tubercle** for attachment of the iliotibial band is located inferior and anterior to the lateral tibial condyle, while the **fibular articular facet** is located on the posterolateral side of the proximal tibia. The patellar ligament inserts on the large **tibial tuberosity** on the proximal midline of the tibia. Projecting inferiorly from the tibial tuberosity along the shaft is the anterior border. It is separated from the **interosseous border**, which faces laterally and is the attachment site for the **interosseous membrane**, by the lateral surface of the tibia. The tibia's medial border is separated from the anterior border by the medial surface and from the interosseous border by the posterior surface. A pronounced **soleal line** is present on the upper, posterior surface of the tibia for attachment of the soleus muscle.

The **fibula** is the slender, lateral companion to the tibia. Its **head** has an articular facet that meets the fibular articular facet of the tibia, while the **apex** of the head of the fibula stretches superiorly as the attachment site for the biceps femoris and lateral collateral ligament. A slight **neck** connects the head to the **body/shaft** of the fibula. For such a small bone, the fibula has many distinct lines extending along its length. The **interosseous border** faces the tibia and is the fibular attachment site for the interosseous membrane. The interosseous border is separated from the anterior border by the medial surface and the lateral surface is bounded by the anterior and posterior borders. Finally, the posterior border is separated from the interosseous border by the posterior surface of the fibula, which has a **medial crest** extending longitudinally along its length (Clinical Correlation 11.3).

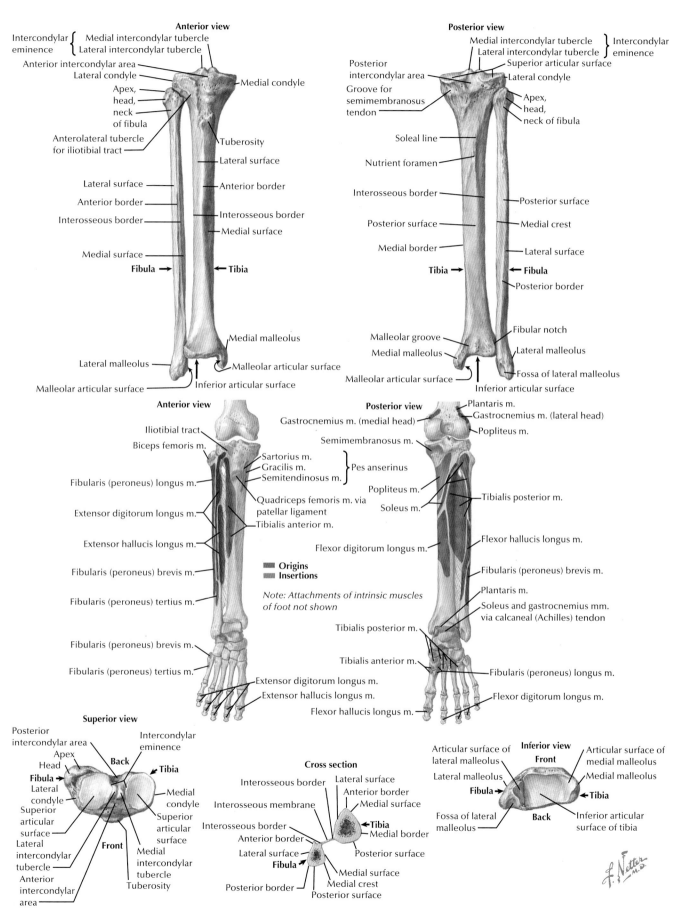

Anterior view

Intercondylar eminence { Medial intercondylar tubercle / Lateral intercondylar tubercle

Anterior intercondylar area

Lateral condyle

Apex, head, neck of fibula

Anterolateral tubercle for iliotibial tract

Lateral surface

Anterior border

Interosseous border

Medial surface

Fibula → ← **Tibia**

Lateral malleolus

Malleolar articular surface

Medial condyle

Tuberosity

Lateral surface

Anterior border

Interosseous border

Medial surface

Medial malleolus

Malleolar articular surface

Inferior articular surface

Posterior view

Medial intercondylar tubercle / Lateral intercondylar tubercle } Intercondylar eminence

Superior articular surface

Lateral condyle

Apex, head, neck of fibula

Posterior intercondylar area

Groove for semimembranosus tendon

Soleal line

Nutrient foramen

Interosseous border

Posterior surface

Medial border

Posterior surface

Medial crest

Lateral surface

Tibia → ← **Fibula**

Posterior border

Fibular notch

Malleolar groove

Medial malleolus

Malleolar articular surface

Lateral malleolus

Fossa of lateral malleolus

Inferior articular surface

Anterior view

Iliotibial tract

Biceps femoris m.

Fibularis (peroneus) longus m.

Extensor digitorum longus m.

Extensor hallucis longus m.

Fibularis (peroneus) brevis m.

Fibularis (peroneus) tertius m.

Fibularis (peroneus) brevis m.

Fibularis (peroneus) tertius m.

Sartorius m.
Gracilis m. } Pes anserinus
Semitendinosus m.

Quadriceps femoris m. via patellar ligament

Tibialis anterior m.

■ Origins
■ Insertions

Note: Attachments of intrinsic muscles of foot not shown

Extensor digitorum longus m.

Extensor hallucis longus m.

Posterior view

Plantaris m.

Gastrocnemius m. (medial head)

Gastrocnemius m. (lateral head)

Popliteus m.

Semimembranosus m.

Popliteus m.

Soleus m.

Flexor digitorum longus m.

Tibialis posterior m.

Flexor hallucis longus m.

Fibularis (peroneus) brevis m.

Plantaris m.

Soleus and gastrocnemius mm. via calcaneal (Achilles) tendon

Tibialis posterior m.

Tibialis anterior m.

Fibularis (peroneus) longus m.

Flexor digitorum longus m.

Flexor hallucis longus m.

Superior view

Posterior intercondylar area

Apex

Head

Fibula

Lateral condyle

Superior articular surface

Lateral intercondylar tubercle

Anterior intercondylar area

Intercondylar eminence

Back

← **Tibia**

Medial condyle

Superior articular surface

Medial intercondylar tubercle

Tuberosity

Front

Cross section

Interosseous border

Interosseous membrane

Interosseous border

Anterior border

Lateral surface

Posterior border

Lateral surface
Anterior border
Medial surface

← **Tibia**
Medial border

Posterior surface

Medial surface

Medial crest

Posterior surface

Fibula

Inferior view

Articular surface of lateral malleolus

Lateral malleolus

Fibula →

Fossa of lateral malleolus

Front

Articular surface of medial malleolus

Medial malleolus

← **Tibia**

Back

Inferior articular surface of tibia

Fig. 11.4 Osteology and Attachments of the Leg and Knee.

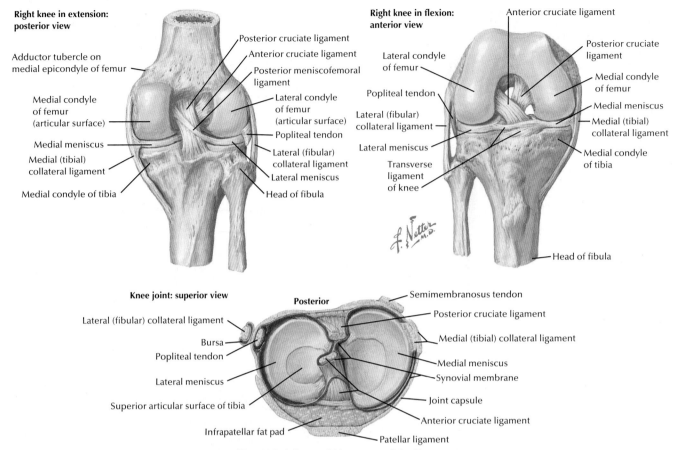

Right knee in extension: posterior view

Adductor tubercle on medial epicondyle of femur

Medial condyle of femur (articular surface)

Medial meniscus

Medial (tibial) collateral ligament

Medial condyle of tibia

Posterior cruciate ligament

Anterior cruciate ligament

Posterior meniscofemoral ligament

Lateral condyle of femur (articular surface)

Popliteal tendon

Lateral (fibular) collateral ligament

Lateral meniscus

Head of fibula

Right knee in flexion: anterior view

Lateral condyle of femur

Popliteal tendon

Lateral (fibular) collateral ligament

Lateral meniscus

Transverse ligament of knee

Anterior cruciate ligament

Posterior cruciate ligament

Medial condyle of femur

Medial meniscus

Medial (tibial) collateral ligament

Medial condyle of tibia

Head of fibula

Knee joint: superior view

Posterior

Lateral (fibular) collateral ligament

Bursa

Popliteal tendon

Lateral meniscus

Superior articular surface of tibia

Infrapatellar fat pad

Semimembranosus tendon

Posterior cruciate ligament

Medial (tibial) collateral ligament

Medial meniscus

Synovial membrane

Joint capsule

Anterior cruciate ligament

Patellar ligament

Fig. 11.5 Joints and Ligaments of the Knee.

CLINICAL CORRELATION 11.3 Fibula and Bone Autografts

When a surgeon carries out a large bony repair, there is sometimes a need for a bone graft to add bulk to the site. Autografting of the patient's own tissue will avert immune rejection of donor bones. The iliac crest is sometimes used, but the middle of the fibula has become a popular donor source because the patient can bear weight on the tibia and walk without a fibula. In addition, the nutrient artery to the bone (arising from the fibular artery) can be harvested alongside the bone and anastomosed to a vessel in the surgical site, making avascular necrosis of the graft less likely.

Knee Joint (Figs. 11.4–11.6)

The knee joint consists of the **patellofemoral** and **tibiofemoral articulations**. The articular surface of the patella is located on its posterior surface and interacts with the patellar surface of the anterior distal femur as the patellofemoral articulation. The ridges on either side of the femur's patellar surface are formed by the most anterior parts of the medial and lateral femoral condyles. These keep the patella from becoming displaced to either side as it is dragged along the patellar surface during flexion and extension of the knee. The patella is held in place by tension between the quadriceps muscles superiorly and the patellar ligament and tibial tuberosity inferiorly.

In contrast, the **tibiofemoral articulation** is tremendously mobile and allows flexion/extension of the knee as the medial and lateral femoral condyles glide across the medial and lateral

condyles of the superior articular surface of the tibia. Because the superior surface of the tibia is relatively flat, this joint requires support from many connective tissue structures. On either side of the intercondylar eminence of the tibia are two ligaments that cross each other to connect the tibia to the femur. The **anterior cruciate ligament** originates from the tibia's anterior intercondylar area and inserts on the posterolateral side of the intercondylar fossa of the femur. Likewise, the **posterior cruciate ligament** originates from the posterior intercondylar area and attaches to the anterolateral side of the intercondylar fossa. These ligaments prevent the tibia from sliding anteriorly (anterior cruciate) or posteriorly (posterior cruciate) relative to the femur.

On either side of the cruciate ligaments are two, C-shaped, fibrocartilage discs: the **medial meniscus** and **lateral meniscus**. The shape of the menisci allows them to deepen the articulations between the femur and the tibia and keep the femoral condyles from becoming displaced. They are triangular in cross-section so that their outer rim is thickest and it gets narrower as one travels deeper in the joint. The inferior rim of each meniscus is tethered to the tibia by the short **coronary ligament of the knee**, also called the meniscotibial ligaments. The lateral meniscus sits on top of the lateral tibial condyle and its two ends insert on the intercondylar eminence of the tibia between the anterior and posterior cruciate ligaments. The lateral meniscus is further stabilized by two ligaments that leave its posterior side and travel alongside the posterior cruciate ligament to reach the medial

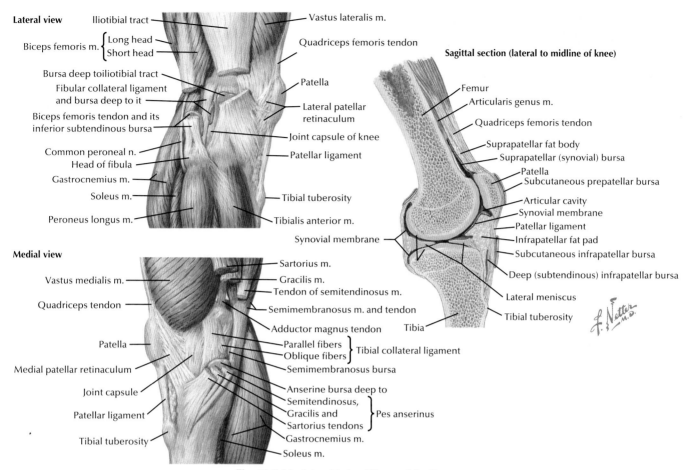

Fig. 11.6 Medial and Lateral Views of the Knee.

femoral condyle, the **anterior meniscofemoral ligament** and **posterior meniscofemoral ligament**. The anterior aspect of the lateral and medial menisci is connected by the **transverse ligament of the knee**, which also inserts onto the anterior intercondylar area. The posterior end of the medial meniscus inserts onto the tibia just anterior to the origin of the posterior cruciate ligament.

The coronary ligaments around the rim of the medial and lateral menisci are continuous with the fibrous capsule of the joint itself. On the medial side, the fibrous layer thickens considerably to create the intracapsular **medial (tibial) collateral ligament** of the knee, which connects the medial tibial plateau and medial meniscus to the medial side of the femoral epicondyle. This ligament prevents lateral (valgus) displacement of the leg relative to the thigh. On the opposite side, the **lateral (fibular) collateral ligament** stretches between the head of the fibula and the lateral femoral epicondyle to prevent medial (varus) displacement of the leg relative to the thigh. The lateral collateral ligament is not an intracapsular ligament because it is located outside of the joint and is separated from the fibrous layer of the capsule by the tendon of the popliteus muscle.

The fibrous layer of the knee joint capsule (see Fig. 11.2) surrounds the upper tibia and inferior femur, attaching to the lateral and medial side of the patella. The synovial layer of the capsule is in close contact with the fibrous layer everywhere except on the posterior side. This **infrapatellar synovial fold**

travels around the cruciate ligaments, excluding them from the synovial space of the knee joint. Two small alar folds of the anterior synovial lining project toward the infrapatellar synovial fold, leaving a small strip of the anterior intercondylar area within the synovial joint space.

On the posteromedial side of the joint capsule is a thickened intracapsular **oblique popliteal ligament** that originates from the fascia covering the popliteus muscle and distal attachment of the semimembranosus muscle. It passes superolaterally, deep to the lateral head of the gastrocnemius muscle and posterior to the lateral femoral condyle. The **posterolateral corner of the knee** hosts an array of structures that stabilize this region. The **arcuate popliteal ligament** arises from the head of the fibula and passes superomedially over the fibrous joint capsule. This ligament may be absent or diminished if the **fabella**, a sesamoid bone found in approximately 23% of people, is present in the overlying lateral head of the gastrocnemius muscle. The **popliteofibular ligament** is an extension of the popliteal tendon that inserts on the head of the fibula, while the rest of the tendon inserts more superiorly on the lateral femoral epicondyle.

The **patellar ligament** connects the apex of the patella to the tibial tuberosity, conveying the contraction of the quadriceps muscles to the leg. On either side of the patellar ligament are two important stabilizers of the anterior knee, the **medial patellar retinaculum** and **lateral patellar retinaculum**, which connect strips of the vastus medialis and vastus lateralis to the

CLINICAL CORRELATION 11.4　Varus and Valgus

When describing the side-to-side motion of body segments (movement in the coronal plane), the terms **varus** and **valgus** are frequently used to denote their movement, the forces applied to them, and associated injuries. These terms describe *motion of a distal segment relative to its proximal segment.* Taking the knee as an example, movement of the leg *medially* when compared with the thigh is called a varus displacement and can occur when lateral stabilizers of the knee such as the lateral collateral ligament are ruptured. Movement of the leg *laterally* in comparison with the thigh results in *valgus* displacement and would result from disruption of the medial stabilizers like the medial collateral ligament. People with knees that are directed laterally (bow-legged) can be described as having **genu varum** because the leg is angled medially compared with the thigh. Even though the knee itself is directed laterally, it is the relationship of the leg (distal segment) compared with the thigh (proximal segment) that matters. Similarly, those with medially directed knees (knock kneed) are described as having **genu valgum** because the leg is angled laterally compared with the thigh.

This terminology applies to joints other than the knee. For example, medial displacement of the forearm relative to the arm (perhaps due to rupture of the lateral collateral ligament of the elbow) would be a varus displacement of the forearm; lateral displacement of the first (big) toe relative to the first metatarsal bone, perhaps due to tight and pointed footwear, is a valgus displacement of the toe, called **hallux valgus**. If the neck of the femur has a decreased angle of inclination (approaches a 90-degree angle relative to the shaft), it is called **coxa vara**. If the angle of inclination is increased (becoming more aligned with the shaft), it is **coxa valga**.

anterior side of the proximal tibia. These convey some contraction of the quadriceps muscles to the leg but are more important in keeping the patella in place as the knee moves through flexion and extension. Deep to the patellar ligament and retinacula is the **infrapatellar fat pad**. This fascinating structure is actually located between the fibrous and synovial layers of the joint and is innervated heavily and acutely sensitive to pain. Inflammation of the knee, accompanied by excessive fluid in the joint space, can cause bulging of the infrapatellar fat pad (Clinical Correlations 11.4 and 11.5).

Superior Tibiofibular Joint (See Figs. 11.4–11.6)

The **superior (proximal) tibiofibular joint** is a synovial joint that allows the fibula a degree of translation superiorly and inferiorly as the ankle moves through dorsiflexion and plantarflexion. The joint is stabilized by **anterior** and **posterior ligaments of the fibular head**. Further inferiorly, the tibia and fibula are connected by the **interosseous membrane of the leg**, a sheet of connective tissue that tethers the medial aspect of the fibular shaft to the lateral tibia. It keeps the two bones connected even when they are fractured.

Distal Tibia and Fibula (See Fig. 11.4)

The **shaft of the tibia** continues inferiorly, ending with a broad depression on its lateral side, the **fibular notch**, and an equally broad bony process on the medial side, the medial malleolus. The posterior side of this process has a **malleolar groove** where tendons of the muscles from the deep posterior compartment of the leg cross the bone. The lateral (inner) aspect of the medial malleolus is smooth and is referred to as the articular facet of the medial malleolus. It is continuous with the smooth **inferior articular surface** that runs along the inferior, distal tibia.

The **shaft of the fibula** continues inferiorly until it terminates as the **lateral malleolus**. The lateral malleolus has a **malleolar groove** for the fibularis longus and brevis tendons, as well as an articular facet. The rectangular articular area formed by the tibia's inferior articular surface and the articular facets of the medial and lateral malleoli all articulate with the talus.

Inferior Tibiofibular Joint (Figs. 11.4 and 11.7)

The **inferior (distal) tibiofibular joint** (also known as the **tibiofibular syndesmosis**) holds the distal fibula within the fibular notch of the tibia, tightly connecting the two bones. This joint is a syndesmosis, consisting entirely of ligaments without articular cartilage or synovial fluid. This articulation is formed by the **anterior tibiofibular ligament** and **posterior tibiofibular ligament**, which are found on the respective sides of the distal leg. The posterior tibiofibular ligament inserts onto a small depression on the posterior lateral malleolus, the fossa of the lateral malleolus.

Tarsal Bones (Fig. 11.8)

The tarsal, or ankle bones, are a collection of seven bones (talus, calcaneus, navicular, cuboid, medial cuneiform, intermediate cuneiform, and lateral cuneiform) that connect the leg to the rest of the foot. The **hindfoot** consists of the talus and calcaneus while the **midfoot** contains the cuboid, navicular, and three cuneiform (medial, intermediate, and lateral) bones. The **forefoot** contains the metatarsals and digits, which will be discussed separately.

Talus

The **talus** has several articulations. The **body of the talus** is the superior proximal portion of the bone that articulates with the tibia, fibula, and calcaneus. The **head of the talus** is the distal portion that articulates with the navicular bone. The two regions are joined by a narrower **neck**. On the superior body is the **trochlea of the talus**, which hosts a superior facet to articulate with the inferior articular surface of the tibia. The trochlea is narrower posteriorly, which gives the foot more mobility when plantarflexed, because less bone is present between the malleoli. The medial and lateral malleolar facets of the trochlea articulate with the medial and lateral malleoli and help to limit inversion and eversion of the foot. There is a pronounced **lateral process** on the lateral side of the talar body. Posterior to the trochlea is the **posterior process** of the talus and its two projections, the **lateral tubercle** and **medial tubercle**, which straddle the groove for the tendon of the **flexor hallucis longus**. The inferior aspect of the talus has posterior, middle, and anterior **calcaneal articular facets**. A very deep **sulcus tali** separates the posterior and middle calcaneal articular facets. The most anterior part of the head of the talus hosts the convex **navicular articular surface**.

Calcaneus (Fig. 11.9)

The **calcaneus** (heel bone) is the largest tarsal bone, and its posterior side is dominated by the **calcaneal tuberosity** with

CLINICAL CORRELATION 11.5 Ligament Rupture of the Knee

Excessive valgus force directed against the leg will stress and possibly rupture the medial (tibial) collateral ligament. To test this ligament, the examiner will conduct the **valgus test** on a supine patient by stabilizing the thigh and pushing the leg laterally. Excessive lateral deflection of the leg without a firm end point is considered a positive test. Because the medial collateral ligament is intracapsular, it tends to heal along with the synovial and fibrous parts of the capsule.

Excessive varus force against the leg will stress and eventually tear the lateral (fibular) collateral ligament. To test this ligament, the examiner will conduct the **varus test** on a supine patient by stabilizing the thigh and pushing the leg medially. Excessive medial deflection of the leg without a firm end point is considered a positive test. Because it is not part of the joint capsule, a complete ligament rupture will not heal without surgical intervention.

The anterior cruciate ligament is frequently injured when the leg rotates externally relative to the femur or during other injuries involving the knee. A complete rupture of the ligament can be demonstrated by the **anterior drawer test**. The patient sits or lays supine with the knee flexed. The examiner stabilizes the foot and then attempts to pull the proximal tibia anteriorly. Excessive anterior translation of the tibia without a firm end point is considered a positive test. Spasm of the thigh muscles can give a false-negative, and these muscles need to be relaxed prior to starting the exam. Another test of the anterior cruciate ligament

is the **Lachman test**. In this case the patient lies supine and the examiner gently pushes the distal thigh down while lifting the proximal tibia with slight lateral rotation. A positive test occurs when there is excessive anterior translation of the tibia with no clear end point.

The posterior cruciate ligament is infrequently inured but can be damaged when the proximal tibia is forcefully driven posteriorly. This may occur when someone in the front seat of a car has his or her knees resting on the dashboard and experiences a head-on collision that forces the dashboard into the passenger. A complete rupture can be demonstrated by a **posterior drawer test**. In this test the patient sits or lays supine with the knee flexed. The examiner stabilizes the foot and then attempts to push the proximal tibia posteriorly. Excessive posterior translation of the tibia without a firm end point is considered a positive test.

Because the structures of the knee are very complex and it is exposed to significant forces, it can be injured in unexpected ways. Because the medial meniscus is attached to the medial collateral ligament, they can be injured together by valgus forces. The classic, **terrible or unhappy triad** of the knee involves linked injury to the medial meniscus, anterior cruciate ligament, and medial collateral ligament. Retrospective studies have demonstrated that injuries to another trio, the **O'Donoghue triad**, are more common. The structures in this triad are the anterior cruciate ligament, medial collateral ligament, and lateral meniscus.

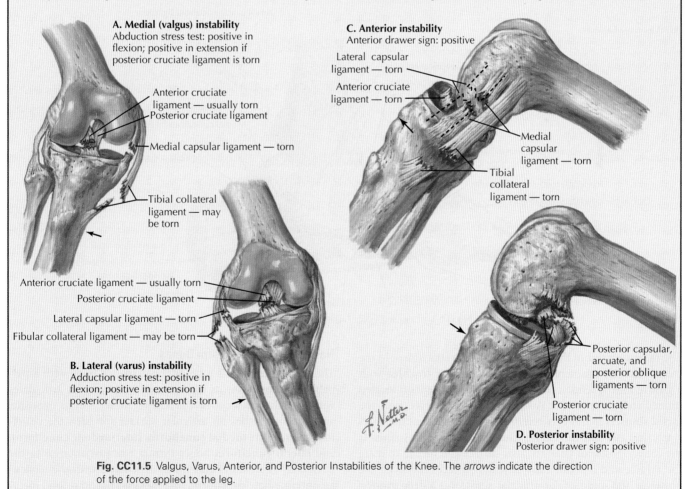

A. Medial (valgus) instability
Abduction stress test: positive in flexion; positive in extension if posterior cruciate ligament is torn

Anterior cruciate ligament — usually torn
Posterior cruciate ligament
Medial capsular ligament — torn
Tibial collateral ligament — may be torn

Anterior cruciate ligament — usually torn
Posterior cruciate ligament
Lateral capsular ligament — torn
Fibular collateral ligament — may be torn

B. Lateral (varus) instability
Adduction stress test: positive in flexion; positive in extension if posterior cruciate ligament is torn

C. Anterior instability
Anterior drawer sign: positive
Lateral capsular ligament — torn
Anterior cruciate ligament — torn
Medial capsular ligament — torn
Tibial collateral ligament — torn

Posterior capsular, arcuate, and posterior oblique ligaments — torn
Posterior cruciate ligament — torn

D. Posterior instability
Posterior drawer sign: positive

Fig. CC11.5 Valgus, Varus, Anterior, and Posterior Instabilities of the Knee. The *arrows* indicate the direction of the force applied to the leg.

pronounced **medial and lateral processes** on its inferior, posterior aspect. The rest of the posterior aspect of the calcaneus is the attachment site for the calcaneal (Achilles) tendon. Anterior to the medial and lateral processes is a rough area on

the inferior surface that terminates in a raised bump, the **calcaneal tubercle**. Anterior to the calcaneal tubercle is a saddle-shaped (bi-concave) **articular surface for the cuboid bone**. The lateral side of the calcaneus hosts two slight bony elevations.

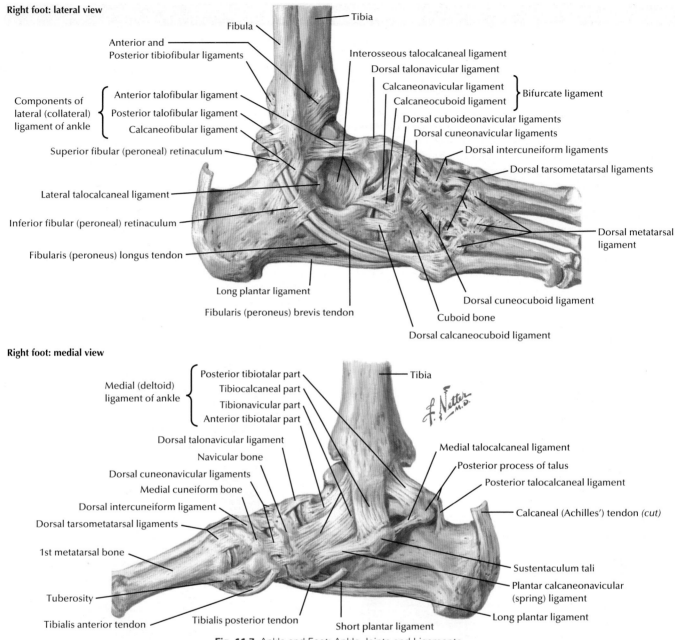

Right foot: lateral view

- Fibula
- Tibia
- Anterior and Posterior tibiofibular ligaments
- Interosseous talocalcaneal ligament
- Dorsal talonavicular ligament
- Calcaneonavicular ligament
- Calcaneocuboid ligament
- Bifurcate ligament
- Components of lateral (collateral) ligament of ankle
  - Anterior talofibular ligament
  - Posterior talofibular ligament
  - Calcaneofibular ligament
- Dorsal cuboideonavicular ligaments
- Dorsal cuneonavicular ligaments
- Dorsal intercuneiform ligaments
- Superior fibular (peroneal) retinaculum
- Dorsal tarsometatarsal ligaments
- Lateral talocalcaneal ligament
- Inferior fibular (peroneal) retinaculum
- Dorsal metatarsal ligament
- Fibularis (peroneus) longus tendon
- Long plantar ligament
- Dorsal cuneocuboid ligament
- Fibularis (peroneus) brevis tendon
- Cuboid bone
- Dorsal calcaneocuboid ligament

Right foot: medial view

- Medial (deltoid) ligament of ankle
  - Posterior tibiotalar part
  - Tibiocalcaneal part
  - Tibionavicular part
  - Anterior tibiotalar part
- Tibia
- *F. Netter M.D.*
- Dorsal talonavicular ligament
- Navicular bone
- Medial talocalcaneal ligament
- Posterior process of talus
- Posterior talocalcaneal ligament
- Dorsal cuneonavicular ligaments
- Medial cuneiform bone
- Dorsal intercuneiform ligament
- Dorsal tarsometatarsal ligaments
- Calcaneal (Achilles') tendon *(cut)*
- 1st metatarsal bone
- Tuberosity
- Sustentaculum tali
- Plantar calcaneonavicular (spring) ligament
- Long plantar ligament
- Tibialis anterior tendon
- Tibialis posterior tendon
- Short plantar ligament

Fig. 11.7 Ankle and Foot: Ankle Joints and Ligaments.

The more superior of the elevations is for the attachment of the calcaneofibular ligament. Inferiorly is a **fibular trochlea** with a groove for the tendon of the fibularis longus tendon located immediately inferior to it. A large interosseous depression, the **tarsal sinus**, is found between the superior aspect of the anterior calcaneus and the lateral talus. Posterior to this sinus is the convex posterior talar articular surface and medial to it are the middle and anterior talar articular surfaces. Between the posterior and middle talar articular surfaces is a deep groove, the **calcaneal sulcus**, which connects with the tarsal sinus. On the medial side of the calcaneus is a prominent shelf of bone, the **sustentaculum tali**, that supports and stabilizes the talus. On its inferior aspect, alongside its connection to the rest of the calcaneus is the groove for the tendon of the flexor hallucis longus tendon.

Navicular and Cuneiform Bones

The **navicular** bone is a broad, boat-shaped bone with a palpable **tuberosity** on its medial side. Posteriorly it articulates with the talus via a concave articular surface. On its opposite, anterior side it has an articular surface for each the cuneiform bones. The **medial cuneiform, intermediate cuneiform,** and **lateral cuneiform** bones form a row just anterior to the navicular. The medial cuneiform articulates with the navicular, intermediate cuneiform, first metatarsal, and second metatarsal bones. The intermediate cuneiform articulates with the navicular, medial cuneiform, lateral cuneiform, and second metatarsal bones. The lateral cuneiform articulates with the navicular, intermediate cuneiform, second metatarsal, third metatarsal, slightly with the fourth metatarsal, and cuboid bones.

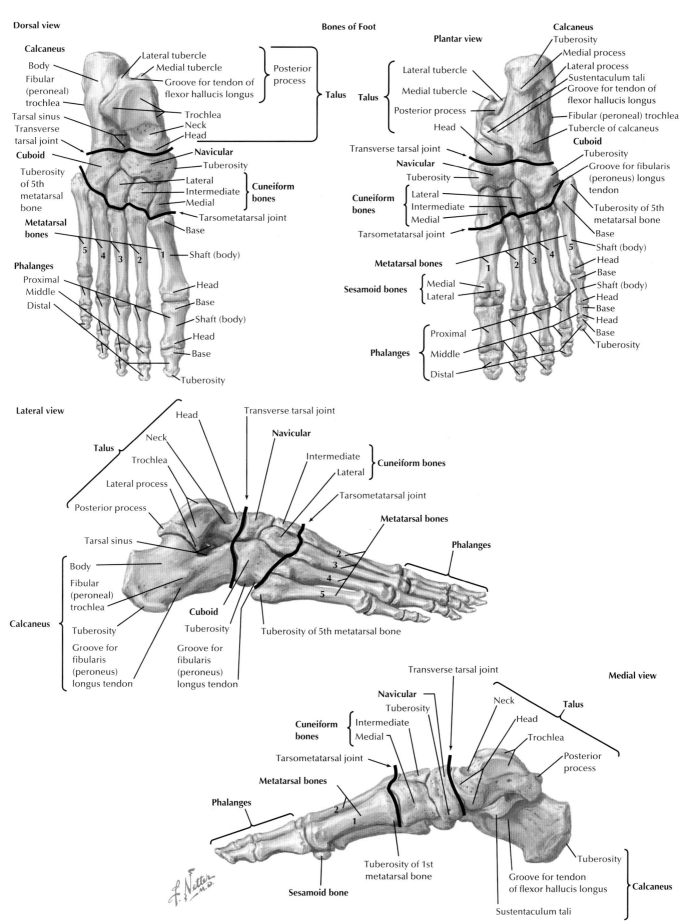

Bones of Foot

Fig. 11.8 Bones of the Foot.

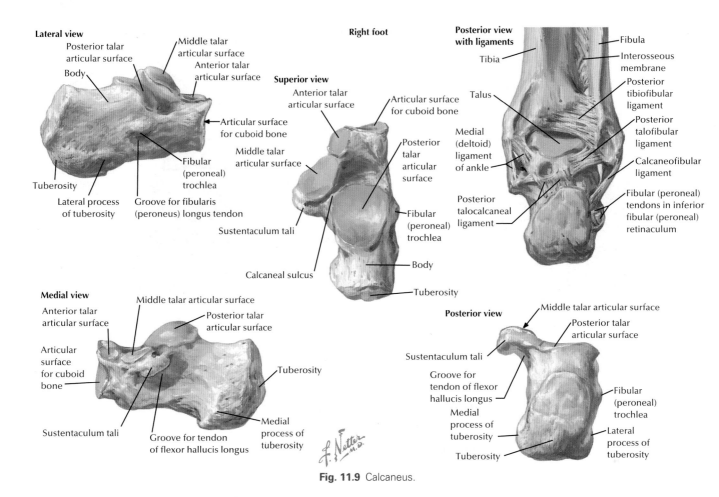

Fig. 11.9 Calcaneus.

Cuboid

On its medial aspect, the **cuboid bone** articulates with the lateral cuneiform and navicular bones. Posteriorly, it has a saddle-shaped **articular surface for the calcaneus**. The inferior aspect of the cuboid has a raised **tuberosity** immediately posterior to the groove for the tendon of the fibularis longus. The cuboid bone's anterior surface has articular surfaces for the fourth and fifth metatarsal bones.

Ankle Joint (See Fig. 11.7)

The **ankle joint** is where the trochlea of the talus articulates with the inferior articular facet of the tibia as well as the articular facets of the medial and lateral malleoli. This allows it to dorsi-flex and plantarflex the foot while being stabilized by ligaments on its medial and lateral side. The **deltoid ligament** is a large, fan-shaped structure that connects the medial malleolus to the nearby tarsal bones. Although the deltoid ligament is made from four other ligaments that are somewhat fused (tibionavicular, tibiocalcaneal, anterior tibiotalar, and posterior tibiotalar parts), they all tend to act together to prevent excessive eversion (valgus deflection) of the foot.

On the lateral side are three separate ligaments that connect the lateral malleolus to the lateral sides of the tarsal bones. The **anterior talofibular ligament** connects the lateral malleolus to the lateral side of the head of the talus, crossing the superior aspect of the tarsal sinus. Posterior to it is the

calcaneofibular ligament that connects the inferior tip of the lateral malleolus to the lateral aspect of the body of the calcaneus. Posteriorly, the **posterior talofibular ligament** extends from the posterior aspect of the lateral malleolus to the lateral tubercle of the posterior process of the talus (Clinical Correlations 11.6 and 11.7).

Subtalar and Transverse Tarsal Joints (Figs. 11.7–11.10)

The articulation between the talar and calcaneal articular facets is technically the **subtalar joint**, where most inversion and eversion occurs. It has a flimsy joint capsule that is reinforced by three ligaments. The **lateral talocalcaneal ligament** extends from the lateral process of the talus to the medial side of the tarsal sinus. Immediately anterior it is the strong **interosseous talocalcaneal ligament**, which stretches from the tarsal sinus and along the length of the calcaneal sulcus. Originating from the lateral and medial tubercles of the posterior process of the talus are **posterior talocalcaneal** and **medial talocalcaneal ligaments**. They insert on the superior aspect of the calcaneal body and the sustentaculum tali, respectively. Clinically, the subtalar joint often includes the **talocalcaneonavicular joint** and the **talonavicular joint** as well, which allows for prona-tion and supination of the foot. Although sometimes treated synonymously, eversion and inversion refer strictly to the sole of the foot facing laterally and medially (the toes remain

CLINICAL CORRELATION 11.6 High Ankle Sprain

When the foot is forced into dorsiflexion, the wide anterior part of the trochlea of the talus can force the medial and lateral malleoli away from each other. If this ruptures the anterior and posterior tibiofibular ligaments, the distal fibula will detach from the tibia, resulting in a **high ankle sprain**. These are graded according to how much of a gap between the distal fibula and tibia is observed on a radiograph.

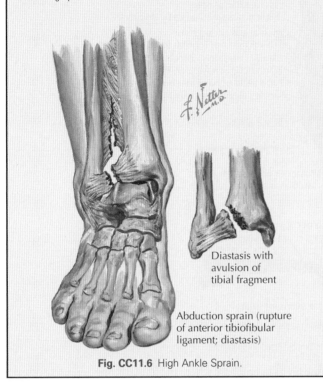

Diastasis with avulsion of tibial fragment

Abduction sprain (rupture of anterior tibiofibular ligament; diastasis)

Fig. CC11.6 High Ankle Sprain.

CLINICAL CORRELATION 11.7 Ligament Rupture of the Ankle

When the foot is forced into eversion/abduction by valgus force, the deltoid ligament is stretched and may undergo a **medial ligament sprain** or rupture. However, the deltoid ligament is very strong, and it will frequently pull on its attachment to the medial malleolus so forcefully that it avulses it from the rest of the tibia. Further eversion is limited by contact with the lateral malleolus, which extends further inferiorly that the medial malleolus. If the valgus force continues, the lateral malleolus will be forced laterally, fracturing the inferior third of the fibular shaft. This combination of medial malleolar avulsion and fibular shaft fracture is known as a **Pott fracture**.

When the foot and ankle are forced into inversion/adduction by varus force, a **lateral ligament sprain** may occur. These ligaments tend to rupture from anterior to posterior: first the anterior talofibular ligament, then the calcaneofibular ligament, and finally the posterior talofibular ligament. The ankle becomes progressively more unstable as more ligaments are ruptured.

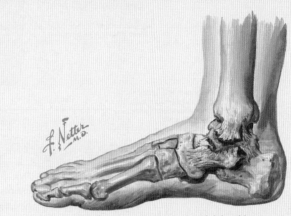

Abduction sprain (rupture of deltoid ligament)

Fig. CC11.7 Abduction Sprain.

directed anteriorly throughout). Pronation involves some external rotation of the foot (toes point laterally), and supination involves some internal rotation of the foot (toes point medially). The two sets of motion are linked and often occur simultaneously.

To make things complicated, the **transverse tarsal joint** is a compound joint that also includes the talocalcaneonavicular joint, specifically the articulation between the talar head and the navicular bone, as well as the **calcaneocuboid joint**. The transverse tarsal joint allows rotation of the distal foot, which supplements the motions of the subtalar joint.

Other Joints and Ligaments of the Tarsus and Foot (See Figs. 11.7, 11.8, and 11.10)

The remaining tarsal bones, the cuboid and three cuneiform bones, form **cuneonavicular, intercuneiform**, and **cuneocuboid articulations**. These joints are less mobile than the others that have been described and are supported by an array of **tarsal ligaments** that keep the bones in place and prevent subluxation. The internal aspects of these bones and their neighbors host several **tarsal interosseous ligaments** (intercuneiform interosseous and cuneocuboid interosseous ligaments). The bones are further stabilized by **dorsal tarsal ligaments**

(dorsal intercuneiform, dorsal cuneocuboid, dorsal cuboidonavicular, dorsal cuneonavicular, dorsal calcaneocuboid ligaments) as well as the **bifurcate ligament** with calcaneonavicular and calcaneocuboid parts that can be injured in inversion injuries. Not surprisingly, there are also a variety of **plantar tarsal ligaments** (plantar cuneonavicular, plantar cuboidonavicular, plantar intercuneiform, plantar cuneocuboid) that also contribute to the stability of these bones.

There are three particularly important ligaments on the plantar side of the foot. The **plantar calcaneonavicular (spring) ligament** stretches between the sustentaculum tali of the calcaneus to the inferior aspect of the navicular bone (including the tuberosity of the navicular) near the insertion of the tibialis posterior tendon. This expansive ligament prevents the navicular and calcaneus from being driven apart by the weight of the body pushing down from the talus. Its superior surface contributes to the articular surface between the head of the talus and the posterior articular facet of the navicular. Just lateral to it is the **short plantar (plantar calcaneocuboid) ligament** that stretches from the calcaneal tubercle to the cuboid bone. Finally, the **long plantar ligament** originates from the calcaneus immediately anterior to the medial and lateral processes of the calcaneal tuberosity.

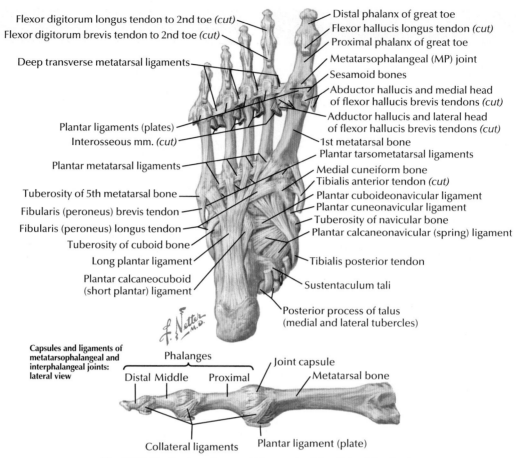

Flexor digitorum longus tendon to 2nd toe *(cut)*
Flexor digitorum brevis tendon to 2nd toe *(cut)*
Deep transverse metatarsal ligaments
Plantar ligaments (plates)
Interosseous mm. *(cut)*
Plantar metatarsal ligaments
Tuberosity of 5th metatarsal bone
Fibularis (peroneus) brevis tendon
Fibularis (peroneus) longus tendon
Tuberosity of cuboid bone
Long plantar ligament
Plantar calcaneocuboid (short plantar) ligament

Distal phalanx of great toe
Flexor hallucis longus tendon *(cut)*
Proximal phalanx of great toe
Metatarsophalangeal (MP) joint
Sesamoid bones
Abductor hallucis and medial head of flexor hallucis brevis tendons *(cut)*
Adductor hallucis and lateral head of flexor hallucis brevis tendons *(cut)*
1st metatarsal bone
Plantar tarsometatarsal ligaments
Medial cuneiform bone
Tibialis anterior tendon *(cut)*
Plantar cuboideonavicular ligament
Plantar cuneonavicular ligament
Tuberosity of navicular bone
Plantar calcaneonavicular (spring) ligament
Tibialis posterior tendon
Sustentaculum tali
Posterior process of talus (medial and lateral tubercles)

Capsules and ligaments of metatarsophalangeal and interphalangeal joints: lateral view

Phalanges
Distal Middle Proximal

Joint capsule
Metatarsal bone
Collateral ligaments
Plantar ligament (plate)

Fig. 11.10 Tendon Insertions and Ligaments of the Sole of the Foot.

It travels anteriorly as a single large bundle to cross the cuboid bone. Thereafter it divides into multiple slips that pass inferior to the fibularis longus tendon and reach as far as the bases of metatarsals 2 to 5. A very strong and broad ligament, the **plantar aponeurosis** (see Fig. 11.20) is found inferior (superficial) to all the intrinsic muscles of the plantar foot. It stretches from the medial and lateral processes of the calcaneal tuberosity and fans outward to the heads of each metatarsal and into the digits themselves. Just proximal to the heads of the metatarsals, the distal extensions of the aponeurosis are bridged by stout **transverse fasciculi**. Distal to (or overlying) the heads of the metatarsals is another transverse band of connective tissue, the **superficial transverse metatarsal ligament**. A smaller (but still significant) **lateral band** of the plantar aponeurosis travels from the calcaneus to the base of the fifth metatarsal (Clinical Correlation 11.8).

Bones, Joints, and Ligaments of the Foot (See Figs. 11.4, 11.7, 11.8, and 11.10)

The rest of the foot, the **forefoot**, consists of the metatarsal bones and phalanges. Like the metacarpal bones in the hand, the **metatarsal bones** form the core of the foot itself. The **base** of each metatarsal bone associates with the cuneiform bones or cuboid. The **body** or **shaft** of each metatarsal extends distally, ending in an enlarged and rounded **head** that articulates with a digit. There is a prominent **tuberosity of the fifth metatarsal**

bone on its lateral base where the fibularis brevis muscle inserts. The first metatarsal has a less pronounced tuberosity of the first metatarsal bone on the inferior aspect of its base. The head of the first metatarsal has medial and lateral articular grooves on its inferior aspect for **sesamoid bones** within the tendon of the flexor hallucis brevis muscle.

The base of the first metatarsal articulates with the medial cuneiform and the base of the second metatarsal. The second metatarsal base articulates with the medial, intermediate, and (barely) lateral cuneiform bones, and the bases of the first and third metatarsals. The base of the third metatarsal articulates with the lateral cuneiform, and bases of the second and fourth metatarsal bones. The base of the fourth metatarsal bone articulates with the cuboid and bases of the third and fifth metatarsals. Finally, the base of the fifth metatarsal articulates with the cuboid and base of the fourth metatarsal bone.

The tarsal bones and the bases of the metatarsals articulate via **tarsometatarsal joints**. These are linked and stabilized by **dorsal and plantar tarsometatarsal ligaments**. A **cuneometatarsal interosseous (Lisfranc) ligament** stretches from the medial cuneiform to the base of the second metatarsal and can be torn or cause avulsion when the foot is rotated excessively. The **intermetatarsal joints** that link the bases of adjacent metatarsal bones are stabilized by **dorsal and plantar metatarsal ligaments** as well as **metatarsal interosseous ligaments** within the joints.

CLINICAL CORRELATION 11.8 Arches of the Foot

The articulations of the tarsal and foot bones are not arrayed in a way that lets the foot sit flat against the ground. Instead, they are arched to absorb the energy they encounter with each step and to make room for the many muscles on the plantar side of the foot. The **longitudinal arch** of the foot is in the sagittal plane and is supported by the plantar aponeurosis and the action of the flexor hallucis longus and flexor digitorum longus muscles. It is subdivided into lateral and medial longitudinal arches. The **lateral longitudinal arch** crosses the talus, cuneiform bones, and metatarsals 4–5 and is maintained by the long and short plantar ligaments as well as superior pull from the fibularis longus tendon. The **medial longitudinal arch** is much higher than the lateral longitudinal arch and spans the calcaneus, cuboid, and metatarsals 1–3. It is maintained by the plantar calcaneonavicular (spring) ligament and superior pull from the tibialis posterior tendon. The **transverse arch of the foot** is in the coronal plane and crosses from the lateral, intermediate, and medial cuneiform bones to the cuboid. The transverse arch is supported by the lateral pull of the fibularis longus tendon and the medial pull of the tibialis posterior tendon.

When these ligaments and tendons are weakened by overuse or poor footwear, the arches can collapse. These **fallen arches** or **pes planus (flat feet)** are painful and make walking less efficient because the springiness of the foot has been lost. This may result is a person walking on the medial side of their tarsal bones when the medial longitudinal arch is obliterated.

Bones, Joints, and Ligaments of the Digits (See Figs. 11.4, 11.7, and 11.10)

The digits themselves are organized around the **phalanges**. The big toe, or **hallux**, (first digit) has two segments, formed by a **proximal phalanx** and **distal phalanx**. The toes (second to fifth digits) have three segments, a **proximal phalanx, middle phalanx,** and **distal phalanx**. Each phalanx has a proximal **base, shaft/body**, and distal **head**. The heads of the proximal and middle phalanges have two rounded ends that form the **trochlea of the phalanx**, which articulates with the bases of the next phalanx. Just like the hand, the distal phalanges host flared-out **tuberosities** just proximal to their heads or, according to some descriptions, in the place of their heads.

At the **metatarsophalangeal** (MTP) joints, the head of each metatarsal is rounded to fit into a shallow depression at the base of each proximal phalanx. There is a stout **medial collateral ligament** and **lateral collateral ligament** on each side, as well as **plantar ligaments,** to protect the joint space, keep movements of the digital flexor tendons smooth, and limit extension. The plantar ligaments (and therefore the heads of the metatarsals) are connected by the **deep transverse metatarsal ligament**, which prevents abduction of the metatarsal heads from each other.

The **proximal interphalangeal** (PIP) and **distal interphalangeal** (DIP) **joints** are very similar to the MTP joint, with **medial collateral, lateral collateral,** and **plantar ligaments** limiting abduction, adduction, and extension. The first digit (hallux, great toe, big toe) has a normal MTP joint but only one interphalangeal joint because it has no middle phalanx (Clinical Correlation 11.9).

CLINICAL CORRELATION 11.9 Mallet, Hammer, and Claw Toes

Common deformities affecting the foot are mallet, hammer, and claw toes. **Mallet toe** occurs when an imbalance between extensors and flexors causes the metatarsophalangeal and proximal interphalangeal joints to be pulled into persistent dorsiflexion and the distal interphalangeal joint into plantarflexion. **Hammer toe** typically affects the second digit; the toe shows dorsiflexion at the metatarsophalangeal joint, plantarflexion at the proximal interphalangeal joint, and dorsiflexion at the distal interphalangeal joint. **Claw toes** typically occur in digits 2–5 and manifest with dorsiflexion at the metatarsophalangeal joint and plantarflexion of both interphalangeal joints.

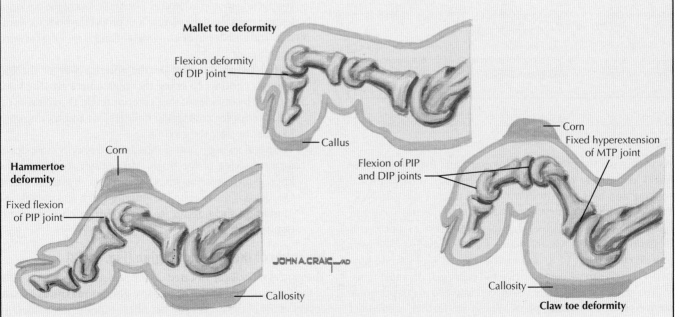

Fig. CC11.9 Lesser Toe Deformities (Claw Toe, Hammertoe, and Mallet Toe). *DIP,* Distal interphalangeal; *MTP,* metatarsophalangeal; *PIP,* proximal interphalangeal.

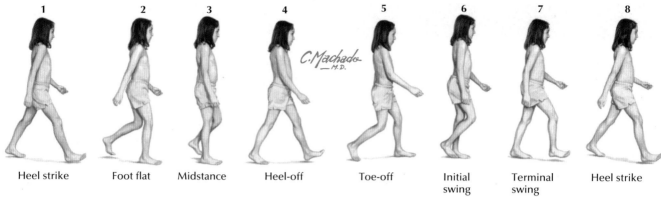

Fig. 11.11 Phases of Gait.

MUSCLE GROUPS OF THE LOWER LIMB

It might be useful to review the section on the lower limb in Chapter 3 or the following table before moving into the detailed anatomy of the muscles in the lower limbs.

Muscle Region	Major Function(s)	Source of Innervation
Gluteal	Abduction and extension of thigh	Superior and inferior gluteal nerves
Iliopsoas	Flexion of thigh	Lumbar anterior rami
Anterior thigh	Extension of leg	Femoral nerve
Medial thigh	Adduction of thigh	Obturator nerve
Posterior thigh	Extension of thigh and flexion of leg	Sciatic nerve
Posterior leg	Plantarflexion of foot, flexion of digits	Tibial nerve
Lateral leg	Eversion of foot	Superficial fibular nerve
Anterior leg	Dorsiflexion of foot, extension of digits	Deep fibular nerve
Plantar foot	Flexion, adduction, abduction of digits	Medial and lateral plantar nerves
Dorsum of foot	Extension of digits	Superficial fibular nerve

Gait

As we discuss the muscles of the lower limb, there will be frequent allusions to how these muscles are used during normal walking and how their dysfunction will disrupt the gait cycle. Problems with the gait cycle can be linked to specific nerve and muscle problems, and observing them can serve as a powerful diagnostic tool. We will introduce gait now, discuss how each muscle contributes to it, and revisit it when we examine how nerve lesions can weaken muscles and cause gait derangements.

The gait cycle (Fig. 11.11) is divided into two major portions: **stance phase** and **swing phase**. These are further subdivided into other phases listed next.

- **Stance:** The limb is bearing weight, either alone or with the other limb.
  - **Heel strike:** Forward swing of the hip is stopped by gluteal muscles. The knee is extended by muscles of the anterior thigh (quadriceps). The foot is dorsiflexed by anterior leg (shin) muscles, and the foot is slightly rotated laterally by the deep gluteal muscles.
  - **Foot flat:** Lateral hip muscles contract to stop the pelvis from dropping toward the swinging leg. The hip is extended by muscles of the posterior thigh (hamstrings). The knee is kept extended by muscles of the anterior thigh that resist flexion under the body's weight. The muscles on the plantar side of the foot (sole) contract to keep the foot bones in place.
  - **Midstance:** Same as flat foot but the dorsiflexion muscles of the anterior leg are countered by the plantarflexion muscles of the posterior leg (calf).
  - **Heel-off (opposite heel strike occurs at this time):** Same as midstance but the plantar flexors of the posterior leg contract strongly to lift the heel and propel the body forward.
  - **Toe-off:** Muscles on the anterior side of the hip (psoas) begin contracting to stop extension. Plantar flexors of the posterior leg and muscles of the plantar foot propel the body forward.
- **Swing:** The limb is not bearing weight and is moving forward through the air.
  - **Initial swing:** Muscles on the anterior side of the hip strongly contract to swing the thigh anteriorly. The knee is flexed by muscles of the posterior thigh. Dorsiflexors on the anterior leg contract to pull the foot and toes upward in order to clear the ground.
  - **Terminal swing:** Gluteal muscles and gravity slow down forward swing of the thigh. Momentum straightens the knee but hamstring muscles prevent hyperextension. Quadriceps muscles on the anterior thigh and dorsiflexor muscles of the anterior leg start contraction in preparation for heel strike.

Muscles of the Gluteal Region (Fig. 11.12)

The gluteal muscles are located on the posterior and lateral sides of the sacrum and ilium. The massive **gluteus maximus** muscle covers many of the others and has fibers running inferolaterally as it descends to insert on the femur and the tough fascia of

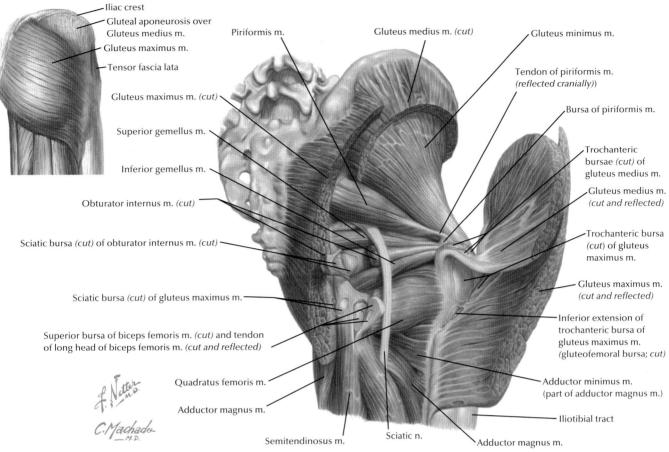

Fig. 11.12 Gluteal Muscles.

the thigh, the **fascia lata**. The gluteus maximus crosses some bony prominences along its course, and repetitive motion or compression against these prominences could cause pain and inflammation. To prevent this, there is a **sciatic bursa of the gluteus maximus** between the muscle and the ischial tuberosity, a **trochanteric bursa of the gluteus maximus** between the muscle and the massive greater trochanter, and several intermuscular gluteal bursae along the gluteal tuberosity and nearby linea aspera. A nearby, superficial subcutaneous trochanteric bursa helps to prevent inflammation as the skin is pushed against the greater trochanter. The superolateral-most part of the gluteus maximus attaches to the iliac crest as the **gluteal aponeurosis**, which also gives rise to part of the gluteus medius. **Gluteal fascia** extends inferiorly from the iliac crest and divides to pass on both sides of the gluteus maximus before blending with the fascia lata. Deep to the gluteus maximus are the **gluteus medius** and **gluteus minimus muscles**. The gluteus medius originates between the posterior and anterior gluteal lines, while the gluteus minimus originates between the anterior and inferior gluteal lines. Both muscles insert onto the greater trochanter of the femur. To prevent irritation of the distal gluteus medius and minimus tendons as they insert into bone, there are **trochanteric bursae of the gluteus medius and minimus** between them and the greater trochanter. Anterior to the gluteus maximus and medius muscles is the last of the superficial gluteal muscles, the **tensor fascia lata**, which is attached to the anterior

aspect of the iliac crest and is actually located within a pocket of the fascia lata itself. This muscle does not have a typical tendon but terminates in a thickened region of the surrounding fascia, the **iliotibial tract**, which extends laterally past the knee to insert on the anterolateral tubercle of the tibia. Because it has to glide across the knee before inserting onto the tibia, there is a **bursa of the iliotibial tract** separating it from the lateral femoral condyle (Clinical Correlation 11.10).

The deep gluteal muscles are all covered by the inferior aspect of the gluteus maximus. Normally they act as external/lateral rotators of the thigh, but they also prevent abduction and distraction of the femoral head from the acetabulum. The **piriformis muscle** originates from the anterior aspect of the sacrum and exits the greater sciatic foramen alongside the gluteal nerves and arteries, the sciatic nerve, and the posterior cutaneous nerve of

---

CLINICAL CORRELATION 11.10
Trochanteric and Sciatic Bursitis

Repetitive flexion and extension of the hip can cause inflammation of the bursae that sit between the gluteal muscles and the greater trochanter. Pain will manifest while ascending stairs and climbing an inclined surface and will be felt superficial to the greater trochanter and may radiate down the lateral thigh. The sciatic bursa between the gluteus maximus and ischial tuberosity can also become inflamed, causing pain over the ischial tuberosity that is worse during hip flexion and while seated with the weight resting on the affected bones.

CLINICAL CORRELATION 11.11 Gluteal Intramuscular Injections

Intramuscular injections are frequently given when the injected material needs to be put into circulation but at a slower rate than intravenous injection. The gluteal muscles are a frequent site for such injections. The inferior gluteal area should be avoided due to the nearby sciatic and posterior cutaneous nerves. Instead, the superolateral quadrant of the gluteal region is used so the injection is placed into the gluteus medius or maximus. However, if there is excessive adipose present or the needle is not advanced far enough, the injection may go into subcutaneous fat and take longer to absorb (or not absorb at all). For this reason, some practitioners prefer to administer intramuscular injections into the deltoid or vastus lateralis muscles.

the thigh. It has a small piriformis bursa that cushions its tendon near its insertion onto the superior part of the greater trochanter. The **obturator internus muscle** also originates from within the pelvis, in this case from the internal aspect of the obturator membrane. Its tendon passes through the lesser sciatic foramen and takes a sharp turn across the ischium, from which it is separated by the sciatic bursa of the obturator internus. Its tendon inserts in the trochanteric fossa and has a subtendinous bursa of the obturator internus near its attachment to the bone. The **superior gemellus muscle** originates from the ischial spine and the **inferior gemellus muscle** from the concavity of the lesser sciatic notch. They both fuse with the tendon of the obturator internus and insert in the trochanteric fossa. The final muscle in this group originates from the ischial tuberosity and inserts on the intertrochanteric crest, the very stout **quadratus femoris muscle** (Clinical Correlation 11.11).

Gluteus Maximus

Proximal attachments	• Posterior iliac crest • Posterior sacrum • Sacrotuberous ligament
Distal attachment	• Gluteal tuberosity of femur and upper linea aspera • Fascia lata of thigh
Functions	• Extension of the thigh from a flexed position, such as rising from a seated position or stepping up • Lateral rotation of thigh
Muscle testing and signs of damage	• Loss of function to the gluteus maximus does not affect normal gait since the hamstring muscles are the primary extensors of the hip during typical walking. • Weakness of the gluteus maximus will prevent a person from ascending the stairs if the affected limb is on the next step up. They will tend to ascend stairs with the affected limb always lagging and never being the limb that ascends to the next step. Likewise, such persons will have difficulty standing from a seated position without an assist from their upper limbs.
Innervation	• Inferior gluteal nerve (L5–S2)
Blood supply	• Superior and inferior gluteal vessels

Gluteus Medius, Gluteus Minimus, and Tensor Fascia Latae

Proximal attachments	• Gluteus medius: Upper half of gluteal surface of ilium, between anterior and posterior gluteal lines • Gluteus minimus: Inferior half of gluteal surface of ilium, between anterior and inferior gluteal lines • Tensor fascia latae: Small strip of gluteal surface of ilium anterior to attachments of gluteus medius and minimus
Distal attachment	• Gluteus medius: Outer, lateral side of greater trochanter of femur • Gluteus minimus: Outer, anterior side of greater trochanter of femur • Tensor fascia latae: Extends to the anterolateral tubercle of the tibia through the iliotibial tract of the fascia lata
Functions	• Gluteus medius and minimus: Bring the greater trochanter and ilium together. This will abduct an unweighted lower limb or elevate the contralateral pelvis when that limb is bearing weight, keeping the pelvis level when standing on a support leg • Tensor fascia latae: Assists in the function of the gluteus medius and minimus, also does actually tense the fascia lata
Muscle testing and signs of dysfunction	• To test gluteus medius, minimus, and tensor fascia latae, have the patient stand on one leg with the body upright. The examiner may need to assist. If these muscles are weak or the superior gluteal nerve is damaged, the patient will fall away from the affected side (Trendelenburg sign) as the pelvis cannot be kept level • To prevent falling while walking, an affected person will sway their upper body toward the affected side as it bears weight (Trendelenburg gait)
Innervation	• Superior gluteal nerve (L5–S1)
Blood supply	• Superior and inferior gluteal vessels

Piriformis

Proximal attachments	• Anterior ala of sacrum between S2 and S4
Distal attachment	• Superior tip of greater trochanter of femur
Functions	• Rotate an extended thigh laterally, abduct a flexed thigh
Muscle testing and signs of dysfunction	• Very slight shortened step due to weakness externally rotating lower limb during heel strike • Spasm or tension of the piriformis can be a cause of gluteal pain and cause the thigh to be persistently laterally rotated
Innervation	• Superior gluteal nerve (L5–S1) or anterior rami of S1–S2
Blood supply	• Superior and inferior gluteal vessels

Obturator Internus, Superior Gemellus, Inferior Gemellus, Quadratus Femoris

Proximal attachments	• Obturator internus: Internal aspect of obturator membrane and surrounding rim of pubis and ischium • Superior gemellus: Ischial spine • Inferior gemellus: Lesser sciatic notch • Quadratus femoris: Between the most posterior part of ischial tuberosity and obturator foramen
Distal attachment	• Obturator internus, superior and inferior gemelli: Trochanteric fossa just inferior to piriformis • Quadratus femoris: Posterior greater trochanter/quadrate tubercle
Functions	• Rotate an extended thigh laterally, abduct a flexed thigh • Resting tone of these muscles helps to keep femoral head within acetabulum
Muscle testing and signs of dysfunction	• Slightly shortened step due to weakness externally rotating lower limb during heel strike
Innervation	• Obturator internus and superior gemellus: Nerve to obturator internus (L5–S1) • Inferior gemellus and quadratus femoris: Nerve to quadratus femoris (L5–S1)
Blood supply	• Inferior gluteal and medial circumflex femoral vessels

Deep Muscles of the Anterior Thigh—Iliopsoas Muscle (Fig. 11.13)

There are several muscles that originate from the torso that function in the lower limb. The **psoas major muscle** is a large muscle hidden deep in the body alongside the vertebral column. It originates from the vertebral bodies and intervertebral discs from T12 to L5 as well as lumbar transverse processes. In the pelvis it fuses with a muscle that originates from the iliac fossa of the ilium, the **iliacus muscle**. The **iliac fascia** on the medial surface of this muscle is very thick, and it fuses with the **psoas fascia** to join the inguinal ligament as the **iliopectineal arch**. This arch creates a muscular space lateral to the arch and a vascular space for the femoral vessels on its medial side. The psoas major and iliacus muscles fuse to create the **iliopsoas muscle**, which crosses the muscular space formed by the inguinal ligament and iliopectineal arch and insets on the lesser trochanter of the femur. To minimize friction as it crosses the iliopubic eminence, the **iliopectineal bursa** (also called iliopsoas bursa) is present just anterior to the coxofemoral joint capsule between the iliofemoral and pubofemoral ligaments. A **subtendinous bursa of the iliacus** is present on the lesser trochanter to help the iliopsoas tendon glide across the bone smoothly as it inserts. The iliopsoas muscle is the major flexor of the thigh at the hip but is powerful enough to reverse the motion and move the torso and upper body when the lower limbs are fixed in place. It also reinforces the hip joint anteriorly. There is often a small **psoas minor muscle** on the surface of the psoas major. It does not enter the lower limb but inserts on the iliopectineal arch and iliac fascia. If present, it will help to control pelvic tilt and flex the pelvis (Clinical Correlation 11.12).

Psoas Major, Iliacus, and Psoas Minor

Proximal attachments	• Psoas major: T12–L5 vertebral bodies and intervertebral discs, lumbar transverse processes • Iliacus: Iliac fossa of ilium, anterior ala of sacrum at S1 level, anterior sacroiliac ligament • Psoas minor: T12–L1 vertebral bodies and intervertebral disc
Distal attachment	• Psoas major and iliacus: Fuse to form iliopsoas muscle and insert on lesser trochanter of femur • Psoas minor: Iliopubic eminence and pectinate line
Functions	• Psoas major and iliacus: Flex the thigh at the hip. If lower limbs are fixed, flex torso at the hip. Stabilize the anterior aspect of the hip joint • Psoas minor: Flex and stabilize the pelvis anteriorly
Muscle testing and signs of dysfunction	• Psoas major and iliacus: Have the patient lay supine. Have patient flex the hip against moderate resistance on each side, and note asymmetry in strength. Spasm of the iliopsoas or psoas major will cause back pain. Shortening of the psoas major can be detected by elevating each lower limb from the table separately. If the contralateral hip lifts off the table, the psoas major on that side has reached its limit. The palm of one hand can be placed under the lumbar vertebrae to note any lordosis to counteract the tension in the psoas major • Psoas minor: Loss of function of the muscle will not be noted. Spasm of it may cause back pain
Innervation	• Psoas major: L1–L3 anterior rami • Psoas minor: L1–L2 anterior rami • Iliacus: L2–L3 anterior rami and/or branches of the femoral nerve
Blood supply	• Lumbar segmental, iliolumbar, deep circumflex iliac, medial circumflex femoral arteries

Muscles of the Anterior Thigh (See Figs. 11.4 and 11.14)

The entire thigh is covered by the **fascia lata**. The muscles of the anterior compartment are separated from the others by divisions of the fascia lata that dive deep and fuse with the femoral periosteum at the medial and lateral lips of the linea aspera, the **lateral femoral intermuscular septum,** and **medial femoral intermuscular septum**. The anterior thigh muscles have multiple functions, but their major action is to extend the leg at the knee and flex the thigh at the hip. The **sartorius muscle** is the longest and most superficial of the muscles in this compartment. It originates from the anterior superior iliac spine and crosses anterior to the hip and medial to the knee as it descends and courses from lateral to medial. The sartorius inserts onto the medial tibial condyle along with the tendons of the gracilis and semitendinosus muscles as a compound tendon, the **pes anserinus**, which stabilizes the medial side of the knee. Because it crosses two joints obliquely, the sartorius muscle has a variety

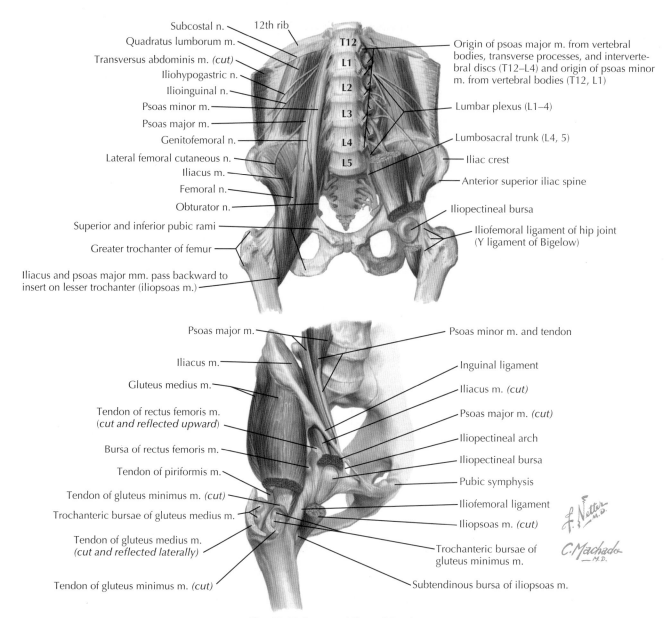

Fig. 11.13 Psoas and Iliacus Muscles.

CLINICAL CORRELATION 11.12   Psoas Abscess

Because of its close association with the vertebral bodies, the psoas major can become involved when infections of the vertebral bodies (possibly a result of tuberculosis) release purulent material. This material may spread deep to the psoas fascia and cause swelling over the entire outline of the psoas major muscle. In the anterior thigh, this can create a prominent swelling just inferior to the inguinal ligament near the attachment of the iliopsoas tendon onto the lesser trochanter. This swelling can be mistaken for other conditions in the area (hernias and swollen lymph nodes) but will be filled with pus and may need to be lanced and drained.

---

of functions. It assists in flexing the hip and knee joints and also laterally rotates the thigh. The **pectineus muscle** originates from the ilium and pubis in the vicinity of the superior pubic ramus and inserts on the pectineal line Cl of the anterior femur just inferior to the lesser trochanter. Functionally it is an adductor of the

thigh and belongs more to the medial compartment. Because it bridges the ilium and pubis, it also bridges the anterior and medial compartments of the thigh.

The majority of the anterior compartment of the thigh is filled by the **quadriceps muscles**. These four muscles stretch from the ilium and femur to the patella via the **quadriceps tendon** and, through it, to the tibial tuberosity via the **patellar ligament**. The patella is a sesamoid bone (a bone found within a muscle tendon), and much ink has been spilled regarding whether or not the patellar ligament should be called the patellar tendon or if the entire assemblage should be called the quadriceps tendon. We will be sticking with the standard terminology (used above) for the time being. The **rectus femoris muscle** is the longest of this group; it originates from the anterior inferior iliac spine (straight head) and the superior rim of the acetabulum (reflected head) and descends on the anterior aspect of the thigh to join the quadriceps tendon. It assists in flexion of the hip and extension of the

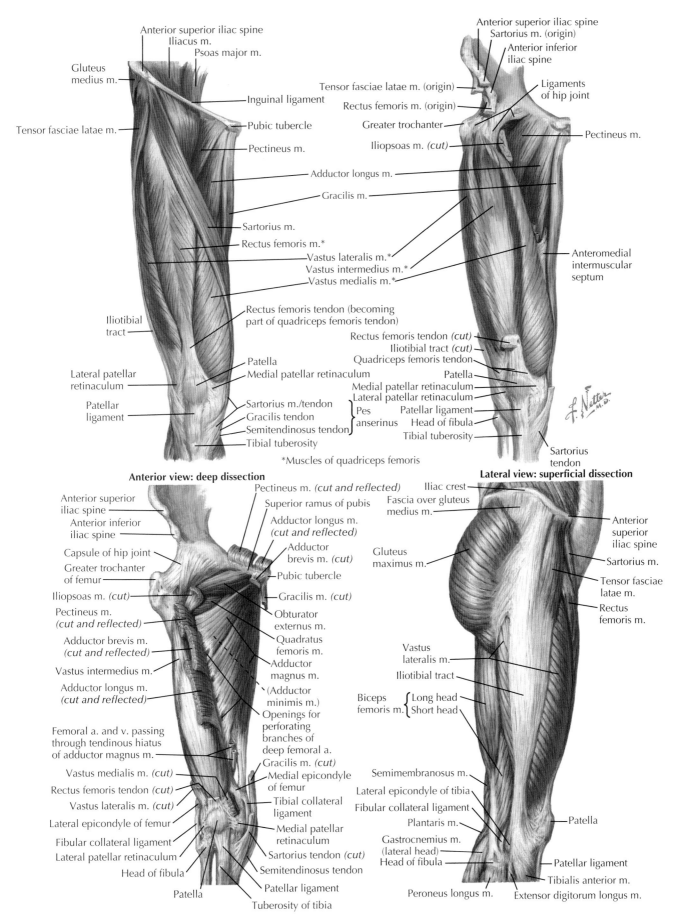

Anterior view: deep dissection

Lateral view: superficial dissection

*Muscles of quadriceps femoris

Fig. 11.14 Muscles of the Front of the Hip and Thigh.

CLINICAL CORRELATION 11.13   Bursitis

Any bursa can become inflamed and swell with fluid (bursitis), but the bursae around the knee are particularly prone to bursitis due to repetitive motion and friction (see Fig. 11.6). The subcutaneous prepatellar or subcutaneous infrapatellar bursae can swell, creating a large, round outline of the anterior knee. The deep infrapatellar bursa can also experience bursitis if weight or impact routinely occurs on the tibial tuberosity. Because priests frequently kneel on hard floors (genuflexion), this condition is also known as clergyman's knee, but it can affect anyone whose knees routinely rest on hard surfaces. Bursitis of the subcutaneous prepatellar bursa can affect those who work on their knees, which is one reason why knee pads are commonly used in certain activities. This used to be known as "washer woman's knee," but this term no longer pertains because few professional cleaners tend to scrub on their hands and knees currently.

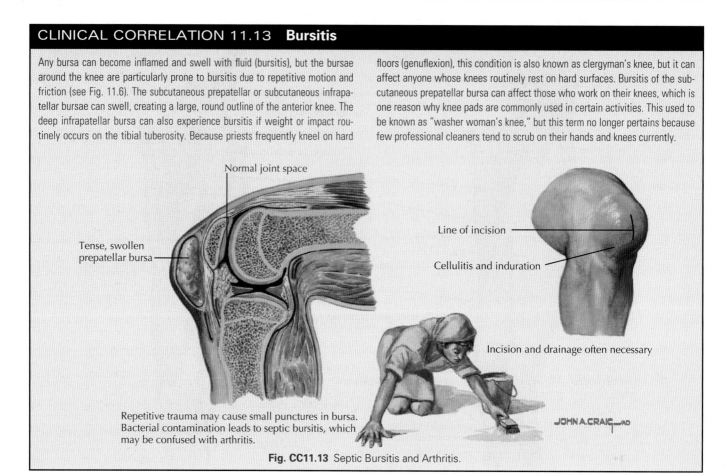

Normal joint space

Tense, swollen prepatellar bursa

Line of incision

Cellulitis and induration

Incision and drainage often necessary

JOHN A. CRAIG—AD

Repetitive trauma may cause small punctures in bursa. Bacterial contamination leads to septic bursitis, which may be confused with arthritis.

Fig. CC11.13 Septic Bursitis and Arthritis.

knee. Because it is less tense during hip flexion, the other quadriceps muscles are the major extensors of the knee when the hip is flexed. The **vastus medialis muscle** is located on the medial side of the femoral shaft with a significant attachment site along the medial lip of the linea aspera. Although it is thickest inferiorly, it actually stretches along the length of the femur from the intertrochanteric line to the quadriceps tendon. Some of its fibers terminate as the **medial patellar retinaculum**, which crosses the knee medial to the patella and patellar ligament, helping to stabilize them during movement. The **vastus lateralis muscle** is a large muscle stretching from the base of the greater trochanter down the lateral aspect of the femur, attaching to the lateral lip of the linea aspera, to just above the lateral supraepicondylar line before contributing to the quadriceps tendon. Some fibers of the vastus lateralis terminate in a **lateral patellar retinaculum** that is lateral to the patella and patellar ligament. The last of the quadriceps muscles, the **vastus intermedius muscle**, originates from the middle third of the anterior femur deep to the rectus femoris and vastus lateralis muscles. Like the others, it also contributes to the quadriceps tendon. The deepest part of the vastus intermedius gives rise to a variable number of slips that insert into the capsule of the knee joint. This **articularis genu muscle** prevents the capsule from becoming slack during extension and getting pinched between the patella and femur.

Deep to the quadriceps tendon (sometimes extending as far superiorly as the middle of the femur!) is the **suprapatellar bursa** (see Fig. 11.6). It is continuous with the synovial space of the knee joint, and infection can pass easily between the two spaces. Because the anterior knee experiences a great deal of impact, there are several true bursae around it: a **subcutaneous prepatellar bursa** that allows the skin to glide smoothly over the patella, a **subcutaneous infrapatellar bursa** between the skin and the patellar ligament, and a **subcutaneous bursa of the tibial tuberosity**. A **deep infrapatellar bursa** sits between the patellar ligament and the area of the tibia just superior to its insertion onto the tibial tuberosity (Clinical Correlations 11.13 and 11.14).

Sartorius

Proximal attachments	• Anterior superior iliac spine
Distal attachment	• Medial tibial condyle as part of the pes anserinus
Functions	• Assists in flexing and laterally rotating thigh at the hip
	• Assists in flexing leg at knee
Muscle testing and signs of dysfunction	• The sartorius contributes to motions (hip flexion and knee flexion) that are carried out by other muscles, making it challenging to isolate
	• To test the sartorius, have the patient flex and externally rotate the hip with the knee flexed against resistance (the hacky-sac kick)
Innervation	• Femoral nerve (L2–L4)
Blood supply	• Branches of femoral, descending genicular, and medial genicular arteries

CLINICAL CORRELATION 11.14 Patellar Dysfunctions

The patella is typically kept in its natural place between the two femoral condyles by the patellar ligament, the medial and lateral patellar retinacula, and the quadriceps muscles. Trauma can cause abnormal positioning of the patella, but this can also occur due to a mismatch between the pull of the vastus medialis versus the vastus lateralis. **Patellar subluxation** occurs when it leaves the groove between the two femoral condyles, and **patellar dislocation** occurs when the patella is completely displaced to one side of a femoral condyle, with lateral displacement being more common. Strengthening the vastus medialis

muscle will often address the problem. **Patellofemoral syndrome** can occur for similar reasons, with the patella grinding against the lateral femoral condyle. However, this syndrome can also occur due to trauma or osteoarthritis affecting the cartilage of the patella and femur. Overuse, trauma, excessive forced extension, and weakening of the tendons in the area can also cause **patellar tendon rupture** between the patella and tibia or **quadriceps tendon rupture** between the quadriceps and patella. Pain and weakness would be immediately evident in either case, with the affected limb being unable to support the body's weight.

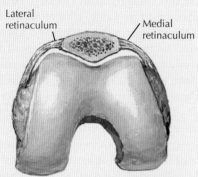

Lateral retinaculum — Medial retinaculum

Skyline view. Normally, patella rides in groove between medial and lateral femoral condyles

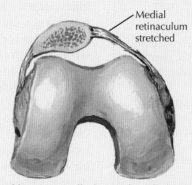

Medial retinaculum stretched

In subluxation, patella deviates laterally because of weakness of vastus medialis muscle, tightness of lateral retinaculum, and high Q angle

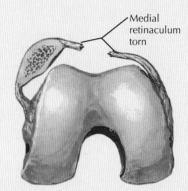

Medial retinaculum torn

In dislocation, patella displaced completely out of intercondylar groove

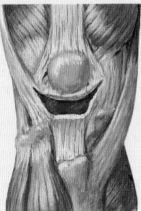

Patellar ligament rupture
Rupture of patellar ligament at inferior margin of patella

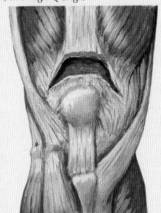

Quadriceps tendon rupture
Rupture of quadriceps femoris tendon at superior margin of patella

Fig. CC11.14 Subluxation and Dislocation of Patella.

Pectineus

Proximal attachments	• Superior pubic ramus and adjacent ilium
Distal attachment	• Pectineal line of femur
Functions	• Assists with adduction, flexion, and medial rotation of the thigh at the hip
Muscle testing and signs of dysfunction	• The pectineus contributes to motions (flexion and adduction of the thigh) that are more strongly carried out by other muscle groups and isolated loss of function of this muscle would be difficult to discern
Innervation	• Portion arising from ilium: Femoral nerve (L2–L4) • Portion arising from pubis: Obturator nerve (L2–L4)
Blood supply	• Branches of obturator, femoral, medial circumflex femoral arteries

Quadriceps Muscle Group

Proximal attachments	• Rectus femoris: Anterior inferior iliac spine and superior rim of acetabulum • Vastus medialis: Medial femoral shaft from intertrochanteric line along medial lip of linea aspera • Vastus lateralis: Base of greater trochanter along lateral lip of linea aspera • Vastus intermedius: Anterior femoral shaft deep to vastus lateralis and rectus femoris
Distal attachment	• Quadriceps tendon converges on the superior aspect of the patella, which sends the patellar ligament to the tibial tuberosity, effectively making it the attachment site of the quadriceps • Anterior sides of medial and lateral tibial condyles via the medial and lateral patellar retinacula from the vastus medialis and lateralis
Functions	• As a group, the quadriceps muscles strongly extend the leg at the knee • The rectus femoris assists in flexion of the thigh at the hip
Muscle testing and signs of dysfunction	• The patient is asked to lay flat with legs dangling unsupported and feet off the ground. Ask the patient to extend each leg against resistance and feel for asymmetry. Weakness of knee extension or atrophy of the quadriceps indicates damage or de-innervation. The same test can be performed with the patient sitting upright, loosening the rectus femoris, and making the other quadriceps muscles carry out the extension of the leg • Spasm of the quadriceps will cause pain in the anterior compartment and a persistently extended knee
Innervation	• Femoral nerve (L2–L4)
Blood supply	• Branches of femoral, medial and lateral circumflex femoral, descending genicular, medial and lateral genicular arteries

Muscles of the Medial Thigh (See Fig. 11.14)

The muscles of the **medial compartment of the thigh** are also surrounded by fascia lata and have investing fascia around each individual muscle. In general, these muscles originate from the inferior aspect of the pubic bone and adjacent parts of the ilium and ischium. Most of them insert on the linea aspera of the femur and adduct the thigh at the hip. The most superficial muscle in this compartment is the **adductor longus muscle**. It originates from a small region of the body of the pubis just anterior to the obturator groove and expands to insert along the middle third of the linea aspera. Posterior to the pectineus and adductor longus is the **adductor brevis muscle**. It originates from a strip of bone along the inferior pubic ramus and inserts onto the inferior pectineal line and upper linea aspera. The obturator nerve splits into anterior and posterior divisions that straddle the adductor brevis and innervate the muscles in this compartment. The large **adductor magnus muscle** lives up to its name, with an **adductor part** originating from the inferior pubic ramus and a **hamstring part** from the ischial ramus and inferior part of the ischial tuberosity. The adductor part inserts along the entire length of the linea aspera, while the hamstring part attaches to the adductor tubercle of the femur. The anterior surface of the adductor magnus is connected to the medial aspect of the vastus medialis by a sheet of connective tissue, the **anteromedial intermuscular septum**. This sheet covers the **adductor canal**, which contains the femoral artery and vein as they descend. The adductor and hamstring parts of the adductor magnus separate from each other to form the adductor hiatus, which allows the femoral vessels to travel into the posterior thigh to become the popliteal vessels. The adductor magnus bridges the medial and posterior compartments of the thigh, and this is reflected by differences in the innervation of the adductor part (obturator nerve) and hamstring part (tibial division of the sciatic nerve). The most anterior and superior part of the adductor magnus sometimes forms a separate and flat **adductor minimus muscle**.

The three other muscles of the medial compartment of the thigh are the pectineus, obturator externus, and gracilis muscles. The pectineus muscle stretches between the anterior and medial compartments and was discussed in the previous section. The **obturator internus muscle** originates from the anterior aspect of the obturator membrane and surrounding pubis and ischium. Its tendon extends laterally, running inferior to the acetabulum and femoral neck to reach the trochanteric fossa of the femur. Despite being in the medial compartment, it functions like a member of the deep gluteal muscle group and laterally rotates the thigh at the hip. The obturator nerve pierces it to enter the medial compartment of the thigh. The **gracilis muscle** is elongated and resembles the sartorius in girth but in a different position. As the most medial thigh muscle, it descends from the body of the pubis and adjacent inferior pubic ramus to join the pes anserinus on the medial side of the knee alongside the distal sartorius and semitendinosus muscles.

Adductor Longus, Adductor Brevis, Adductor Magnus

Proximal attachments	• Adductor longus: Body of pubic bone anterior to obturator groove
	• Adductor brevis: Inferior pubic ramus
	• Adductor magnus:
	  • Adductor part: Inferior pubic ramus and ischial ramus
	  • Hamstrings part: Ischial ramus and inferior ischial tuberosity

Distal attachment	• Adductor longus: Middle third of linea aspera
	• Adductor brevis: Inferior pectineal line, superior part of linea aspera
	• Adductor magnus:
	  • Adductor part: Linea aspera
	  • Hamstrings part: Adductor tubercle of femur

Functions	• When the lower limb is not bearing weight, these muscles will adduct the thigh at the hip. When the lower limb is weighted, they assist in keeping the pelvis level • The hamstring portion of the adductor magnus helps to extend the thigh at the hip
Muscle testing and signs of dysfunction	• Loss of adductor muscle function can be difficult to diagnose but may result in balance issues as the pelvis has difficulty staying level • Spasm or injury to these muscles (groin pull) will cause weakness in adduction but also pain, often near the muscle's attachment to the pelvis
Innervation	• Adductor longus, adductor brevis, adductor part of adductor magnus: Obturator nerve (L2–L4) • Hamstring part of adductor magnus: Tibial division of sciatic nerve (L4–S3)
Blood supply	• Branches of femoral, deep femoral, medial circumflex femoral, descending genicular, medial genicular arteries

Obturator Externus

Proximal attachments	• External aspect of obturator membrane and surrounding pubis and ischium
Distal attachment	• Trochanteric fossa just inferior to obturator internus attachment
Functions	• Rotate an extended thigh laterally, abduct a flexed thigh • Helps to keep femoral head within acetabulum
Muscle testing and signs of dysfunction	• Very slight shortened step due to weakness externally rotating lower limb during heel strike.
Innervation	• Obturator nerve (L2–L4)
Blood supply	• Obturator and medial circumflex femoral arteries

Gracilis

Proximal attachments	• Body of pubis and adjacent inferior pubic ramus
Distal attachment	• Medial tibial condyle as part of the pes anserinus
Functions	• Adducts the thigh at the hip • Slight internal rotation of the thigh, flexion of the leg at the knee
Muscle testing and signs of dysfunction	• Isolated loss of gracilis function would be difficult to detect • Spasm or injury to the gracilis would will cause weakness in adduction but also pain, often near the muscle's attachment to the inferior pubic bone.
Innervation	• Obturator nerve (L2–L4)
Blood supply	• Obturator, descending genicular, and medial genicular arteries

Muscles of the Posterior Thigh (See Figs. 11.4, 11.6, 11.12, 11.14, and 11.15)

The three muscles of the **posterior compartment of the thigh**, the semitendinosus, semimembranosus, and biceps femoris, with a long and short head, are also surrounded by the fascia lata. These muscles sit posterior to the femur and posterior to the medial and lateral femoral intermuscular septae as they insert on the linea aspera. As a group, these muscles are called the hamstring muscles, but technically only the three that originate from the ischial tuberosity are true hamstring muscles, excluding the short head of the biceps brachii that originates from the posterior femur. All of the muscles in the posterior compartment have a distal insertion on the tibia or fibula. Because of this, when the lower limb is unweighted, they will strongly flex the leg at the knee, which is important during the initial swing segment of the gait cycle. When a leg is supporting weight, the true hamstring muscles (attaching to the ischial tuberosity) extend the thigh at the hip, which is important during the foot flat and midstance segments of the gait cycle. Because muscles are most efficient when they are somewhat stretched, the hamstring muscles are effective at either flexing the knee or extending the hip but not both simultaneously.

The **semitendinosus muscle** originates from the posterior aspect of the ischial tuberosity alongside the long head of the biceps femoris muscle. The semitendinosus descends on the medial side of the posterior thigh. It gets its name from its strong, ropy tendon that lays posterior to the semimembranosus muscle on the medial side of distal thigh. This tendon joins the sartorius and gracilis muscles on the medial side of the tibia as the pes anserinus. The three tendons are separated from the medial condyle of the tibia by the **anserine bursa**. When the knee is flexed, muscles of the pes anserinus as well as the semimembranosus are lined up in a way that allows them to medially rotate the leg at the knee.

Superficial dissection — Iliac crest   **Deeper dissection**

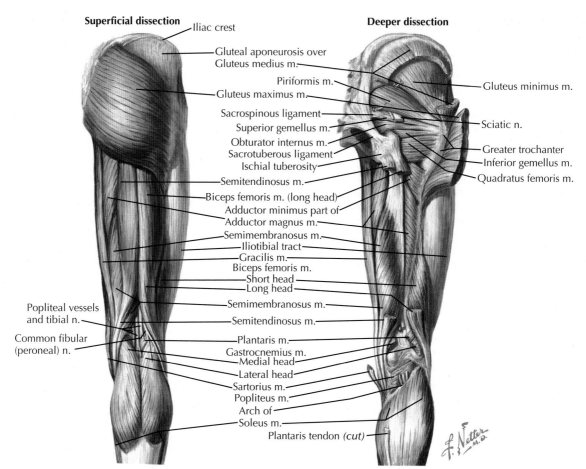

- Gluteal aponeurosis over
- Gluteus medius m.
- Piriformis m.
- Gluteus maximus m.
- Sacrospinous ligament
- Superior gemellus m.
- Obturator internus m.
- Sacrotuberous ligament
- Ischial tuberosity
- Semitendinosus m.
- Biceps femoris m. (long head)
- Adductor minimus part of
- Adductor magnus m.
- Semimembranosus m.
- Iliotibial tract
- Gracilis m.
- Biceps femoris m.
- Short head
- Long head
- Semimembranosus m.
- Semitendinosus m.
- Plantaris m.
- Gastrocnemius m.
- Medial head
- Lateral head
- Sartorius m.
- Popliteus m.
- Arch of
- Soleus m.
- Plantaris tendon *(cut)*

- Gluteus minimus m.
- Sciatic n.
- Greater trochanter
- Inferior gemellus m.
- Quadratus femoris m.

Popliteal vessels and tibial n.

Common fibular (peroneal) n.

Fig. 11.15 Muscles of the Back of the Hip and Thigh: Posterior View.

The **semimembranosus muscle** originates slightly lateral to the common origin of the semitendinosus and long head of biceps brachii. In fact, there is a superior bursa of the biceps femoris between them. It descends on the medial aspect of the posterior thigh, expanding into a broad muscular belly in the inferior thigh and then to a broad tendon that flattens to insert in three spots: the fascia of the popliteus, the oblique popliteal ligament on the posterior side of the knee joint capsule, and the medial tibial condyle, underneath which is a semimembranosus bursa.

Originating alongside the semitendinosus muscle is the **long head of the biceps femoris muscle**. It crosses from medial to lateral as it descends and inserts laterally on the head of the fibula. It is joined by the **short head of the biceps femoris muscle**. Despite being short, it is still a substantial muscle and its origin stretches from the inferior half of the linea aspera to the lateral supracondylar line of the femur. It fuses with the long head and both insert onto the fibular head. The tendon of the biceps femoris inserts near the attachment site of the lateral (fibular) collateral ligament of the knee and can be used to locate that ligament during physical exam or dissection. The tendon of the biceps femoris is

separated from the lateral collateral ligament and lateral tibial condyle by the **inferior subtendinous bursa of the biceps femoris**. The short head of the biceps femoris is the only muscle in the posterior compartment that is not innervated by the tibial division of the sciatic nerve; instead it is innervated by the common fibular division of the sciatic nerve. When the knee is flexed, the biceps femoris is able to laterally rotate the leg at the knee, acting as the counterpart of the pes anserinus and semitendinosus muscles on the medial side tuberosity (Clinical Correlation 11.15).

CLINICAL CORRELATION 11.15 **Injury to the Hamstring Muscles**

Hamstring muscle injuries can occur anywhere along the length of each muscle, but they are most common at the tendinous origin of the muscles from the ischial tuberosity. Hurdling, kicking a ball, or other forms of exercise where the hip is forcefully flexed and the knee is forcefully extended at the same time puts tremendous stress on the hamstring muscles. A partial or full tear of the tendon at this site will produce gluteal pain and a reluctance (or inability) to walk. Occasionally, the pull of the muscles may avulse part of the ischial tuberosity.

Hamstring (Semitendinosus, Semimembranosus, and Biceps Femoris)

Proximal attachments	• Semitendinosus: Common tendon with long head of biceps femoris from posterior ischial tuberosity
	• Semimembranosus: Lateral aspect of ischial tuberosity
	• Biceps femoris
	  • Long head: Common tendon with semitendinosus from ischial tuberosity
	  • Short head: Inferior linea aspera and lateral supracondylar line of femur

Distal attachment	• Semitendinosus: Medial tibial condyle as part of the pes anserinus • Semimembranosus: Medial tibial condyle, popliteal muscle fascia, oblique popliteal ligament • Biceps femoris: Tendons of both heads fuse as insert on the lateral aspect of the fibular head
Functions	• Flex leg at the knee—initial swing phase of gait cycle • Semitendinosus, semimembranosus, long head of biceps femoris: Extend thigh at the hip—foot flat and midstand phases of gait cycle
Muscle testing and signs of dysfunction	• With the patient lying prone, bring the patient's knee into flexion with their foot in the air. The examiner asks the patient to resist as the knee is gently but firmly brought into extension. Look for strength asymmetry, you may also rest your palm on the patient's hamstring muscles to palpate them during the procedure • Tightness, weakness, and cramping of hamstring muscles are very common. This is common in sedentary cultures, where people such as textbook authors spend many hours each day seated with their knees flexed and hamstrings passively shortened
Innervation	• Semitendinosus, semimembranosus, long head of biceps femoris: Tibial division of sciatic nerve (L4–S3) • Short head of biceps femoris: Common fibular division of sciatic nerve (L4–S2)
Blood supply	• Perforating branches of deep femoral, lateral genicular, and medial genicular arteries

Muscles of the Posterior Leg

Like the other limb compartments, the muscles in the posterior leg are each covered by the own investing fascia while the **deep fascial of the leg (crural fascia)** surrounds the entire leg and fuses with the periosteum of the tibia and fibula. It is connected to the fascial lata by the **popliteal fascia**, a tough sheet of connective tissue that covers the popliteal vessels and accompanying nerves of the posterior knee. Divisions of the deep fascia of the leg and the **interosseous membrane** create four compartments: anterior, lateral, deep posterior, and superficial posterior. We will begin with the superficial posterior compartment of the leg due to its continuity with the posterior thigh.

Superficial Posterior Compartment of Leg (Figs. 11.4, 11.6, and 11.15–11.18)

The **superficial posterior compartment of the leg** is covered posteriorly by the deep fascia of the leg and is separated from the lateral and deep posterior compartments by the posterior intermuscular septum of the leg. The muscles in this compartment are almost exclusively dedicated to strong plantarflexion of the foot at the ankle and all fuse to form the **calcaneal (Achilles) tendon** that attaches to the posterior aspect of the calcaneal tuberosity.

The muscle that takes up most of the space in this compartment is the **soleus muscle**. It has a broad, horseshoe-shaped origin stretching from the medial border and soleal line on the posterior side of the superior tibia, crossing over the interosseous membrane and onto the superior third of the posterior fibula. Medially there is a **tendinous arch of the soleus**, a gap that allows the tibial nerve and posterior tibial vessels to enter the deep posterior compartment of the leg. This broad muscle provides the majority of the collagen fibers that form the calcaneal tendon, especially its medial side; this makes it a strong plantar flexor of the ankle.

The most superficial muscle in this compartment is the **gastrocnemius muscle**, with a lateral head and a medial head. The **lateral head of the gastrocnemius** originates from the lateral femoral condyle, just above the attachment to the lateral (fibular) collateral ligament of the knee. The **medial head of the gastrocnemius** arises from the popliteal surface of the femur, immediately superior to the medial femoral condyle. To prevent friction and irritation during contraction, there are lateral and medial subtendinous bursae of the gastrocnemius sitting between the origin of each head and the underlying femoral epicondyles. The two heads form a common tendon as they descend that joins the calcaneal tendon, biased a bit toward its lateral side. Because the gastrocnemius crosses the knee and ankle joint, it affects both; it can flex the knee and plantar flex the ankle, but it can only do one of those motions strongly at one time. Occasionally (approximately 23% of people) a sesamoid bone is present on the deep surface of the lateral head of the gastrocnemius muscle, the **fabella** bone.

Because of their common tendon, similar functions, and close proximity, the soleus and two heads of the gastrocnemius muscles are often referred to collectively as the **triceps surae muscle**. To stretch the gastrocnemius, one can lean against a wall with the knee extended while pushing the heel toward (but not quite in contact with) the ground. Doing the same stretch with the knee flexed will specifically target the soleus because flexion of the knee has relaxed the gastrocnemius muscles somewhat. The subtendinous **bursa of the calcaneal tendon** cushions the tendon it as it approaches the

Superficial dissection

Semitendinosus m.
Semimembranosus m.
Gracilis m.
Popliteal a. and v.
Sartorius m.
Superior medial genicular a.
Gastrocnemius m. (medial head)
Nerve to soleus m.
Small saphenous v.
Gastrocnemius m.

Iliotibial tract
Biceps femoris m.
Tibial n.
Common fibular (peroneal) n.
Superior lateral genicular a.
Plantaris m.
Gastrocnemius m. (lateral head)
Lateral sural cutaneous n. (cut)
Medial sural cutaneous n. (cut)

Soleus m.
Plantaris tendon

Soleus m.

Flexor digitorum longus tendon
Tibialis posterior tendon
Posterior tibial a. and v.
Tibial n.
Medial malleolus
Flexor hallucis longus tendon
Flexor retinaculum
Calcaneal branch of posterior tibial a.

Fibularis (peroneus) longus tendon
Fibularis (peroneus) brevis tendon
Calcaneal (Achilles) tendon
Lateral malleolus
Superior fibular (peroneal) retinaculum
Fibular (peroneal) a.
Calcaneal branches of fibular (peroneal) a.
Calcaneal tuberosity

Intermediate dissection

Adductor magnus tendon
Popliteal a. and v.
Superior medial genicular a.
Gastrocnemius m. (medial head) (cut)
Tibial collateral ligament
Plantaris m.
Semimembranosus tendon (cut)
Inferior medial genicular a.
Popliteus m.
Nerve to soleus m.
Tendinous arch of Soleus m.
Soleus m.
Plantaris tendon
Gastrocnemius m. (cut)

Tibial n.
Common fibular (peroneal) n. (cut)
Superior lateral genicular a.
Lateral and medial sural cutaneous nn. (cut)
Gastrocnemius m. (lateral head) (cut)
Fibular collateral ligament
Biceps femoris tendon (cut)
Inferior lateral genicular a.
Head of fibula
Common fibular (peroneal) n. (cut)
Fibularis (peroneus) longus m.

Soleus m. inserting into calcaneal (Achilles) tendon
Flexor digitorum longus tendon
Tibialis posterior tendon
Posterior tibial a. and v.
Tibial n.
Medial malleolus
Flexor hallucis longus tendon
Flexor retinaculum
Calcaneal (Achilles) tendon
Calcaneal branch of posterior tibial a.

Fibularis (peroneus) longus tendon
Fibularis (peroneus) brevis tendon
Lateral malleolus
Superior fibular (peroneal) retinaculum
Fibular (peroneal) a.
Calcaneal branches of fibular (peroneal) a.
Calcaneal tuberosity

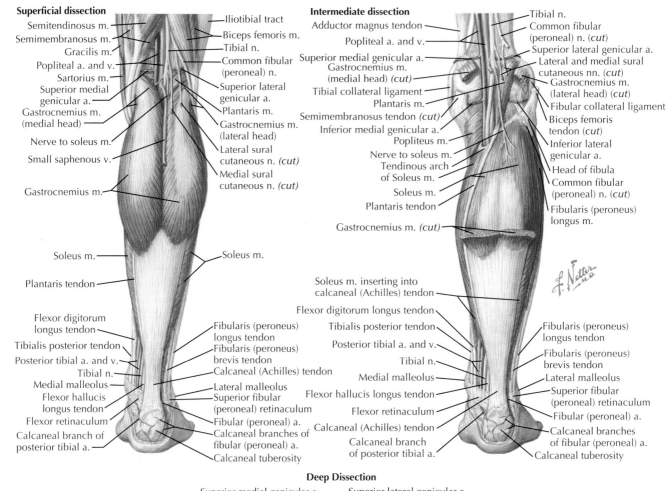

Deep Dissection

Superior medial genicular a.
Gastrocnemius m. (medial head) (cut)
Popliteal a. and tibial n.
Tibial collateral ligament
Semimembranosus tendon (cut)
Inferior medial genicular a.
Popliteus m.
Posterior tibial recurrent a.
Tendinous arch of soleus m.
Posterior tibial a.
Flexor digitorum longus m.
Tibial n.
Tibialis posterior m.

Superior lateral genicular a.
Plantaris m. (cut)
Sural (muscular) branches
Gastrocnemius m. (lateral head) (cut)
Fibular collateral ligament
Biceps femoris tendon (cut)
Inferior lateral genicular a.
Head of fibula
Common fibular (peroneal) n.
Soleus m. (cut and reflected)
Anterior tibial a.
Fibular (peroneal) a.

Flexor hallucis longus m. (retracted)

Fibular (peroneal) a.
Interosseous membrane
Perforating branch
Communicating branch } of fibular (peroneal) a.
Fibularis (peroneus) longus tendon
Fibularis (peroneus) brevis tendon
Lateral malleolus and posterior lateral malleolar branch of fibular (peroneal) a.
Superior fibular (peroneal) retinaculum
Lateral calcaneal branch of fibular (peroneal) a.
Lateral calcaneal branch of sural n.
Inferior fibular (peroneal) retinaculum
Fibularis (peroneus) brevis tendon
Fibularis (peroneus) longus tendon
Flexor digitorum longus tendon
5th metatarsal bone

Calcaneal (Achilles) tendon (cut)
Flexor digitorum longus tendon
Tibialis posterior tendon
Medial malleolus and posterior medial malleolar branch of posterior tibial a.
Flexor retinaculum
Medial calcaneal branches of posterior tibial a. and tibial n.
Tibialis posterior tendon
Medial plantar a. and n.
Lateral plantar a. and n.
Flexor hallucis longus tendon
1st metatarsal bone

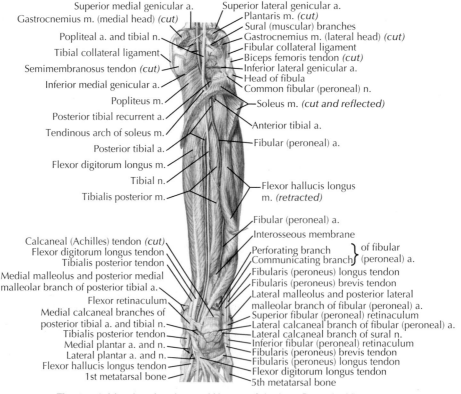

Fig. 11.16 Muscles, Arteries, and Nerves of the Leg: Posterior View.

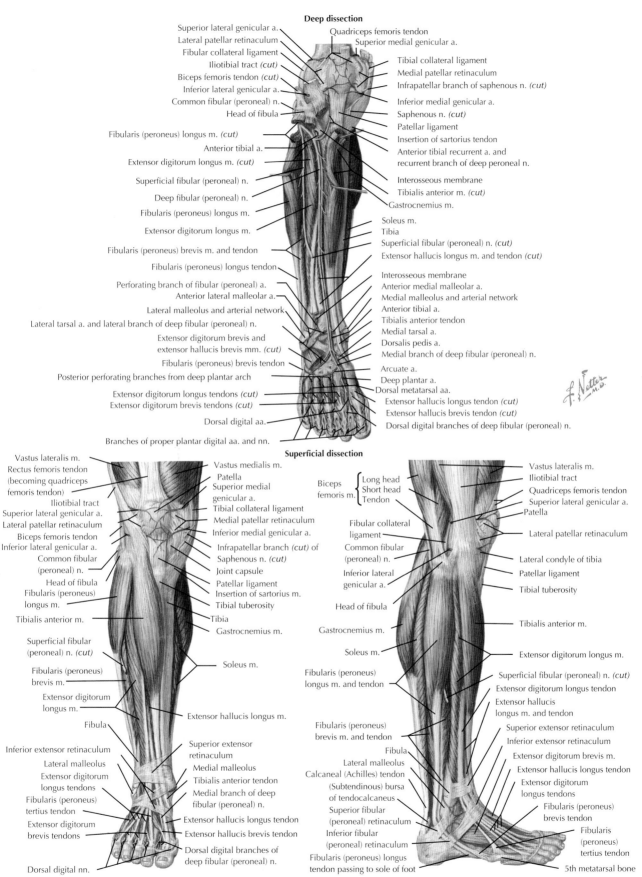

Deep dissection

Superior lateral genicular a.
Lateral patellar retinaculum
Fibular collateral ligament
Iliotibial tract *(cut)*
Biceps femoris tendon *(cut)*
Inferior lateral genicular a.
Common fibular (peroneal) n.
Head of fibula

Fibularis (peroneus) longus m. *(cut)*
Anterior tibial a.
Extensor digitorum longus m. *(cut)*
Superficial fibular (peroneal) n.
Deep fibular (peroneal) n.
Fibularis (peroneus) longus m.
Extensor digitorum longus m.
Fibularis (peroneus) brevis m. and tendon
Fibularis (peroneus) longus tendon
Perforating branch of fibular (peroneal) a.
Anterior lateral malleolar a.
Lateral malleolus and arterial network
Lateral tarsal a. and lateral branch of deep fibular (peroneal) n.
Extensor digitorum brevis and
extensor hallucis brevis mm. *(cut)*
Fibularis (peroneus) brevis tendon
Posterior perforating branches from deep plantar arch
Extensor digitorum longus tendons *(cut)*
Extensor digitorum brevis tendons *(cut)*
Dorsal digital aa.
Branches of proper plantar digital aa. and nn.

Quadriceps femoris tendon
Superior medial genicular a.
Tibial collateral ligament
Medial patellar retinaculum
Infrapatellar branch of saphenous n. *(cut)*
Inferior medial genicular a.
Saphenous n. *(cut)*
Patellar ligament
Insertion of sartorius tendon
Anterior tibial recurrent a. and
recurrent branch of deep peroneal n.
Interosseous membrane
Tibialis anterior m. *(cut)*
Gastrocnemius m.
Soleus m.
Tibia
Superficial fibular (peroneal) n. *(cut)*
Extensor hallucis longus m. and tendon *(cut)*
Interosseous membrane
Anterior medial malleolar a.
Medial malleolus and arterial network
Anterior tibial a.
Tibialis anterior tendon
Medial tarsal a.
Dorsalis pedis a.
Medial branch of deep fibular (peroneal) n.
Arcuate a.
Deep plantar a.
Dorsal metatarsal aa.
Extensor hallucis longus tendon *(cut)*
Extensor hallucis brevis tendon *(cut)*
Dorsal digital branches of deep fibular (peroneal) n.

Superficial dissection

Vastus lateralis m.
Rectus femoris tendon
(becoming quadriceps
femoris tendon)
Iliotibial tract
Superior lateral genicular a.
Lateral patellar retinaculum
Biceps femoris tendon
Inferior lateral genicular a.
Common fibular
(peroneal) n.
Head of fibula
Fibularis (peroneus)
longus m.
Tibialis anterior m.
Superficial fibular
(peroneal) n. *(cut)*
Fibularis (peroneus)
brevis m.
Extensor digitorum
longus m.
Fibula
Inferior extensor retinaculum
Lateral malleolus
Extensor digitorum
longus tendons
Fibularis (peroneus)
tertius tendon
Extensor digitorum
brevis tendons
Dorsal digital nn.

Vastus medialis m.
Patella
Superior medial
genicular a.
Tibial collateral ligament
Medial patellar retinaculum
Inferior medial genicular a.
Infrapatellar branch *(cut)* of
Saphenous n. *(cut)*
Joint capsule
Patellar ligament
Insertion of sartorius m.
Tibial tuberosity
Tibia
Gastrocnemius m.
Soleus m.
Extensor hallucis longus m.
Superior extensor
retinaculum
Medial malleolus
Tibialis anterior tendon
Medial branch of deep
fibular (peroneal) n.
Extensor hallucis longus tendon
Extensor hallucis brevis tendon
Dorsal digital branches of
deep fibular (peroneal) n.

Biceps
femoris m. { Long head
Short head
Tendon
Fibular collateral
ligament
Common fibular
(peroneal) n.
Inferior lateral
genicular a.
Head of fibula
Gastrocnemius m.
Soleus m.
Fibularis (peroneus)
longus m. and tendon
Fibularis (peroneus)
brevis m. and tendon
Fibula
Lateral malleolus
Calcaneal (Achilles) tendon
(Subtendinous) bursa
of tendocalcaneus
Superior fibular
(peroneal) retinaculum
Inferior fibular
(peroneal) retinaculum
Fibularis (peroneus) longus
tendon passing to sole of foot

Vastus lateralis m.
Iliotibial tract
Quadriceps femoris tendon
Superior lateral genicular a.
Patella
Lateral patellar retinaculum
Lateral condyle of tibia
Patellar ligament
Tibial tuberosity
Tibialis anterior m.
Extensor digitorum longus m.
Superficial fibular (peroneal) n. *(cut)*
Extensor digitorum longus tendon
Extensor hallucis
longus m. and tendon
Superior extensor retinaculum
Inferior extensor retinaculum
Extensor digitorum brevis m.
Extensor hallucis longus tendon
Extensor digitorum
longus tendons
Fibularis (peroneus)
brevis tendon
Fibularis
(peroneus)
tertius tendon
5th metatarsal bone

Fig. 11.17 Muscles, Arteries, and Nerves of the Leg: Anterior View.

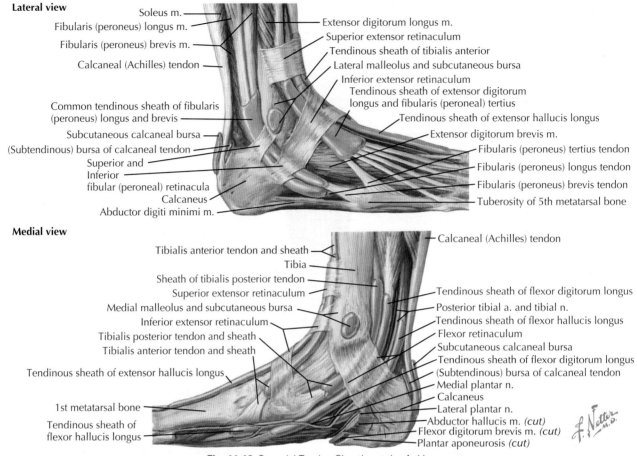

Lateral view

Soleus m.
Fibularis (peroneus) longus m.
Fibularis (peroneus) brevis m.
Calcaneal (Achilles) tendon

Common tendinous sheath of fibularis (peroneus) longus and brevis
Subcutaneous calcaneal bursa
(Subtendinous) bursa of calcaneal tendon
Superior and Inferior fibular (peroneal) retinacula
Calcaneus
Abductor digiti minimi m.

Extensor digitorum longus m.
Superior extensor retinaculum
Tendinous sheath of tibialis anterior
Lateral malleolus and subcutaneous bursa
Inferior extensor retinaculum
Tendinous sheath of extensor digitorum longus and fibularis (peroneal) tertius
Tendinous sheath of extensor hallucis longus
Extensor digitorum brevis m.
Fibularis (peroneus) tertius tendon
Fibularis (peroneus) longus tendon
Fibularis (peroneus) brevis tendon
Tuberosity of 5th metatarsal bone

Medial view

Tibialis anterior tendon and sheath
Tibia
Sheath of tibialis posterior tendon
Superior extensor retinaculum
Medial malleolus and subcutaneous bursa
Inferior extensor retinaculum
Tibialis posterior tendon and sheath
Tibialis anterior tendon and sheath
Tendinous sheath of extensor hallucis longus
1st metatarsal bone
Tendinous sheath of flexor hallucis longus

Calcaneal (Achilles) tendon
Tendinous sheath of flexor digitorum longus
Posterior tibial a. and tibial n.
Tendinous sheath of flexor hallucis longus
Flexor retinaculum
Subcutaneous calcaneal bursa
Tendinous sheath of flexor digitorum longus
(Subtendinous) bursa of calcaneal tendon
Medial plantar n.
Calcaneus
Lateral plantar n.
Abductor hallucis m. *(cut)*
Flexor digitorum brevis m. *(cut)*
Plantar aponeurosis *(cut)*

Fig. 11.18 Synovial Tendon Sheaths at the Ankle.

calcaneal tuberosity. Another, more superficial structure, the **subcutaneous calcaneal bursa**, prevents friction as the skin and subcutaneous tissues glide across the calcaneal tuberosity. Inflammation of these bursae can be mistaken for tendon injury (Clinical Correlation 11.16).

Also originating from the lateral supraepicondylar line of the femur and oblique popliteal ligament is the odd **plantaris muscle**. It commonly has a stout muscle belly near its superior origin that quickly gives off a long, thin tendon that descends on the medial side of the calcaneal tendon and sometimes fuses with it. Because it crosses the knee and ankle joints, it could theoretically flex the knee and plantarflex the ankle, but because it is much smaller than the other muscles in this compartment, it has a negligible contribution to both motions. Due to its high density of muscle spindle fibers, it is more likely to be proprioceptive in nature. However, its functional insignificance makes its long tendon an excellent source for autografts to repair other tendons or ligaments.

Gastrocnemius.

Proximal attachments	• Medial head: Popliteal surface of femur superior to medial femoral condyle • Lateral head: Lateral femoral condyle
Distal attachment	• Attaches to posterior aspect of calcaneus in the lateral part of calcaneal tendon
Functions	• Strongly plantar flexes the foot at the ankle, particularly when the ankle is already somewhat plantarflexed and the knee is extended, such as the toe-off phase of gait • Assists the muscles of the posterior compartment of the thigh in flexing the knee, particularly when the ankle is dorsiflexed
Muscle testing and signs of dysfunction	• Loss of the gastrocnemius without loss of the soleus would weaken toe-off but not completely compromise the motion of plantarflexion • Action of both the gastrocnemius and soleus muscles would be lost during a rupture of the calcaneal tendon. This makes walking very difficult and would result in a shortened stance phase due to the loss of flat foot, heel-off, and toe-off phases
Innervation	• Tibial nerve (L4–S3)
Blood supply	• Genicular arteries, sural arteries from popliteal artery

CLINICAL CORRELATION 11.16   Calcaneal Tendonitis and Rupture

Overuse of the calcaneal tendon can cause pain due to microtrauma of the tendon as it inserts onto the calcaneal tuberosity. This pain is exacerbated by contraction or stretch of the triceps surae (see Fig. 11.18). If the trauma or stretch is too severe for the tendon to withstand, it can rupture. This often happens when the triceps surae are stretched while contracting strongly (eccentric contraction). If the rupture is complete, then the gastrocnemius and soleus will retract into the top of the posterior leg and the heel of the foot will fall to the ground, unable to plantarflex. This injury requires surgical repair in any patient who wishes to maintain activity thereafter. The integrity of the calcaneal tendon can be tested by having a patient lie supine on a table with the foot unsupported and relaxed. The examiner gently but firmly squeezes the gastrocnemius muscles. If the calcaneal tendon is intact, some plantarflexion will occur.

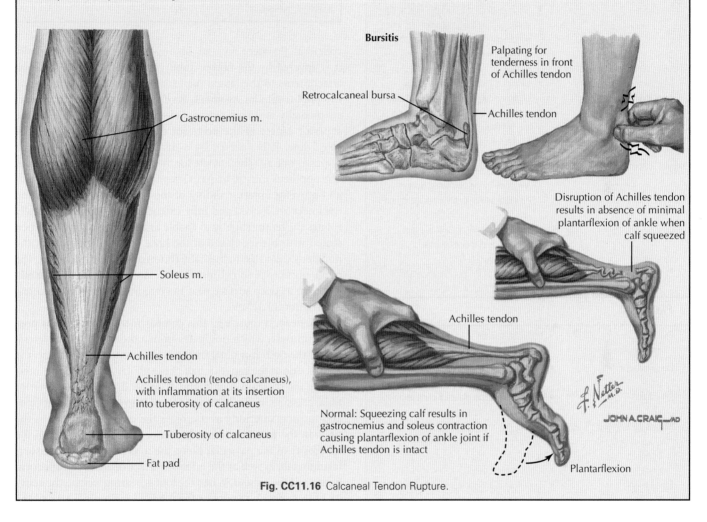

Fig. CC11.16 Calcaneal Tendon Rupture.

Soleus.

Proximal attachments	• Soleal line and medial border of tibia, superior portion of the posterior fibula
Distal attachment	• Attaches to posterior aspect of calcaneus as the medial part of calcaneal tendon
Functions	• Strongly plantar flexes the foot at the ankle. Unlike the gastrocnemius, the soleus can strongly plantarflex the foot at the ankle while the knees are flexed
Muscle testing and signs of dysfunction	• Loss of the soleus muscle would compromise plantarflexion, making jumping difficult and compromising the flat foot, heel-off, and toe-off phases of gait • Action of both the gastrocnemius and soleus muscles would be lost during a rupture of the calcaneal tendon. This makes walking very difficult and would result in a shortened stance phase due to the loss of flat foot, heel-off, and toe-off phases
Innervation	• Tibial nerve (L4–S3)
Blood supply	• Branches of the popliteal, posterior tibial, and fibular arteries

Plantaris.

Proximal attachments	• Popliteal surface of femur immediately superior to lateral femoral condyle
Distal attachment	• Posteromedial aspect of calcaneal tuberosity medial to calcaneal tendon
Functions	• Weakly assists in plantarflexion of ankle • Primarily proprioceptive
Muscle testing and signs of dysfunction	• Loss of this muscle would have no noticeable effect on plantarflexion or gait
Innervation	• Tibial nerve (L4–S3)
Blood supply	• Superior lateral genicular and sural arteries from popliteal artery

Deep Posterior Compartment of the Leg (See Figs. 11.4, 11.5, 11.16, and 11.18)

The **deep posterior compartment of the leg** is bounded posteriorly by the posterior intermuscular septum and anteriorly by the fibula, tibia, and interosseous membrane. The four muscles of this compartment (popliteus, tibialis posterior, flexor digitorum longus, flexor hallucis longus) are in close contact with the tibia, fibula, and interosseous membrane. They are all innervated by branches of the tibial nerve and receive their blood supply from the genicular, posterior tibial, or fibular arteries.

The **popliteus muscle** originates from a small region immediately superior to the lateral femoral condyle but just inferior to the femoral attachment of the lateral (fibular) collateral ligament. It is separated from the lateral femoral condyle by a bursa or extension of the synovial lining of the knee joint, the subpopliteal bursa or recess, and is separated from the lateral

CLINICAL CORRELATION 11.17 Popliteal (Baker) Cysts

Effusion (excessive fluid) in the knee joint can cause the synovial lining of the joint to herniate through the fibrous joint capsule or through some of the bursae that communicate with the synovial space of the knee. These **popliteal (Baker) cysts**, filled with synovial fluid, extend from the posterior knee superior to the popliteus muscle. They can become quite large and impede full flexion of the knee.

collateral ligament by the fibulopopliteal bursa. Proximally it is covered by the fibrous joint capsule of the knee and has attachments to the lateral meniscus and head of the fibula via the popliteofibular ligament. As the muscle descends, it travels medially and fans out considerably before attaching to the superior aspect of the posterior tibia, immediately above the soleal line. It is covered by a distinct popliteal fascia, which serves as one attachment site for the semimembranosus muscle. The popliteus muscle helps to keep the lateral meniscus in place and prevents anterior sliding of the femur on the tibia. When the knees are locked and fully extended, the popliteus laterally rotates the femur slightly to enable knee flexion to begin. When seated with the leg flexed at the knee and swinging freely, the popliteus will assist in medially (internally) rotating the leg. The popliteus muscle sometimes has a sesamoid bone, the **cyamella** bone, on its deep surface near the femoral attachment (Clinical Correlation 11.17).

The deepest muscle in this compartment is the **tibialis posterior muscle**, which originates from a broad area of the lateral side of the posterior tibial shaft just inferior to the soleal line, the medial side of the superior half of the fibular shaft, and the intervening interosseous membrane. It descends along the posterior tibia, crossing medially to run posterior to the medial malleolus and turning anteriorly as it crosses the malleolar groove to the tibia. In the foot, the tibialis posterior fans out to insert on the tuberosity of the navicular bone, the inferior side of the sustentaculum tali, as well as the inferior surface of all three cuneiform bones and the cuboid. When the foot is bearing weight, the activity of this muscle maintains the medial longitudinal arch of the foot. If the foot is unweighted, it will act with its anterior counterpart, the tibialis anterior muscle, to invert the foot at the ankle.

The **flexor digitorum longus muscle** is the most medial muscle in this compartment as it originates from the posterior middle third of the tibia, just inferior to the soleal line. It descends along the posterior tibia, passes posterior to the tibialis anterior muscle, turns anteriorly, and crosses inferior to the medial malleolus and the tendon of the tibialis posterior. Once it enters the medial side of the foot, the tendon passes laterally and divides to create individual tendons to each of the digits 2 to 5. Each tendon of the flexor digitorum longus crosses the MTP, PIP, and DIP joints to insert on the plantar side of the base of the distal phalanx of digits 2 to 5. The quadratus plantae and four lumbrical muscles (to be discussed with the muscles of the foot) attach to the tendons of the flexor digitorum longus. The flexor digitorum longus assists in plantarflexion of the foot at the ankle, helps to support the medial longitudinal arch of the foot, and is the only muscle that flexes the DIP joint. Flexion of the distal phalanx is especially important during the toe-off phase of gait to propel the body forward.

The **flexor hallucis longus muscle** is the most lateral muscle in the deep posterior compartment of the leg, which is somewhat interesting since its tendon crosses to the first digit (hallucis) on the medial side of the foot. It originates from the inferior half of the posterior shaft of the fibula and a small portion of the adjacent interosseous membrane. Close to the ankle, its tendon crosses medially and inferior to the medial malleolus, tibialis posterior tendon, flexor digitorum longus tendon, tibial nerve, and posterior tibial artery. As it enters the foot, it passes posteriorly along a groove in the talus and inferior to its own groove on the inferior surface of the sustentaculum tali. The large tendon of the flexor hallucis longus attaches to the plantar side of the base of the first distal phalanx. It is the only muscle that flexes the interphalangeal joint of the first digit. As the tendon extends toward the first digit, it is straddled by the two heads of the flexor hallucis brevis muscle, which contain sesamoid bones at the level of the MTP joint that keep the tendon from being displaced.

The tibialis posterior tendon, flexor digitorum longus tendon, posterior tibial vessels, tibial nerve, and flexor hallucis longus tendon pass posterior to the medial malleolus in that order. They are each surrounded by separate **tendon sheaths** that appear at the level of the medial malleolus and continue along their respective tendons to the tarsal bones and into the foot. The whole assemblage is covered by a **flexor retinaculum** that extends from the inferior aspect of the medial malleolus to the medial side of the calcaneus, just inferior to the sustentaculum tali. A nearby **subcutaneous bursa of the medial malleolus** prevents friction as the skin and subcutaneous tissues glide across the medial ankle.

Popliteus.

Proximal attachments	• Lateral epicondyle of femur deep to fibrous layer of knee joint capsule • Small but important connections to the lateral meniscus and head of fibula
Distal attachment	• Posterior tibia between medial condyle, intercondylar area, and soleal line
Functions	• Prevents anterior displacement of the distal femur • Retracts the lateral meniscus during flexion of the leg at the knee to prevent injury • "Unlocks" knee from a fully extended position by laterally rotating the distal femur on the tibial condyles • Medially rotate an unsupported and flexed leg
Muscle testing and signs of dysfunction	• Tendon rupture or avulsion can occur when the leg is forcefully rotated laterally (externally) relative to the femur • Damage to the muscle, tendon, or attachments to the fibular head and lateral meniscus can occur during injuries involving the posterolateral corner of the knee • Dysfunction of the popliteus muscle can be difficult to diagnose
Innervation	• Tibial nerve (L4–S3)
Blood supply	• Inferior lateral genicular, middle genicular, posterior tibial arteries

Tibialis posterior.

Proximal attachments	• Lateral side of posterior tibial shaft, inferior to soleal line • Medial side of the fibular shaft • Interosseous membrane
Distal attachment	• Tuberosity of navicular bone • Inferior side of sustentaculum tali • Inferior side of the medial, intermediate, lateral cuneiform bones and the cuboid
Functions	• Supports medial longitudinal arch of foot during weight bearing • Inverts the foot at the ankle in conjunction with the tibialis anterior muscle
Muscle testing and signs of dysfunction	• Dysfunction of the tibialis posterior muscle commonly causes a falling of the medial longitudinal arch of the foot that is more pronounced when standing • Weakness in inverting the foot due to loss of the tibialis posterior muscle may eventually result in persistent eversion of the foot due to uncompensated pull from the fibularis muscles
Innervation	• Tibial nerve (L4–S3)
Blood supply	• Branches from posterior tibial, fibular, medial plantar arteries

Flexor digitorum longus.

Proximal attachments	• Middle third of posterior tibial shaft inferior to soleal line
Distal attachment	• Plantar aspects of base of the distal phalanx of digits 2–5
Functions	• Four individual tendons flex the distal interphalangeal joints of digits 2–5 • Assists in plantarflexion of the foot at the ankle • Assists in maintaining the medial longitudinal arch of the foot
Muscle testing and signs of dysfunction	• Dysfunction of the flexor digitorum longus would result in weakness flexing digits 2–5 and profound loss of flexion at the distal interphalangeal joint. This would noticeably weaken the toe-off phase of the gait cycle • The function of this muscle can specifically be assessed by asking patient to curl the toes while the examiner stabilizes the middle phalanx of each digit 2–5. If the distal phalanx flexes, the tendon to that digit is intact and the muscle is functional
Innervation	• Tibial nerve (L4–S3)
Blood supply	• Branches from posterior tibial, medial, and lateral plantar arteries

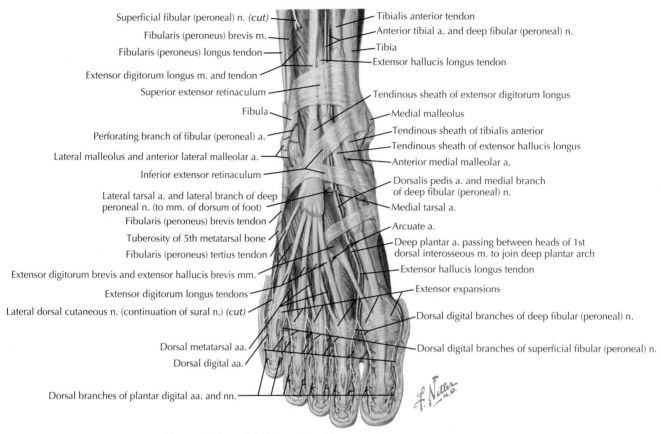

Superficial fibular (peroneal) n. *(cut)*
Fibularis (peroneus) brevis m.
Fibularis (peroneus) longus tendon
Extensor digitorum longus m. and tendon
Superior extensor retinaculum
Fibula
Perforating branch of fibular (peroneal) a.
Lateral malleolus and anterior lateral malleolar a.
Inferior extensor retinaculum
Lateral tarsal a. and lateral branch of deep peroneal n. (to mm. of dorsum of foot)
Fibularis (peroneus) brevis tendon
Tuberosity of 5th metatarsal bone
Fibularis (peroneus) tertius tendon
Extensor digitorum brevis and extensor hallucis brevis mm.
Extensor digitorum longus tendons
Lateral dorsal cutaneous n. (continuation of sural n.) *(cut)*
Dorsal metatarsal aa.
Dorsal digital aa.
Dorsal branches of plantar digital aa. and nn.

Tibialis anterior tendon
Anterior tibial a. and deep fibular (peroneal) n.
Tibia
Extensor hallucis longus tendon
Tendinous sheath of extensor digitorum longus
Medial malleolus
Tendinous sheath of tibialis anterior
Tendinous sheath of extensor hallucis longus
Anterior medial malleolar a.
Dorsalis pedis a. and medial branch of deep fibular (peroneal) n.
Medial tarsal a.
Arcuate a.
Deep plantar a. passing between heads of 1st dorsal interosseous m. to join deep plantar arch
Extensor hallucis longus tendon
Extensor expansions
Dorsal digital branches of deep fibular (peroneal) n.
Dorsal digital branches of superficial fibular (peroneal) n.

Fig. 11.19 Superficial Dissection of Muscles of the Dorsum of the Foot.

Flexor hallucis longus.

Proximal attachments	• Inferior half of posterior shaft of fibula and adjacent interosseous membrane
Distal attachment	• Plantar aspect of base of the distal phalanx of digit 1
Functions	• Flexes the interphalangeal joint of digit 1
	• This is the major muscle involved in the toe-off phase of gait that propels a person forward at the end of stance phase
Muscle testing and signs of dysfunction	• Dysfunction of the flexor hallucis longus would result in weakness flexing digit 1, particularly at the interphalangeal joint. This would severely weaken the toe-off phase of the gait cycle
	• The function of this muscle can specifically be assessed by asking patient to flex the big toe while the examiner stabilizes the proximal phalanx. If the distal phalanx flexes, the tendon to that digit is intact and the muscle is functional
Innervation	• Tibial nerve (L4–S3)
Blood supply	• Branches from fibular, medial plantar arteries

Lateral Compartment of the Leg (See Figs. 11.4 and 11.17–11.19)

The **lateral compartment of the leg** is bounded anteriorly by the anterior intermuscular septum, laterally by the deep fascia of the leg, posteriorly by the posterior intermuscular septum of the leg, and medially by the fibula. The muscles in this compartment, the fibularis longus and brevis (sometimes called the peroneal muscles), are innervated by the superficial fibular nerve that branches from the common fibular nerve. There is no artery within the lateral compartment; muscles within it receive perforating branches from the anterior tibial artery (anterior compartment) and fibular artery (deep posterior compartment).

The **fibularis longus muscle** originates from the lateral aspect of the head of the fibula and the superior half of the fibular shaft. The **fibularis brevis muscle** originates just inferior to it along the lateral aspect of the inferior half of the fibular shaft. As they descend, the fibularis longus covers and obscures the fibularis brevis, which can be seen if the tendon of the fibularis longus is displaced. The tendons of the fibularis longus and brevis pass posterior and inferior to the lateral malleolus, which has a malleolar groove to host the tendons as they descend. A nearby subcutaneous bursa of the lateral malleolus prevents friction as the skin and subcutaneous tissues glide across the lateral ankle. A **superior fibular retinaculum** covers the space between the lateral malleolus and calcaneus and tethers the tendons together in a single **common tendinous sheath of the** fibularis tendons. The **inferior fibular retinaculum** covers the fibular trochlea on the lateral aspect of the calcaneus and keeps the fibularis tendons and their individual tendon sheaths in place as they diverge.

The tendon of the fibularis brevis is located superior to the fibular trochlea, and the fibularis longus passes inferior to it as they pass lateral to the calcaneus. The fibularis brevis tendon continues lateral to the cuboid bone and attaches to the tuberosity of the base of the fifth metatarsal. The tendon of the fibularis longus has a more elaborate route within the **plantar tendinous sheath of the fibularis longus** that passes inferior to the cuboid bone within its own groove, deep to the long plantar ligament, before finally inserting onto the lateral aspect of the medial cuneiform bone and the medial base of the first metatarsal. Because the fibularis longus uses the cuboid bone as a pulley, it acts to maintain the lateral longitudinal arch of the foot. Both fibularis muscles evert the foot, which allows us to maintain contact with uneven ground as we walk. Damage to these muscles or the superficial fibular nerve will make eversion difficult and may lead to more frequent inversion injuries to the ankle.

Fibularis Longus and Fibularis Brevis

Proximal attachments	• Fibularis longus: Superior half of lateral fibular shaft • Fibularis brevis: Inferior half of lateral fibular shaft
Distal attachment	• Fibularis longus: Lateral aspects of medial cuneiform and base of first metatarsal • Fibularis brevis: Tuberosity of the base of the fifth metatarsal
Functions	• Eversion of the foot at the ankle • Minor contribution to plantarflexion
Muscle testing and signs of dysfunction	• Rupture of a tendon of the fibularis longus or fibularis brevis or damage to the superficial fibular nerve will cause weakness in eversion of the foot at the ankle and an inability to resist inversion. This may manifest as more frequent inversion falls or sprains (rolling the ankle) • With patient seated and the leg unsupported, the examiner will stabilize the distal leg in one hand and the foot in the other. The patient is asked to evert the foot (turn the sole outward) while the examiner gently tries to invert the foot. Asymmetry in strength may indicate damage or de-innervation affecting the fibularis muscles
Innervation	• Superficial fibular nerve (L5–S2)
Blood supply	• Superiorly: Perforating branches from anterior tibial artery • Inferiorly: Perforating branches from fibular artery

Anterior Compartment of the Leg (See Figs. 11.4 and 11.17–11.19)

The **anterior compartment of the leg** is bounded anteriorly by an especially thick deep fascia of the leg, laterally by the anterior intermuscular septum of the leg, medially by the tibia, and posteriorly by the interosseous membrane. The muscles in this compartment (tibialis anterior, extensor digitorum longus, extensor hallucis longus) are innervated by the deep fibular nerve, a branch of the common fibular nerve. Structures of the anterior compartment of the leg receive blood from the anterior tibial artery, which reaches the compartment by branching off the popliteal artery and passing through the interosseous membrane.

The large **tibialis anterior muscle** originates from the lateral aspect of the anterior tibia, stretching from the lateral tibial condyle just below the insertion of the iliotibial tract to the middle of the shaft, including the adjacent interosseous membrane. The muscle descends along the lateral side of the anterior border of the tibia and crosses anterior to the medial malleolus before inserting onto the medial, inferior aspects of the distal medial cuneiform bone and the base of the first metatarsal. There is a subtendinous bursa of the tibialis anterior present between its tendon and the tarsal bones just proximal to its insertion site. It is the major dorsiflexor of the foot at the ankle, which is essential during the swing phase of gait to prevent dragging of the toes, and also during the heel strike part of the stance phase. In conjunction with the tibialis posterior, it inverts the foot.

The **extensor digitorum longus muscle** is the most lateral muscle in this compartment as it originates from a small region of the lateral tibial condyle, fibular head, and adjacent interosseous membrane before extending inferiorly along the superior two-thirds of the anterior fibular shaft. A small and inconstant part of the extensor digitorum muscle, the **fibularis tertius muscle**, originates from the anterior shaft of the fibula a few centimeters superior to the lateral malleolus. As the extensor digitorum tendon approaches the ankle, it splits into five distinct tendons. Four of these cross the dorsum of the foot and create **extensor expansions** that attach to the dorsal sides of the bases of the middle and distal phalanges of digits 2 to 5. Because of this, the extensor digitorum longus muscle extends MTP joints of digits 2 to 5 and assists in dorsiflexion. The fifth tendon, if it is present, comes from the fibularis tertius portion of the muscle and inserts on the superolateral aspect of the shaft of the 5th (and sometimes 4th) metatarsal. It assists in dorsiflexion and eversion of the foot and may act as a proprioceptive muscle to sense sudden stretch during inversion.

The **extensor hallucis longus muscle** originates from the middle third of the fibula and adjacent interosseous membrane, deep to the tibialis anterior and extensor digitorum longus muscles. Its tendon descends between the other two muscles as it crosses the ankle and dorsum of the foot and attaches strongly to the dorsal side of the base of the distal phalanx. It extends the first digit, or hallux, at the MTP and interphalangeal joints and assists in dorsiflexion of the foot.

A **superior extensor retinaculum** crosses between the distal fibula and tibia to cover the (from lateral to medial) extensor digitorum longus, extensor hallucis longus, and tibialis anterior tendons. As the same tendons cross the ankle, they are covered by a Y-shaped **inferior extensor retinaculum** that begins on the superior body of the calcaneus. Medially, it divides into two sheets that cover the anterior and posterior surfaces of the extensor digitorum longus and fibularis tertius tendons. Thereafter the layers rejoin and then split into a superior band that attaches to the medial malleolus and an inferior band that reaches the medial cuneiform and base of the first metatarsal and fuses with the plantar aponeurosis. The tendons of the muscles of the anterior compartment of the leg are covered by individual **tendon sheaths**. The tendon sheath of the tibialis anterior begins in the distal leg and is present deep to the superior extensor retinaculum and the superior band of the inferior extensor retinaculum. The tendon sheath of the extensor hallucis longus begins distal to the superior extensor retinaculum and covers its tendon as it travels deep to the superior and inferior bands of the inferior extensor retinaculum. Finally, the tendon sheath of the extensor digitorum longus surrounds the common tendon of this muscle as it passes deep to the inferior extensor retinaculum and divides to surround the very proximal parts of the individual digital extensor tendons and the tendon of the fibularis tertius.

Tibialis Anterior

Proximal attachments	• Lateral condyle and lateral aspect of the superior half of the tibial shaft and adjacent interosseous membrane
Distal attachment	• Medial, inferior aspect of distal medial cuneiform bone and base of the first metatarsal
Functions	• Strong dorsiflexion of the foot at the ankle • In conjunction with the tibialis posterior, inversion of the foot at the ankle
Muscle testing and signs of dysfunction	• The patient sits with the legs unsupported, while the examiner stabilizes the distal leg. The examiner plantarflexes the foot, while the patient attempts to resist the motion by dorsiflexing. Asymmetry in strength or pain during the motion may indicate damage to the muscle or the deep fibular nerve • Loss of function of the tibialis anterior will result in the toes of the affected foot being dragged on the ground during swing phase of gait or when ascending stairs. A patient may compensate by adopting a "high steppage" gait to ensure the foot clears the ground
Innervation	• Deep fibular (L4–L5)
Blood supply	• Anterior tibial artery

Extensor Digitorum Longus and Fibularis Tertius

Proximal attachments	• Lateral condyle of tibia, nearby fibular head and interosseous membrane • Superior two thirds of anterior shaft of fibula • Fibularis tertius: Anterior fibula superior to the lateral malleolus
Distal attachment	• Extensor expansions on the dorsum of digits 2–5 • Fibularis tertius: Superolateral shaft of metatarsals 4–5
Functions	• Strong extension of digits 2–5, which is helpful during swing phase of gait • Assists in dorsiflexion • Fibularis tertius: Assists the fibularis longus and brevis in eversion, assists other anterior compartment muscles in dorsiflexion
Muscle testing and signs of dysfunction	• The patient sits with the legs unsupported while the examiner stabilizes the foot. The examiner then gently but firmly flexes the toes while the patient attempts to resist and extend them. Asymmetry in strength or pain during the motion may indicate damage to the muscle, one of the tendons, or the deep fibular nerve • Loss of function may result in the affected toes being dragged during swing phase or when ascending stairs. This will likely not be noted unless tibialis anterior is also dysfunctional • Fibularis tertius: This tendon is frequently damaged during inversion sprains of the foot and may cause avulsion of the tuberosity of the base of the fifth metatarsal when it experiences sudden, violent strain
Innervation	• Deep fibular (L4–L5)
Blood supply	• Anterior tibial artery

Extensor Hallucis Longus

Proximal attachments	• Middle one third of anterior fibula and adjacent interosseous membrane
Distal attachment	• Dorsal aspect of the base of distal phalanx of digit 1 (hallux)
Functions	• Strong extension of digit 1 at the metatarsophalangeal and interphalangeal joints, which is helpful during swing phase of gait • Assists in dorsiflexion
Muscle testing and signs of dysfunction	• The patient sits with the legs unsupported while the examiner stabilizes the foot. The examiner then flexes the large toe while the patient attempts to resist the motion by extending it. Asymmetry in strength or pain during the motion may indicate damage to the muscle, its tendon, or the deep fibular nerve
Innervation	• Deep fibular (L4–L5)
Blood supply	• Anterior tibial artery

Fascial Structures and Muscles of the Dorsum of the Foot (See Figs. 11.17–11.19)

Deep to the thin skin on the dorsum of the foot is a distinct **dorsal fascia of the foot** that contains the muscles, vessels, and nerves in this area within a thin **dorsal compartment of the foot**. The dorsal fascia fuses laterally and medially with fibers of the plantar aponeurosis. The two small muscles in this **dorsal compartment of the foot** are the **extensor digitorum brevis muscle** and **extensor hallucis brevis muscle**. Both muscles share a fused origin on the anterior superior calcaneus within the tarsal sinus. Their tendons diverge as they project medially. The three tendons of the extensor digitorum extend distally and join the lateral aspect of the extensor expansion on the dorsum of digits 2 to 4, excluding the fifth digit. The tendon of the extensor hallucis longus projects medially to digit 1 (hallux) and attaches to the dorsal side of the base of the proximal phalanx. Both muscles are innervated by the lateral branch of the deep fibular nerve after it leaves the anterior compartment of the leg.

Extensor Digitorum Brevis (EDB) and Extensor Hallucis Brevis (EHB)

Proximal attachments	• EDB and EHB: Anterior aspect of tarsal sinus on anterior calcaneus
Distal attachment	• EDB: Extensor expansions on the dorsum of digits 2–4 • EHB: Dorsal base of the proximal phalanx of digit 1 (hallux)
Functions	• EDB: Assists in extension of digits 2–4 at the metatarsophalangeal and interphalangeal joints. • EHB: Assists in extension of digit 1 at the metatarsophalangeal joint
Muscle testing and signs of dysfunction	• Dysfunction of these muscles would be very difficult to detect if the extensor hallucis longus and extensor digitorum longus muscles were intact • These muscles may be hypertrophied in dancers, martial artists, gymnasts, and others who strongly extend their toes for a prolonged time. Loss of innervation to these muscles may produce noticeable atrophy in such people on the affected side
Innervation	• Lateral branch of deep fibular nerve (L5–S1)
Blood supply	• Lateral tarsal artery

Fascial Structures and Muscles of the Plantar Foot (Fig. 11.20)

Deep to the thick skin of the plantar foot is a layer of superficial fascia and adipose tissue. This layer is especially dense on the heel, with a deep layer of adipose tissue confined in fibrous compartments by skin ligaments. These serve as compressible units that absorb the force of each heel strike. Deep to the adipose tissue is a very strong sheet of connective tissue that covers the majority of the plantar foot, the **plantar aponeurosis**. It has a **lateral band** that begins on the lateral process of the calcaneal tuberosity that stretches toward the base of the fifth metatarsal. The larger, more central part of the plantar aponeurosis begins on the posterior aspect of the calcaneal tuberosity and stretches distally, splitting into separate slips for each digit. These slips fuse with the underlying fibrous layer of the tendon sheaths of the flexor tendons and are also connected to adjacent digital slips by **transverse fascicles**. Over the heads of the metatarsals and just proximal to the digits is another collection of connective tissue fibers that connect and reinforce the slips of the plantar aponeurosis, the **superficial transverse metatarsal ligaments**. The **deep transverse metatarsal ligament** connects the heads of the metatarsals and fuses to the plantar side of each MTP joint capsule (Clinical Correlation 11.18).

The medial and lateral sides of the plantar aponeurosis meet the dorsal fascia of the foot but are also continuous with connective tissue septae that extend deeply to create several compartments in the foot itself. The number of compartments present in the foot is controversial. In this book we will use the scheme presented in Lugo-Pico et al. (2019). The lateral, medial, and superficial central compartments stretch across the hindfoot, midfoot, and forefoot. The deep central compartment is located in the hindfoot, while the adductor and interosseous compartments are in the forefoot. Superior to the metatarsals is the dorsal compartment of the foot, which was described in the preceding section. As we discuss the muscles on the plantar side of the foot, their individual functions will be listed; however, these muscles tend to function as a unit to bind the bones of the foot together and prevent displacement of the tarsal and metatarsal bones throughout all parts of the stance phase of gait and during other activities that put stress on the foot.

Lateral Compartment of the Foot

The **lateral compartment of the foot** contains the abductor digiti minimi and flexor digiti minimi brevis muscles. The **abductor digiti minimi muscle** originates from the lateral process of the calcaneus and a short strip of bone just anterior to the medial process. Some fibers also originate from the overlying lateral band of the plantar aponeurosis. It wraps around the plantar side of the base of the fifth metatarsal just medial to the tuberosity of that bone. Some fibers from the base of the fifth metatarsal join the muscle and extend distally to insert on the lateral side of the base of the fifth digit's proximal phalanx. The angle at which it approaches its insertion allows it to abduct and flex the fifth digit at the MTP joint. The **flexor digiti minimi brevis muscle** originates from the middle region of the base of the fifth metatarsal on its plantar side. It then travels distally, just medial to the abductor digiti minimi, to insert on the plantar base of the proximal phalanx of the fifth digit. This allows it to flex the fifth digit at the MTP joint.

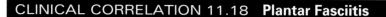

CLINICAL CORRELATION 11.18   Plantar Fasciitis

Connective tissue structures tend to be well-innervated but poorly perfused with blood. This makes them painful when traumatized and slow to heal. The plantar aponeurosis is particularly prone to injury due to the large amounts of weight it must endure with each step. Overuse or excessive impact on the heel can result in microtrauma and inflammation that lead to plantar fasciitis. The pain associated

with this condition is worse after significant time spent with seated or laying down, such as first thing in the morning. Because the plantar aponeurosis can be retraumatized easily, it is important to prevent excessive impact or stretching of it during treatment. Long-standing inflammation can lead to a bone spur (calcaneal spur) at the site where the traumatized aponeurosis attaches to the calcaneus.

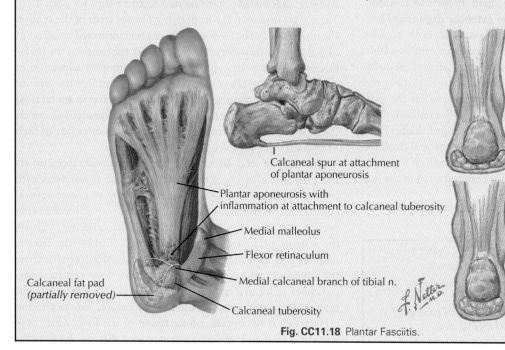

Calcaneal spur at attachment of plantar aponeurosis

Plantar aponeurosis with inflammation at attachment to calcaneal tuberosity

Medial malleolus

Flexor retinaculum

Calcaneal fat pad (partially removed)

Medial calcaneal branch of tibial n.

Calcaneal tuberosity

Loose-fitting heel counter in running shoe allows calcaneal fat pad to spread at heel strike, increasing transmission of impact to heel.

Firm, well-fitting heel counter maintains compactness of fat pad, which buffers force of impact.

Fig. CC11.18 Plantar Fasciitis.

Abductor digiti minimi (AbDM) and flexor digiti minimi brevis (FDMB).

Proximal attachments	• AbDM: Lateral process of calcaneus and area just anterior to medial process, plantar aspect of base of fifth metatarsal • FDMB: Middle, plantar side of base of the fifth metatarsal
Distal attachment	• AbDM: Lateral side of base of proximal phalanx of fifth digit • FDMB: Plantar side of base of proximal phalanx of fifth digit
Functions	• Stabilize bones of the foot during stance phase of gait and other motions • AbDM: Abduct and flex the metatarsophalangeal joint of the fifth digit • FDMB: Flex the metatarsophalangeal joint of the fifth digit
Muscle testing and signs of dysfunction	• Atrophy of these muscles could be noted if they were de-innervated • Weakness in abduction or flexion of the fifth digit may be noted during an extremely thorough physical exam
Innervation	• Lateral plantar nerve (S2–S3)
Blood supply	• Lateral plantar artery

Medial Compartment of the Foot

The **medial compartment of the foot** acts on the first digit similarly to how the lateral compartment acts on the fifth digit. It contains the abductor hallucis and flexor hallucis brevis muscles. The **abductor hallucis muscle** originates from the medial process of the calcaneus and extends along the medial side of the foot to reach the medial side of the base of the first digit's proximal phalanx. This arrangement allows it to slightly abduct the hallux and also to flex it at the first MTP joint. The **flexor hallucis brevis muscle** has a small site of origin from the medial side of the cuboid and lateral side of the lateral cuneiform bones. In the forefoot, it divides into **medial** and **lateral heads** that straddle the flexor hallucis longus tendon. The medial and lateral heads of the muscle insert on the medial and lateral sides of the base of the proximal phalanx on the plantar side. The tendon of each head of the flexor hallucis brevis has a **sesamoid bone** in its tendon at the level of the MTP joint. This muscle is a strong flexor of the first digit at the MTP joint, making it a key component in the toe-off phase of gait.

Superficial dissection

Superficial transverse metatarsal ligaments

Proper plantar digital aa. and nn.

Superficial branch of medial plantar a.

Transverse fasciculi

Digital slips of plantar fascia

Cutaneous branches of lateral plantar a. and n.

Cutaneous branches of medial plantar a. and n.

Plantar fascia

Lateral band of plantar fascia (calcaneometatarsal ligament)

Tuberosity of calcaneus with overlying fatpad (partially cut away)

Medial calcaneal branches of tibial n. and posterior tibial a.

First layer

Proper digital branches of medial plantar n.

Proper digital branches of lateral plantar n.

Proper plantar digital aa.

Common plantar digital aa. from plantar metatarsal aa.

Lumbrical mm.

Lateral and medial head of flexor hallucis brevis m.

Flexor hallucis longus tendon

Abductor hallucis m. and tendon

Flexor digitorum brevis m.

Fibrous sheaths of flexor tendons

Tendons of flexor digitorum brevis m. overlying tendons of flexor digitorum longus m.

Metatarsal branch of lateral plantar a.

Flexor digiti minimi brevis m.

Abductor digiti minimi m.

Plantar fascia *(cut)*

Tuberosity of calcaneus

Second layer

Flexor digitorum longus tendons

Flexor digitorum brevis tendons

Sesamoid bones

Lumbrical mm.

Lateral head and Medial head of flexor hallucis brevis m.

Flexor hallucis longus tendon

Abductor hallucis tendon and m. *(cut)*

Flexor digitorum longus tendon

Superficial and deep branches of medial plantar a.

Medial plantar a. and n.

Tibialis posterior tendon

Flexor hallucis longus tendon

Flexor retinaculum

Abductor hallucis m. *(cut)*

Flexor digiti minimi brevis m.

Lateral plantar n. and a.

Quadratus plantae m.

Abductor digiti minimi m. *(cut)*

Nerve to abductor digiti minimi m.

Flexor digitorum brevis m. and plantar aponeurosis *(cut)*

Third layer

Tendons of lumbrical mm. *(cut)*

Transverse head and Oblique head of adductor hallucis m.

Flexor hallucis brevis m. (medial and lateral heads)

Flexor hallucis longus tendon *(cut)*

Abductor hallucis m. *(cut)*

Tibialis posterior tendon

Flexor digitorum longus tendon *(cut)*

Flexor hallucis longus tendon

Flexor retinaculum

Abductor hallucis m. *(cut)*

Plantar interosseous mm.

Tuberosity of 5th metatarsal bone

Peroneus brevis tendon

Peroneus longus tendon and fibrous sheath

Quadratus plantae m. *(cut and slightly retracted)*

Abductor digiti minimi m. *(cut)*

Flexor digitorum brevis m. and plantar aponeurosis *(cut)*

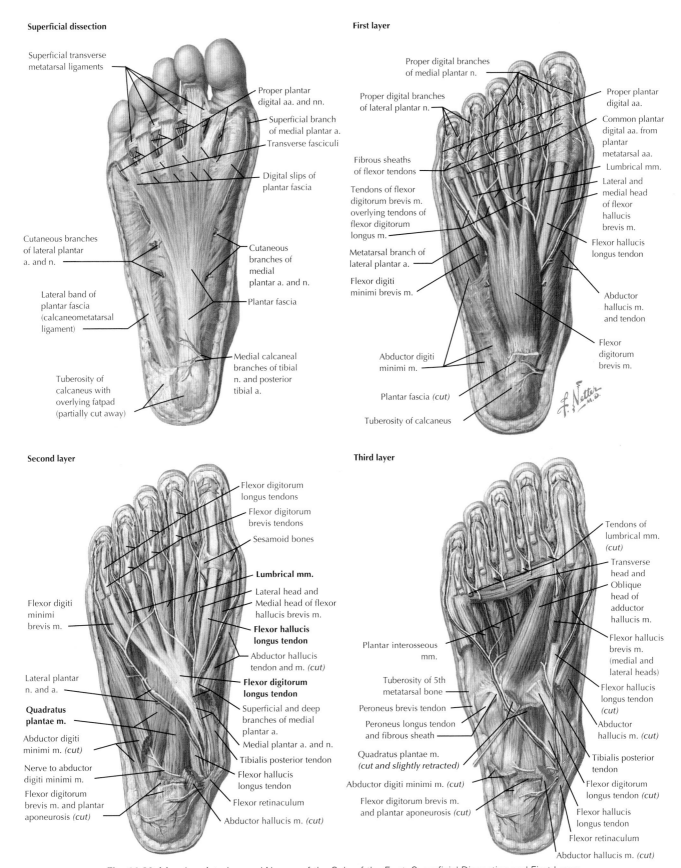

Fig. 11.20 Muscles, Arteries, and Nerves of the Sole of the Foot: Superficial Dissection and First Layer.

Abductor hallucis (AbH) and flexor hallucis brevis (FHB).

Proximal attachments	• AbH: Medial process of calcaneus • FHB: Medial side of cuboid and lateral side of lateral cuneiform bones
Distal attachment	• AbH: Medial, plantar side of base of proximal phalanx of first digit • Flexor digiti minimi brevis inserts on the plantar base of first digit's proximal phalanx • Medial head: Medial side of base • Lateral head: Lateral side of base
Functions	• Stabilize bones of the foot during stance phase of gait and other motions • AbH: Abduct and flex the metatarsophalangeal joint of the first digit • FHB: Flex the metatarsophalangeal joint of the first digit, which happens strongly during the toe-off portion of the stance phase of gait
Muscle testing and signs of dysfunction	• Weakness in these muscles would result in difficulty abducting or flexing the metatarsophalangeal joint of the first digit. Due to the size of these muscles, atrophy may actually be noted during physical exam • Weakness of the FHB muscle would make the toe-off segment of the stance phase of gait weak
Innervation	• Medial plantar nerve (S2–S3)
Blood supply	• Medial plantar artery

Central Compartment of the Foot

The **central compartment of the foot** is covered and protected by the plantar aponeurosis. The **flexor digitorum brevis muscle** is a stout muscle that originates from the area between the lateral and medial processes of the calcaneus as well as the overlying plantar aponeurosis. It extends distally, giving off four distinct tendons that travel to digits 2 to 5, inserting on the medial and lateral sides of the shaft of the middle phalanx of each digit. This makes it a strong flexor of the MTP and PIP joints for digits 2 to 5 during the toe-off part of stance phase. Deep to the flexor digitorum brevis muscle are the **tendon(s) of the flexor digitorum longus muscle**, which leaves the deep posterior compartment of the leg, travels inferior to the medial malleolus, and enters the foot from the medial side. As it crosses laterally, deep to the flexor digitorum brevis muscle, the single tendon of that muscle splits into individual tendons to the distal phalanges of digits 2 to 5. **Lumbrical muscles** arise from the medial side of each digital tendon of the flexor digitorum longus. These run parallel to the tendons from which they originate and insert on the extensor expansion of digits 2 to 5. Along the way, they pass inferior to the MTP joint and exert their contraction superior to the proximal and DIP joints. This allows the lumbricals of the foot to act similarly to those in the hand, flexing the MTP and extending the interphalangeal joints but in a less pronounced way. The **quadratus plantae muscle** originates from the body of the calcaneus and inserts onto the posterior aspect of the tendon of the flexor digitorum longus. Contraction of this muscle aligns the lateral tendons of the flexor digitorum longus with the digits to which they run. Some sources place this muscle in a separate compartment (deep central), but the physiologic validity of this compartment has been questioned.

As they approach each digit, the flexor digitorum longus and brevis tendons enter a **tendon sheath** that is made of a **fibrous sheath** surrounding a **synovial sheath** that lubricates the movement of these tendons as they contract. The fibrous sheath has fibers arrayed in a variety of directions, with some anular fibers making a ring around the synovial sheath and other cruciform fibers that cross each other. Tendon sheaths are anchored to the digital aspects of the plantar aponeurosis. Within the tendon sheaths the tendons are connected to the overlying phalanges by **vincula** (singular is vinculum) that bring small but essential blood vessels to the tendons. There are also **plantar (volar) plates** of fibrocartilage on the inferior side of each MTP, PIP, and DIP joint that reinforce them and help the tendons to glide during flexion and extension.

Flexor digitorum brevis (FDB), lumbricals, and quadratus plantae (QP).

Proximal attachments	• FDB: Between medial and lateral processes of the calcaneus and plantar aponeurosis • Lumbricals: Medial aspect of each tendon of the flexor digitorum longus • QP: Body of calcaneus
Distal attachment	• FDB: Medial and lateral aspects of the shaft of the middle phalanges of digits 2–5 • Lumbricals: Medial aspect of extensor expansions of digits 2–5 • QP: Posterior aspect of flexor digitorum longus tendon
Functions	• Stabilize bones of the foot during stance phase of gait and other motions • FDB: Flex metatarsophalangeal (MTP) and proximal interphalangeal (PIP) joints of digits 2–5, assisting during the toe-off portion of the stance phase of gait • Lumbricals: Flex MTP and extend the associated PIP and distal interphalangeal joints • QP: Align the tendons of the flexor digitorum longus
Muscle testing and signs of dysfunction	• Weakness of the FDB muscle or rupture of one of its tendons would result in difficulty flexing the affected MTP and PIP joints of digits 2–5. This would result in weakness during the toe-off segment of the stance phase of gait • Weakness of the quadratus plantae and lumbricals of the foot would be difficult to diagnose by physical exam or gait assessment
Innervation	• FDB and lumbrical to digit 2: Medial plantar nerve (S2–S3) • Lumbricals to digits 3–5 and QP: Lateral plantar nerve (S2–S3)
Blood supply	• Medial and lateral plantar arteries

Adductor Compartment of the Foot

The **adductor compartment of the foot** is located in the forefoot and is described as containing (at least part of) the adductor hallucis muscle. This muscle has two heads. An **oblique head** arises from the bases of metatarsals 2 to 4 and runs distally next to the lateral head of the flexor hallucis brevis muscle. The **transverse head** originates from the deep transverse metatarsal ligament in the vicinity of the heads of the metatarsals 3 to 5. The two heads of the adductor hallucis muscle converge on the lateral side of the base of the proximal phalanx of the first digit. Like the other muscles of the plantar foot, it helps to keep the bones connected but can also adduct the hallux laterally at the MTP joint.

Adductor hallucis.

Proximal attachments	• Oblique head: Plantar sides of the bases of metatarsals 2–4
	• Transverse head: Deep transverse metatarsal ligament and underlying connective tissue structures
Distal attachment	• Lateral side of the base of the proximal phalanx of the first digit
Functions	• Stabilize bones of the foot during stance phase of gait and other motions
	• Maintain the transverse arch of the foot
	• Adduct the hallux (move laterally) at the metatarsophalangeal joint
Muscle testing and signs of dysfunction	• It would be very difficult to diagnose isolated injury to this muscle.
Innervation	• Lateral plantar nerve (S2–S3)
Blood supply	• Medial and lateral plantar arteries

Interosseous Compartments

Between each metatarsal bone is an **interosseous compartment** that is separate from adjacent interosseous compartments, although this description is not universal. There are three, unipennate **plantar interossei** that arise from the medial aspects of metatarsals 3 to 5 and insert onto the medial side of the bases of their own proximal phalanges. Their contraction brings digits 3, 4, and 5 toward the second digit, adducting them (mnemonic: **PAD** = **P**lantar **AD**duct). The neutral midline of the second digit is the frame of reference for ad/abduction, therefore the second digit can only abduct because it cannot move closer to its own neutral midline. The first plantar interosseous muscle originates from the medial side of the third metatarsal and inserts on the medial base of the third digit's proximal phalanx. The other two plantar interosseous muscles are similar, arising from the medial side of metatarsals 4 and 5 and inserting on the medial side of the base of their proximal phalanges.

There are four, bipennate **dorsal interossei,** and they abduct digits 2, 3, and 4 away from the midline of the second digit (mnemonic: **DAB** = **D**orsal **AB**duct). Both medial and lateral motions of the second digit are called abduction because both motions move it away from its neutral position's midline. The first dorsal interosseous muscle originates from the first and second metatarsals, while the second dorsal interosseous comes from between the second and third metatarsals. They insert on the medial and lateral aspects, respectively, of the base of the proximal phalanx of the second digit. The third dorsal interosseous originates between the third and fourth metatarsals and inserts on the lateral aspect of the base of the proximal phalanx of the third digit. Finally, the fourth dorsal interosseous comes from between the fourth and fifth metatarsals and inserts on the lateral aspect of the base of the proximal phalanx of the fourth digit. Recall that the abductor digiti minimi abducts the fifth digit. No interosseous muscles attach to the hallux because it has dedicated adductor hallucis and abductor hallucis muscles.

Plantar and dorsal interosseous muscles.

Proximal attachments	• Plantar
	• First: Medial aspect of metatarsal 2
	• Second and third: Lateral aspect of metatarsals 4 and 5
	• Dorsal
	• First: Between metatarsals 1 and 2
	• Second: Between metatarsals 2 and 3
	• Third: Between metatarsals 3 and 4
	• Fourth: Between metatarsals 4 and 5
Distal attachment	• Plantar: First, second, and third plantar interossei insert on the medial aspects of the base of the proximal phalanges of digits 3–5
	• Dorsal:
	• First and second insert on medial and lateral sides of base of proximal phalanx of second digit
	• Third and fourth insert on lateral sides of base of proximal phalanx of third and fourth digits
Functions	• Stabilize bones of the foot during stance phase of gait and other motions
	• Plantar interossei adduct digits 3, 4, 5 toward the second digit
	• Dorsal interossei abduct digits 2, 3, and 4 away from the second digit's neutral midline
	• Both sets of interossei also flex the digits at the metatarsophalangeal joint
Muscle testing and signs of dysfunction	• Weakness of these muscles would be difficult to diagnose since the toes do not have a wide range of motion in abduction/adduction. There might be some weakness in the toe-off part of the stance phase of gait.
Innervation	• Lateral plantar nerve (S2–S3)
Blood supply	• Medial and lateral plantar arteries

Another way to describe the muscles of the plantar foot is to describe how they form (somewhat) distinct layers from superficial to deep. Deep to the plantar aponeurosis, there are four layers:

1. Abductor hallucis, flexor digitorum brevis, abductor digiti minimi
2. Tendons of flexor digitorum longus, quadratus plantae, lumbricals 1 to 4
3. Flexor hallucis brevis (medial and lateral heads), adductor hallucis (oblique and transverse heads, flexor digiti minimi brevis, tendon of flexor hallucis longus
4. Tendon of fibularis longus, plantar interossei, dorsal interossei

If we were to proceed further, we would reach the dorsum of the foot, with the extensor hallucis brevis, extensor digitorum brevis, tendon of extensor hallucis longus, and tendons of extensor digitorum longus (Clinical Correlation 11.19).

INNERVATION OF THE LOWER LIMB

The Spinal Nerves to the Lower Limb and Dermatomes (Fig. 11.21)

The L1–S3 anterior rami innervate the muscles of the lower limb and convey sensation from the overlying skin. Injury to a peripheral nerve will result in a distinctive set of motor and sensory losses, whereas more proximal compression of a lumbosacral spinal nerve or anterior ramus will manifest as sensory aberration along a dermatome. Like the upper limb, dermatomes associated with the lower limb begin segmentally near the vertebrae on the back and extend on the dorsal side of the lower limbs. The

---

CLINICAL CORRELATION 11.19   Traction Apophysitis

The site of a muscle attachment on a bone sometimes includes cartilage growth plates. Very active children and adolescents can develop **traction apophysitis**, where the pull of a tendon causes enlargement of the cartilage of the growth plate and fragmentation of the ossification centers and the eventual bone. Although this can occur in the upper limbs, it is most prominent in the lower limb due to the larger size of the muscles and prolonged use of those muscles in many types of athletics.

- **Iselin syndrome** is a traction apophysitis of the tuberosity of the base of the fifth metatarsal by the pull of the fibularis brevis tendon.

- **Sever disease** is enlargement of the calcaneal tuberosity by the pull of the calcaneal tendon.
- **Osgood-Schlatter disease** is enlargement of the tibial tuberosity by traction of the patellar ligament and quadriceps.
- **Sinding-Larsen-Johansson syndrome** involves enlargement of the inferior apex of the patella by the pull of the patellar ligament and quadriceps.
- Traction apophysitis of the anterior superior iliac spine and anterior inferior iliac spine can result from the pull of the sartorius and rectus femoris muscles, respectively.

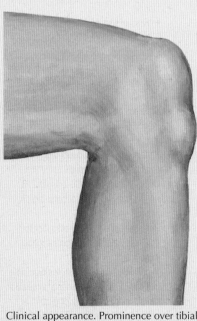

Clinical appearance. Prominence over tibial tuberosity due partly to soft tissue swelling and partly to avulsed fragments.

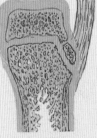

Normal insertion of patellar ligament of ossifying tibial tuberosity

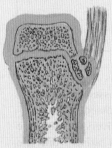

In Osgood-Schlatter disease, superficial portion of tuberosity pulled away, forming separate bone fragments.

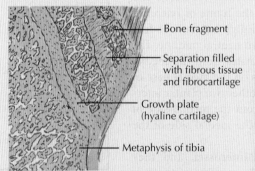

Bone fragment

Separation filled with fibrous tissue and fibrocartilage

Growth plate (hyaline cartilage)

Metaphysis of tibia

High-power magnification of involved area

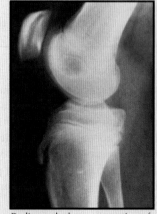

Radiograph shows separation of superficial portion of tibial tuberosity.

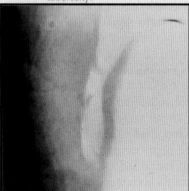

Focal radiograph shows fragment at site of insertion of patellar ligament.

Fig. CC11.19 Osgood-Schlatter Lesion.

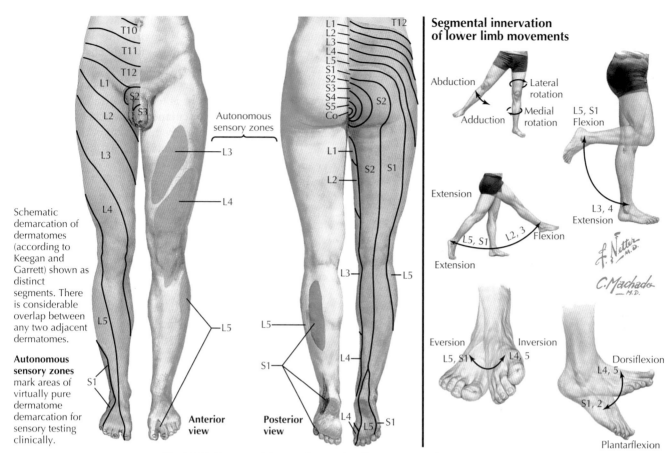

Fig. 11.21 Segmental Sensory Innervation (Dermatomes) of the Lower Limb.

dermatomes converge on a ventral axial line that disrupts this clear arrangement. Starting from the back, the L1 dermatome covers the skin of the inguinal area, including the inferior abdomen and the upper thigh to the ventral axial line. Similarly, the L2 dermatome stretches across skin superior to the greater trochanter across the upper thigh, while the L3 dermatome covers the area lateral to the trochanter and the middle of the anterior thigh before reaching the ventral axial line. The L4 dermatome runs along the middle thigh laterally, the anterior inferior thigh, patella, and anteromedial leg and foot, including the medial malleolus, and medial side of the hallux. The L5 dermatome travels along the posterolateral thigh, knee, and upper leg before moving to the anterior leg and foot, including the dorsal and plantar aspects of digits 2 to 4. The S1 dermatome begins just superior to the gluteal crease and descends across the buttock just lateral to the midline of the posterior thigh, leg, ankle, and foot. S1 includes the lateral malleolus and the dorsal and plantar aspects of the lateral foot and fifth digit. The S2 dermatome also travels across the buttock but turns inferomedially to include the upper part of the medial thigh and some of the external genitalia. The rest of the S2 dermatome descends just medial to the midline along the posterior thigh, leg, ankle, and foot, including part of the medial, plantar heel. The S3 dermatome does not extend into the lower limb (although S3 does contribute to the motor activity in the limb) but carries sensation from the genitalia and forms a "bullseye" pattern of circular dermatomes around the anus in conjunction with S4, S5, and one coccygeal dermatome.

Posterior Rami and the Lower Limb (Fig. 11.22)

Each lumbar and sacral spinal nerve gives off a posterior ramus that will travel to the muscles and skin of the back. In the lower limb, the posterior rami create the cluneal nerves that supply the skin overlying the gluteal muscles. The **superior cluneal nerves** come from the posterior rami of L1 to L3, while the **medial cluneal nerves** arise from posterior rami of S1 to S3. A set of **inferior cluneal nerves** are also present but come from the posterior cutaneous nerve of the thigh, which arises from an anterior ramus.

The Lumbar Plexus and Sacral Plexus (Fig. 11.23)

The anterior rami from L1 to L4 will combine to form the **lumbar plexus**, and L5 to S4 anterior rami will create the **sacral plexus**. Because the sacral plexus has some inputs from lumbar anterior rami, it is sometimes called the lumbosacral plexus. The anterior ramus of T12, the **subcostal nerve**, as well as the branches from L1, the **iliohypogastric** and **ilioinguinal nerves**, innervate the muscles and skin of the lower abdomen. These will be discussed in the next chapter.

Lumbar Plexus Contributions to the Lower Limb (See Fig. 11.23A)

Branches of the anterior rami of L1 and L2 fuse to become the **genitofemoral nerve**, which passes through the psoas muscle and descends along its anterior surface before it splits into two branches before leaving the abdomen. The **genital branch of the genitofemoral nerve (L1)** conveys sensations from the anterior

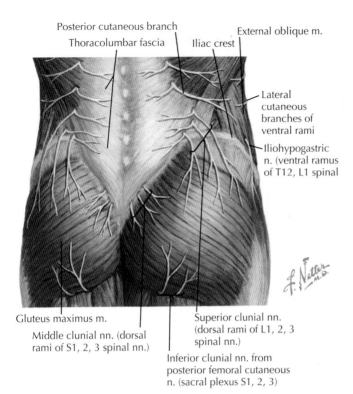

Posterior cutaneous branch

Thoracolumbar fascia

External oblique m.

Iliac crest

Lateral cutaneous branches of ventral rami

Iliohypogastric n. (ventral ramus of T12, L1 spinal

Gluteus maximus m.

Middle clunial nn. (dorsal rami of S1, 2, 3 spinal nn.)

Superior clunial nn. (dorsal rami of L1, 2, 3 spinal nn.)

Inferior clunial nn. from posterior femoral cutaneous n. (sacral plexus S1, 2, 3)

Fig. 11.22 Nerves of the Back.

genitalia and innervates the cremaster muscle in the spermatic cord, which can elevate the testes. The **femoral branch of the genitofemoral nerve (L2)** innervates a small region of anteromedial skin immediately inferior to the inguinal ligament overlying the femoral triangle. The remaining anterior rami of the lumbar and sacral plexuses split into **posterior** and **anterior divisions** that will innervate muscles derived from the embryonic dorsal and ventral muscle masses of the lower limb, respectively. The dorsal muscle mass will differentiate into muscles of the gluteal region, anterior thigh, lateral leg, anterior leg, and dorsum of the foot, while the ventral muscle mass gives rise to muscles of the pelvis, medial thigh, posterior thigh, posterior leg, and plantar foot.

The posterior divisions (NOT posterior rami) of L2 and L3 pass through the psoas major muscle and contribute to the **lateral cutaneous nerve of the thigh (L2–L3)** (Fig. 11.24). This nerve exits laterally from the psoas major, descends along the medial surface of the iliacus muscle, and exits the abdomen by passing through the inguinal ligament near the anterior superior iliac spine. It innervates a significant area of skin on the anterolateral thigh, extending from the iliac crest to the lateral knee (Clinical Correlation 11.20).

The posterior divisions of L2–L4 anterior rami that pass through the psoas major contribute to the **femoral nerve (L2–L4)** (see Fig. 11.24). This very large nerve descends in the crease between the psoas major and iliacus muscles and exits inferior to the inguinal ligament and lateral to the iliopectineal arch on the anterior surface of the iliopsoas muscle. The femoral nerve ramifies tremendously just after it enters the anterior compartment of the thigh. A very proximal articular branch of the femoral nerve conveys sensation from the anterior aspect of

the coxofemoral (hip) joint capsule. Many muscular branches innervate the sartorius, rectus femoris, and pectineus muscles. Other muscular branches to the vastus lateralis, vastus intermedius, vastus medialis, and articularis genu descend a significant distance to reach their target muscles. These branches also supply a sensory branch to the anterior joint capsule of the knee. There are several **anterior cutaneous branches of the femoral nerve** that convey sensation from the skin of the anteromedial thigh between the lateral femoral cutaneous nerve and the cutaneous branch of the obturator nerve.

The **saphenous nerve (L3–L4)** (see Fig. 11.24) is a medial continuation of the femoral nerve that descends along the medial knee, leg, ankle, and heel; it conveys sensation from all the skin along its course. Immediately inferior to the knee it gives off an **infrapatellar branch** that extends laterally, crossing the patellar ligament and the tibial tuberosity. The **medial cutaneous nerves of the leg** are branches of the saphenous nerve covering the medial aspect of the leg from the anterior midline to posterior midline. The saphenous nerve terminates as several branches over the medial ankle and heel, sometimes including a small bit of skin on the medial, plantar foot (Clinical Correlation 11.21).

The anterior divisions of L2–L4 descend within the psoas major and form the **obturator nerve (L2–L4)** (Fig. 11.25), which descends along the medial aspect of the psoas major muscle and into the pelvis. It passes medial to the obturator internus muscle and leaves the pelvis through the obturator canal into the medial compartment of the thigh. In the thigh, the obturator nerve divides into an anterior and posterior branch that can be found on either side of the adductor brevis muscle. The anterior branch innervates the adductor brevis, adductor longus, and gracilis muscles, and it often innervates part of the pectineus muscle. It has an articular branch that is sensory to part of the coxofemoral joint and has a cutaneous branch that conveys sensation from a patch of skin on the medial thigh, just superior to the knee. The posterior branch innervates the obturator externus and adductor brevis muscles, as well as the adductor portion of the adductor magnus muscle. It has an inconstant articular branch to the posterior aspect of the knee capsule. There may be (approximately 10%) an **accessory obturator nerve (L3–L4)** that enters the medial compartment of the thigh by passing deep to the inguinal ligament near the femoral vein (Clinical Correlation 11.22).

The lumbar plexus ends with part of the L4 anterior ramus and all of the L5 anterior ramus descending into the pelvis and fusing with each other as they pass along the anterior aspect of the ala of the sacrum. This is the **lumbosacral trunk**, and it is an important contributor to the sacral plexus.

Sacral Plexus Contributions to the Lower Limb (See Fig. 11.23B and 11.26)

The lumbosacral trunk enters the pelvis and joins the anterior rami of S1 to S4 to create the sacral plexus. Nerves arising from the **posterior division** of the sacral plexus innervate the muscles of the gluteal area, posterior thigh (minor), lateral leg, anterior leg, and the dorsum of the foot. Nerves from the **anterior division** innervate muscles of the pelvis, posterior thigh (major), posterior leg, and plantar foot.

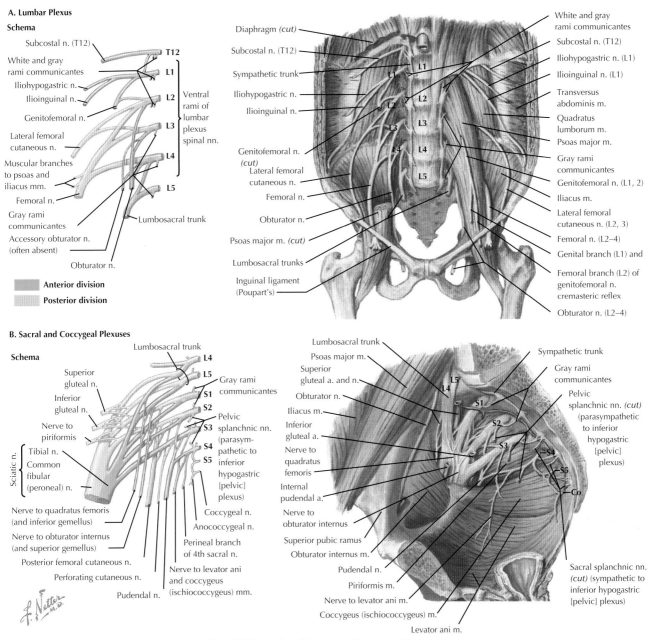

Fig. 11.23 Lumbar, Sacral, and Coccygeal Plexuses.

The **posterior division** (see Fig. 11.26A) of the sacral plexus gives off the **superior gluteal nerve (L4–S1)** that exits the greater sciatic foramen superior to the piriformis muscle. It travels in a plane between the gluteus medius and gluteus minimus muscles before reaching the tensor fascia latae muscle, which it also innervates. The superior gluteal nerve has no cutaneous branches. The superior gluteal nerve or distinct branches of S1 and S2 most commonly innervate the piriformis muscle (Iwanaga et al., 2019), but many texts list a separate nerve to the piriformis (S1–S2) as innervating this muscle. The **inferior gluteal nerve (L5–S2)** arises from the posterior division of the sacral plexus and exits through the greater sciatic foramen, running along the inferior aspect of the piriformis muscle. It sends out many branches to innervate the overlying gluteus maximus muscle and has no cutaneous branches. The final nerve from

the posterior division is the **common fibular nerve (L4–S2)**, and it will be discussed as part of the sciatic nerve (Clinical Correlation 11.23).

The sacral plexus's **anterior division** (see Fig. 11.26A) gives off small branches to pelvic muscles and the **pudendal nerve (S2–S4)** and all of its branches; it also contributes to the coccygeal plexus and anococcygeal nerves. These will be discussed in the next chapter. Pertinent to the lower limb, the anterior division of the sacral plexus gives off the **nerve to the quadratus femoris (L4–S1)**, which also innervates the inferior gemellus muscle, and the **nerve to the obturator internus (L5–S2)**, which also innervates the superior gemellus muscle. A **perforating cutaneous nerve (S2–S3)** leaves the sacral plexus, pierces the sacrotuberous ligament, and supplies the inferomedial skin of the buttocks. The **tibial nerve (L4–S3)** is the last nerve to come

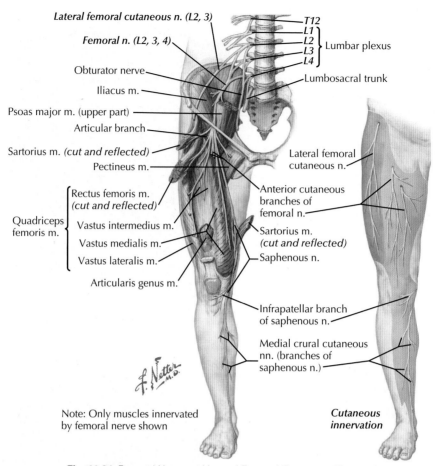

Fig. 11.24 Femoral Nerve and Lateral Femoral Cutaneous Nerves.

CLINICAL CORRELATION 11.20 Damage to Lateral Cutaneous Nerve of Thigh

Compression of the lateral cutaneous nerve of the thigh can occur when it is pinched by traction of the inguinal ligament (caused by pendulous belly fat, late pregnancy) or by direct compression around the waist (heavy tool belts or overly tight pants). This manifests as tingling or pain along the course of this nerve, sometimes covering nearly the entire lateral thigh.

from the anterior division of the sacral plexus and contributes to the sciatic nerve.

The **posterior cutaneous nerve of the thigh (S1–S3)** (see Fig. 11.26) receives contributions from the posterior and anterior divisions of the sacral plexus. It exits via the greater sciatic foramen just inferior to the piriformis muscle and descends between the gluteus maximus and deep gluteal muscles to reach the posterior thigh, where it travels posterior to the hamstring muscles, innervating the overlying skin and contributing to the S1 and S2 dermatomes of the posterior thigh and popliteal area. Near the gluteus maximus it gives off several **inferior cluneal nerves** to the inferolateral gluteal area and some perineal branches to the superior aspect on the medial thigh.

Sciatic Nerve (See Figs. 11.23 and 11.26)

The common fibular and tibial nerves arise from the posterior and anterior divisions of the sacral plexus and bundle together

to form the **sciatic nerve (L4–S3)**. Although it is considered to be the largest nerve in the body, it is a compound of its two contributors rather than a single, unified nerve. The sciatic nerve exits the pelvis through the greater sciatic foramen inferior to the piriformis muscle and descends between the gluteus maximus and deep gluteal muscles. In the posterior thigh it travels deep the to the hamstring muscles, with the tibial portion of the sciatic nerve giving off muscular branches to the semitendinosus, semimembranosus, hamstring part of the adductor magnus, and long head of the biceps femoris muscles. The common fibular portion of the sciatic nerve innervates the short head of the biceps femoris muscle. Occasionally the sciatic nerve is divided as it leaves the pelvis, with the tibial contribution to the sciatic nerve exiting inferior to the piriformis while the common fibular contribution exits superior to, or through, the piriformis.

In the distal thigh or upper part of the popliteal fossa, the **common fibular nerve** and **tibial nerve** separate from each other. Both nerves give off articular branches that innervate the knee joint capsule and structures within the joint. The common fibular nerve gives off a cutaneous branch, the **lateral sural cutaneous nerve**, that conveys sensation from the skin of the lateral knee and superior lateral leg. A similar **medial sural cutaneous nerve** comes from the tibial nerve and conveys sensation from a small patch of skin on the superior, posterior leg. Sometimes these two cutaneous nerves remain separate, but frequently, the lateral sural cutaneous nerve sends a communicating branch to its medial

CLINICAL CORRELATION 11.21 Damage to the Femoral Nerve

Damage to the femoral nerve in the pelvis or near its exit inferior to the inguinal ligament would disrupt practically all motor and sensory activity associated with the nerve. The anterior compartment muscles would undergo atrophy and flaccid paralysis, making flexion of the knee weaker (assuming the iliopsoas is unaffected despite sharing some of the same L2–L4 anterior rami that form the femoral nerve) due to loss of rectus femoris and sartorius activity. Active extension of the leg at the knee would be lost due to absence of quadriceps activity. Sensory loss over the anterior thigh as well as the anteromedial knee, leg, ankle, and heel would occur due to disruption of the anterior cutaneous branches of the femoral nerve and all branches of the saphenous nerve. A person with this injury will be unable to keep their knee extended during the entirety of stance phase and would likely need crutches to ambulate. Some patients with femoral nerve palsy use momentum at the end of swing phase to hyperextend the knee and then plant the straightened limb like a stilt during a modified stance phase.

Damage to any of the muscular branches of the femoral nerve would result in flaccid paralysis of the muscles it innervates, but the muscles innervated by other branches would be unaffected. The saphenous nerve parallels the greater saphenous vein and may be damaged if that vein is harvested for a coronary artery bypass graft. This would manifest as altered or absent sensation of the anteromedial knee, leg, ankle, and heel inferior to the lesion. The infrapatellar branch of the saphenous nerve is frequently cut during surgical procedures to the knee, leaving a patch of numb skin over the lateral knee.

CLINICAL CORRELATION 11.22 Damage to the Obturator Nerve

The obturator nerve can be damaged during pelvic fractures or compressed by tumors. Proximal injuries to the obturator nerve will cause atrophy and flaccid paralysis of the muscles of the medial compartment of the thigh. This makes adduction of the thigh against resistance much weaker and would be associated with sensory losses from a patch of skin on the medial thigh. If an accessory obturator nerve is present, some of the anterior muscles in the medial compartment (e.g., the adductor longus) would be spared. Penetrating trauma to the medial thigh could affect the anterior or posterior branch, which would result in weakness in a subset of the muscles in the medial compartment of the thigh. A person with obturator nerve palsy would likely have slight instability of the pelvis during stance phase, particularly if the patient's upper body shifts laterally during stance phase. However, instability would likely develop as the patient attempts side-to-side movements while switching from one foot to the other.

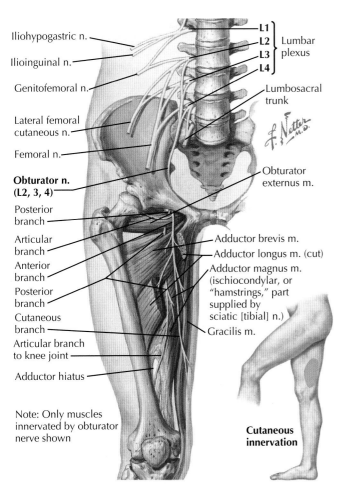

Iliohypogastric n.

Ilioinguinal n.

Genitofemoral n.

Lateral femoral cutaneous n.

Femoral n.

Obturator n. (L2, 3, 4)

Posterior branch

Articular branch

Anterior branch

Posterior branch

Cutaneous branch

Articular branch to knee joint

Adductor hiatus

L1 L2 L3 L4 Lumbar plexus

Lumbosacral trunk

Obturator externus m.

Adductor brevis m.

Adductor longus m. (cut)

Adductor magnus m. (ischiocondylar, or "hamstrings," part supplied by sciatic [tibial] n.)

Gracilis m.

Note: Only muscles innervated by obturator nerve shown

Cutaneous innervation

Fig. 11.25 Obturator Nerve.

counterpart to form the **sural nerve**, which descends along the posterior midline of the leg and innervates the skin of the posterolateral leg. Inferiorly it gives off **lateral calcaneal branches** to the heel as well as the **lateral dorsal cutaneous nerve** to the dorsum of the lateral foot, including the lateral aspect of the fifth digit.

The **common fibular nerve (L4–S2)** (Fig. 11.27) leaves the sciatic nerve and travels along the medial aspect of the biceps femoris muscle before crossing posterior to the head of the fibula and lateral to the neck of the fibula. At this point it typically splits into superficial and deep fibular nerves. The **superficial fibular nerve (L5–S2)** enters the lateral compartment of the leg and gives off muscular branches to innervate the fibularis longus and brevis muscles. It also has several cutaneous branches that supply the skin overlying the lateral compartment. In the distal leg, the superficial fibular nerve ends as it divides into two sensory branches, the **intermediate dorsal cutaneous nerve** and the **medial dorsal cutaneous nerve**. The intermediate dorsal cutaneous nerve conveys sensation from the area dorsal to metatarsals 3 to 4 and divides into **dorsal digital nerves** spanning the lateral side of digit 3 to the medial side of digit 5. The medial dorsal cutaneous nerve mediates sensation from the dorsum of the foot near metatarsals 1 to 3 and divides into dorsal digital nerves from the medial side of digit 1 to the medial side of digit 3, but excluding the space between digits 1 and 2.

The **deep fibular nerve (L4–L5)** descends in the anterior compartment of the leg, giving off muscular branches to the tibialis anterior, extensor digitorum longus, and extensor hallucis longus muscles. After crossing the talus, it splits into a **lateral branch** that innervates the extensor digitorum brevis and extensor hallucis brevis muscles. Its **medial branch** travels along the dorsum of the foot, where it splits into two **dorsal digital nerves**, covering the medial and lateral aspects of digit 1 and the medial aspect of digit 2. The branches of the superficial and deep fibular nerves innervate at least some of the joint capsules of any articulations they cross or that are crossed by the muscles they innervate.

The other major branch of the sciatic nerve is the **tibial nerve (L4–S3)** (Fig. 11.28). In the superior popliteal fossa, it is found

A. Nerves of the buttock

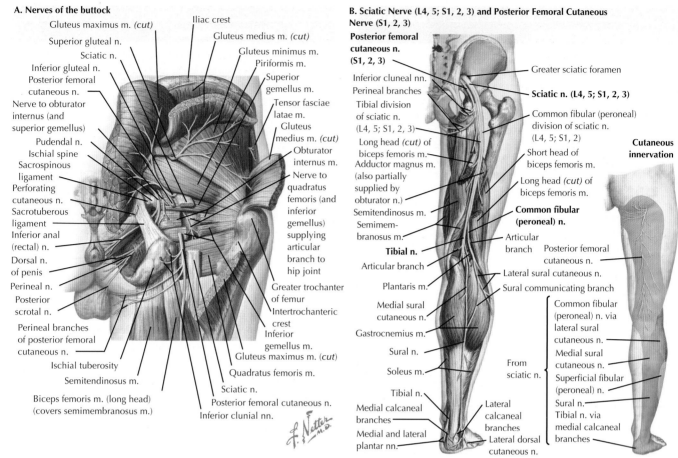

B. Sciatic Nerve (L4, 5; S1, 2, 3) and Posterior Femoral Cutaneous Nerve (S1, 2, 3)

Fig. 11.26 (A) Nerves of the buttock and (B) sciatic nerve and posterior femoral cutaneous nerve.

between the semimembranosus and biceps femoris muscles, giving off an articular branch to the knee joint. Lower, it travels posterior to the popliteus muscle and between the two heads of the gastrocnemius and deep to the tendinous arch of the soleus. Thereafter it travels in the deep posterior compartment of the leg. It gives off muscular branches to the muscles in the posterior leg, including the popliteus. The **interosseous nerve of the leg** comes off the tibial nerve and travels toward the posterior aspect of the interosseous membrane to innervate deep muscles like the tibialis posterior. In the inferior leg the tibial nerve gives off several **medial calcaneal branches** that travel along the medial aspect of the calcaneal tendon to convey sensation from the posteromedial and inferior heel region.

The tibial nerve travels posterior and inferior to the medial malleolus, covered by the flexor retinaculum. In this area it runs alongside the posterior tibial artery and inferior to the tendons of the tibialis posterior, and flexor digitorum longus, but superior to the tendon of the flexor hallucis longus. Upon reaching the planter foot, the tibial nerve terminates as the medial and lateral plantar nerves. The **medial plantar nerve (L4–L5)** (see Fig. 11.28) travels deep (superior) to the abductor hallucis and flexor digitorum brevis muscles. It innervates both of those muscles as well as the flexor hallucis brevis and first lumbrical muscles. It gives off several sensory branches to the medial skin of the plantar foot as well as **common plantar**

digital nerves that run parallel to the metatarsals before splitting into **proper plantar digital nerves** to the medial and lateral aspects of digits 1 to 3 and the medial side of digit 4. The **lateral plantar nerve (S1–S2)** (see Fig. 11.28) innervates the quadratus plantae, abductor digiti minimi, and flexor digiti minimi brevis muscles before giving off deep and superficial branches. The deep branch innervates the remaining muscles of the plantar foot, the adductor hallucis, lumbricals 2 to 4, and interossei. The superficial branch innervates the skin of the lateral plantar foot, dividing into a common plantar digital nerve and then proper plantar digital nerves to the lateral and medial aspects of digit 5 and the lateral aspect of digit 4 (Clinical Correlations 11.24 and 11.25).

Autonomic Innervation of the Lower Limb (Figs. 11.23A and 11.29)

In the upper and lower limbs, the sympathetic nervous system innervates sweat glands in the skin as well as the smooth muscle sphincters that regulate blood flow to skeletal muscle and skin. For the lower limbs, preganglionic sympathetic axons from intermediolateral cell columns of the T12–L2(3) spinal cord project their axons through anterior roots, spinal nerves, and anterior rami. These axons leave each anterior ramus as a white rami communicans to reach the sympathetic chain and distribute themselves into paravertebral ganglia between T12

Injury to the superior and inferior gluteal nerves can result from hip dislocation, needle-stick, pelvic fracture, pelvic tumors or following hip arthroplasty. If the **superior gluteal nerve** is compressed or lesioned, the gluteus medius, minimus, and tensor fascia latae will be weakened or paralyzed. This most strikingly manifests as an inability to keep the pelvis level when standing upright on one leg. To test the superior gluteal nerve, have the patient stand on one leg with the body upright. If the gluteus medius and minimus are weak, the patient will fall away from the affected side (Trendelenburg sign) because the pelvis cannot be kept level against the pull of gravity. To prevent falling while walking, an affected person will sway the upper body toward the affected side as it bears weight (Trendelenburg gait) to keep his or her center of gravity over the standing limb.

If the inferior gluteal nerve is compressed or lesioned, the gluteus maximus will be weakened or paralyzed. This does not affect normal gait because the hamstring muscles are the primary extensors of the hip during relaxed walking; however, there will be profound weakness extending the hip from a flexed position. This makes it impossible (or very difficult) to ascend the stairs with the affected foot leading; instead the patient will ascend with the opposite limb and the affected one will be brought up thereafter. There will also be difficulty standing from a seated position without a push-off from the upper limbs.

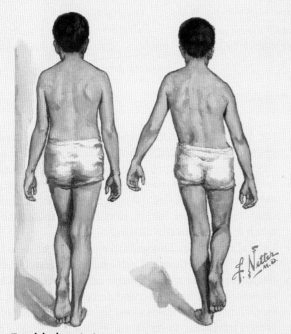

Trendelenburg test
Left: Patient demonstrates negative Trendelenburg test of normal right hip. **Right:** positive test of involved left hip. When patient is standing on the affected side, the pelvis on the opposite side drops. The trunk shifts to the left as patient attempts to decrease biomechanical stresses across involved hip and thereby maintain balance.
Fig. CC11.23 Trendelenburg Test.

and S5. Within these ganglia are the postganglionic sympathetic nerve cells with which they synapse. The postganglionic neurons send their axons through gray rami communicantes to reach the T12–S5 spinal nerves. Thereafter postganglionic axons may travel to the back via posterior rami or to the lower limb via the anterior rami of the lumbar and sacral plexus. These axons travel along all the peripheral nerves to innervate smooth muscle precapillary sphincters in skeletal muscle as well as sweat glands, arrector pili muscles, and precapillary sphincters in the skin.

THE BLOOD SUPPLY TO THE LOWER LIMB

Proximal Arteries of the Lower Limb and Thigh

The **abdominal aorta** gives off four **lumbar segmental arteries** that supply the muscles of the posterior abdominal wall, including the psoas major and minor muscles, as well as the back and the lumbar spinal nerves. The aorta bifurcates into a left and right **common iliac artery** (Figs. 11.30 and 12.25), which splits into internal and external iliac arteries. The **median sacral artery** is a small midline artery that continues along the aorta's original course across the anterior lumbar and sacral vertebrae.

The **internal iliac artery (Fig. 12.25)** descends into the true pelvis, where it splits into many arteries to the pelvic organs and several branches that leave the pelvis to reach the lower limb. Branches to the pelvic organs will not be discussed in this section, just those impacting the lower limb.

- **Obturator**: Leaves the anterior division of the internal iliac artery and travels inferior to the arcuate line. It then leaves the pelvis alongside the obturator nerve by passing through the obturator foramen to reach the medial compartment of the thigh, where it divides into anterior and posterior branches that circle the obturator foramen. The posterior branch gives off an **acetabular branch** that travels through the ligament of the head of the femur. The anterior and posterior branches anastomose with each other and the medial circumflex femoral artery. In the pelvis it provides a pubic branch to the posterior body of the pubis.
- **Iliolumbar**: Discussed in detail in the Torso chapter.
- **Lateral sacral**: Discussed in detail in the Torso chapter.
- **Superior gluteal**: Exits the greater sciatic notch superior to the piriformis muscle, parallel to the superior gluteal nerve. It divides into a superficial branch that runs between the gluteus maximus and medius muscles and a very large deep branch between the gluteus medius and minimus to reach the tensor fascia latae muscle.
- **Inferior gluteal**: Exits the greater sciatic notch inferior to the piriformis muscles, along with the inferior gluteal nerve. It supplies all muscles in the inferior gluteal region and the superior part of the posterior thigh and gives off the important **artery to the sciatic nerve.** It anastomoses with the medial circumflex femoral artery.
- **Internal pudendal**: Discussed in detail in Chapter 12.

The **external iliac artery (11.30, 11.31, 12.25)** travels along the superior edge of the arcuate line, giving off two major branches immediately before exiting the pelvis.
- **Deep circumflex iliac**: Discussed in detail in the Torso chapter.
- **Inferior epigastric**: Discussed in detail in the Torso chapter. Once the external iliac artery passes inferior to the inguinal ligament via the vascular space (medial to the iliopectineal

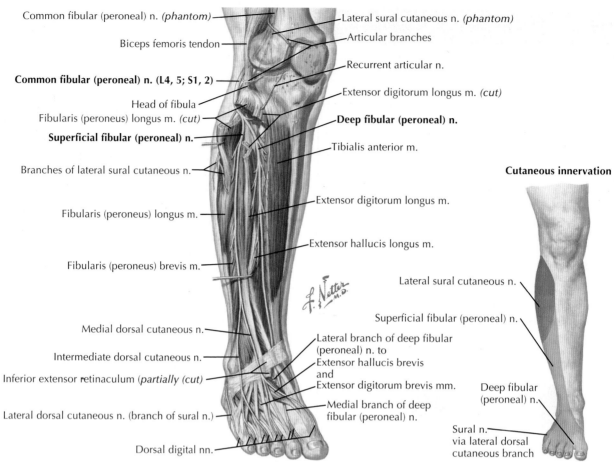

Common fibular (peroneal) n. *(phantom)*

Biceps femoris tendon

Common fibular (peroneal) n. (L4, 5; S1, 2)

Head of fibula

Fibularis (peroneus) longus m. *(cut)*

Superficial fibular (peroneal) n.

Branches of lateral sural cutaneous n.

Fibularis (peroneus) longus m.

Fibularis (peroneus) brevis m.

Medial dorsal cutaneous n.

Intermediate dorsal cutaneous n.

Inferior extensor retinaculum *(partially (cut)*

Lateral dorsal cutaneous n. (branch of sural n.)

Dorsal digital nn.

Lateral sural cutaneous n. *(phantom)*

Articular branches

Recurrent articular n.

Extensor digitorum longus m. *(cut)*

Deep fibular (peroneal) n.

Tibialis anterior m.

Extensor digitorum longus m.

Extensor hallucis longus m.

Lateral branch of deep fibular (peroneal) n. to Extensor hallucis brevis and Extensor digitorum brevis mm.

Medial branch of deep fibular (peroneal) n.

Cutaneous innervation

Lateral sural cutaneous n.

Superficial fibular (peroneal) n.

Deep fibular (peroneal) n.

Sural n. via lateral dorsal cutaneous branch

Fig. 11.27 Common Fibular (Peroneal) Nerve.

arch) it enters the anterior compartment of the thigh and becomes the femoral artery (Clinical Correlation 11.26).

The **femoral artery** (Figs. 11.31 and 11.32) is the direct continuation of the external iliac artery and is the blood supply to almost all of the lower limb, excluding the gluteal region. The femoral artery enters the anterior thigh inferior to the inguinal ligament and medial to the iliopectineal arch. It descends anterior to the pectineus and adductor longus muscles and medial to the vastus medialis and deep to the sartorius muscle. The femoral artery travels within the adductor canal, deep to the anteromedial intermuscular septum, before piercing the adductor hiatus. In the anterior thigh it gives off several important branches.

- **Superficial epigastric artery:** Discussed in detail in Chapter 12.
- **Superficial circumflex iliac artery:** Discussed in detail in Chapter 12.
- **Superficial and deep external pudendal arteries:** Discussed in detail in Chapter 12.
- **Deep artery of the thigh/profunda femoris artery:** Leaves the posterolateral side of its parent, the femoral artery, and descends anterior to the pectineus but posterior to the adductor longus. This large artery supplies blood to muscles of the medial compartment of the thigh and has several important branches of its own.
  - **Medial circumflex femoral artery:** Leaves the deep femoral artery (sometimes femoral artery) and loops around

the medial and posterior aspect of the iliopsoas tendon, giving off a superficial branch to the medial thigh muscles. Its deep branch wraps around the inferior femoral neck to provide the majority of blood to the **retinacular arteries** around the femoral neck that perfuse the femoral head. Its acetabular branch runs through the acetabular notch to perfuse nearby tissues.

- **Lateral circumflex femoral artery:** Leaves the deep femoral artery (sometimes femoral artery) and travels deep to the sartorius and rectus femoris muscles before splitting into ascending, transverse, and descending branches. The ascending branch travels along the anterior aspect of the greater trochanter to supply the gluteal muscles and contributes slightly to the retinacular arteries. The transverse and descending branches supply the gluteal and quadriceps muscles and the descending branch anastomoses with the superior lateral genicular artery near the knee.
- **Perforating arteries (see Fig. 11.32B):** Three to four arteries leave the deep artery of the thigh and pass through the adductor brevis and magnus, across the medial side of the femur to perfuse the muscles of the posterior thigh. It also provides a nutrient artery to the femur.
- **Descending genicular artery:** Leaves the femoral artery and descends deep to the sartorius. It has an **articular branch** that travels into the vastus medialis to the knee joint and anastomoses with branches of the superior medial genicular

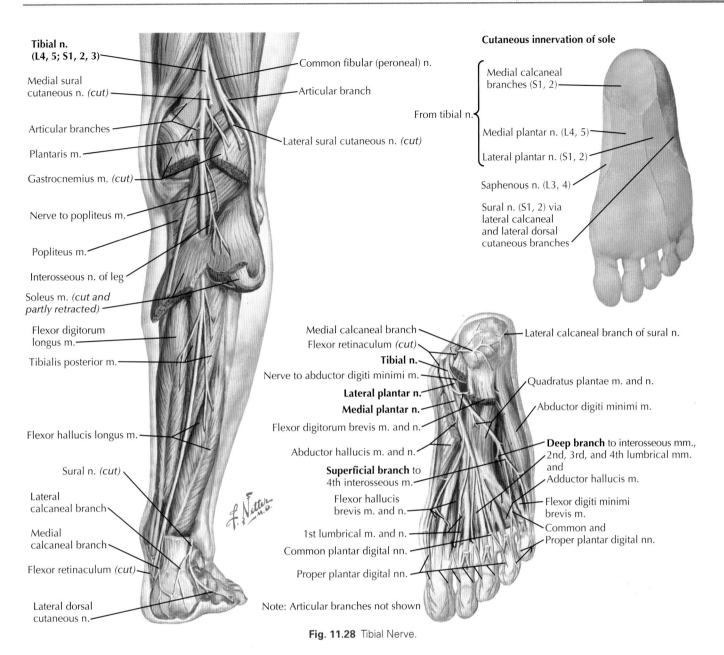

Fig. 11.28 Tibial Nerve.

artery and the patellar anastomosis. There is also a **saphenous branch** that travels alongside the saphenous nerve toward the gracilis muscle and into the medial leg to contribute to the genicular anastomosis.

Once the femoral artery passes through the adductor hiatus of the adductor magnus muscle and enters the popliteal fossa, its name changes to the popliteal artery (Clinical Correlation 11.27).

The **popliteal artery (Figs. 11.16, 11.32, and 11.33)** enters the superior aspect of the popliteal fossa between the semimembranosus and biceps femoris muscles and descends along the popliteal surface of the distal femur. Alongside the tibial nerve, it descends between the medial and lateral heads of the gastrocnemius, medial to the plantaris muscle and posterior to the popliteus muscle. In the popliteal fossa, it has several branches related to the knee, the **genicular arteries**. The superficial branches of the genicular arteries supply nearby

muscles while their deep branches contribute to an arterial network around the knee, the **genicular anastomosis**, as well as a more anterior **patellar anastomosis**. These linked anastomotic networks maintain blood flow to the leg when the knee is flexed.

- **Superior lateral genicular artery:** Leaves the popliteal artery and travels superior to the tendon of the lateral head of the gastrocnemius. It frequently anastomoses with the descending branch of the lateral circumflex femoral artery.
- **Superior medial genicular artery:** Travels superior to the tendon of the medial head of the gastrocnemius. It may anastomose directly with the saphenous branch of the descending genicular artery or into the genicular anastomosis.
- **Inferior lateral genicular artery:** Runs between the lateral head of the gastrocnemius and popliteus muscles before coursing deep to the lateral collateral ligament.

CLINICAL CORRELATION 11.24   Damage to the Branches of the Sciatic Nerve

Damage to the sciatic nerve and its branches can be very debilitating because of the many nerves that arise from it and the muscles innervated by them. We will work through how damage to individual nerves would manifest clinically and then ascend to examine how damage to more proximal branches of the sciatic nerve would create more deficits.

Isolated damage to the **deep fibular nerve** is somewhat unusual due to its protected location. If it were compressed or lesioned, the muscles of the anterior compartment of the leg and dorsum of the foot would be weakened or flaccidly paralyzed, resulting in weakness in dorsiflexion of the foot and extension of the digits. This would cause "foot drop" and dragging of the foot during the swing phase of gait. Patients with this issue often compensate by adopting a high-steppage gait with the knee lifted high so that the foot clears the ground as it swings. This issue would also make the heel strike phase of stance phase difficult, and the patient would need to "tip toe" as the foot reaches the ground. Some patients compensate for this by flicking the foot forward as the swing phase ends so that the heel can contact the ground. There would also be an isolated loss of sensation from the area between digits 1 and 2.

Injury to the **superficial fibular nerve** may occur during trauma to the lateral leg and would manifest with weakness or paralysis of the fibularis longus and brevis muscles in the lateral compartment. This would cause weakness in eversion of the foot, which might manifest in subtle ways with the patient having more frequent inversion sprains of the ankle or difficulty walking on uneven ground. There would also be loss of sensation on the anterolateral leg and the dorsum of the foot, excluding the space between digits 1 and 2.

Damage to the **common fibular nerve** is relatively common due to its superficial location and potential for compression against the head of the fibula. Trauma to it will manifest as damage to both deep and superficial fibular nerves. This will result in foot drop, weakness in eversion, and a loss of sensation from the anterolateral leg and entire dorsum of the foot. High-steppage gait and frequent inversion sprains of the foot may be noted. If the common fibular nerve is damaged proximal to the branching of the lateral sural cutaneous nerve, there will be an accompanying loss of sensation on the posterolateral leg and knee.

The **medial and lateral plantar nerves** can be injured by penetrating trauma to the foot. This can de-innervate any plantar muscles distal to the site of damage. This will cause weakness and atrophy of the affected muscles, making weight bearing during stance phase and toe-off more difficult. Any skin innervated by the affected nerves will lose sensation distal to the injury. Damage to the **tibial nerve** can occur due to penetrating trauma of the popliteal fossa or posterior leg. This will result in weakness or paralysis of muscles of the plantar foot as well as the deep and superficial posterior compartments. Note that muscles that are innervated proximal to the site of damage will be unaffected. Loss of tibial nerve function results in profound weakness during the midstance, heel-off, and toe-off stages of gait as the weakened muscles cannot plantarflex or resist dorsiflexion. Damage to the tibial nerve will also result in a loss of sensation over the majority of the plantar foot. If the nerve is damaged proximal to the branching of the medial sural cutaneous nerve, there will be an accompanying loss of sensation on the posterior leg.

Damage to the **sciatic nerve** in the mid-to-lower posterior thigh would manifest as loss of function to both common fibular and tibial nerves with sparing of the hamstring muscles in the posterior thigh itself. This would result in weakness or flaccid paralysis of all muscles of the leg and foot and loss of sensation on the anterolateral and posterior sides of the leg as well as the entire foot. Such an injury would make unassisted walking impossible, and crutches, prostheses, or a wheelchair would be required for mobility. Damage to the **sciatic nerve superior to the posterior thigh** would be absolutely debilitating because the muscles of the posterior thigh and all muscles of the leg and foot would be weak or flaccidly paralyzed. This would manifest in the same manner as aforementioned but would also include paralysis of the hamstring muscles, making flexion of the knee against resistance weak or impossible. This may occur during hip replacement or by compression of the nerve against bone during surgical procedures. Sensory losses from the posterior, lateral, and anterior leg would be noted, but the saphenous nerve on the medial side would not be affected. Depending on the exact mechanism of trauma, the posterior cutaneous nerve of the thigh may be unaffected, but its close proximity to the sciatic nerve may make it vulnerable.

CLINICAL CORRELATION 11.25   Plantar Reflex and Babinski Sign

This test is conducted by taking a blunt object and firmly (but not painfully) moving it from the lateral heel across the plantar foot toward the hallux. If the upper motor neurons to the muscles on the plantar side of the foot are intact, the patient's toes will flex in a normal **plantar reflex**. However, if there is an upper motor neuron lesion, then the toes will extend and abduct, known as the **Babinski sign**. Note that the Babinski sign is abnormal in adults but normal in infants because their upper motor neuron tracts are not fully myelinated. By 1 year of age, a normal plantar reflex is typically present.

- **Inferior medial genicular artery:** Courses medially in the area of the semimembranosus tendon to anastomose directly with the saphenous branch of the descending genicular artery or via the genicular anastomosis.
- **Middle genicular artery:** This vessel does not contribute significantly to the genicular anastomosis but pierces the posterior aspect of the joint capsule of the knee through a gap in the oblique popliteal ligament to supply the structures within the joint.
- **Sural arteries:** Leave the medial and lateral sides of the popliteal artery and perfuse the triceps surae muscles: the gastrocnemius, plantaris, and soleus.

The popliteal artery then travels through the tendinous arch of the soleus and divides to become the anterior and posterior tibial arteries (Clinical Correlation 11.28).

Arteries of the Leg and Foot

The **anterior tibial artery** (see Figs. 11.16, 11.17, 11.19, 11.32B, and 11.33) travels through the interosseous membrane to reach that anterior compartment of the leg. It is joined by the deep fibular nerve and supplies blood to the muscles of the compartment as it descends along the lateral aspect of the tibialis anterior muscle. It also gives off perforating branches that reach the lateral compartment. It has two proximal branches and two distal branches.

- **Posterior tibial recurrent artery:** Leaves the anterior tibial artery just before it travels through the interosseous membrane and runs superiorly, deep to the popliteus muscle.
- **Anterior tibial recurrent artery:** Leaves the anterior tibial artery just after it travels through the interosseous membrane and ascends lateral to the patellar ligament to contribute to the patellar anastomosis.
- **Anterior medial malleolar artery:** Leaves the distal anterior tibial artery and contributes to an arterial network across the medial malleolus.

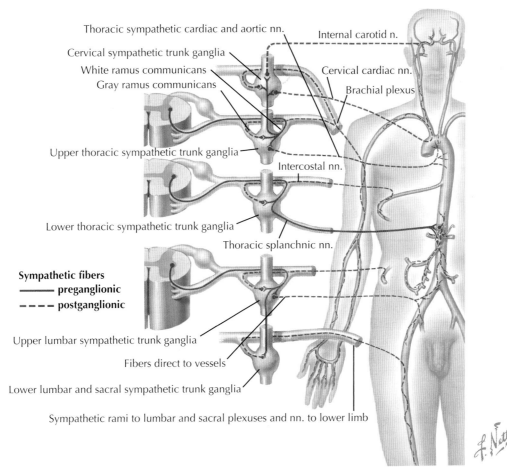

Thoracic sympathetic cardiac and aortic nn.

Internal carotid n.

Cervical sympathetic trunk ganglia

White ramus communicans

Cervical cardiac nn.

Gray ramus communicans

Brachial plexus

Upper thoracic sympathetic trunk ganglia

Intercostal nn.

Lower thoracic sympathetic trunk ganglia

Thoracic splanchnic nn.

Sympathetic fibers
—— preganglionic
- - - postganglionic

Upper lumbar sympathetic trunk ganglia

Fibers direct to vessels

Lower lumbar and sacral sympathetic trunk ganglia

Sympathetic rami to lumbar and sacral plexuses and nn. to lower limb

Fig. 11.29 Innervation of Blood Vessels: Schema.

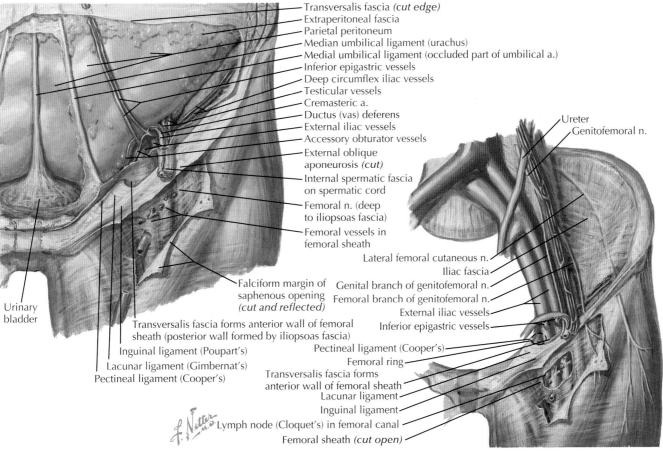

Transversalis fascia *(cut edge)*
Extraperitoneal fascia
Parietal peritoneum
Median umbilical ligament (urachus)
Medial umbilical ligament (occluded part of umbilical a.)
Inferior epigastric vessels
Deep circumflex iliac vessels
Testicular vessels
Cremasteric a.
Ductus (vas) deferens
External iliac vessels
Accessory obturator vessels
External oblique aponeurosis *(cut)*
Internal spermatic fascia on spermatic cord
Femoral n. (deep to iliopsoas fascia)
Femoral vessels in femoral sheath

Ureter
Genitofemoral n.

Lateral femoral cutaneous n.
Iliac fascia
Genital branch of genitofemoral n.
Femoral branch of genitofemoral n.
External iliac vessels
Inferior epigastric vessels

Urinary bladder

Falciform margin of saphenous opening *(cut and reflected)*

Transversalis fascia forms anterior wall of femoral sheath (posterior wall formed by iliopsoas fascia)

Inguinal ligament (Poupart's)

Lacunar ligament (Gimbernat's)

Pectineal ligament (Cooper's)

Pectineal ligament (Cooper's)
Femoral ring
Transversalis fascia forms anterior wall of femoral sheath
Lacunar ligament
Inguinal ligament
Lymph node (Cloquet's) in femoral canal
Femoral sheath *(cut open)*

Fig. 11.30 Femoral Sheath and Inguinal Canal.

CLINICAL CORRELATION 11.26
Accessory Obturator Artery

The obturator artery typically arises from the anterior division of the internal iliac artery. However, an accessory obturator artery may branch from either the inferior epigastric or external iliac arteries and descend along the lacunar ligament and posterior pubis to reach the obturator foramen. Sometimes the entire obturator artery arises from the inferior epigastric or external iliac artery. The high incidence of this variation (approximately 20%–30%) and its position make it important to consider when dealing with femoral hernias or pelvic fractures. The vascular ring formed by the internal iliac, obturator, accessory obturator, and external iliac arteries has the charming name, **corona mortis**, or crown of death.

- **Anterior lateral malleolar artery:** Leaves the distal anterior tibial artery and anastomoses with the perforating branch of the fibular artery to form a lateral malleolar network.

As the anterior tibial artery crosses the talus, it becomes the **dorsalis pedis artery/dorsal artery of the foot**, which travels lateral to the tendon of the extensor hallucis longus as far as the base of the first metatarsal. This artery gives off several branches across the dorsum of the foot.

- **Medial tarsal arteries:** Branch off the dorsalis pedis across the navicular and medial cuneiform bones to anastomose with medial malleolar arteries.

- **Lateral tarsal artery:** Runs laterally across the navicular and lateral cuneiform bones to supply the muscles of the dorsum of the foot.
- **Arcuate artery:** Formed by an additional anastomotic connection between the lateral tarsal and dorsalis pedis arteries. It runs along the bases of metatarsals 2 to 4.
- **Dorsal metatarsal arteries:** Come off the dorsalis pedis or arcuate arteries to travel between metatarsal bones and give off **dorsal digital arteries** that provide blood to the dorsal side of each digit.
  - The first dorsal metatarsal artery (dorsalis pedis) branches into dorsal digital arteries on the medial and lateral sides of digit 1 and the medial side of digit 2.
  - The second dorsal metatarsal artery (arcuate artery) branches into dorsal digital arteries on the lateral side of digit 2 and medial side of digit 3.
  - The third dorsal metatarsal artery (arcuate artery) branches into dorsal digital arteries on the lateral side of digit 3 and medial side of digit 4.
  - The fourth dorsal metatarsal artery (arcuate artery) branches into dorsal digital arteries on the lateral side of digit 4 and the medial and lateral sides of digit 5.
- **Deep plantar artery:** Terminal branch of the dorsalis pedis artery, it travels inferiorly (deep) between metatarsals 1 and 2, just proximal to the first dorsal interosseous muscle. It

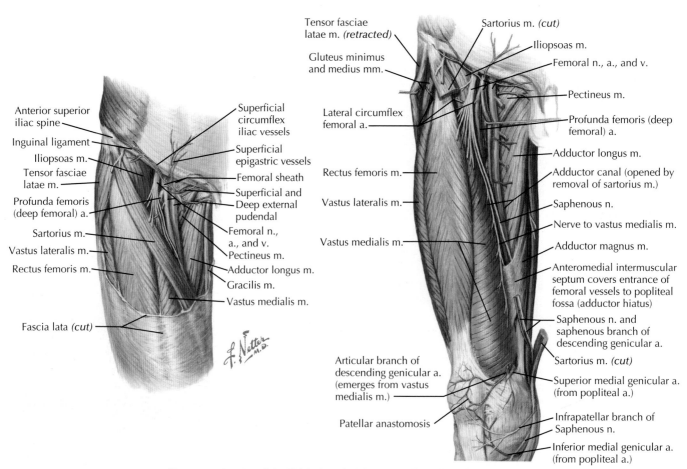

Fig. 11.31 Arteries of the Thigh: Anterior Views with Superficial Dissections.

A. Anterior view: deep dissection

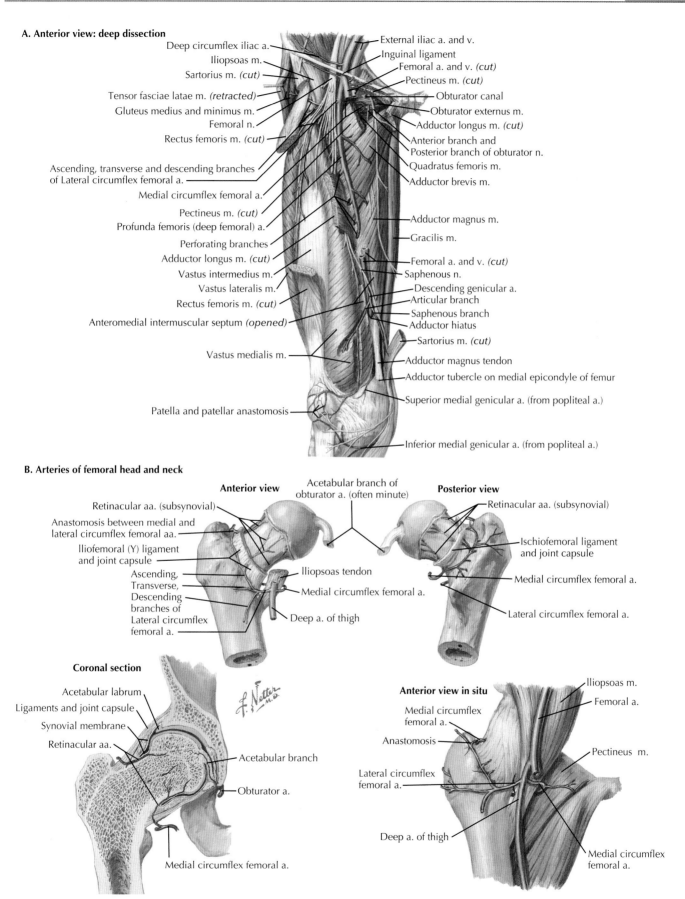

Deep circumflex iliac a.
Iliopsoas m.
Sartorius m. *(cut)*
Tensor fasciae latae m. *(retracted)*
Gluteus medius and minimus m.
Femoral n.
Rectus femoris m. *(cut)*
Ascending, transverse and descending branches of Lateral circumflex femoral a.
Medial circumflex femoral a.
Pectineus m. *(cut)*
Profunda femoris (deep femoral) a.
Perforating branches
Adductor longus m. *(cut)*
Vastus intermedius m.
Vastus lateralis m.
Rectus femoris m. *(cut)*
Anteromedial intermuscular septum *(opened)*
Vastus medialis m.
Patella and patellar anastomosis

External iliac a. and v.
Inguinal ligament
Femoral a. and v. *(cut)*
Pectineus m. *(cut)*
Obturator canal
Obturator externus m.
Adductor longus m. *(cut)*
Anterior branch and Posterior branch of obturator n.
Quadratus femoris m.
Adductor brevis m.
Adductor magnus m.
Gracilis m.
Femoral a. and v. *(cut)*
Saphenous n.
Descending genicular a.
Articular branch
Saphenous branch
Adductor hiatus
Sartorius m. *(cut)*
Adductor magnus tendon
Adductor tubercle on medial epicondyle of femur
Superior medial genicular a. (from popliteal a.)
Inferior medial genicular a. (from popliteal a.)

B. Arteries of femoral head and neck

Anterior view
Acetabular branch of obturator a. (often minute)
Posterior view

Retinacular aa. (subsynovial)
Anastomosis between medial and lateral circumflex femoral aa.
Iliofemoral (Y) ligament and joint capsule
Ascending, Transverse, Descending branches of Lateral circumflex femoral a.
Iliopsoas tendon
Medial circumflex femoral a.
Deep a. of thigh

Retinacular aa. (subsynovial)
Ischiofemoral ligament and joint capsule
Medial circumflex femoral a.
Lateral circumflex femoral a.

Coronal section
Acetabular labrum
Ligaments and joint capsule
Synovial membrane
Retinacular aa.
Acetabular branch
Obturator a.
Medial circumflex femoral a.

Anterior view in situ
Iliopsoas m.
Femoral a.
Medial circumflex femoral a.
Anastomosis
Lateral circumflex femoral a.
Pectineus m.
Deep a. of thigh
Medial circumflex femoral a.

Fig. 11.32 (A) Arteries of the thigh: anterior view with deep dissection and schema. (B) Arteries of the femoral head and neck.

anastomoses with the deep plantar arch (primarily from the lateral plantar artery) in the deep plantar foot.

The **posterior tibial artery** (see Figs. 11.16, 11.20, and 11.33) continues inferiorly from the popliteal artery into the deep posterior compartment of the leg, descending between the flexor digitorum longus and tibialis posterior muscles. The posterior tibial artery supplies the muscles of the posterior compartment, gives off a nutrient artery to the tibia, and has several other important branches.

- **Circumflex fibular branch:** Arises very proximally from the posterior tibial or anterior tibial artery and courses laterally around the neck of the fibula and joins the inferior lateral genicular artery and genicular anastomosis.

CLINICAL CORRELATION 11.27
Avascular Necrosis of the Femoral Head

As mentioned briefly in Chapter 5, disruption of the medial circumflex femoral artery will deprive the femoral head of its blood supply, causing avascular necrosis. This can result from a fracture of the proximal femur or disruption of the vessel itself. While there are other arteries in the area (acetabular branch of the obturator and lateral circumflex femoral), they rarely provide enough blood to the head of the femur to compensate for loss of the medial circumflex femoral artery. The affected bone is often painful and may eventually collapse.

- **Fibular artery:** Leaves the posterior tibial artery laterally and descends along (or through) the flexor hallucis longus muscle, giving off a nutrient artery to the fibula as well as daughter arteries.
  - **Posterior lateral malleolar branch:** Crosses the lateral side of the lateral malleolus and anastomoses with corresponding anterior branches from the anterior tibial and perforating branch of the fibular arteries.
  - **Communicating branch:** Crosses the distal tibia medially to anastomose with distal posterior tibial artery.
  - **Perforating branch:** Passes through the distal interosseous membrane to run across the anterior surface of the lateral malleolus and contribute to the lateral malleolar network.
  - **Lateral calcaneal branch:** Crosses inferior to the attachment site of the calcaneal tendon. It contributes to the calcaneal anastomosis on the posterior and inferior aspect of the calcaneal tuberosity.
- **Posterior medial malleolar branches:** Cross the medial malleolus to anastomose with anterior branches from the anterior tibial artery to create a medial malleolar network of arteries.
- **Medial calcaneal branches:** Pass through the flexor retinaculum and contribute to the calcaneal anastomosis on the posterior and inferior aspect of the calcaneal tuberosity.

The tibial artery leaves the posterior leg by crossing inferior to the medial malleolus, deep to the flexor retinaculum. In this location it passes inferior to the tendons of the tibialis posterior

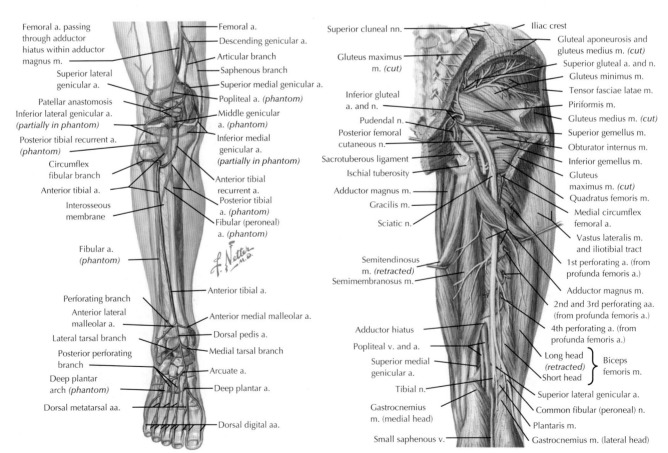

Fig. 11.33 Arteries of the Knee, Leg, and Foot.

CLINICAL CORRELATION 11.28 Popliteal Aneurysm and Hemorrhage

Aneurysm of the popliteal artery was once fairly common due to the repeated flexion/extension of the knee experienced during horseback riding. If the popliteal artery is weakened and expands, it can create a pulsatile mass in the popliteal fossa that expands posteriorly, putting pressure on the tibial nerve. This aneurysm can be ligated and removed because the genicular anastomosis is frequently sufficient to bypass the dysfunctional segment. The popliteal artery passes immediately posterior to the distal femur, making it vulnerable during trauma to the femur or during total knee replacement surgeries. Hemorrhage from the popliteal artery must be controlled quickly and can result in necrosis of the leg and foot if they are deprived of blood for too long a period.

CLINICAL CORRELATION 11.29 Anastomoses Around the Knee

There are several routes that arterial blood can follow around the knee (see Figs. 11.32 and 11.33). This is particularly important when the knee is in full flexion and the popliteal artery is bent. Four of the genicular arteries (superior lateral, superior medial, inferior lateral, inferior medial) create the genicular anastomosis around the knee. The patellar anastomosis is continuous with the genicular anastomosis and refers specifically to the arterial network on the anterior patella.

Contributing arteries that originate superior to the knee
- Descending branch of lateral circumflex femoral artery to the superior lateral genicular artery
- Articular branch of descending genicular artery to the superior medial genicular artery and patellar anastomosis
- Saphenous branch of descending genicular artery to the inferior medial genicular artery

Contributing arteries that originate inferior to the knee
- Anterior tibial artery
  - Posterior tibial recurrent artery to the inferior genicular arteries
  - Anterior tibial recurrent artery to the patellar anastomosis
- Posterior tibial artery
  - Circumflex fibular branch to the inferior lateral genicular artery

If the popliteal artery is damaged, ligated, or compressed for a prolonged period, one or more of these channels may enlarge to carry blood past the blockage to perfuse the leg and foot.

CLINICAL CORRELATION 11.30 Locating Pulses in the Lower Limb

There are a few typical sites at which the pulse can be checked in each of the lower limbs (Fig. 5.2). Weaker pulses in the lower limb when compared with those of the upper limbs or neck may signify narrowing of the aorta or iliac arteries. Increased pressure in a compartment of the lower limb that puts pressure on an artery traveling through it can also weaken pulses distal to the compartment.
- Femoral artery: The pulse can be felt as the artery is compressed just inferior to the inguinal ligament within the femoral triangle. Diminished pulses here may indicate problems with the aorta or iliac arteries. Excessive adipose tissue in the area may create difficulties in palpating it.
- Popliteal artery: This pulse can be palpated but is more difficult due to the deep position of the artery within the popliteal fossa. Diminished pulses here compared with the femoral pulse may indicate occlusion of the vessel in the anterior compartment of the thigh or as it crosses through the adductor canal.
- Posterior tibial artery: Can be palpated by compressing the vessel against the medial malleolus and tarsal bones. Diminished pulse here compared with the popliteal and dorsalis pedis pulses may indicate excessive pressure or compartment syndrome in the posterior leg.
- Dorsalis pedis artery: Palpable on the anterior aspect of the ankle/dorsum of the foot between the tibialis anterior and extensor hallucis longus tendons. Diminished pulse here compared with popliteal and posterior tibial pulses may indicate excessive pressure or compartment syndrome of the anterior leg.

and 3, 3 and 4, and 4 and 5 to reach the dorsal metatarsal arteries on the opposite side.
- **Plantar metatarsal arteries:** Stretch anteriorly from the deep plantar arch and run along the plantar interosseous muscles. Once they cross deep to the deep transverse metatarsal ligament, they are referred to as **common plantar digital arteries**, and these in turn will give off **plantar digital arteries proper** to the digits themselves.
- **Medial plantar artery** (see Fig. 11.20): Runs alongside the medial plantar nerve before splitting into a superficial and deep branch to supply muscles and skin of the medial, plantar foot.
  - **Superficial branch:** Travels along the medial surface of the foot to reach the medial side of the hallux and contribute to the **plantar digital artery proper.**
  - **Deep branch:** Runs along the lateral head of the flexor hallucis brevis to contribute to the common plantar digital artery between the heads of metatarsals 1 and 2 (Clinical Correlations 11.29–11.31).

Deep Veins of the Lower Limbs (Fig. 11.34)

In the following section, only the largest deep veins of the lower limb will be mentioned by name, but any artery that was listed previously will almost certainly have an accompanying vein that travels alongside it and drains into one of the larger deep veins. However, venous pathways are far more variable than arterial pathways, and there are frequently multiple veins running along a large artery, known as **venae comitantes** (accompanying veins). Veins of the lower limb tend to have valves in their lumen to prevent the retrograde flow of venous blood, which is particularly important because venous return from these limbs frequently needs to operate against gravity.

and flexor digitorum longus and superior to the tibial nerve and tendon of the flexor hallucis longus. Deep to the abductor hallucis muscle it splits into the lateral and medial plantar arteries.
- **Lateral plantar artery** (see Fig. 11.20): Travels with the lateral plantar nerve between flexor digitorum brevis and quadratus plantae muscles. It supplies blood to nearby muscles and skin as it continues laterally, terminating as a **plantar digital artery proper** on the lateral fifth digit.
  - **Deep branch:** This large branch of the lateral plantar artery dives deep to the quadratus plantae and oblique head of the adductor hallucis muscles. Thereafter it stretches medially as the **deep plantar arch**, which anastomoses with the deep plantar artery, a terminal branch of the dorsalis pedis artery. **Posterior perforating branches**: small vessels that pass through the spaces between metatarsals 2

CLINICAL CORRELATION 11.31   **Compartment Syndromes**

The compartments of the lower limb are encased in tough, inelastic fascial sheets that both surround the muscles of the limb and fuse to the underlying bone. When the muscles within the compartments contract, they increase the pressure in the compartment. This is helpful in propelling venous blood and lymphatic fluid superiorly since muscular contractions will propel the blood proximally and valves in their walls prevent retrograde flow. However, excessive pressure in a compartment can occur due to acute overuse, bone fracture, and other reasons (e.g., snakebite). The excessive pressure in the compartment is painful and limits the amount of active contraction or passive stretch that muscles in the compartment can tolerate. If the pressure meets or exceeds diastolic blood pressure, it will compromise blood return through the compartment. If it climbs higher and exceeds systolic blood pressure, it will prevent arterial blood from reaching the tissues of the compartment, including the small arteries supplying peripheral nerves. In general, an intracompartmental pressure at or greater than 30 mm Hg is considered a good benchmark to diagnose acute compartment syndrome. While this can occur in any compartment, the compartments of the leg are frequently affected.

- Anterior compartment: Extreme pain will be evident during attempted dorsiflexion (muscles contract) or plantarflexion (muscles stretched). Decreased

dorsalis pedis pulse may be evident due to compression of anterior tibial artery, as well as loss of sensation from the space between digits 1 and 2 caused by compression of the deep fibular nerve.
- Lateral compartment: Pain will be evident as the foot is everted (contract) or inverted (stretched).
- Superficial and deep posterior compartments: Extreme pain will be evident during attempted plantarflexion (contract) or dorsiflexion (stretched). Decreased tibialis posterior pulse at the medial malleolus may be evident due to compression of the artery, as well as loss of motor activity and sensation from the plantar foot caused by compression of the tibial nerve in the leg.

Treatment of compartment syndrome is straightforward. The fascia surrounding the compartment is sliced open (fasciotomy) so that the muscle can expand and relieve the pressure, which allows blood to flow. Once swelling has subsided, the compartment and overlying skin are sutured. The anterior and lateral compartments are opened with an incision on the anterolateral leg to ensure that both compartments have been exposed. The posterior compartments are reached via an incision along the medial tibia.

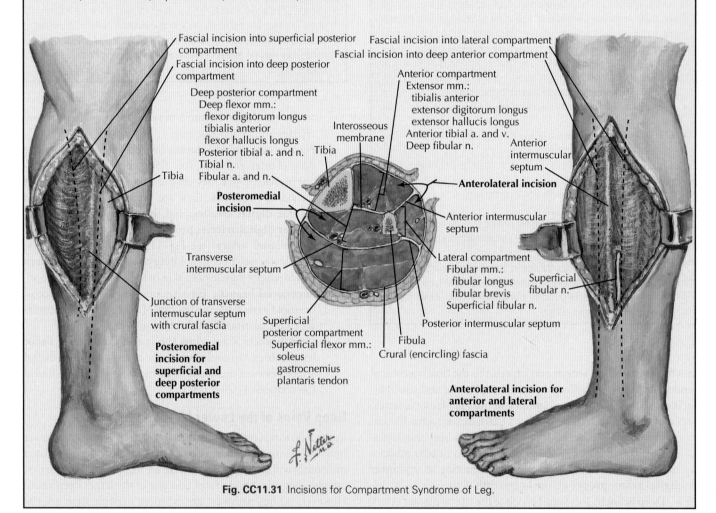

Fig. CC11.31 Incisions for Compartment Syndrome of Leg.

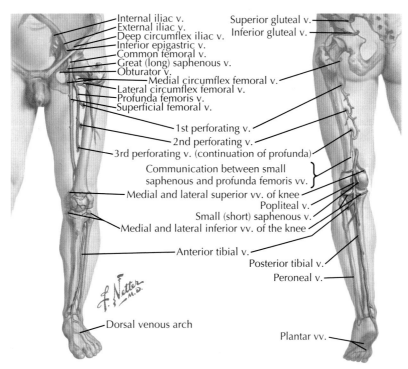

Fig. 11.34 Deep Veins of the Lower Extremity.

In the plantar foot, **plantar digital veins** drain proximally into **plantar metatarsal veins**, reaching a **plantar venous arch** that runs alongside the deep plantar arterial arch. Venous blood will then drain to the **medial or lateral plantar veins**, which come together to form the **posterior tibial vein**. The **fibular vein** will drain to the posterior tibial vein, which unites with the **anterior tibial vein** (from the anterior compartment of the leg) to form the **popliteal vein**. The popliteal vein collects blood from the **genicular veins** that surround the knee as well as large **sural veins** from the muscles of the superficial posterior compartment of the leg. It travels superiorly through the adductor hiatus and enters the anterior thigh as the **femoral vein**. Venous blood from the posterior compartment of the thigh drains anteriorly via **perforating veins** to the **deep femoral vein**, which also receives blood from the **medial and lateral circumflex femoral veins**. The deep femoral vein then joins the femoral vein. The femoral vein ascends into the abdomen by passing inferior to the inguinal ligament and medial to the femoral artery. Once inside the pelvis it is called the **external iliac vein**.

The **internal iliac vein** receives venous blood from the genitalia and internal pelvic structures. In addition, the **superior gluteal, inferior gluteal, lateral sacral**, and **obturator veins** drain to the internal iliac vein. The internal and external iliac veins fuse to create the common iliac vein. The common iliac veins also receive some blood from the iliolumbar and (on the left side) the median sacral veins before the right and left common iliac veins join to become the **inferior vena cava**.

Superficial Veins of the Lower Limb (Fig. 11.35)

In the lower limb, there are some subcutaneous veins of special significance. They do not have an arterial partner and can often be visualized or seen protruding from the skin in people with low body fat. **Dorsal digital veins** collect blood from the digits and

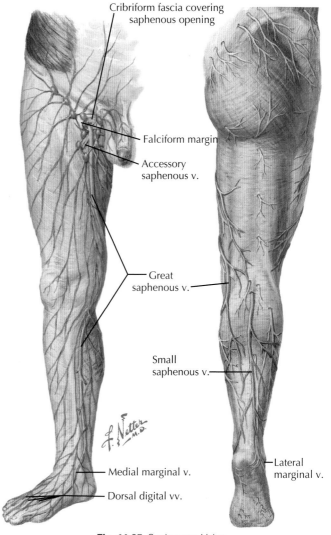

Fig. 11.35 Saphenous Veins.

CLINICAL CORRELATION 11.32 Varicose Veins

Varicosities occur when the valves inside veins become incompetent and are no longer able to close, causing blood to become static within the vessel. Increased pressure in the veins of the pelvis or reversal of blood flow from the deep veins of the lower limb into the superficial veins may predispose patients to varicosities. The increased volume of blood in varicose veins may cause them to become swollen and tortuous. This may cause **thrombophlebitis**, inflammation, and pain in the vein and surrounding tissues. Varicosities of the medial leg and thigh may be associated with dilation of the superior aspect of the greater saphenous vein, a **saphenous varix**, which results in a bulge near the femoral triangle that can be confused with lymph node enlargement or a femoral hernia.

drain to **dorsal metatarsal veins** that then drain into a large **dorsal venous arch of the foot**. The lateral side of this arch is the lateral **marginal vein**, which carries venous blood from the superficial tissues on the lateral dorsum of the foot into the **small saphenous vein**, located superficial to the crural fascia of the leg and receives many veins from the posterior leg. It pierces the fascia over the popliteal fossa to dive deep and fuse with the popliteal vein.

The medial side of the dorsal venous arch of the foot ends as the **medial marginal vein**, which continues superiorly along the medial aspect of the leg, knee, and thigh as the massive **greater saphenous vein**. Many veins in the superficial tissues of the lower limb drain to the greater saphenous vein, a particularly large **accessory saphenous vein** drains the anterior lateral thigh, sometimes extending as far inferiorly as the lateral leg. Just inferior to the inguinal ligament, the greater saphenous vein and some of its tributaries, such as the **external pudendal, superficial circumflex iliac, superficial epigastric**, pierce a flimsy **cribriform fascia** that overlies a gap in the fascia lata, the **saphenous opening**, and join the femoral vein. The lateral side of the saphenous opening is the strong **falciform margin**, with **superior and inferior horns** extending onto their respective sides of the saphenous opening (Clinical Correlations 11.32–11.34).

LYMPHATIC DRAINAGE OF THE LOWER LIMB (FIG. 11.36)

There are deep lymphatic vessels that run alongside the arteries and veins of the foot, leg, thigh, and gluteal region. Superficial lymphatic vessels of the plantar foot dive deep to meet the deep lymphatic vessels around the deep plantar arch. Lymphatic fluid from the digits drains through small superficial lymphatic vessels toward the dorsum of the foot. These small vessels enlarge as they travel proximally and fuse with one another. As the vessels get larger, they tend to run parallel to the superficial veins such as the small saphenous and greater saphenous veins. Lymphatic vessels from the lateral dorsum of the foot and posterior leg tend to run alongside the small saphenous vein, carrying lymphatic fluid to **superficial** and **deep popliteal lymph nodes** that are located in the popliteal fossa. Some lymph nodes (anterior tibial, posterior tibial, fibular nodes) may be named for the nearby vessels in the popliteal fossa. After passing through the popliteal lymph nodes, lymphatic fluid joins the deep lymphatics alongside the popliteal and femoral vessels.

Lymphatic fluid and vessels from the medial aspect of the foot, anterior leg, and anterior thigh tend to run parallel to the greater saphenous vein and ascend toward the inguinal ligament.

CLINICAL CORRELATION 11.33 Deep Venous Thromboses and Embolism

Deep venous thromboses are clots that occur when venous blood becomes static within a large vein, commonly in the lower limbs. Clots form more easily in slow-moving blood, and these can block the lumen of the vessel. This impedes blood flow and causes swelling, warmth, and pain in the affected limb distal to the thrombus. This can happen when a person sits still for a prolonged time during travel, after a surgical procedure, following a video game or entertainment binge or due to incompetent valves or loose fascia surrounding a compartment prevents blood return. More seriously, the clot or parts of the clot may break loose and travel proximally. These traveling clots are called **emboli** (sing: embolus), and in systemic veins they are carried to the right side of the heart and into branches of the pulmonary arteries. Small **pulmonary emboli** can block branches of the pulmonary arteries, causing pain and shortness of breath. Large pulmonary emboli can block one or both pulmonary arteries, causing sudden death.

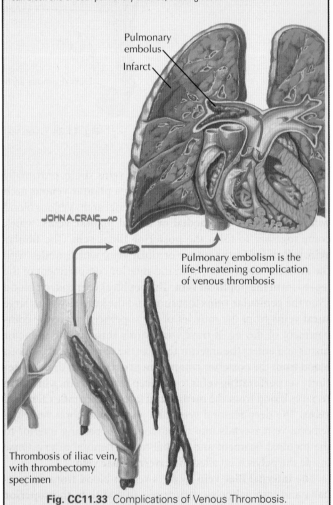

Fig. CC11.33 Complications of Venous Thrombosis.

CLINICAL CORRELATION 11.34 Autograft of the Greater Saphenous Vein

Because of its large size and accessible position, the greater saphenous vein is frequently harvested from the medial thigh and leg as an autograft to bypass blocked vessels or create peripheral anastomoses. Loss of a greater saphenous vein does not typically cause major problems and increases the amount of blood traveling in the deep veins of the lower limb. Due to the valves in its lumen, the vein must be reversed prior to implantation so that the flow of blood pushes the valves against the walls of the vessel, rather than being impeded by them.

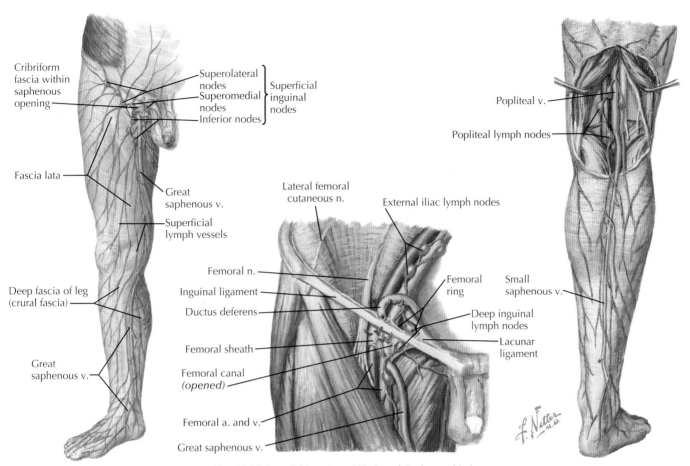

Fig. 11.36 Lymph Vessels and Nodes of the Lower Limb.

In the medial groin, this fluid encounters the **superficial inguinal nodes**. The **inferior group** of superficial inguinal lymph nodes sits along the proximal greater saphenous vein, a **superomedial group** is located superior to the saphenous opening, and a **superolateral group** extends laterally along the inguinal ligament. The lymphatic fluid from these nodes overwhelmingly tends to drain through the saphenous opening, where it encounters **deep inguinal lymph nodes** medial to the femoral vein. The most proximal node in this group is located immediately deep to the inguinal ligament and is known as **Cloquet node**. Enlargement of this node may be a sign of infection or cancer of the lower limb or pelvic viscera. Thereafter the lymphatic fluid will enter the pelvis, passing through **external iliac** and **common iliac lymph nodes**.

There are **inferior gluteal and superior gluteal lymph nodes** sitting near the base of the corresponding arteries. These drain to **internal iliac lymph nodes**. Internal iliac lymph nodes also receive lymphatic fluid from the pelvic organs and passes it superiorly to the common iliac lymph nodes. Thereafter the lymphatic fluid moves superiorly and encounters **preaortic** and **lumbar lymph nodes** before reaching the **cisterna chyli** in the upper lumbar region. Lymphatic fluid from both lower limbs and the abdominopelvic organs tends to collect in the cisterna chyli before passing up the **thoracic duct**, a large lymph vessel that passes through the posterior aspect of the diaphragm into the posterior mediastinum of the thorax, and finally arches posterior to the left internal jugular vein to empty into the **left subclavian vein**. Thereafter the lymphatic fluid becomes part of the blood plasma (Clinical Correlation 11.35).

CLINICAL CORRELATION 11.35
Peripheral Edema

An accumulation of intercellular fluid can cause peripheral edema (swelling) of the limbs, particularly the lower limbs due to the difficulty moving the fluid superiorly against gravity. It can occur due to disruption of lymphatic drainage (**lymphedema**), but cardiovascular conditions that cause the backup of blood into the systemic veins (e.g., congestive heart failure) can also result in peripheral edema. One common test is to push a fingertip into the anterior leg for several seconds. If the impression remains for a significant time after the finger is removed, it is referred to as **pitting edema**.

NEUROVASCULAR BUNDLES

There are several locations in the lower limb where large vessels run alongside nerves. Injuries in these areas will tend to damage the vessels and the nerves together, causing hemorrhage and de-innervation injuries. Hemorrhage from veins will tend to seep out, although the volume of blood in these veins can be massive. Hemorrhage involving arteries will have a pulsatile nature, spurting in time with the pulse. Although the hemorrhage may be immediately life-threatening, the neurologic deficits may take much longer to rehabilitate, if possible.

Gluteal Region and Pelvis

- **Superior gluteal nerve and vessels:** This bundle exits the greater sciatic foramen superior to the piriformis muscle.

Thereafter the superior gluteal vessels (deep branch) and nerve travel alongside each other in the plane between the gluteus medius and minimus muscles. Injury to this bundle would result in hemorrhage and weakness keeping the pelvis level when standing on the ipsilateral leg and abducting the thigh at the hip.

- **Inferior gluteal nerve and vessels:** This bundle exits the greater sciatic foramen inferior to the piriformis muscle alongside the sciatic, posterior femoral cutaneous, and pudendal nerves. The bundle quickly ceases to exist as the inferior gluteal nerve moves superficially to reach the gluteus maximus. Injury to this bundle would result in hemorrhage and weakness in extending the hip from a flexed position, such as ascending the stairs or standing up when seated.
- **Obturator nerve and vessels:** This bundle converges in the lateral pelvis and passes through the obturator foramen to reach the medial thigh. The vessels do not travel far in the compartment, but the nerve continues inferiorly, splitting in an anterior and medial branch. Injury to this bundle in the pelvis or near the pubis would result in hemorrhage and weakness keeping the pelvis level and adducting the thigh at the hip.

Thigh

- **Femoral nerve and vessels:** From medial to lateral, the femoral vein, artery, and nerve (V.A.N.) are located in the femoral triangle of the anterior thigh. This bundle exists only briefly before the femoral nerve arborizes into many motor and sensory branches and the femoral vessels descend deep to the sartorius muscle. Trauma to this bundle near the inguinal ligament would cause massive arterial and venous hemorrhage made worse by retraction of the lacerated vessels into the abdomen. There would also be profound weakness of the anterior thigh muscles, causing an inability to extend the knee or resist flexion of the joint, as well as loss of sensation from the anterior thigh, medial knee, leg, ankle, and heel.
- **Saphenous nerve, saphenous branch of descending genicular artery, and greater saphenous vein:** The greater saphenous vein is present on the medial side of the ankle, leg, and thigh. Around the knee it is joined by the saphenous branch of the descending genicular artery, a branch off the femoral artery, as well as the saphenous nerve, a cutaneous branch of the femoral nerve. This bundle is vulnerable when the greater saphenous vein is harvested as a vascular autograft. Overly enthusiastic removal at or below the knee may traumatize the saphenous branch of the descending genicular artery, causing arterial hemorrhage, or the saphenous nerve, resulting in loss of sensation along the medial leg, ankle, and heel.
- **Tibial nerve and popliteal vessels:** This is a relatively loose bundle, with the vessels located deep in the popliteal fossa and the tibial nerve more superficially. Compression of the structures by a popliteal cyst may result in diminished posterior tibial and dorsalis pedis pulses and weakness in the muscles of the posterior leg and plantar foot. Trauma to the knee from the posterior side would likely encounter the tibial nerve first and cause flaccid paralysis of muscles in the posterior leg and plantar foot. During knee surgery, the popliteal vessels can be injured from an anterior approach because they are directly in contact with the distal femur. This would

result in arterial and venous hemorrhage because the artery and vein are very closely connected in a fibrous sheath.

Leg

- **Sural nerve and small saphenous vein:** The small saphenous vein runs alongside the sural nerve in the superficial fascia of the posterior leg. Trauma to the posterior leg or lower popliteal region can result in venous hemorrhage and loss of sensation from the posterolateral leg, lateral ankle, heel, and foot.
- **Tibial nerve and posterior tibial vessels:** The tibial nerve leaves the popliteal fossa and enters the posterior leg alongside the posterior tibial vessels, which continue from the popliteal vessels. This bundle is well protected from trauma because it runs in the deep posterior compartment but not in contact with the tibia or fibula; however, it can be affected by compartment syndrome. The bundle is more vulnerable as it approaches the medial malleolus. Trauma to it near the ankle would cause hemorrhage from the artery and vein as well as flaccid paralysis of the muscles of the plantar foot and loss of sensation from the plantar foot. Due to their proximity, the tendons of the tibialis posterior, flexor digitorum longus, and flexor hallucis longus may also be injured.
- **Deep fibular nerve and anterior tibial vessels:** The anterior tibial artery and deep fibular vessels meet in the anterior compartment of the leg and descend between the tibialis anterior and extensor digitorum longus muscles. This bundle can be injured by outside trauma, a tibial fracture, or compartment syndrome. Hemorrhage or compression of the vessels would weaken the tibialis anterior pulse and might cause flaccid paralysis of the muscles of the anterior leg if the nerve is damaged prior to releasing motor branches but would certainly result in absent or altered sensation from the skin between the first and second digits.

Foot

- **Medial plantar nerve and vessels:** This bundle is present in the plantar foot, deep to the abductor hallucis before dividing into superficial and deep branches. Injury to this bundle before it divides would result in hemorrhage and weakness of the abductor hallucis, flexor digitorum brevis, flexor hallucis brevis, and first lumbrical and loss of sensation to the medial plantar foot and plantar aspect of digits 1 to 3 and the medial half of digit 4.
- **Lateral plantar nerve and vessels:** This bundle is also present in the plantar foot, deep to the abductor hallucis before traveling laterally and dividing into superficial and deep branches. Injury to this bundle before it divides would result in hemorrhage and weakness of the quadratus plantae, abductor digiti minimi, flexor digiti minimi brevis, adductor hallucis, interossei, and lumbricals 2 to 4 and loss of sensation to the lateral plantar foot and plantar aspect of digit 5 and the lateral half of digit 4.
- **Common plantar digital nerves and vessels:** The common plantar digital vessels (from the deep plantar artery and vein) and the common plantar digital nerves (from medial and lateral plantar nerves) are located deep in the plantar foot but can be injured by penetrating trauma. This will cause

CLINICAL CORRELATION 11.36   Femoral Triangle and Sheath

The **femoral triangle** is an anatomic landmark bounded by the inguinal ligament, the sartorius muscle, and the lateral border of the adductor longus muscle (see Figs. 11.30–11.32). The floor of the triangle is formed by the adductor brevis and iliopsoas muscles. The femoral nerve enters the femoral triangle by passing deep to the inguinal ligament and lateral to the iliopectineal arch, alongside the iliopsoas in the muscular compartment. On the medial side of the iliopectineal arch is the vascular space that conveys the femoral artery and vein into the femoral triangle as well as the **femoral canal**, which contains lymphatic vessels.

The fascia lata and cribriform fascia form the roof of the femoral triangle, with a layer of subcutaneous fat and skin overlying them. Injuries to the femoral triangle can be very severe due to the large vessels and nerves within it, coupled by the very thin layer of tissue protecting it. The femoral artery, vein, and canal are surrounded by the **femoral sheath**, a funnel-shaped sheet of connective tissue that is continuous with the transversalis fascia of the abdomen and surrounds the vessels and contributes to their adventitial layer. Each vessel within the femoral sheath is separated from its neighbor by fibrous septae.

CLINICAL CORRELATION 11.37   Femoral Canal and Femoral Hernias

The femoral canal is not a large space; it extends from the level of the saphenous opening in the thigh to end superiorly as the **femoral ring** just deep to the inguinal ligament. It contains adipose tissue and loose fibers, as well as lymphatic vessels and (occasionally) lymph nodes that allow lymphatic fluid from the lower limbs and external genitalia to reach deep lymph vessels. The femoral canal can collapse readily when the femoral vein distends, but the canal itself cannot expand because it is bounded posteriorly by the pubic bone and pectineus muscle, laterally by septae of the femoral sheath, anteriorly by the inguinal ligament, and medially by the lacunar ligament. It is covered by a thin, fatty **femoral septum** and the parietal peritoneum. This weak spot in the abdominal wall predisposes it to being a site

where loops of the bowel can herniate when intra-abdominal pressure rises excessively. If such a **femoral hernia** occurs, the bowel will push a layer of parietal peritoneum (the hernia sac) ahead of it as it migrates through the femoral canal and into the femoral triangle. This will often cause a bulging or lump in the groin that is inferior to the inguinal ligament, unlike direct or indirect inguinal hernias, which are located superior to it. Due to the tight and inelastic nature of the femoral canal, hernias in this space can become incarcerated (stuck) and/or strangulated (deprived of blood) as they are pushed against the lacunar ligament. Surgical treatment of a femoral hernia often involves incision of the lacunar ligament, which can be complicated if an accessory obturator artery is present.

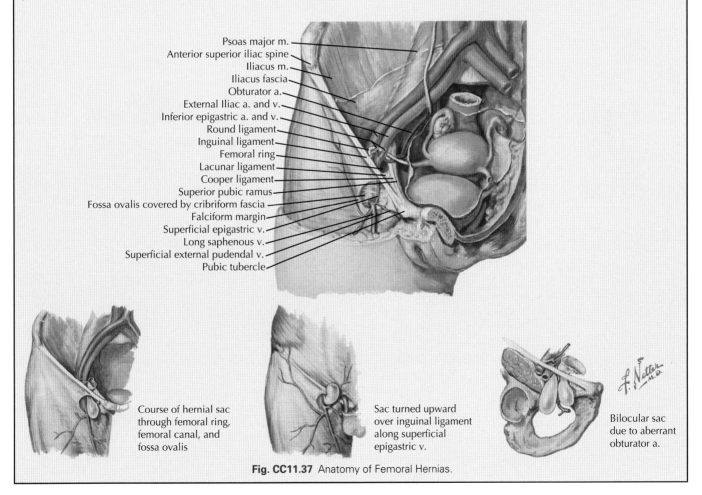

Psoas major m.
Anterior superior iliac spine
Iliacus m.
Iliacus fascia
Obturator a.
External Iliac a. and v.
Inferior epigastric a. and v.
Round ligament
Inguinal ligament
Femoral ring
Lacunar ligament
Cooper ligament
Superior pubic ramus
Fossa ovalis covered by cribriform fascia
Falciform margin
Superficial epigastric v.
Long saphenous v.
Superficial external pudendal v.
Pubic tubercle

Course of hernial sac through femoral ring, femoral canal, and fossa ovalis

Sac turned upward over inguinal ligament along superficial epigastric v.

Bilocular sac due to aberrant obturator a.

Fig. CC11.37 Anatomy of Femoral Hernias.

hemorrhage and sensory loss along the digits that are innervated by the specific common plantar digital nerve.

- **Plantar digital vessels and nerves proper:** The proper plantar digital nerves and arteries are located on the lateral and

medial plantar sides of the digits. They can be injured by lacerations that cause hemorrhage and loss of sensation distal to the injury on the affected side of the digit (Clinical Correlations 11.36 and 11.37).

REFERENCES

Iwanaga J, Eid S, Simonds E, Schumacher M, Loukas M, Tubbs RS. The majority of piriformis muscles are innervated by the superior gluteal nerve. *Clinical Anatomy*. 2019;32:282–286.

Lugo-Pico JG, Aiyer A, Kaplan J, Kadakia AR. Foot Compartment Syndrome Controversy. In: Mauffrey C, Hak D, Martin III M, eds. *Compartment Syndrome*. Cham: Springer; 2019.

Clinical Anatomy of the Torso

INTRODUCTION

When health professionals discuss the musculoskeletal system, the focus typically falls on the back, upper limbs, and lower limbs. However, the anterior neck, thorax, abdomen, and pelvis (hereafter collectively referred to as the torso, or the body without head and limbs) have important musculoskeletal components that contribute to movements of the body. We will focus the discussion primarily on the bones, muscles, nerves, and vessels that have not been discussed in detail in earlier chapters but will call out previously mentioned structures of the back, upper limbs, and lower limbs when appropriate.

BONES AND CARTILAGE STRUCTURES OF THE TORSO

The vertebral column extends along the entire length of the torso, from the cervical vertebrae to the sacrum. Review Chapter 9 for details of the cervical, thoracic, lumbar, sacral, and coccygeal vertebrae.

Anterior Neck (Fig. 12.1)

In addition to the cervical vertebrae, the hyoid bone and laryngeal cartilages are located in the anterior neck and there are skeletal muscles associated with them. The laryngeal cartilages are located inferior to the hyoid bone and create several prominences on the anterior neck. These are made of hyaline cartilage but parts of them may ossify with age. I will describe the cartilages and some of their anatomical relationships related to the muscles of the anterior neck; however, I will not discuss them in detail since the larynx is not primarily a structure of the skeletal system. The **laryngeal muscles** move the laryngeal cartilages and the true vocal cords and are involved in respiration and phonation (speech). Similarly, the **muscles of the tongue, soft palate, pharynx, and esophagus** are most directly involved in the gastrointestinal and respiratory systems.

The small **hyoid bone** is a U-shaped bone with its convexity facing anteriorly at the level of the C3 vertebral body. It has a central **body** with a **lesser horn** extending superiorly from it on the left and right, as well as a **greater horn** that extends further posterolaterly. Each lesser horn is connected to the styloid process of the temporal bone by the **stylohyoid ligament**, which helps prevent anterior displacement of the bone. Suprahyoid muscles connect it to the temporal bone, mandible, and tongue, while infrahyoid muscles connect it to the sternum, scapula, and thyroid cartilage. The greater horn of the hyoid also serves as the origin for the middle pharyngeal constrictor muscle, which fans out posteriorly. These connections allow the hyoid bone to "float" in the anterior neck, serving as a nexus point for all of those muscles. The inferior surface of the hyoid bone is linked to the superior border of the thyroid cartilage by the **thyrohyoid membrane**. When the hyoid bone is elevated, this membrane elevates the laryngeal cartilages to help seal off the airway during swallowing (Clinical Correlation 12.1).

There are many **laryngeal cartilages** that serve as a skeleton of sorts for the muscles and connective tissue structures of the larynx, also known as the voice box.

- **Thyroid cartilage**: a large cartilage formed by a right and left lamina that meet on the anterior midline, where it projects forward at the C5 level as the laryngeal prominence, or "Adam's apple" in men. It is very broad anteriorly but discontinuous posteriorly, giving it a shape like a shield. An **oblique line** is notable on its lateral side that curves superiorly toward the **superior horn** that extends from its posterior superior edge to the posterior end of the greater horn of the hyoid bone. Separate cartilages may be found between the thyroid's superior horn and the greater horn of the hyoid bone, thickening that region of the thyrohyoid membrane. An **inferior horn** projects from its posterior inferior edge and meets the lateral side of the cricoid cartilage, forming the synovial **cricothyroid joint** and capsule. This allows the

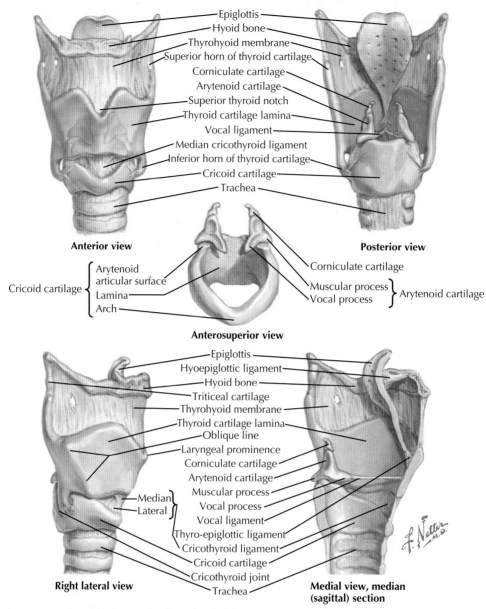

Fig. 12.1 Cartilages of the Larynx.

thyroid cartilage to "rock" anteriorly and posteriorly with the cricothyroid joint as the pivot point.

- **Cricoid cartilage**: forms a complete ring with a narrow anterior arch and a much thicker posterior lamina. In addition to the cricothyroid joint, it is connected to the inferior border of the thyroid cartilage by the **cricothyroid membrane.** It also connects to the first C-shaped tracheal cartilage via the cricotracheal ligament.

- **Arytenoid cartilages**: articulate with the superior aspect of the cricoid cartilage and have the **vocal ligament** extending anteriorly to reach the posterior side of the thyroid cartilage near the midline. The vocal ligament forms the core of the true vocal fold and most laryngeal muscles are devoted to adjusting the degree of abduction/adduction and tension on the ligament to change the vibrations that it makes as air flows past, allowing us to speak and make other noises. Smaller corniculate cartilages are located atop the arytenoids.

- **Epiglottic cartilage**: posterior to the hyoid bone and thyroid cartilage, this spoon-shaped cartilage is covered by mucosa and connected to nearby cartilages by an array of ligaments, muscles, and mucosal folds. Its posterior surface helps to close the laryngeal opening during swallowing.

The inferior larynx terminates as the trachea, which conveys air to and from the lungs in the thorax. The thyroid gland is found on the anterior surface of the trachea shortly before it enters the thorax.

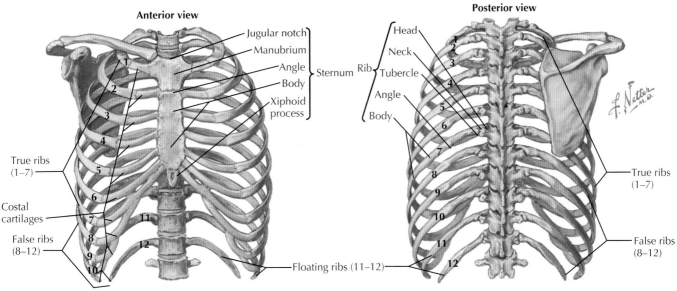

Fig. 12.2 Osteology: Thorax.

Thorax (Fig. 12.2)

The thoracic vertebrae, ribs, and sternum are the bony components of the thorax. They protect the organs (lungs, heart, and thymus) in the **thoracic cavity** and serve as attachment sites for muscles of the thorax, back, abdomen, and upper limbs. From a superior view, the first ribs, first thoracic vertebra, and manubrium surround the **superior thoracic aperture** where the carotid arteries, jugular veins, subclavian vessels, esophagus, trachea enter or exit the thoracic cavity. Likewise, the inferior ribs, costal arch, and xiphoid process surround the much larger **inferior thoracic aperture**, which is associated with the thoracic diaphragm and has the esophagus, aorta, inferior vena cava (IVC), and thoracic duct passing through it.

Twelve **ribs** (Fig. 12.3, see also Fig. 12.2) extend laterally from the thoracic vertebrae and wrap around the lungs and heart to form the **thoracic cage**. **Costal cartilages** continue from the bony ribs, forming costochondral joints with them. Only the costal cartilages of ribs 1 to 7 (**true ribs**) actually reach the sternum directly. The costal cartilages of ribs 8 to 12 (**false ribs**) fuse to the costal cartilages of their superior neighbors at interchondral joints, creating the **costal arch/margin**. The angle formed by the left and right costal arches as they approach the inferior sternum is the infrasternal angle. Ribs 11 and 12 (**floating ribs**) do not reach the sternum at all; they and their costal cartilages have no anterior bony connections. The space between neighboring ribs is the **intercostal space** and is where several muscles and a neurovascular bundle are found.

Each rib has a **costal head** that articulates with its associated thoracic vertebral bodies via a single **articular facet** (ribs 1, 11, and 12, and sometimes 10) or paired **articular demifacets** (ribs 2 to 9, or sometimes 10) that are separated by an interarticular crest. Each **joint of the head of the rib** is stabilized by the **radiate ligament of the head of the rib** as it forms a circular ligament that holds the head of each rib in the joint. Within the radiate ligament is a small intra-articular ligament of the head of the rib that anchors the costal head to the center of the vertebral facet or demifacet.

Just lateral to the head is the narrower costal **neck**, which sometimes hosts its own crest along its posterior side. Lateral to the neck is the prominent **costal tubercle** and its articular facet, marking where it articulates with the transverse costal facets of the associated thoracic vertebrae. The **costotransverse ligament** extends between the costal neck and the vertebral transverse process at the same level. A **superior costotransverse ligament** connects the costal neck to the transverse process of its superior neighbor while the **lateral costotransverse ligament** connects the lateral end of the transverse process to the tubercle of the rib, effectively becoming a capsular ligament for the **costotransverse joint**.

The costal tubercle is the first part of the costal **body** or **shaft**, which initially projects posteriorly but undergoes an anterior turn that creates a bend that is convex posteriorly, the **costal angle**. Along the inferomedial aspect of the entire costal body is a shallow **costal groove** that protects the intercostal neurovascular bundle that travels medial and inferior to each rib.

The central ribs (3 to 10) have all the typical features of a rib described above. The **1st rib** is very short, broad, and flat, lacking a costal groove. Its superior surface has a **groove for the subclavian vein** and a slightly more posterior **groove for the subclavian artery** that are separated by the **scalene tubercle**, where the anterior scalene muscle attaches. The 2nd rib is longer than the 1st but is still fairly flat and has a very slight costal groove. Its superior surface has a roughened area anterior to the costal tubercle, the **tuberosity for the serratus anterior**. The **11th rib** has a distinct costal head but the remaining features, including the costotransverse joint and ligaments, are diminished and indistinct. The **12th rib** is similar to the 11th but even smaller. It is connected to the transverse processes of the L1 and L2 vertebrae by the **lumbocostal ligament** (Clinical Correlations 12.2 and 12.3).

Typically when people speak of the breastbone or **sternum** (see Fig. 12.3), they are referring to an assembly of three fused

Rib Characteristics and Costovertebral Articulations

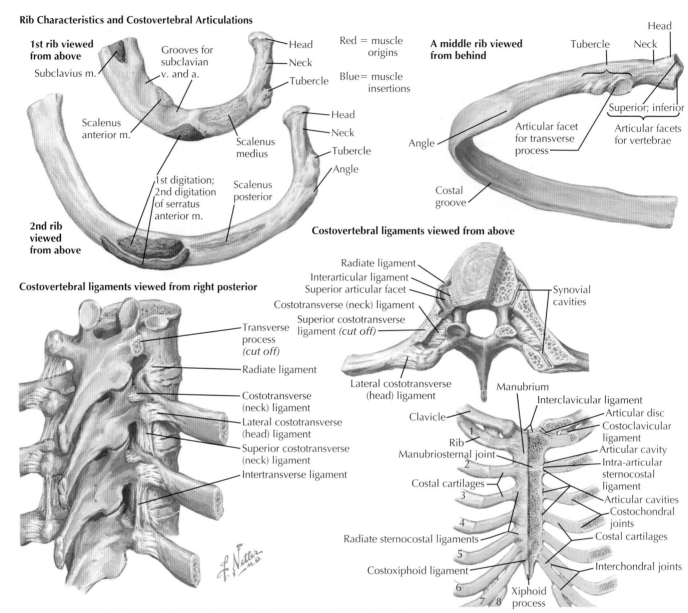

Fig. 12.3 Rib Characteristics and Costovertebral Articulations. Ribs and sternocostal joints; costovertebral joints.

bones of the anterior thorax, the **manubrium, sternal body,** and **xiphoid process**. The superior aspect of the manubrium has a midline depression, the **jugular notch**, located just anterior to the infrahyoid muscles and trachea. On either side of the jugular notch are the left and right **clavicular notches** where the manubrium articulates with the left and right clavicles via a fibrocartilage disc. The manubrium meets the sternal body at the **sternal angle**, where the **manubriosternal joint** is located. The inferior aspect of the sternal body joins the cartilaginous xiphoid process, which slowly ossifies with age, at the **xiphisternal joint**. Continuing inferiorly along the manubrium and sternum's lateral sides are **costal notches** that articulate with the costal cartilages of ribs 1 to 7 to form **sternocostal joints**. The 1st sternocostal joint is on the lateral side of the manubrium and is notable for being a **synchondrosis**, a joint formed only by hyaline cartilage, whereas the others are synovial joints. The

2nd sternocostal joint is on the lateral side of the manubriosternal joint and the 3rd to 7th sternocostal joints are on the lateral aspect of the sternal body. These joints are stabilized by outer **radiate sternocostal ligaments** as well as **intra-articular sternocostal ligaments**. The anterior aspect of the radiate sternocostal ligaments fan out to form a sternal membrane. The 7th rib is also linked to the xiphoid process by costoxiphoid ligaments (Clinical Correlations 12.4 and 12.5).

Bones of the Abdomen and Pelvis

The lumbar vertebrae, ilium, ischium, and pubic bones are the skeletal supports for the muscles of the abdomen and pelvis. These have already been described in detail in Chapters 9 and 11. Regarding the pelvic girdle as a whole, a distinction is often made between the greater and lesser pelvis. The **greater (false) pelvis** is made of the upper sacrum and wings of the ilium, making it

CLINICAL CORRELATION 12.2 Fractures of the Ribs

Rib fractures are relatively common during trauma, falls, and athletic injuries. While they are painful, nondisplaced rib fractures will often heal with conservative treatment. To identify a fracture radiographically, the patient may need to be imaged during both inhalation and exhalation to find the fracture line. The jagged ends of fractured ribs can injure the nearby intercostal nerve and vessels causing sensory and motor losses as well as hemorrhage. Fractured ribs can also lacerate the lungs, diaphragm, liver, or spleen. These injuries are emergencies and require immediate treatment.

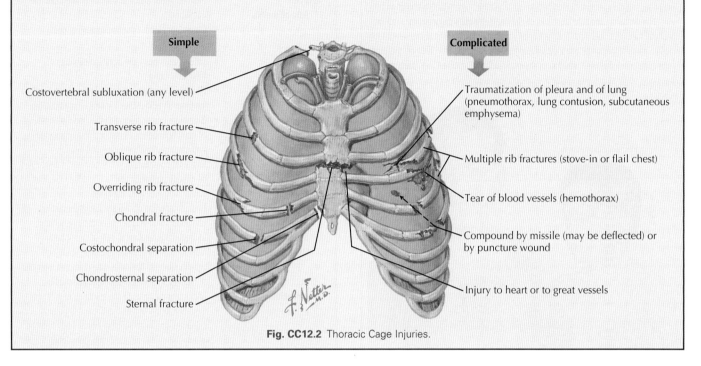

Simple

Costovertebral subluxation (any level)

Transverse rib fracture

Oblique rib fracture

Overriding rib fracture

Chondral fracture

Costochondral separation

Chondrosternal separation

Sternal fracture

Complicated

Traumatization of pleura and of lung (pneumothorax, lung contusion, subcutaneous emphysema)

Multiple rib fractures (stove-in or flail chest)

Tear of blood vessels (hemothorax)

Compound by missile (may be deflected) or by puncture wound

Injury to heart or to great vessels

Fig. CC12.2 Thoracic Cage Injuries.

CLINICAL CORRELATION 12.3 Rib Subluxation, Dislocation, and Separation

The ribs have limited mobility and are generally very stable. In a **costovertebral subluxation**, the head of the rib can shift from its position alongside the vertebral body, stretching the radiate ligament of the head of the rib and causing pain from the displaced rib and accompanying muscle spasms. In contrast, a **chondrosternal separation** (called a rib dislocation by some clinicians) occurs when the costal cartilage becomes displaced from the sternum. This type of separation can involve costal cartilages of the true ribs on the sternum or the cartilages of the false ribs onto the costal arch. Finally, a **costochondral separation** (also known just as rib separation) occurs when the bony and cartilaginous parts of a rib are separated from each other. Traumatic separations can be very pronounced but even small shifts involving the costal cartilages can cause significant discomfort and localized swelling (see Fig. CC12.1).

discontinuous anteriorly. The **lesser (true) pelvis** is a continuous bony ring made of the inferior sacrum, the part of the ilium inferior to the arcuate line, and the pubis and ischium.

MUSCLES AND FASCIAL LAYERS OF THE TORSO

Muscles and Fascia of the Anterior Neck (Fig. 12.4)

In addition to muscles of the back in the cervical region, there are several muscles in the anterior neck that maneuver the head and neck and attach to the hyoid bone. The thin **platysma muscle** is the most superficial muscle of the anterior neck. It originates in the **superficial cervical fascia** (subcutaneous tissue) near the body and angle of the mandible and continues inferiorly past the clavicle. Since it is a muscle of facial expression, innervated by cranial nerve VII (the facial nerve) and does not significantly move the neck, we will not discuss it further in this text.

Deep to the platysma is the **superficial (investing) layer of deep cervical fascia** that surrounds the entire cervical region. Superiorly, this layer of fascia stretches from the occipital bone, across the mastoid and styloid processes of the temporal bones, zygomatic bone, angle and body of the mandible, and hyoid bone. Posteriorly, it attaches to the cervical spinous processes via the nuchal ligament. Inferiorly it attaches to the spine and acromion of the scapula, the clavicle, and sternum. In the neck the fascia splits and surrounds the anterior and posterior sides of the trapezius and sternocleidomastoid muscles. The anterior and posterior sheets of the investing layer on either side of the left and right sternocleidomastoid muscles meet just superior to the manubrium, creating a **suprasternal space**.

Sternocleidomastoid

Like the **trapezius muscle**, which was discussed in detail in Chapter 9, the **sternocleidomastoid muscle** (Fig. 12.5, see also Figs. 12.4) is innervated by the spinal accessory nerve (cranial nerve XI). It has two heads that originate from the superior manubrium and proximal clavicle and fuse quickly as they ascend. A small depression between the two heads, the lesser supraclavicular fossa, can be palpated when the muscle is contracted and serves as a landmark for locating the subclavian vein deep to the muscle. The sternocleidomastoid

CLINICAL CORRELATION 12.4 Pectus Excavatum and Pectus Carinatum

For reasons that may be genetic, the anterior chest and sternum can sometimes be misshapen. **Pectus excavatum** describes a "caved-in" chest with the sternum and costal cartilages concave anteriorly. Mild cases may be treated with exercise, but very severe malformations may require surgical intervention to prevent compression and displacement of the heart. **Pectus carinatum** describes a chest that juts outward in an anteriorly convex shape. This is thought to be due to an overgrowth of the xiphoid and costal cartilages that pushes the sternum forward. While this can occur during childhood, it often manifests during a growth spurt at puberty under the influence of signals like growth hormone.

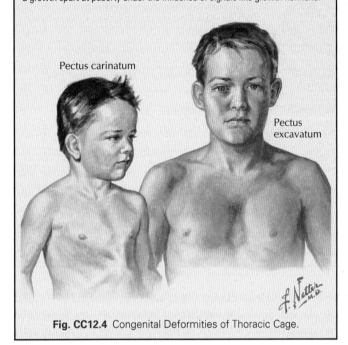

Pectus carinatum

Pectus excavatum

Fig. CC12.4 Congenital Deformities of Thoracic Cage.

CLINICAL CORRELATION 12.5 Bone Marrow and the Sternum

During early life, the inner aspect of many bones contains **red marrow** that creates new circulating blood cells and platelets, a process called hematopoiesis. As people age, this red marrow is largely replaced by adipose-rich **yellow marrow**, particularly in the long limb bones. Hematopoietic red marrow remains in the vertebral bodies, iliac crest, and sternum (see Fig. 12.3). Because these cells proliferate continuously and rapidly, these areas must be protected during imaging procedures involving radiation. Bone marrow from the sternal body is often harvested by needle biopsy when the marrow needs to be examined.

ascends posterolaterally to insert onto the lateral portion of the mastoid process of the temporal bone and a small portion of the adjacent occipital bone. Due to its oblique course it has several actions. Unilateral contraction will side-bend the head ipsilaterally but rotate it contralaterally. Bilateral contraction will flex the head and neck, bringing the chin toward the chest. However, since the sternocleidomastoid crosses the "tipping point" of the occipital condyles, if the head and neck are already extended, bilateral contraction will strongly extend

them even further. In addition to the motor innervation from the spinal accessory nerve, sensory branches from the anterior rami of C3–C4 also enter the sternocleidomastoid in the neck (Clinical Correlation 12.6).

Inferior Attachments	• Sternal head: anterior aspect of the superior manubrium
	• Clavicular head: superior aspect of the proximal clavicle
Superior Attachment	• Lateral aspect of the mastoid process of temporal bone
Functions	• Unilateral contraction will side-bend the head ipsilaterally and rotate the head contralaterally.
	• Bilateral contraction with the head's center of gravity anterior to the occipital condyles will strongly flex the head and neck.
	• Bilateral contraction with the head's center of gravity posterior to the occipital condyles will strongly extend the head.
Muscle Testing and Signs of Dysfunction	• Flaccid paralysis of one sternocleidomastoid can occur when the spinal accessory nerve is injured. The unbalanced pull of the opposite, healthy sternocleidomastoid will cause side-bending (lateral flexion) away from, and rotation of the head toward, the weakened muscle.
Innervation	• Motor: cranial nerve XI, the spinal accessory nerve
	• Sensory: branches of the C3 and C4 spinal nerves along with sensory nerve cells located along the spinal accessory nerve roots.
Blood Supply	• Branches from the suprascapular artery inferiorly, branches from the superior thyroid and external carotid arteries in the mid portion, and branches from the occipital artery more superiorly.

Suprahyoid Muscles (Geniohyoid, Mylohyoid, Stylohyoid, Digastric)

The **suprahyoid muscles** (Fig. 12.6, see also Fig. 12.5) (mylohyoid, geniohyoid, stylohyoid, and digastric muscles) are located deep to the superficial layer of deep cervical fascia. They link the hyoid bone to the mandible and temporal bone, which allows them to elevate the hyoid during swallowing. Elevation of the hyoid also elevates the larynx via the thyrohyoid membrane, which closes the larynx so that food and fluid are directed posteriorly toward the esophagus. The **geniohyoid muscle** attaches to the anterior body of the hyoid bone and travels anteriorly to insert onto the genu of the mandible. Inferior to the geniohyoid, the **mylohyoid muscle** originates from the anterior body of the hyoid and fans out to the left and right, attaching to the medial aspect of the mandible, the mylohyoid line. In addition to the hyoid bone, fibers of the mylohyoid also originate from the **mylohyoid raphe**, a midline connective tissue band that stretches between the hyoid and genu of the mandible. The geniohyoid and mylohyoid both elevate and anteriorly shift the hyoid during swallowing and form the muscular floor of the oral cavity. The **stylohyoid muscle** stretches from the styloid process of the temporal bone to the superior hyoid bone in the vicinity of the lesser horn. The **digastric muscle** has a

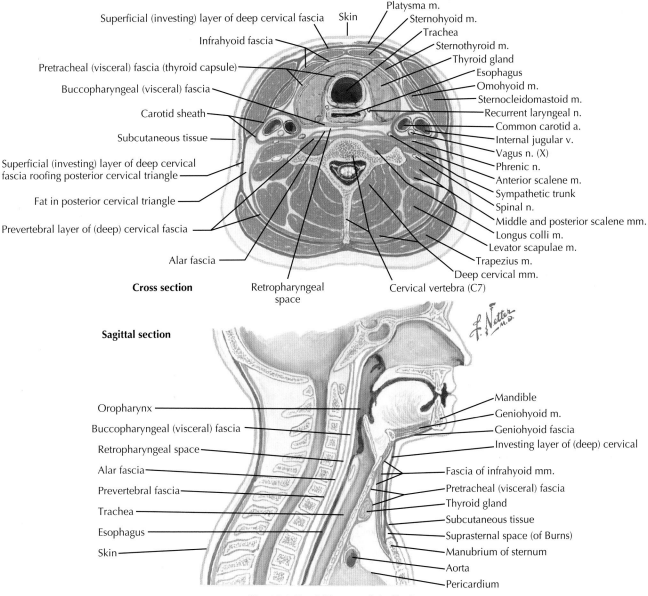

Fig. 12.4 Fascial Layers of the Neck.

posterior belly that attaches to the medial aspect of the mastoid process of the temporal bone and an **anterior belly** that attaches to the posterior aspect of the mandible near the genu and body of the bone, inferior to the mylohyoid muscle. The two bellies are connected by an **intermediate tendon** that is tethered to the superior, lateral aspect of the hyoid body by a connective tissue sling. In addition to the sling, the stylohyoid muscle splits so that its fibers straddle the intermediate tendon of the digastric muscle as they insert on the hyoid bone. Contraction of the stylohyoid and digastric muscles will elevate and posteriorly shift the hyoid bone during swallowing.

Two muscles of the tongue also originate from the superior aspect of the hyoid bone but a detailed description of them is better suited to a book on the digestive or nervous systems. In short, part of the **genioglossus muscle**, which protrudes the tongue, attaches to the superior aspect of the body of the hyoid and inserts into the muscles and connective tissues of the tongue. The **hyoglossus muscle** originates from a broad line extending across almost the entire length of the greater horn of the hyoid bone. The sheet-like muscle inserts into the muscles at the base of the tongue and helps to depress it.

Inferior Attachments	• Geniohyoid: anterior body of hyoid • Mylohyoid: anterior body of hyoid • Stylohyoid: superior hyoid near the lesser horn • Digastric: intermediate tendon of digastric muscle is tethered to superior body of hyoid by a connective tissue sling and the stylohyoid muscle

Superior Attachment	• Geniohyoid: genu of mandible near its posterior midline
	• Mylohyoid: mylohyoid line along the medial side of the body of mandible and mylohyoid raphe where the left and right sides meet
	• Stylohyoid: styloid process of temporal bone
	• Digastric:
	  • Posterior belly attaches to the medial side of mastoid process of temporal bone.
	  • Anterior belly attaches to the posterior aspect of genu and part of body of mandible.

Functions	• All suprahyoid muscles elevate the hyoid bone and larynx (through the thyrohyoid membrane). This closes the laryngeal opening against the epiglottis during swallowing and prevents aspiration. • Contraction of the mylohyoid and geniohyoid will shift the hyoid anteriorly; contraction of the stylohyoid and digastric muscles will shift the hyoid posteriorly. • The suprahyoid muscles are also active during wide opening of the mouth, pulling the mandible inferiorly toward the hyoid bone.
Muscle Testing and Signs of Dysfunction	• Dysfunction of a single suprahyoid muscle may not be very noticeable if the others are able to compensate for its loss. • Loss of more than one suprahyoid muscle can result in coughing and aspiration due to failure of the larynx to fully close when swallowing. • Asymmetry of the hyoid bone can sometimes be detected by gently palpating the bone while asking the patient to swallow.

Innervation	• Geniohyoid: C1 branch traveling with hypoglossal nerve/cranial nerve XII
	• Mylohyoid: nerve to mylohyoid, a branch of trigeminal nerve/cranial nerve V
	• Stylohyoid: facial nerve/cranial nerve VII
	• Digastric:
	  • Anterior belly: nerve to mylohyoid, a branch of trigeminal nerve/cranial nerve V
	  • Posterior belly: facial nerve/cranial nerve VII

Blood Supply	• Facial, lingual, inferior alveolar, occipital, and posterior auricular arteries all of which arise from external carotid artery

Infrahyoid Muscles (Sternohyoid, Omohyoid, Sternothyroid, Thyrohyoid)

Deep to the superficial layer of deep cervical fascia in the anterior neck are the **infrahyoid muscles**, sometimes called the "strap" muscles (see Figs. 12.4–12.6), which are each covered by their own surface fascia. The infrahyoid muscles (sternohyoid, sternothyroid, thyrohyoid, and omohyoid) are long, strap-like muscles that all attach to the inferior aspect of the hyoid bone and depress it when they contract. The **sternohyoid muscle** originates from the posterior side of the manubrium and inserts on the inferior body of the hyoid bone. The **omohyoid muscle** has a **superior belly** that is attached to the hyoid bone immediately lateral to the sternohyoid. An **intermediate tendon** connects it to the **inferior belly**, which veers posterolaterally to insert onto the superior border of the scapula, just medial to the scapular notch. The intermediate tendon is tethered to the proximal clavicle and first rib by a fascial sling within the nearby deep cervical fascia. Deep to the sternohyoid and omohyoid are two muscles that follow a similar course to the sternohyoid but do it in two steps with the thyroid cartilage as an intermediate insertion point. The **sternothyroid muscle** originates from the posterior manubrium and inserts on the anterolateral side of the thyroid cartilage, just inferior to the oblique line. Thereafter the **thyrohyoid muscle** completes the journey, originating superior to the oblique line and inserting along the inferior body and greater horn of the hyoid bone. These muscles are innervated by anterior rami from C1 to C3 that create the ansa cervicalis, a part of the cervical plexus that forms a loop on the anterior aspect of the carotid sheath.

Inferior Attachments	• Sternohyoid: posterior manubrium • Omohyoid: superior border of scapula immediately medial to scapular notch, the intermediate tendon is tethered to the medial clavicle • Sternothyroid: posterior manubrium • Thyrohyoid: oblique line on the lateral side of thyroid cartilage
Superior Attachment	• Sternohyoid: inferior side of the body of hyoid • Omohyoid: inferior aspect of body and greater horn of hyoid • Sternothyroid: oblique line on the lateral side of thyroid cartilage • Thyrohyoid: inferior aspect of body and greater horn of hyoid

Functions	• All infrahyoid muscles depress the hyoid bone. This returns the hyoid to its normal position after swallowing and also stabilizes it during movements of the tongue.
	  • Omohyoid: also pulls the hyoid posteriorly.
	  • Sternothyroid: depresses larynx
	  • Thyrohyoid: depresses the hyoid in concert with the sternothyroid, can also elevate the larynx when the hyoid is elevated during swallowing.

Muscle Testing and Signs of Dysfunction	• Dysfunction of a single muscle may not be noticeable. • Loss of several infrahyoid muscles, perhaps due to injury to the ansa cervicalis or cervical spinal nerves, would result in difficulty swallowing and tilting of the hyoid bone as the suprahyoid muscles elevate the affected side without any resistance from the dysfunctional infrahyoid muscles. • Asymmetry of the hyoid bone can sometimes be detected by gently palpating the bone while asking the patient to swallow.
Innervation	• Sternohyoid: ansa cervicalis (C1–C3) • Omohyoid: ansa cervicalis (C1–C3) • Sternothyroid: ansa cervicalis (C2–C3) • Thyrohyoid: C1 branch traveling with hypoglossal nerve/cranial nerve XII
Blood Supply	• Superior thyroid artery from external carotid artery • Inferior thyroid artery from thyro-cervical trunk of subclavian artery • Internal thoracic artery from subclavian artery

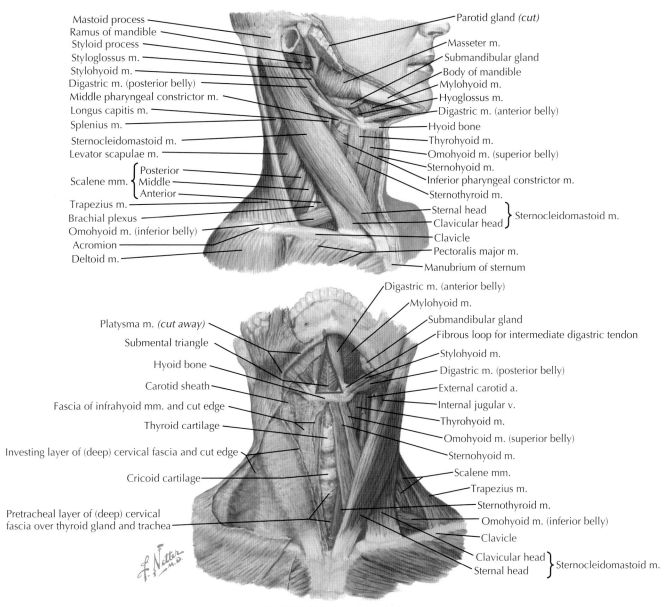

Mastoid process
Ramus of mandible
Styloid process
Styloglossus m.
Stylohyoid m.
Digastric m. (posterior belly)
Middle pharyngeal constrictor m.
Longus capitis m.
Splenius m.
Sternocleidomastoid m.
Levator scapulae m.
Scalene mm. { Posterior / Middle / Anterior }
Trapezius m.
Brachial plexus
Omohyoid m. (inferior belly)
Acromion
Deltoid m.

Parotid gland (cut)
Masseter m.
Submandibular gland
Body of mandible
Mylohyoid m.
Hyoglossus m.
Digastric m. (anterior belly)
Hyoid bone
Thyrohyoid m.
Omohyoid m. (superior belly)
Sternohyoid m.
Inferior pharyngeal constrictor m.
Sternothyroid m.
Sternal head }
Clavicular head } Sternocleidomastoid m.
Clavicle
Pectoralis major m.
Manubrium of sternum

Digastric m. (anterior belly)
Mylohyoid m.
Submandibular gland
Fibrous loop for intermediate digastric tendon
Stylohyoid m.
Digastric m. (posterior belly)
External carotid a.
Internal jugular v.
Thyrohyoid m.
Omohyoid m. (superior belly)
Sternohyoid m.
Scalene mm.
Trapezius m.
Sternothyroid m.
Omohyoid m. (inferior belly)
Clavicle
Clavicular head }
Sternal head } Sternocleidomastoid m.

Platysma m. (cut away)
Submental triangle
Hyoid bone
Carotid sheath
Fascia of infrahyoid mm. and cut edge
Thyroid cartilage
Investing layer of (deep) cervical fascia and cut edge
Cricoid cartilage
Pretracheal layer of (deep) cervical fascia over thyroid gland and trachea

Fig. 12.5 Muscles of the Neck.

Longus Colli and Longus Capitis Muscles

Posterior to the infrahyoid muscles, the **pretracheal layer of the deep cervical fascia** surrounds the trachea, thyroid gland, esophagus, and recurrent laryngeal nerves (see Fig. 12.4). This layer of fascia is continuous with the buccopharyngeal fascia that covers the pharynx more superiorly. Laterally, the **carotid sheath** covers the common carotid artery (and its branches, the external and internal carotid arteries), internal jugular vein, and vagus nerve on each side. The left and right carotid sheaths are connected to each other by **alar fascia**, which is found immediately posterior to the pretracheal layer of deep cervical fascia. Posterior to the alar fascia is the **retropharyngeal space**, a potential space that can sometimes convey purulent material from the posterior pharynx into the mediastinum of the thorax.

The next layer is the **prevertebral layer of the deep cervical fascia** surrounding the cervical vertebrae and many of the muscles that attach to them (Fig. 12.7). The longus coli, longus capitis, and rectus capitis anterior attach primarily to the anterior aspect of the cervical vertebra. The anterior scalene, middle scalene, posterior scalene, levator scapulae, and rectus capitis lateralis muscles attach primarily to the lateral aspect of the cervical vertebrae. Finally, the erector spinae, splenius, transversospinalis, and suboccipital muscles attach primarily to the posterior aspect of the cervical vertebrae. The erector spinae, splenius, and transversospinalis muscles were described in detail in Chapter 9; the levator scapulae were described in Chapter 10.

The **longus colli muscles** are shaped like a parenthesis with (from inferior to superior) inferior fibers originating from the

CLINICAL CORRELATION 12.6   Torticollis

Injury to the sternocleidomastoid muscle during the birthing process can result in bleeding and fibrous connective tissue forming in the muscle. This results in shortening of the affected sternocleidomastoid and persistent side-bending toward, and rotation away from, the affected side. This is known as torticollis (wry neck) and may require surgical release of the muscle from its proximal attachments. Torticollis can also occur prior to birth, because of trauma to the muscle, or idiopathically.

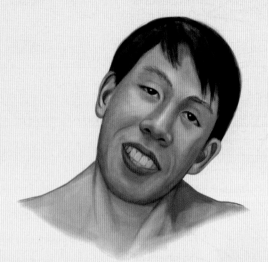

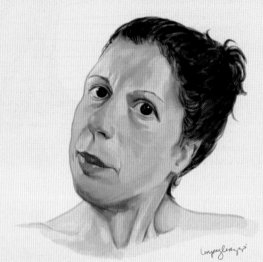

Young man with muscular torticollis. Head tilted to left with chin turned slightly to right because of contracture of left sternocleidomastoid muscle.

Untreated torticollis in middle-aged woman. Thick, fibrotic, tendon-like bands have replaced sternocleidomastoid muscle, making head appear tethered to clavicle. Two heads of left sternocleidomastoid muscle are prominent.

Fig. CC12.6 Torticollis.

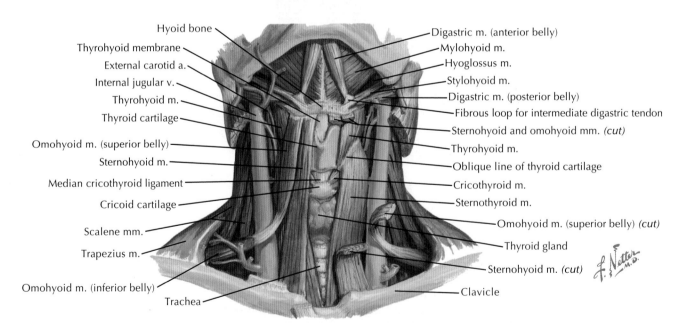

Hyoid bone
Thyrohyoid membrane
External carotid a.
Internal jugular v.
Thyrohyoid m.
Thyroid cartilage
Omohyoid m. (superior belly)
Sternohyoid m.
Median cricothyroid ligament
Cricoid cartilage
Scalene mm.
Trapezius m.
Omohyoid m. (inferior belly)
Trachea

Digastric m. (anterior belly)
Mylohyoid m.
Hyoglossus m.
Stylohyoid m.
Digastric m. (posterior belly)
Fibrous loop for intermediate digastric tendon
Sternohyoid and omohyoid mm. *(cut)*
Thyrohyoid m.
Oblique line of thyroid cartilage
Cricothyroid m.
Sternothyroid m.
Omohyoid m. (superior belly) *(cut)*
Thyroid gland
Sternohyoid m. *(cut)*
Clavicle

Fig. 12.6 Infrahyoid and Suprahyoid Muscles.

anterior bodies of vertebrae T3 up to C5, traveling in a superolateral direction to insert on the C6–C3 transverse processes. More superior members of this muscle group arise from the C5–C3 transverse processes and ascend superomedially to insert on the C4–C2 vertebral bodies and area lateral to the anterior tubercle of C1. The nearby **longus capitis muscle** originates from the anterior tubercles of the transverse processes of the C6–C3 vertebrae and ascends superomedially to insert on the occipital bone just anterior to the occipital condyles. The longus capitis and colli will flex the neck and head (respectively) when contracted bilaterally. When contracted unilaterally, they side-bend the neck and head ipsilaterally. Both are innervated by branches from the nearby anterior rami of C1–C6.

Inferior Attachments	• Longus colli
	  • Lower, superolateral group: anterior T3–C5 vertebral bodies
	  • Upper, superomedial group: C5–C3 transverse processes
	• Longus capitis: anterior tubercles of transverse processes of C3–C6 vertebrae

Superior Attachment	• Longus colli
	  • Lower, superolateral group: C6–C3 transverse processes
	  • Upper, superomedial group: anterior C4–C2 vertebral bodies, lateral to C1 anterior tubercle
	• Longus capitis: base of occipital bone anterior to occipital condyles

Functions	• Longus colli: Bilateral contraction will cause flexion of the neck. Unilateral contraction will cause ipsilateral side-bending and minor contralateral rotation. • Longus capitis: Bilateral contraction will cause flexion of the head. Unilateral contraction will cause ipsilateral side-bending.
Muscle Testing and Signs of Dysfunction	• Dysfunction of these muscles would be very difficult to diagnose and has no distinctive clinical signs. • Hyperextension injuries of the head and neck can injure these muscles and nearby connective tissue structures. This would result in deep cervical pain during active flexion or passive extension of the head and neck.
Innervation	• Longus colli: anterior rami of C2–C6 • Longus capitis: anterior rami of C1–C3
Blood Supply	• Inferior thyroid and ascending cervical arteries arising from thyro-cervical trunk of subclavian artery

Inferior Attachments	• Rectus capitis anterior: anterior aspect of lateral mass of C1 • Rectus capitis lateralis: most lateral aspect of lateral mass of C1
Superior Attachment	• Rectus capitis anterior: base of occipital bone anterior to occipital condyle • Rectus capitis lateralis: occipital bone posterior to jugular foramen
Functions	• Rectus capitis anterior and lateralis both flex the head on the atlas. The rectus capitis lateralis may also contribute in a minor way to side-bending of the head.
Muscle Testing and Signs of Dysfunction	• Dysfunction of these muscles would be very difficult to diagnose and has no distinctive clinical signs. • Hyperextension or side-bending injuries involving the head can injure these muscles and nearby connective tissue structures. This would result in deep cervical pain during active flexion or passive extension of the head and neck.
Innervation Blood Supply	• Branches from anterior rami of C1–C2 • Vertebral artery • Ascending pharyngeal artery from external carotid artery

Rectus Capitis Anterior and Rectus Capitis Lateralis Muscles

Two small but stout muscles connect the anterior and lateral aspects of the atlas to the base of the occipital bone and complement the suboccipital muscles of the posterior neck. The **rectus capitis anterior** runs from the anterior aspect of the lateral mass of C1 to the base of the occipital bone near the occipital condyles alongside the longus capitis muscle. The **rectus capitis lateralis muscle** originates from the lateral mass of C1 and inserts on the jugular process of the occipital bone, which is on the posterior side of the jugular foramen.

Anterior Scalene, Middle Scalene, and Posterior Scalene Muscles

The three scalene muscles (see Figs. 12.5–12.7) stretch between the cervical transverse processes and extend inferolaterally to insert onto the first two ribs at the base of the neck. The **anterior scalene muscle** begins at the transverse processes of C3–C6 and descends to attach to the scalene tubercle on the superior surface of the 1st rib, located between the groove for the subclavian vein (anteriorly) and the groove for the subclavian artery (posteriorly). The phrenic nerve, which innervates the thoracic diaphragm, comes together from the anterior rami of C3–C5 on the anterior surface of the anterior scalene muscle where it is vulnerable to injury. The **middle scalene muscle** is similar but begins on the posterior tubercles of the transverse processes of the C5–C7 vertebrae and inserts on the superior surface of the first rib immediately posterior to the groove for the subclavian artery. The subclavian artery and roots of the brachial plexus pass through the **scalene triangle**, formed by the 1st rib, anterior scalene muscle, and middle scalene muscle. The **posterior scalene muscle** arises from the same transverse processes as the middle scalene but stretches further inferiorly to insert on the superior side of the middle part of the 2nd rib's body. Unilateral contraction of the scalene muscles will side-bend the cervical vertebrae ipsilaterally when the ribs are fixed in place. However, if the cervical vertebrae are held rigidly straight, contraction of the scalene muscles can elevate the 1st and 2nd ribs during inspiration. This becomes more pronounced in conditions like emphysema where the muscles of respiration must work harder during inspiration. The scalene muscles are innervated by branches from the anterior rami of C3–C8. There is a great deal of disagreement about exactly which levels innervate each

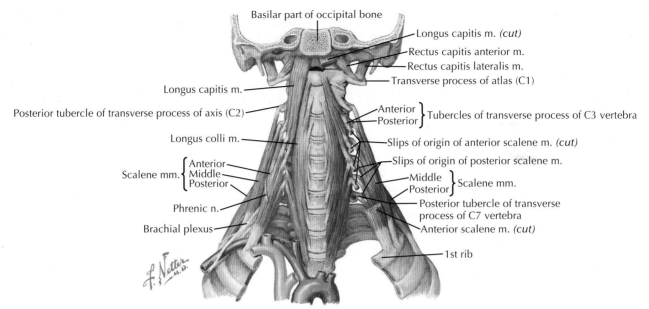

Fig. 12.7 Scalene and Prevertebral Muscles.

muscle, and this likely reflects significant variation between individuals (Clinical Correlation 12.7).

Superior Attachment	• Anterior scalene: lateral aspects of C3–C6 transverse processes • Middle and posterior scalene: posterior tubercles of transverse processes of C5–C7 vertebrae
Inferior Attachments	• Anterior scalene: scalene tubercle of the 1st rib • Middle scalene: posterior to groove for subclavian artery on the 1st rib • Posterior scalene: superolateral body of the 2nd rib
Functions	• Unilateral contraction of the scalene muscles will side-bend the cervical vertebrae ipsilaterally when the ribs are fixed in place. • If the cervical vertebrae are held rigidly straight, contraction of the scalene muscles will elevate ribs 1 and 2 during inspiration. • Bilateral contraction of the anterior scalene may assist with flexion of the neck.
Muscle Testing and Signs of Dysfunction	• Spasm of the scalene muscles can result in pain at the base of the neck or persistently elevated 1st or 2nd ribs. They can be palpated lateral to the sternocleidomastoid at the base of the neck.
Innervation Blood Supply	• Branches from C3 to C8 anterior rami • Ascending cervical and inferior thyroid arteries from thyrocervical trunk of subclavian artery

Muscles and Fascia of the Thorax

The skin and superficial fascia covering the thorax is much like it is elsewhere, with a variable amount of adipose tissue within the superficial fascia. One unique feature of the thorax is the breast, a modified sweat gland that expands into the superficial fascia from its opening at the nipple. The breast is a clinically

CLINICAL CORRELATION 12.7
Interscalene Nerve Block

The roots of the brachial plexus pass between the anterior and middle scalene muscles, making this an excellent area to inject anesthetic to block motor and sensory activity of the upper limb in preparation for a surgical procedure. Since these nerves are large and the subclavian vessels are located nearby, this block is often done with ultrasound guidance. An interscalene nerve block will affect the superior and middle trunks of the brachial plexus to a greater degree than the inferior trunk, so other blocks may be used when the hand is being treated surgically. As with a cervical plexus nerve block, the phrenic nerve is often affected due to its proximity on the anterior surface of the anterior scalene muscle.

important structure for a variety of reasons related to the reproductive and integumental (skin) systems and the development of cancer.

Deep to the skin and superficial fascia are the muscles and fasciae that surround the thoracic cage, consisting of the manubrium, sternal body, xiphoid process, ribs, and thoracic vertebrae. The thoracic cage is truly a versatile structure. It protects the thoracic organs, acts as an anchor for muscles of the proximal upper limb, and expands and contracts during breathing. Several muscles found in the thoracic region have their major effects on the upper limb and were discussed in detail in Chapter 10. These include the pectoralis major, pectoralis minor, latissimus dorsi, subclavius, levator scapulae, rhomboid major, rhomboid minor, and serratus anterior muscles. Other muscles found in the thoracic region, such as the trapezius, erector spinae, levatores costarum, serratus posterior superior, and serratus posterior inferior muscle were previously described in Chapter 9. Without making things more confusing than they need to be, there are also several muscles of the abdominal wall that attach to parts of the thoracic cage such as the rectus abdominis, external abdominal oblique, internal abdominal oblique, transversus abdominis, quadratus lumborum. These will be discussed in the next section on the

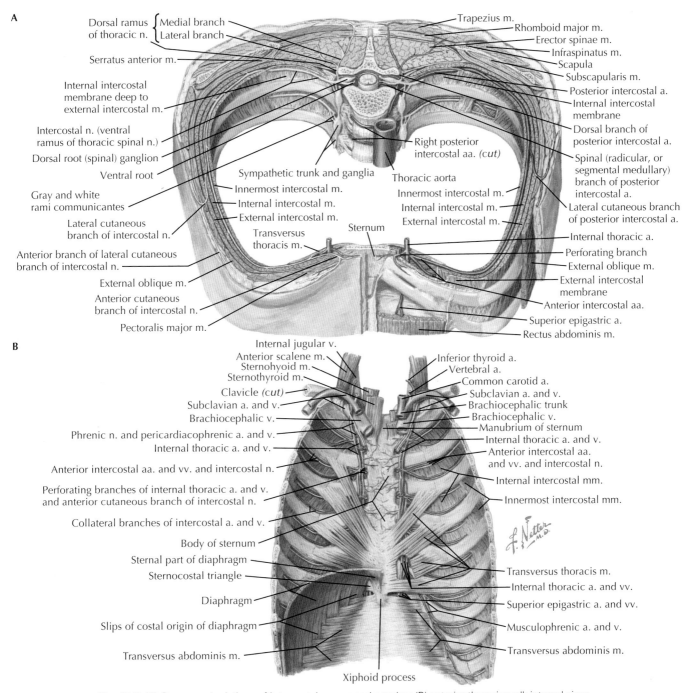

A

Dorsal ramus { Medial branch
of thoracic n. { Lateral branch

Serratus anterior m.

Internal intercostal
membrane deep to
external intercostal m.

Intercostal n. (ventral
ramus of thoracic spinal n.)

Dorsal root (spinal) ganglion

Ventral root

Gray and white
rami communicantes

Lateral cutaneous
branch of intercostal n.

Anterior branch of lateral cutaneous
branch of intercostal n.

External oblique m.

Anterior cutaneous
branch of intercostal n.

Pectoralis major m.

Trapezius m.
Rhomboid major m.
Erector spinae m.
Infraspinatus m.
Scapula
Subscapularis m.
Posterior intercostal a.
Internal intercostal
membrane
Dorsal branch of
posterior intercostal a.
Spinal (radicular, or
segmental medullary)
branch of posterior
intercostal a.
Lateral cutaneous branch
of posterior intercostal a.
Internal thoracic a.
Perforating branch
External oblique m.
External intercostal
membrane
Anterior intercostal aa.
Superior epigastric a.
Rectus abdominis m.

Sympathetic trunk and ganglia
Innermost intercostal m.
Internal intercostal m.
External intercostal m.
Transversus
thoracis m.

Right posterior
intercostal aa. (cut)
Thoracic aorta
Innermost intercostal m.
Internal intercostal m.
External intercostal m.
Sternum

B

Internal jugular v.
Anterior scalene m.
Sternohyoid m.
Sternothyroid m.
Clavicle (cut)
Subclavian a. and v.
Brachiocephalic v.
Phrenic n. and pericardiacophrenic a. and v.
Internal thoracic a. and v.
Anterior intercostal aa. and vv. and intercostal n.
Perforating branches of internal thoracic a. and v.
and anterior cutaneous branch of intercostal n.
Collateral branches of intercostal a. and v.
Body of sternum
Sternal part of diaphragm
Sternocostal triangle
Diaphragm
Slips of costal origin of diaphragm
Transversus abdominis m.

Inferior thyroid a.
Vertebral a.
Common carotid a.
Subclavian a. and v.
Brachiocephalic trunk
Brachiocephalic v.
Manubrium of sternum
Internal thoracic a. and v.
Anterior intercostal aa.
and vv. and intercostal n.
Internal intercostal mm.
Innermost intercostal mm.
Transversus thoracis m.
Internal thoracic a. and vv.
Superior epigastric a. and vv.
Musculophrenic a. and v.
Transversus abdominis m.

Xiphoid process

Fig. 12.8 (A) Course and relations of intercostal nerves and arteries; (B) anterior thoracic wall: internal view.

abdomen. We are left with a group of muscles that have their primary effect on movement of the ribs and expansion of the lungs: the external intercostal, internal intercostal, innermost intercostal, subcostal, transversus thoracis muscles, and the diaphragm.

Intercostal, Subcostal, and Transversus Thoracis Muscles

The intercostal muscles (Fig. 12.8) are found between adjacent ribs and, as a group, run from the back to the sternum. However, no one member of the intercostal muscle group runs the entire

length of the intercostal space and each member of this group is separated from each other and overlying muscles by a thin layer of **thoracic fascia**. They receive innervation and blood from the intercostal nerve and vessels within each intercostal space. The 11 pairs of **external intercostal muscles** are the most superficial muscles within the intercostal spaces, connecting adjacent ribs. Starting near the tubercle of each rib, their fibers run in an inferoanterior ("hands in pocket") direction before reaching the costochondral junction of the ribs. At this point the muscle fibers disappear but an **external intercostal membrane** continues in the same plane to reach the sternum. These muscles are most active during inspiration. Using the first rib as a fixed structure (with likely assistance from the scalene muscles), each external intercostal muscle pulls its inferior rib superiorly, expanding the thoracic cage.

Just deep to the external intercostal muscles are 11 pairs of **internal intercostal muscles** with fibers running in an inferoposterior direction, perpendicular to the external intercostal fibers. The internal intercostal muscles extend posteriorly in the intercostal spaces from the sternum to the costal angle, where they give off an **internal intercostal membrane** in the same plane. The internal intercostal muscle fibers near the sternum and costal cartilages are active during inspiration, complementing the action of the external intercostal muscles. However, the lateral part of each internal intercostal muscle is active during expiration, pulling the ribs inferiorly toward the abdominal muscles. Since elastic recoil of the lungs is responsible for most exhalation when a person is relaxed, these muscles only become active during rapid, forced expiration in order to pump air out of the lungs faster and more forcefully than elastic recoil would allow on its own. Deep to the internal intercostals are the **innermost intercostal muscles**. The fibers of these muscles run the same direction as the internal intercostals and they are only seen in the most lateral part of the intercostal space, somewhere between the costal angle and costochondral junction. The intercostal nerve and vessels travel between the internal and innermost intercostal muscles, serving as a valuable landmark during dissection. Additionally, a variable number of **subcostal muscles** may be present in the inferior thoracic cage. These appear similar to the internal and innermost intercostal muscles but typically span two intercostal spaces. The innermost and subcostal muscles are thought to assist the internal intercostal muscle during expiration. Lastly, the fan-shaped **transversus thoracis muscle** originates from the inferior, internal side of the sternum and xiphoid process and spreads out superolaterally to insert on the costal cartilages. It is thought to assist in depression of the ribs during exhalation but may be proprioceptive or even prevent excessive expansion during inspiration (Clinical Correlations 12.8 and 12.9).

Inferior Attachments	• All intercostal muscles connect the ribs enclosing a single intercostal space.
	  • External intercostal: muscle fibers begin posteriorly near tubercles of the rib
	  • Internal intercostal: between costal angles and tubercles is the internal intercostal membrane; muscle fibers begin near costal angles.
	  • Innermost intercostal: fibers begin near costal angles
	• Subcostal: found in inferior, posterior portion of thoracic cage originating from internal aspect of ribs
	• Transversus thoracis: posterior aspect of sternal body and xiphoid process

Superior Attachment	• All intercostal muscles connect the ribs enclosing an intercostal space.
	  • External intercostal: fibers run inferoanteriorly; end near costochondral junctions, extending a membrane to sternum thereafter.
	  • Internal intercostal: fibers run inferoposteriorly; end at sternum
	  • Innermost intercostal: fibers directed inferoposteriorly; end prior to the costochondral junction
	• Subcostal: ascends superolaterally to insert on internal aspect of rib 2 levels higher
	• Transversus thoracis: a variable number of fibers insert on posterior aspects of costal cartilages 2 to 6.

Functions	• External intercostal: elevate the ribs toward the 1st rib during inspiration. • Internal intercostal: anterior part elevates the anterior ribs and costal cartilages during inspiration. Lateral part depresses the ribs during forced expiration. • Innermost intercostal: depress ribs during forced expiration • Subcostal: likely depress ribs during forced expiration • Transversus thoracis: likely to depress anterior ribs and costal cartilages toward xiphoid process during forced expiration.
Muscle Testing and Signs of Dysfunction	• Loss of one member of the intercostal muscle group is very rare. • If an intercostal nerve were damaged proximally, all muscles in that intercostal space would become flaccidly paralyzed, causing some difficulty breathing but would be compensated for by other respiratory muscles. • Getting a "stitch in your side" is a cramp or soreness of the intercostal muscles experienced during strenuous activity or exercise.
Innervation	• Intercostal nerves (anterior rami from T1 to T11)
Blood Supply	• Superior thoracic artery from axillary artery (1st and 2nd intercostal spaces) • Posterior intercostal arteries from thoracic aorta • Anterior intercostal arteries from internal thoracic artery

CLINICAL CORRELATION 12.8 Pneumothorax

Pneumothorax refers to the presence of air within the pleural cavities, which will compress the lung and push it away from its intimate contact with the parietal pleura. A **spontaneous pneumothorax** can occur when "blebs" on the surface of a lung rupture but can also happen when the thoracic wall is disrupted, opening a pathway from the outside into the pleural space. Since a path through a traumatized thoracic wall has a much lower resistance than the normal pathway through the airway and into the spongy tissues of the lungs, air will readily enter the pleural cavity and compress the lung toward the mediastinum. In an **open**

pneumothorax, air can move in and out of this gap as the patient breathes. **Tension pneumothorax** is a particularly dangerous condition in which the traumatized thoracic wall forms a flap that opens when the patient inhales, allowing air into the pleural space; however, the flap is pushed closed during exhalation, trapping air. Therefore, each inhalation raises pressure in the affected pleural space and compresses the lung further. This can eventually shift the mediastinum and heart away from the affected side, even compressing the opposite lung. A needle can be introduced into the affected pleural space to vent the air.

Open pneumothorax pathophysiology

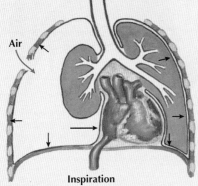

Air

Inspiration

Air enters pleural cavity through an open, sucking chest wound. Negative pleural pressure is lost, permitting collapse of ipsilateral lung and reducing venous return to heart. Mediastinum shifts, compressing opposite lung

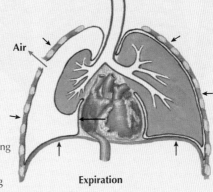

Air

Expiration

As chest wall contracts and diaphragm rises, air is expelled from pleural cavity via wound. Mediastinum shifts to affected side, and mediastinal flutter further impairs venous return by distortion of venae cavae

Tension pneumothorax pathophysiology

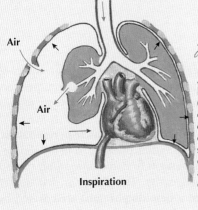

Air

Air

Inspiration

Air enters pleural cavity through lung wound or ruptured bleb (or occasionally via penetrating chest wound) with valvelike opening. Ipsilateral lung collapses, and mediastinum shifts to opposite side, compressing contralateral lung and impairing its ventilating capacity

Pressure

Expiration

Intrapleural pressure rises, closing valvelike opening, preventing escape of pleural air. Pressure is thus progressively increased with each breath. Mediastinal and tracheal shifts are augmented, diaphragm is depressed, and venous return is impaired by increased pressure and vena caval distortion

Fig. CC12.8 Pneumothorax.

Deep to the intercostal, subcostal, and transversus thoracis muscles is a thin but important layer of **endothoracic fascia** that lines the inner surface of the thoracic cage. It attaches the parietal pleura to the thoracic cage so that as the ribs and diaphragm move, the parietal pleura and lungs expand and contract along with them. The endothoracic fascia becomes thicker in the uppermost part of the pleural space, forming a **suprapleural membrane** (Sibson fascia) between the first rib and mediastinum of the thorax. At the inferior limit of the thoracic cage the endothoracic fascia reflects onto the superior surface of the diaphragm as the **diaphragmatic fascia**.

Diaphragm

The **diaphragm** (Fig. 12.9) (also known as respiratory or thoracic diaphragm) is located between the thoracic cavity and the peritoneal cavity of the abdomen. The diaphragm has muscle fibers along its periphery, running from the lumbar vertebrae, lower ribs, and xiphoid process, which are all connected to a **central tendon**. The muscles of the diaphragm are divided into sternal, costal, and lumbar parts. The **sternal part** consists of two small slips of muscle that originate from the xiphoid process and pass posteriorly toward the central tendon. The costal part arises from the deep aspects of ribs 6 to 12 and their costal cartilages. The costal part contributes the

CLINICAL CORRELATION 12.9   Flail Chest

When significant trauma occurs to the thorax a segment of the sternum or an area of the ribcage may become completely detached from other bony elements of the thorax (see Fig. CC12.2). This can occur even if the fracture does not break the skin. The segment will undergo **paradoxical motion** during breathing.

During inhalation it moves deeper due to the drop in pressure in the pleural cavity as the diaphragm drops and the intact part of the ribcage expands. During exhalation the pressure in the pleural cavity increases, which will force the detached, flail segment outward as the rest of the ribcage contracts.

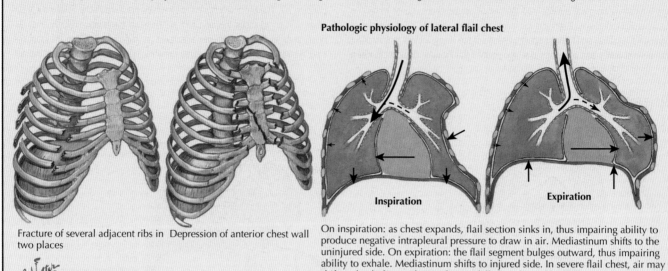

Pathologic physiology of lateral flail chest

Inspiration

Expiration

Fracture of several adjacent ribs in two places   Depression of anterior chest wall

On inspiration: as chest expands, flail section sinks in, thus impairing ability to produce negative intrapleural pressure to draw in air. Mediastinum shifts to the uninjured side. On expiration: the flail segment bulges outward, thus impairing ability to exhale. Mediastinum shifts to injured side. In severe flail chest, air may shift uselessly from side to side (pendelluft) indicated by broken lines

Fig. CC12.9 Flail Chest.

---

majority of muscle to the diaphragm and sweeps laterally and posteriorly from the sternum and chondral arch. Anteriorly it meets the sternal part at the fibrous **sternocostal triangle**, another weak spot in the diaphragm that can allow abdominal contents to herniate superiorly. The costal part meets the lumbar part in the vicinity of the 12th rib, forming the fibrous **lumbocostal triangle**. The **lumbar part** also contributes a significant amount of muscle to the diaphragm. It arises from a **left crus** and larger **right crus** that arise from the anterior L1–L3 vertebral bodies and ascend toward the central tendon. The connection between the left crus and right crus is the **median arcuate ligament**, which covers the aorta. Moving laterally from the diaphragmatic crura, the left and right **medial arcuate ligaments** cross over the psoas major muscles in the posterior abdominal wall and fuse with the psoas fascia. Posterior to the lumbocostal triangle, **lateral arcuate ligaments** cover the quadratus lumborum muscles and fuse with the anterior layer of thoracolumbar fascia on their surface. Muscle fibers arising from the medial and lateral arcuate ligaments fan out

superiorly toward the central tendon. The superior aspect of the central tendon is firmly adherent to the parietal pericardium, the fibrous connective tissue structure that surrounds and protects the heart.

The diaphragm is the most important muscle in respiration. When it is relaxed during expiration, pressure from the abdominal organs causes the diaphragm to dome upward on the left and right into the pleural cavity. The right and left domes (each is sometimes called a **hemidiaphragm**) are covered by the diaphragmatic fascia and then by a layer of diaphragmatic pleura that is in contact with the basal surface of each lung. The left hemidiaphragm reaches the level of the 5th intercostal space during expiration and the right reaches a bit higher to the 5th rib due to the underlying liver. When the diaphragm contracts, it flattens to expand the pleural space and compress the abdominal organs. The muscles of the diaphragm are innervated by the phrenic nerve, which arises from the anterior rami of C3–C5 before traveling along an extended course to reach the diaphragm.

Peripheral Attachments	• Sternal part: posterior xiphoid process
	• Costal part: deep aspect of ribs 6–12 and their costal cartilages
	• Lumbar part:
	  • Left and right crus originating from anterior L1–L3 vertebral bodies and intervertebral discs.
	  • Medial arcuate ligament
	  • Lateral arcuate ligament

Central Attachment	• Central tendon of diaphragm
Functions	• Contraction will cause the diaphragm to flatten and descend. This expands the pleural cavities during inspiration and increases pressure in the abdominal cavity. • Relaxation of the diaphragm will result in it doming upward, pulled by recoil of the lungs in the pleural cavity and pressure from the abdominal cavity below.
Muscle Testing and Signs of Dysfunction	• Flaccid paralysis of ½ of the diaphragm will cause profound difficulty breathing during inspiration that is only partially compensated for by other muscles. • A flaccid diaphragm will dome upward, moving more superiorly during inspiration (paradoxical movement) due to pressure from abdominal organs that are compressed by the healthy ½ of the diaphragm. This can be seen radiographically. • Spasm of the diaphragm results in hiccups.
Innervation	• Motor and sensory activity of the diaphragm is via left and right phrenic nerves from C3 to C5 anterior rami. • Some sensation on the diaphragm and its overlying diaphragmatic pleura is conveyed by nearby intercostal and subcostal nerves.

Blood Supply	• Superior phrenic artery (thoracic aorta) to posterior superior aspect
	• Inferior phrenic artery (abdominal aorta) to its posterior inferior aspect
	• Internal thoracic artery gives off two branches that supply the diaphragm
	  • Pericardiacophrenic artery supplies lateral aspect
	  • Musculophrenic artery supplies anterior and lateral aspect
	• Intercostal arteries supply some of the lateral aspect of the diaphragm

The diaphragm has three large openings within it. The **caval opening**, located at the T8 vertebral level during expiration, allows the IVC to enter the thorax and reach the right atrium of the heart. The **esophageal hiatus** is located slightly to the left of the T10 vertebral level during expiration and it conveys the esophagus from the mediastinum of the thorax into the abdomen. Despite being on the left side, the esophageal hiatus is within the right diaphragmatic crus, a large muscle bundle that shifts strongly to the right as it inserts onto the lumbar vertebral bodies. The median arcuate ligament, formed by the meeting of the left and right diaphragmatic crura, covers the aorta (without compressing it) as it exits the thorax through the **aortic hiatus** at the T12 vertebral level to enter the abdomen (Clinical Correlation 12.10).

Muscles and Fascia of the Abdomen

The muscles of the abdominal wall are anchored to the thoracic cage, lumbar vertebrae, and pelvis, with no bony support on their anterior side. The latissimus dorsi, erector spinae, and serratus posterior inferior muscles are located in close proximity to the muscles that make up the abdominal wall and they have been described in detail in Chapters 9 and 10. Posteriorly, the psoas major described in Chapter 11 forms part of the muscular abdominal wall along with the quadratus lumborum. The external abdominal oblique, internal abdominal oblique, and transversus abdominis muscles sweep across the lateral and anterior sides of the abdomen and give off flat aponeurotic tendons that reach the anterior midline. The rectus abdominis and pyramidalis muscles are oriented vertically and are located on the anterior abdominal wall.

The fascial layers of the abdomen (Figs. 12.10 and 12.11) begin deep to the skin. The **subcutaneous tissue** of the abdomen has a variable amount of adipose within its **fatty layer** (Camper fascia). Immediately underlying it is the **membranous layer** (Scarpa fascia) that is in contact with the abdominal wall muscles. The membranous layer becomes thicker as it approaches the pelvis, where it becomes the superficial perineal fascia. The external abdominal oblique, internal abdominal oblique, and transversus abdominis muscles are found on the anterolateral side of the abdominal wall, deep to the membranous layer of subcutaneous tissue. The superficial and deep aspect of each muscle is covered by its own **investing fascia** (the superficial investing fascia covers the external oblique, the intermediate investing fascia covers the internal oblique, and the deep investing fascia covers the transversus abdominis), which are separated from each other by a thin layer of loose (areolar) connective tissue. This is what allows these layers to slide across each other during flexion, extension, and rotation of the trunk. Each of these muscles gives off a thin but broad aponeurotic tendon that passes across the rectus abdominis muscle. The point where they transition from muscle fibers to aponeurotic tendons is called the **linea semilunaris**. The aponeuroses pass anterior and posterior to the rectus abdominis to form the **rectus sheath**. At the midline, all the aponeuroses insert into a vertical band of connective tissue, the **linea alba**, that is sandwiched between the left and right rectus abdominis muscles. Because the linea alba is located on the anterior midline of the abdomen, it is interrupted by the umbilicus at the **umbilical ring**. Posterior to the transversus abdominis and its deep investing fascia is the **transversalis fascia** (endoabdominal fascia), a layer that lines the inside of the abdominal wall. A variably thick layer of **extraperitoneal fat/fascia** is located between the transversalis fascia and the final layer, the **parietal peritoneum**. The parietal peritoneum lines the inside of the abdominopelvic cavity and is in direct contact with many of the abdominal organs (Clinical Correlation 12.11).

External and Internal Abdominal Oblique and Transversus Abdominis Muscles

The **external abdominal oblique muscle** (see Figs. 12.10A and 12.11B) forms from muscular slips that arise from the

Thoracic surface

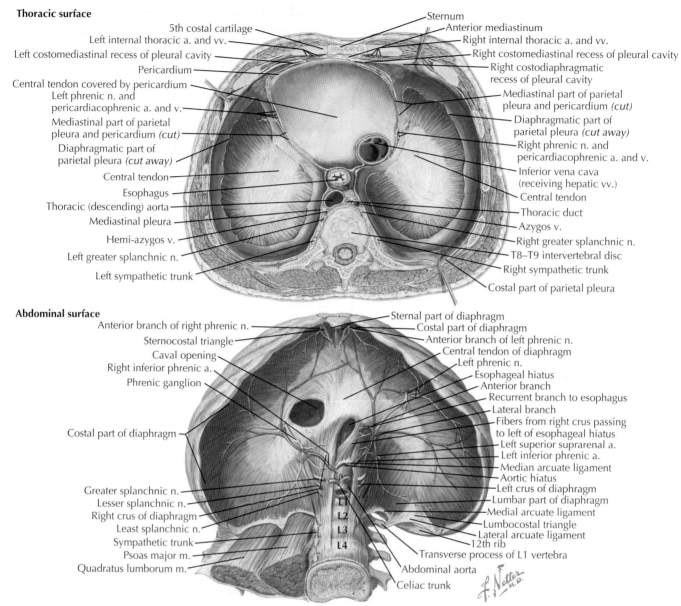

Sternum
Anterior mediastinum
5th costal cartilage
Left internal thoracic a. and vv.
Right internal thoracic a. and vv.
Left costomediastinal recess of pleural cavity
Right costomediastinal recess of pleural cavity
Pericardium
Right costodiaphragmatic recess of pleural cavity
Central tendon covered by pericardium
Left phrenic n. and pericardiacophrenic a. and v.
Mediastinal part of parietal pleura and pericardium (cut)
Mediastinal part of parietal pleura and pericardium (cut)
Diaphragmatic part of parietal pleura (cut away)
Diaphragmatic part of parietal pleura (cut away)
Right phrenic n. and pericardiacophrenic a. and v.
Central tendon
Inferior vena cava (receiving hepatic vv.)
Esophagus
Central tendon
Thoracic (descending) aorta
Thoracic duct
Mediastinal pleura
Azygos v.
Hemi-azygos v.
Right greater splanchnic n.
Left greater splanchnic n.
T8–T9 intervertebral disc
Left sympathetic trunk
Right sympathetic trunk
Costal part of parietal pleura

Abdominal surface

Sternal part of diaphragm
Anterior branch of right phrenic n.
Costal part of diaphragm
Sternocostal triangle
Anterior branch of left phrenic n.
Caval opening
Central tendon of diaphragm
Right inferior phrenic a.
Left phrenic n.
Phrenic ganglion
Esophageal hiatus
Anterior branch
Recurrent branch to esophagus
Lateral branch
Fibers from right crus passing to left of esophageal hiatus
Costal part of diaphragm
Left superior suprarenal a.
Left inferior phrenic a.
Median arcuate ligament
Aortic hiatus
Greater splanchnic n.
Left crus of diaphragm
Lesser splanchnic n.
Lumbar part of diaphragm
Right crus of diaphragm
Medial arcuate ligament
Least splanchnic n.
Lumbocostal triangle
Sympathetic trunk
Lateral arcuate ligament
Psoas major m.
12th rib
Quadratus lumborum m.
Transverse process of L1 vertebra
Abdominal aorta
Celiac trunk
L1
L2
L3
L4

Fig. 12.9 Thoracic and Abdominal Surfaces of the Diaphragm.

superficial aspect of the ribs 5 to 12. Like the serratus anterior muscle, these slips fuse to create a large, flat, powerful muscle. The muscle fibers mimic the appearance of the external intercostal muscles, descending primarily in an inferoanterior direction, which becomes anteromedial as the muscle reaches the anterior side of the abdomen. As it descends, the external abdominal oblique muscle inserts onto the outer lip of the iliac crest starting at or near the tuberculum. Inferiorly, the **external abdominal oblique aponeurosis** inserts from the anterior superior iliac spine, across the superior aspect of the pubic bone, to reach the pubic tubercle. It also passes across the anterior side of the rectus abdominis muscle and contributes to the anterior layer of the rectus sheath. As the aponeurosis inserts between the anterior superior iliac spine and pubic tubercle, it thickens and turns slightly posteriorly. In this area, the aponeurosis is called the **inguinal ligament** and its attachment to

the pelvis marks the separation of the abdomen from the thigh. Medially the inguinal ligament divides to insert on several areas of the pubic bone, creating the pectineal ligament, the lacunar ligament, and the reflected inguinal ligament on the anterior aspect of the rectus sheath. Near the pubic tubercle in males, the external abdominal oblique aponeurosis splits widely to create the **superficial inguinal ring** (see Fig. 12.10A) that allows the spermatic cord to pass into the scrotum and reach the testes. The external abdominal oblique aponeurosis also contributes a layer to the outside of the spermatic cord, the **external spermatic fascia**. The spilt in the aponeurosis creates a **lateral crus** and **medial crus** on either side of the superficial inguinal ring, the two crura are joined and reinforced by **intercrural fibers**. Despite this reinforcement, this gap in the aponeurosis creates a weak spot in the abdominal wall, which predisposes the area to hernias.

CLINICAL CORRELATION 12.10 Diaphragmatic Hernias

The complex anatomy of the diaphragm and the large pressure changes it has to mediate make it a structure that is vulnerable to herniation. **Congenital diaphragmatic hernias** occur during embryonic development and result in gaps in the lateral diaphragm. This allows abdominal organs to move into the left pleural space (the liver typically blocks such a herniation on the right side), which compresses the lungs and other thoracic contents. If not diagnosed prior to birth, this will lead to lung failure and death when the neonate attempts to breathe. A similar presentation may occur when the phrenic nerve is damaged, causing the diaphragm to manifest flaccid paralysis. This can result in **eventration of the diaphragm**, wherein the abdominal contents push the paralyzed diaphragm into the thorax, compressing the lung. A less severe congenital hernia is the **retrosternal (Morgagni) hernia** that results from a gap or weakness in the diaphragm's attachments to the xiphoid process, allowing abdominal organs to push into the inferior mediastinum, just posterior to the sternum. **Hiatal hernias** involve a portion of the stomach being pulled through the esophageal hiatus by the esophagus (sliding hiatal hernia) or being pushed through the hiatus alongside the esophagus (paraesophageal hiatal hernia).

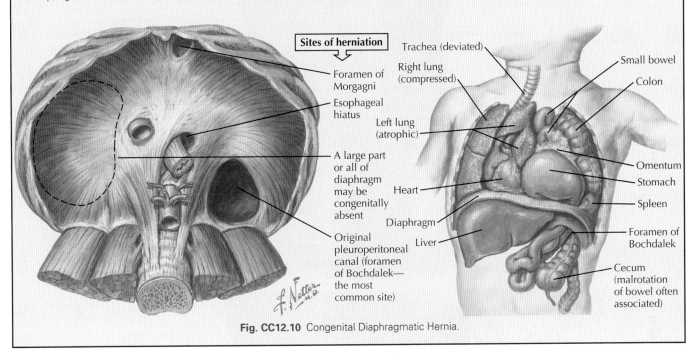

Fig. CC12.10 Congenital Diaphragmatic Hernia.

Deep to the external abdominal oblique is the **internal abdominal oblique muscle** (see Fig. 12.10B and 12.11B), which originates posteriorly from the middle layer of the thoracolumbar fascia, the intermediate zone of the iliac crest, and a small part of the lateral, deep inguinal ligament. Its fibers run in a superomedial direction, perpendicular to those of the external abdominal oblique, and its **internal abdominal oblique aponeurosis** inserts onto the superficial aspects of ribs 10 to 12, contributes to the rectus sheath, then inserts onto the linea alba. Inferiorly, it fuses with the aponeurosis of the transversus abdominis to form a **conjoint tendon** (inguinal falx) that inserts onto the pectineal line of the pubis. As the spermatic cord passes through the internal abdominal oblique muscle, some of the muscle fibers join the cord and form the **cremaster muscle** that (see Fig. 12.10B and 12.11A) elevates the testes when it contracts.

Deep to the internal abdominal oblique is the **transversus abdominis muscle** (see Fig. 12.11). Muscle slips that form this muscle come from the internal aspect of ribs 7 to 12 (alongside fibers that contribute to the diaphragm), the middle layer of thoracolumbar fascia, the inner lip of the iliac crest, as well as a small part of the lateral, deep inguinal ligament. This muscle travels horizontally across the abdomen and gives off the **transversus abdominis aponeurosis** that contributes to the rectus sheath and inserts onto the linea alba. Inferolaterally, the fibers of this muscle may fuse somewhat with those of the internal abdominal oblique since it shares a common origin from the ilium and deep aspect of the ilioinguinal ligament. Inferomedially, the aponeuroses of these two muscles will fuse into a conjoint tendon that inserts onto the pubic bone just posterior to the medial crus of the superficial inguinal ring. Lateral

A. Superficial dissection anterolateral abdominal wall

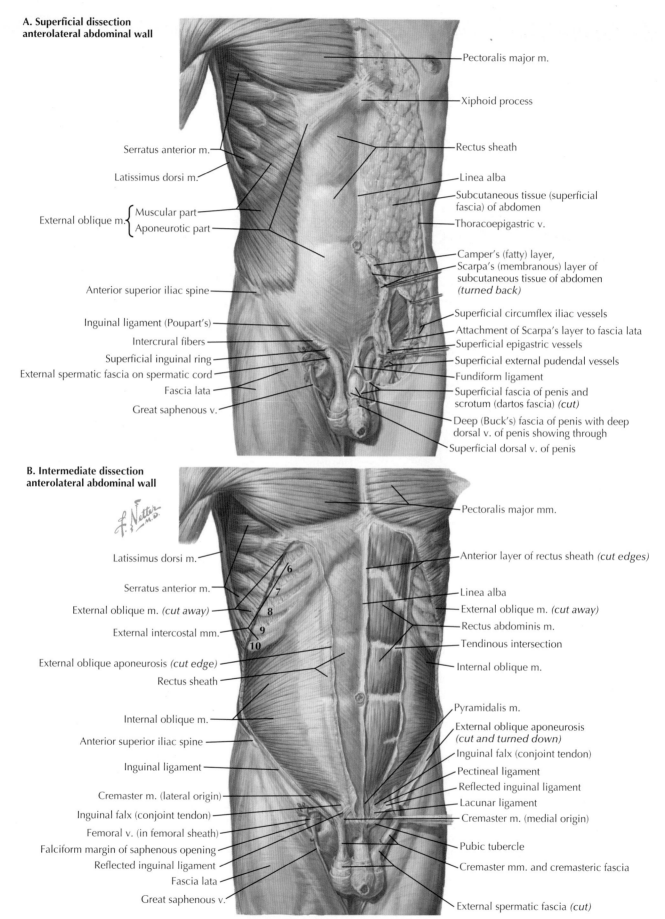

Pectoralis major m.

Xiphoid process

Rectus sheath

Linea alba

Subcutaneous tissue (superficial fascia) of abdomen

Thoracoepigastric v.

Camper's (fatty) layer, Scarpa's (membranous) layer of subcutaneous tissue of abdomen *(turned back)*

Superficial circumflex iliac vessels

Attachment of Scarpa's layer to fascia lata

Superficial epigastric vessels

Superficial external pudendal vessels

Fundiform ligament

Superficial fascia of penis and scrotum (dartos fascia) *(cut)*

Deep (Buck's) fascia of penis with deep dorsal v. of penis showing through

Superficial dorsal v. of penis

Serratus anterior m.

Latissimus dorsi m.

External oblique m. { Muscular part / Aponeurotic part }

Anterior superior iliac spine

Inguinal ligament (Poupart's)

Intercrural fibers

Superficial inguinal ring

External spermatic fascia on spermatic cord

Fascia lata

Great saphenous v.

B. Intermediate dissection anterolateral abdominal wall

Pectoralis major mm.

Anterior layer of rectus sheath *(cut edges)*

Linea alba

External oblique m. *(cut away)*

Rectus abdominis m.

Tendinous intersection

Internal oblique m.

Pyramidalis m.

External oblique aponeurosis *(cut and turned down)*

Inguinal falx (conjoint tendon)

Pectineal ligament

Reflected inguinal ligament

Lacunar ligament

Cremaster m. (medial origin)

Pubic tubercle

Cremaster mm. and cremasteric fascia

External spermatic fascia *(cut)*

Latissimus dorsi m.

Serratus anterior m.

External oblique m. *(cut away)*

External intercostal mm.

External oblique aponeurosis *(cut edge)*

Rectus sheath

Internal oblique m.

Anterior superior iliac spine

Inguinal ligament

Cremaster m. (lateral origin)

Inguinal falx (conjoint tendon)

Femoral v. (in femoral sheath)

Falciform margin of saphenous opening

Reflected inguinal ligament

Fascia lata

Great saphenous v.

6
7
8
9
10

f. Netter m.d.

Fig. 12.10 Anterior Abdominal Wall.

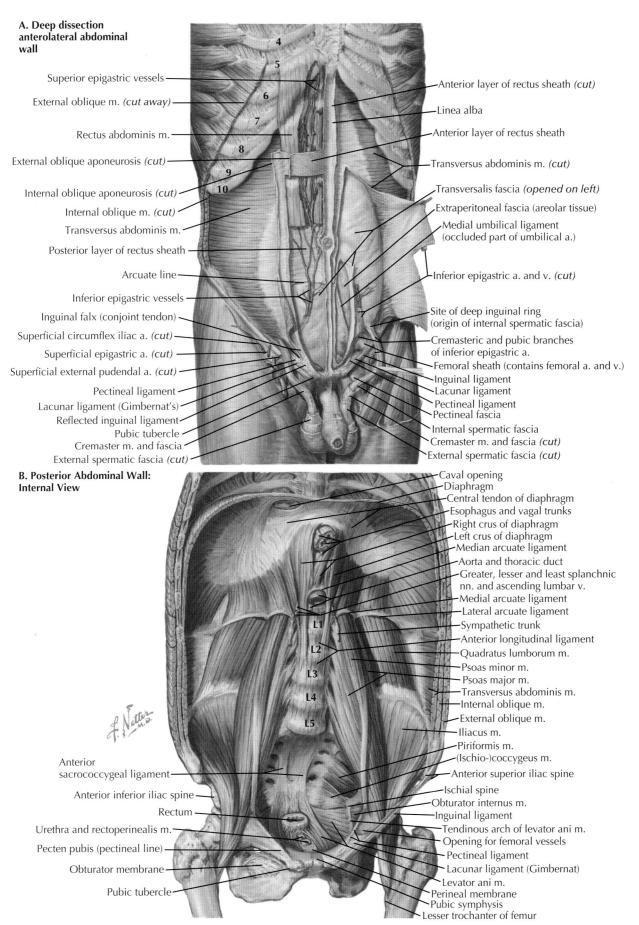

A. Deep dissection anterolateral abdominal wall

Superior epigastric vessels

External oblique m. *(cut away)*

Rectus abdominis m.

External oblique aponeurosis *(cut)*

Internal oblique aponeurosis *(cut)*

Internal oblique m. *(cut)*

Transversus abdominis m.

Posterior layer of rectus sheath

Arcuate line

Inferior epigastric vessels

Inguinal falx (conjoint tendon)

Superficial circumflex iliac a. *(cut)*

Superficial epigastric a. *(cut)*

Superficial external pudendal a. *(cut)*

Pectineal ligament

Lacunar ligament (Gimbernat's)

Reflected inguinal ligament

Pubic tubercle

Cremaster m. and fascia

External spermatic fascia *(cut)*

Anterior layer of rectus sheath *(cut)*

Linea alba

Anterior layer of rectus sheath

Transversus abdominis m. *(cut)*

Transversalis fascia *(opened on left)*

Extraperitoneal fascia (areolar tissue)

Medial umbilical ligament (occluded part of umbilical a.)

Inferior epigastric a. and v. *(cut)*

Site of deep inguinal ring (origin of internal spermatic fascia)

Cremasteric and pubic branches of inferior epigastric a.

Femoral sheath (contains femoral a. and v.)

Inguinal ligament

Lacunar ligament

Pectineal ligament

Pectineal fascia

Internal spermatic fascia

Cremaster m. and fascia *(cut)*

External spermatic fascia *(cut)*

B. Posterior Abdominal Wall: Internal View

Caval opening

Diaphragm

Central tendon of diaphragm

Esophagus and vagal trunks

Right crus of diaphragm

Left crus of diaphragm

Median arcuate ligament

Aorta and thoracic duct

Greater, lesser and least splanchnic nn. and ascending lumbar v.

Medial arcuate ligament

Lateral arcuate ligament

Sympathetic trunk

Anterior longitudinal ligament

Quadratus lumborum m.

Psoas minor m.

Psoas major m.

Transversus abdominis m.

Internal oblique m.

External oblique m.

Iliacus m.

Piriformis m.

(Ischio-)coccygeus m.

Anterior superior iliac spine

Ischial spine

Obturator internus m.

Inguinal ligament

Tendinous arch of levator ani m.

Opening for femoral vessels

Pectineal ligament

Lacunar ligament (Gimbernat)

Levator ani m.

Perineal membrane

Pubic symphysis

Lesser trochanter of femur

Anterior sacrococcygeal ligament

Anterior inferior iliac spine

Rectum

Urethra and rectoperinealis m.

Pecten pubis (pectineal line)

Obturator membrane

Pubic tubercle

Fig. 12.11 Anterior and Posterior Abdominal Wall.

CLINICAL CORRELATION 12.11   Tension Lines of the Skin/Langer Lines

The skin and underlying fascial layers are connected by bands of tissue that take on a distinctive orientation in each region of the body. When an incision is made parallel to these tension (Langer) lines, the wound does not tend to open. When an incision is made across these lines, it will gape and be more difficult to suture. In the forearm, thigh, and leg these lines primarily run from proximal to distal, with some transverse lines around the anterior knee and posterior elbow. On the posterior neck, upper posterior thorax, arm, lower back, abdomen, and lateral thigh the lines are mostly horizontal. The upper chest has lines running inferomedially while the lines in the pectoral region are mostly vertical and the middle back has lines running inferolaterally. Tension lines in the inguinal and gluteal regions run inferomedially.

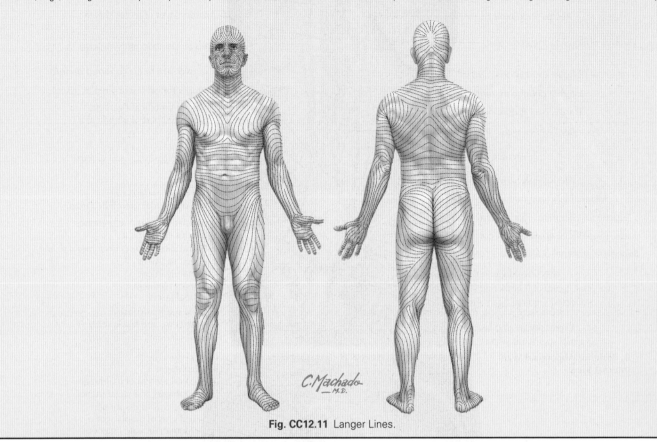

Fig. CC12.11 Langer Lines.

CLINICAL CORRELATION 12.12   Inguinal Canal

The **inguinal canal** is a channel through the anteroinferior abdominal wall that conveys the ductus deferens and testicular vessels toward the testes in males and the round ligament of the uterus into the connective tissues of the labia majora in females (see Fig. 12.12). Hereafter, I will discuss how the spermatic cord is formed and not focus on the round ligament of the uterus. This is not out of latent sexism (or so I hope) but because the round ligament is a connective tissue remnant of the gubernaculum with minimal clinical problems related to it, while the spermatic cord is a large structure that is involved in several common clinical problems. The ductus deferens and testicular vessels develop posterior/deep to the peritoneal cavity, so as they leave the abdomen, they do not pierce the parietal peritoneum. However, they do pierce the transversalis fascia immediately lateral to the inferior epigastric artery at the deep inguinal ring. As they do so, they pick up a layer called the **internal spermatic fascia** that bundles them together as the spermatic cord. The spermatic cord passes inferior to the transversus abdominis muscle and then passes through the internal abdominal oblique muscle, from which it picks up slips of skeletal muscle (and accompanying nerve and vessels), creating the **cremaster muscle,** which also contains bundles of smooth muscle interspersed alongside the skeletal muscle fibers. As the spermatic cord passes through the external abdominal oblique aponeurosis at the superficial inguinal ring, it picks up the **external spermatic fascia.** The cord then descends into the scrotum and testes.

to the conjoint tendon is a gap in the inferior border of the muscle that allows the spermatic cord to pass through. This gap is located near the **deep inguinal ring** that is formed as the ductus deferens and testicular vessels pierce the transversalis fascia to create the spermatic cord (Clinical Correlations 12.12 and 12.13).

Superior/ Posterior Attachments	• External abdominal oblique: superficial aspects of ribs 5–12 • Internal abdominal oblique: middle layer of thoracolumbar fascia, intermediate zone of iliac crest, lateral aspect of inguinal ligament • Transversus abdominis: internal aspects of ribs 7–12, middle layer of thoracolumbar fascia, inner lip of anterior iliac crest, lateral aspect of inguinal ligament
Inferior/Anterior Attachments	• External abdominal oblique: outer lip of anterior iliac crest, superior pubic bone and tubercle (as the inguinal ligament), and linea alba (as part of the rectus sheath) • Internal abdominal oblique: superficial aspects of ribs 10–12, linea alba (as part of the rectus sheath) and pectineal line of pubis (as the conjoint tendon) • Transversus abdominis: linea alba (as part of the rectus sheath) and pectineal line of pubis (as the conjoint tendon)
Functions	• Bilateral contraction of the abdominal oblique and transversus abdominis muscles will compress the abdominal contents and slightly flex the torso. • External abdominal oblique: unilateral contraction rotates torso contralaterally (e.g., contraction of right external oblique rotates the upper body to the left) • Internal abdominal oblique: unilateral contraction rotates the torso ipsilaterally (e.g., contraction of right internal oblique rotates the upper body to the right) • Transversus abdominis: compresses abdominal contents
Muscle Testing and Signs of Dysfunction	• Loss of innervation due to injury to one nerve (possibly during surgery) would be compensated for by the nearby muscles but would leave a strip of flaccidly paralyzed muscle, possibly resulting in a weak spot that may be prone to herniation.
Innervation	• External abdominal oblique: T7–T11 intercostal and subcostal T12 nerves • Internal abdominal oblique and transversus abdominis: T6–T11 intercostal nerves, T12 subcostal nerve, branches from L1 anterior ramus
Blood Supply	• Intercostal arteries 10–11 • Subcostal artery • Musculophrenic artery • Deep circumflex iliac artery • Superficial circumflex iliac artery • Superficial epigastric artery

Rectus Abdominis and Pyramidalis Muscles

The **rectus abdominis muscle** (Fig. 12.12, see also Figs. 12.10B and 12.11A) is one of the most famous muscles in the body and many people spend a great deal of effort to develop this muscle and get "6-pack abs." The reason for the distinctive appearance of the rectus abdominis is that its individual muscle bellies, which hypertrophy with consistent exercise, are separated from each other by **tendinous intersections** that are adherent to the overlying rectus sheath. These distinct muscle bellies are one of the few places we can see evidence of the separate myotomes that were derived from the segmented somites. Superiorly, the rectus abdominis attaches broadly to the costal cartilages of ribs 5 to 7 and the xiphoid process. As it descends, it has between 4 and 5 muscular bellies separated by its tendinous intersections before it inserts onto the superior pubic bone and pubic symphysis. The left and right rectus sheaths are separated by the linea alba on the median plane of the abdomen, while the linea semilunaris is located on the lateral side of each rectus sheath. The most anterior parts of the T6–T11 intercostal nerves and subcostal nerves innervate the rectus abdominis and also give off anterior cutaneous nerves to the overlying skin. Two vessels supply the rectus abdominis within the sheath: the superior epigastric artery leaves the internal thoracic artery and supplies the superior portion of the muscle, while the large inferior epigastric artery arises from the external iliac artery and ascends within the rectus sheath to supply the inferior part of the muscle and anastomose with the superior epigastric artery. When this muscle contracts it will strongly flex the torso and lumbar vertebrae, bringing the ribs closer to the pelvis and compressing the contents of the abdominopelvic cavity. If the lower limbs are not bearing weight, then contraction of the rectus abdominis tilts the pelvis anterosuperiorly, as is done in leg-lifts.

A very small, triangular **pyramidalis muscle** (see Figs. 12.10B and 12.12) is often (~92%) present anterior to the rectus abdominis in the inferior abdomen. This muscle is not a major mover of the body as it extends from the most inferior part of the linea alba to the pubic bones, attaching just anterior to the rectus abdominis. Contraction of this muscle may tense the anterior body wall and assist the rectus abdominis in a very minor way (Biomechanics Box 12.1 and Clinical Correlation 12.14).

Superior Attachment	• Rectus abdominis: costal cartilages of ribs 5–6 and xiphoid process
	• Pyramidalis: inferior linea alba
Inferior Attachments	• Rectus abdominis: superior pubic bones, pubic crest, pubic symphysis
	• Pyramidalis: pubic crest immediately anterior to rectus abdominis muscle
Functions	• Flexes the torso and lumbar vertebrae, bringing the ribs and pelvis closer. If the pelvis is fixed in place, the upper body will curl inferiorly. If the thorax is fixed in place, then the pelvis and lower limbs will move superiorly.
	• Like the abdominal oblique and transversus abdominis muscles, contraction of the rectus abdominis muscle compresses the organs of the abdominopelvic cavity.
Muscle Testing and Signs of Dysfunction	• Weakness of the rectus abdominis due to de-innervation or atrophy will result in protrusion of the inferior abdominal wall when standing, even in slender people. This is due to anterior settling of the abdominal organs, which are not held back by the rectus abdominis.
	• Patients with weak or atrophied rectus abdominis muscles may be unable to do a sit-up without assistance from the upper limbs or rolling to one side. Hip flexors may be used to compensate and the examiner should watch to ensure that the torso is "curling" during the exercise.
Innervation	• Rectus abdominis: T6–T11 intercostal and T12 subcostal nerves
	• Pyramidalis: T12 subcostal nerve
Blood Supply	• Superior epigastric artery from the internal thoracic artery
	• Inferior epigastric artery from the external iliac artery

Inferior Attachments	• Internal lip of posterior iliac crest
	• Iliolumbar ligaments
Superior Attachment	• Medial inferior aspect of 12th rib
	• Tips of lumbar transverse processes
Functions	• Ipsilateral side bending of the lumbar vertebrae
	• Depression of the 12th rib
	• Weak extension of the lumbar vertebrae
Muscle Testing and Signs of Dysfunction	• The quadratus lumborum may become tight or spastic due to atrophy or postural issues. It is an underappreciated source of lower back pain and spasm may persistently side-bend the back toward the tightened muscle.
	• It can be stretched by having a patient sit with the hip stable. He or she then reaches the upper limb over the head and side-bends the body away from the quadratus lumborum muscle that is being stretched.
Innervation	• T12 subcostal nerve
	• Anterior rami of L1–L4
Blood Supply	• Iliolumbar artery
	• Subcostal and lumbar arteries

Quadratus Lumborum

The **quadratus lumborum muscle** (see Fig. 12.11) is located on the posterior abdominal wall, medial to the origin of the internal abdominal oblique and transversus abdominis muscles from the middle layer of the thoracolumbar fascia. The quadratus lumborum is sandwiched by the middle and anterior layers of the thoracolumbar fascia as they fold medially to insert onto the lumbar transverse processes. The quadratus lumborum attaches to the medial, inferior aspect of the 12th rib, the tips of the lumbar transverse processes, and the internal lip of the iliac crest on the posterior ilium and the nearby iliolumbar ligaments. It is innervated by all the nerves that are near it, the subcostal (T12) nerve, and the anterior rami of L1–L4. The quadratus lumborum is a weak extender of the back but is significant in side-bending/lateral flexion of the lumbar vertebrae. It depresses the 12th rib during expiration and fixes it in place so that internal intercostal muscles have a solid anchor point to depress the more superior ribs.

Muscles and Fascia of the Pelvis

The pelvic muscles and fascia form complex structures that are linked to the ilium, ischium, and pubis as well as the pelvic organs themselves. The psoas major, iliacus, piriformis, obturator internus, and obturator externus muscles (see Fig. 12.11) are prominent in the pelvis but they exert their action primarily in the lower limb and they have been discussed in detail in that chapter. The **psoas major** and **iliacus muscles** are found in the greater pelvis as they descend anteriorly to reach the anterior thigh. The **piriformis muscle** is located in the lesser pelvis on the anterior surface of the sacrum but exits laterally through the greater sciatic foramen to reach the greater trochanter. The **obturator internus muscle** forms the lateral wall of the lesser pelvis as it sits on the medial side of the obturator foramen and sends its tendon posteriorly to turn across the lesser sciatic notch to the greater trochanter.

The **pelvic diaphragm** forms a bowl that supports the pelvic organs within the lesser pelvis but through which the urethra, vagina, and rectum pass on their way to the external environment. More inferiorly is a (mostly) triangular sheet of muscle and fascia, the **urogenital triangle**, which anchors and surrounds the erectile tissues of the external genitalia and through which the urethra and vagina pass. A more posterior **anal triangle** has fewer muscles but those that are present surround the distal rectum and anus as they reach the outside. Together, the urogenital and anal triangles are called the **perineum**.

Pelvic Diaphragm—Levator Ani and Coccygeus Muscles

The **pelvic diaphragm** (Fig. 12.13, see also Fig. 12.11) originates from the lateral wall of the lesser pelvis and descends as it approaches the body's midline. Unlike the thoracic diaphragm, which domes upward and descends on contraction,

Since the abdominal muscles surround the abdominal organs, weakness of the abdominal muscles coupled with increased abdominal pressure can cause the abdominal organs, frequently the small intestines, to push through weak spots in the body wall, called **herniation**. There are several areas that are particularly prone to herniation. Lumbar hernias were discussed in Chapter 9 and femoral hernias in Chapter 11. Since the spermatic cord pierces the abdominal wall via the inguinal canal, it creates a weak spot in that location. If intra-abdominal pressure is too great, the small intestine can be pushed through this weak spot

(shoving a layer of parietal peritoneum ahead of it, called a hernia sac) to create an **indirect inguinal hernia**. Since this hernia parallels the spermatic cord, it can extend into the scrotum or (rarely in women) the labia majora. Another weak spot, the **inguinal triangle,** exists in the lower abdomen **and** is bounded by the lateral aspect of the rectus abdominis muscle, the inferior epigastric artery, and the inguinal ligament. A **direct inguinal hernia** may push through this space and protrude directly through the abdominal wall above the pubic bone. These hernias do not descend into the scrotum or labia majora.

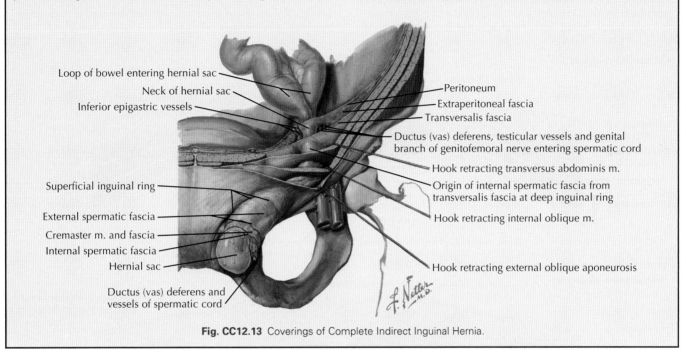

Fig. CC12.13 Coverings of Complete Indirect Inguinal Hernia.

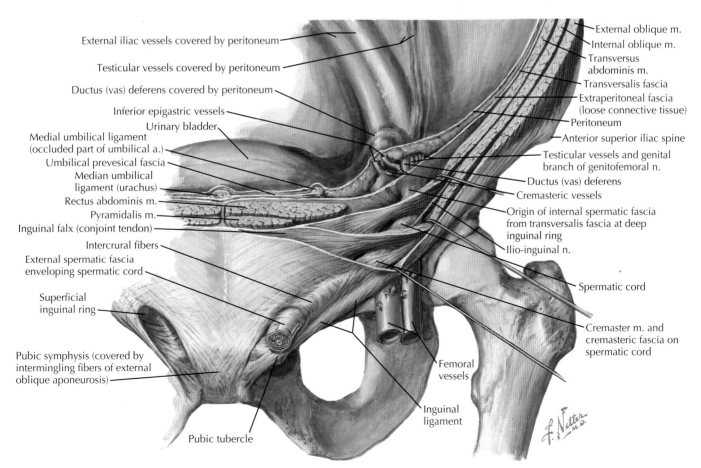

Fig. 12.12 Inguinal Canal and Spermatic Cord.

BIOMECHANICS BOX 12.1   **The Rectus Sheath**

The **rectus sheath** surrounds the rectus abdominis and pyramidalis muscles, isolating them from the other muscles and acting as a compression sleeve that helps the muscles contract more efficiently (see Fig. 12.10). Posterior to the sheath is the transversalis fascia, extraperitoneal fat, and parietal peritoneum. The layering of the rectus sheath is complex, with an **anterior layer** and a **posterior layer** that shifts to become thicker anteriorly at a point approximately 3 cm inferior to the umbilicus, called the **arcuate line**. Superior to the arcuate

line, the anterior layer of the rectus sheath is formed by the aponeurosis of the external abdominal oblique and ½ of the internal abdominal oblique aponeurosis; the posterior layer is formed by the other ½ of the internal abdominal oblique aponeurosis and the transversus abdominis aponeurosis. Inferior to the arcuate line the anterior layer of the rectus sheath is formed by the aponeurosis of the external abdominal oblique, the internal abdominal oblique aponeurosis, and the transversus abdominis aponeurosis.

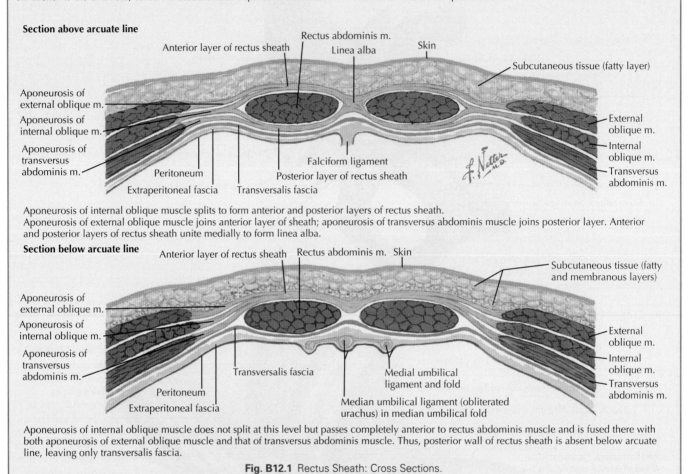

Section above arcuate line

Anterior layer of rectus sheath — Rectus abdominis m. — Linea alba — Skin — Subcutaneous tissue (fatty layer)

Aponeurosis of external oblique m.
Aponeurosis of internal oblique m.
Aponeurosis of transversus abdominis m.

Peritoneum — Extraperitoneal fascia — Transversalis fascia — Posterior layer of rectus sheath — Falciform ligament

External oblique m. — Internal oblique m. — Transversus abdominis m.

Aponeurosis of internal oblique muscle splits to form anterior and posterior layers of rectus sheath.
Aponeurosis of external oblique muscle joins anterior layer of sheath; aponeurosis of transversus abdominis muscle joins posterior layer. Anterior and posterior layers of rectus sheath unite medially to form linea alba.

Section below arcuate line

Anterior layer of rectus sheath — Rectus abdominis m. Skin — Subcutaneous tissue (fatty and membranous layers)

Aponeurosis of external oblique m.
Aponeurosis of internal oblique m.
Aponeurosis of transversus abdominis m.

Transversalis fascia — Medial umbilical ligament and fold

Peritoneum — Extraperitoneal fascia — Median umbilical ligament (obliterated urachus) in median umbilical fold

External oblique m. — Internal oblique m. — Transversus abdominis m.

Aponeurosis of internal oblique muscle does not split at this level but passes completely anterior to rectus abdominis muscle and is fused there with both aponeurosis of external oblique muscle and that of transversus abdominis muscle. Thus, posterior wall of rectus sheath is absent below arcuate line, leaving only transversalis fascia.

Fig. B12.1 Rectus Sheath: Cross Sections.

CLINICAL CORRELATION 12.14   **Other Abdominal Hernias**

While the abdominal wall is a fairly stout sleeve of muscle, there are some additional areas that are prone to herniation when intra-abdominal pressure exceeds its ability to resist the push of the abdominal organs. The linea alba is a tough band of connective tissue but **epigastric hernias of the linea alba** can occur through its superior half (between the xiphoid process and umbilicus) and **umbilical hernias** may push through the linea alba in the vicinity of the umbilicus itself. Umbilical hernias occur regularly in newborns and can be repaired if they do not reduce on their own. More laterally, the gut tube can herniate through a weakness of the linea semilunaris, causing a **Spigelian hernia**. Umbilical, epigastric, and Spigelian hernias can occur in adults and are associated with obesity and muscle atrophy.

the pelvic diaphragm domes inferiorly and ascends when it contracts. This arrangement makes it such that contraction of both diaphragms will raise the pressure in the abdominopelvic cavity. This is common during labored breathing, sneezing, and defecation. The pelvic diaphragm consists of two muscles, the levator ani (which is further subdivided) and the coccygeus muscle. The **levator ani muscle** begins on the posterior surface of the pubic bone and continues laterally across the fascia of the obturator internus muscle, passing from the pubis to the ilium and toward the ischial spine. This attachment is strengthened by a thickened region of the obturator fascia, the **tendinous arch of the levator ani**. From its fixed position on the lateral wall of the pelvis, the levator ani descends medially, wrapping around the vagina and/or rectum before it attaches to its counterpart from the opposite side or to the inferior sacrum and coccyx. There are three muscles that contribute to the levator ani muscle. The left and right **puborectalis muscles** originate from the posterior body of the pubis and extend their fibers around the posterior aspect of the distal rectum, forming a **puborectal sling** that bends the rectum anterosuperiorly. The tone of this muscle helps to maintain rectal continence. Anterior to the rectum is a space between the left and right puborectalis muscles, the **urogenital hiatus**, which allows the vagina and/or urethra to pass through the levator ani. Originating a bit more laterally from the pubic body and tendinous arch, the left and right **pubococcygeus muscles** fan out more broadly and meet each other on the midline just posterior to the rectum, as thin tendons that form a fibrous raphe, the **anococcygeal body**. Along its length the pubococcygeus also gives off discrete slips of muscle that pass superior to the puborectalis muscle and surround the anus (puboanalis muscle), vagina in females (pubovaginalis muscle), or prostate in males (puboprostaticus muscle). Between the vagina or prostate anteriorly and the anus posteriorly is a thin sheet (puboperinealis muscle) that surrounds the **perineal body**, a midline knot of connective tissue that helps anchor and stabilize structures of the perineum. The final member of the levator ani is the thin **iliococcygeus muscle**, which originates from the posterior aspect of the tendinous arch and extends fibers medially to meet its counterpart at the midline raphe that creates part of the anococcygeal body as well as the coccyx and possibly inferior sacrum.

Posterior to the levator ani is the **coccygeus (ischiococcygeus) muscle**, the other contributor to the pelvic diaphragm. It stretches between the ischial spine and the coccyx and inferior sacrum. In humans this muscle pushes upward against the abdominopelvic organs when it contracts and may move the coccyx to a small degree. In dogs, this stout muscle wags the tail. As the most inferior muscles of the body, the muscles of the pelvic diaphragm are innervated by the lowest spinal levels, the S4–S5 anterior rami as well the coccygeal plexus. The pudendal nerve (S2–S4) travels near the levator ani (within the fascia of the obturator internus) and may contribute some axons originating from the S4 anterior ramus.

Anterior/Lateral Attachments	• Levator ani
	  • Puborectalis: posterior body of pubis
	  • Pubococcygeus: posterior body of pubis and anterior tendinous arch of levator ani on obturator fascia
	  • Iliococcygeus: posterior part of tendinous arch of levator ani
	• Coccygeus: ischial spine

Posterior/Medial Attachments	• Levator ani
	  • Puborectalis: meets opposite puborectalis posterior to rectum
	  • Pubococcygeus: anococcygeal body and coccyx, also midline perineal structures
	  • Iliococcygeus: anococcygeal body, coccyx, and inferior sacrum
	• Coccygeus: inferior sacrum and coccyx

Functions	• Levator ani—maintains rectal continence and supports the pelvic viscera, especially when pressure in the abdominopelvic cavity is increased.
	  • Puborectalis: forms puborectal sling between the left and right pubic bones and the posterior rectum. Tone of this muscle "kinks" the rectum and discourages defecation.
	  • Pubococcygeus: elevates pelvic diaphragm to support and compress pelvic viscera. Additional slips (puboanalis, pubovaginalis, puboprostatic, puboperinealis muscles) exist superior to the puborectalis and surround midline structures of the perineum, compressing and elevating them.
	  • Iliococcygeus: elevates pelvic diaphragm, supports and compresses pelvic viscera
	• Coccygeus: elevates pelvic diaphragm to support and compress pelvic viscera, also slight movement of the coccyx.

Muscle Testing and Signs of Dysfunction	• Weakness of the pelvic diaphragm can occur for several reasons: nerve damage, atrophy from lack of use, trauma due to laceration or childbirth, or hernia. Rectal incontinence may occur since the rectum is no longer strongly supported. • Weakness of the pelvic diaphragm can predispose a person to hernias or prolapse of organs through their openings into the perineal region.
Innervation	• S4–S5 anterior rami, possibly via the pudendal nerve (S2–S4) • Coccygeal plexus
Blood Supply	• Branches of inferior vesical, internal pudendal, inferior gluteal arteries, which arise from internal iliac artery

A. Pelvic diaphragm: female

Medial view

Pubic bone (*cut surface*)

Obturator canal
Urethra
Vagina
Pubococcygeus m.
Tendinous arch of levator ani m.
Rectum
Iliococcygeus m.
Ischial spine
Coccygeus
Coccyx
Piriformis m.

Obturator internus m. and obturator fascia (*cut*)
Arcuate line of ilium

Inferior view
Musculofascial extensions to urethra
Pubic symphysis
Deep dorsal v. of clitoris
Musculofascial extensions to vagina
Inferior (arcuate) pubic ligament
Puborectalis m.
Urethra
Pubococcygeus m.
Inferior pubic ramus
Iliococcygeus m.
Vagina
Tendinous arch of levator ani m.
Interdigitating fibers of perineum
Obturator internus m.
Rectum
Ischial tuberosity
Levator plate (median raphe) of levator ani m.
Ischial spine
(Ischio-)coccygeus m.
Piriformis m. (*cut*)
Sacrospinous ligament (*cut*)
Sacrotuberous ligament (*cut*)
Sacrum
Obturator internus tendon
Ischial spine
Sacrospinous ligament
Piriformis m.
Sacrotuberous ligament
Anococcygeal body (ligament) (attachment of external anal sphincter m.)
Tip of coccyx

Superior view
Inferior (arcuate) pubic ligament
Pubic symphysis
Inguinal ligament (Poupart's)
Urethra
Vagina
Rectum
Levator plate (median raphe) of levator ani m.
Coccyx
Anterior sacrococcygeal ligament
Sacral promontory
Deep dorsal v. of clitoris
Transverse perineal ligament
Fascia of deep perineal mm.
Obturator canal
Obturator fascia (over obturator internus m.)
Tendinous arch of levator ani m.
Pubococcygeus m.
Ischial spine
Iliococcygeus m.
Piriformis m.
Coccygeus (ischiococcygeus) m.

B. Ischioanal fossae

Ureter
Extraperitoneal (supralevator) space (fibrofatty tissue)
Submucous space (internal venous plexus)
Fat body of ischio-anal fossa
Transverse fibrous septum of ischio-anal fossa
Peri-anal space (external venous plexus)
Intersphincteric groove (anocutaneous line)

Sigmoid colon
Iliacus m. and fascia
External iliac vessels
Iliopectineal line
Sacrogenital fold (uterosacral in female)
Peritoneum (*cut edge*) forming floor of pararectal fossa
Tendinous arch of levator ani m.
Obturator internus m. and fascia
Levator ani m. and superior and inferior fascia of pelvic diaphragm
Pudendal canal (Alcock's) contains internal pudendal vessels, pudendal n., and perineal n.
Rectal fascia
Ischial tuberosity
External anal sphincter m.
Conjoined longitudinal m.
Internal anal sphincter m.

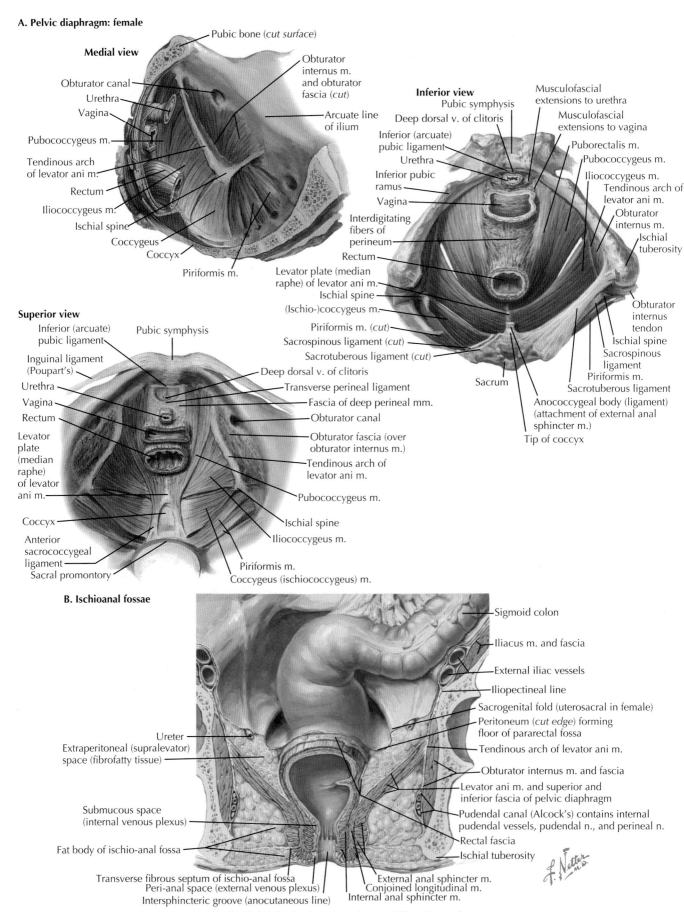

Fig. 12.13 (A) Pelvic diaphragm: female; (B) ischioanal fossae.

Muscles of the Deep Perineal Space—Superior to Perineal Membrane

The walls of the abdominopelvic cavity (Fig. 12.14, see also Fig. 12.13B) are covered by **parietal peritoneum** that releases an aqueous fluid that allows the abdominopelvic organs to glide across each other and the body wall and discourages adhesions from forming. The organs of the abdomen and pelvis are covered by **visceral peritoneum** and an underlying layer of **visceral pelvic fascia** that anchors each organ to its mesentery or the body wall. As the rectum, vagina, and urethra pierce the pelvic diaphragm, the visceral pelvic fascia reflects onto the muscles of the pelvic diaphragm, becoming **parietal pelvic fascia**. This fascia can be further classified by the structures that it covers (piriformis fascia, obturator internus fascia, superior and inferior fascia of the pelvic diaphragm, pre-sacral fascia) and it is continuous with the transversalis fascia of the abdomen and the psoas fascia of the greater pelvis. The visceral and parietal pelvic fascia thicken along the area where they meet and organs pierce the pelvic diaphragm. This thickened line of fascia extending from the pubis to the sacrum is called the **tendinous arch of the pelvic fascia** (NOT to be confused with the nearby but different tendinous arch of the levator ani) and it anchors the pelvic organs in place. Between the parietal pelvic fascia and the overlying parietal peritoneum is a variable layer, the **extraperitoneal fascia**, which may be thin and indistinct or contain a significant amount of adipose tissue.

The **perineum** (see Fig. 12.14) is the inferior region of the pelvis where the anus and external genitalia are found. The perineum is covered by skin and is composed of the urogenital and anal triangles. The **urogenital triangle** has one apex at the pubic symphysis and the other two at the left and right ischial tuberosities. The two lateral borders of the triangle are formed by the medial aspect of both the inferior pubic and ischial rami (often called the ischiopubic ramus) on each side of the pelvis. The posterior border of the triangle is formed by an imaginary line between the two ischial tuberosities with the perineal body at or near the midpoint of the line. Note that the perineal body does not always lie on the line between the two ischial tuberosities, so the posterior border of the urogenital triangle is sometimes a bit convex anteriorly.

The posterior border of the urogenital triangle is also the anterior border of the **anal triangle**. The lateral borders of the anal triangle are the left and right sacrotuberous ligaments and its apices are the left and right ischial tuberosities and the coccyx. Deep to the skin of the anal triangle are two large areas filled with adipose tissue, the **ischioanal fossae**, the external anal sphincter, as well as the vessels and nerves to structures of the perineum. The ischioanal fossae continue anteriorly toward the pubic bones; however, along the way they are covered inferiorly by the fascia, muscles, and erectile tissues of the urogenital triangle. This creates the left and right **anterior recesses of the ischioanal fossa**, with the fascia of the urogenital triangle as the inferior border, the levator ani muscle as the superomedial border, and the obturator internus muscle as the lateral border on each side. Inferior to the tendinous arch of the levator ani, the fascia of the obturator membrane contains the pudendal nerve and internal pudendal vessels within the pudendal (Alcock) canal. Branches of this neurovascular bundle supply the muscles and skin of the perineum.

The structures of the urogenital triangle (Fig. 12.15, see also Fig. 12.14B) have their major effects in the urinary and reproductive systems, so I will only discuss them briefly. The **perineal membrane** extends across the urogenital triangle, with midline openings for the urethra and/or vagina. The perineal body is located on the midline of its posterior border. Superior to the perineal membrane is the **deep perineal space** and that surface of the perineal membrane is covered by a thin (usually) **deep transverse perineal muscle**. This muscle is best developed along the posterior border of the perineal membrane but has stronger bands that surround the urethra and/or vagina. The **external urethral sphincter** is part of the deep transverse perineal muscle that is present in both females and males and surrounds a significant length of the urethra after it exits the bladder or prostate. It is typically contracted until we willfully relax it during urination and is a major structure involved in urinary continence. The **compressor urethrae muscle** extends from the ischial ramus to fuse with fibers of the external urethral sphincter. In females, there is also a circular band of muscle that surrounds the urethra and vagina, the **sphincter urethrovaginalis**.

Lateral Attachments	• All parts of the deep transverse perineal muscle originate from the ischial and inferior pubic rami. As it travels medially it will subdivide into the external urethral sphincter, compressor urethrae, and sphincter urethrovaginalis.
Medial Attachment	• Posterior fibers travel from ischial tuberosities to the perineal body. • External urethral sphincter: surrounds urethra inferior to bladder (female) or inferior prostate (male) • Compressor urethrae: anterior external urethral sphincter muscle • Sphincter urethrovaginalis: encircles the urethra and vagina (female only)
Functions	• Stabilizes the perineum and pushes superiorly against the pelvic organs. • External urethral sphincter: major muscle of urinary continence, relaxes to allow urination to occur willfully. • Compressor urethrae: assists the external urethral sphincter muscle in preventing urination when contracted. • Sphincter urethrovaginalis: compresses urethra and vagina when contracted.
Muscle Testing and Signs of Dysfunction	• Dysfunction of this muscle would manifest in urinary incontinence or due to difficulty contracting or relaxing the external urethral sphincter. • Weakness of the perineal muscles can result in perineal pain, sexual dysfunction, or make a patient more prone to prolapse of organs.
Innervation	• Perineal nerve and dorsal nerves of the penis or clitoris. Both are branches of the pudendal nerve (S2–S4).
Blood Supply	• Perineal and dorsal arteries of the penis or clitoris. Both are branches of the internal pudendal artery

A

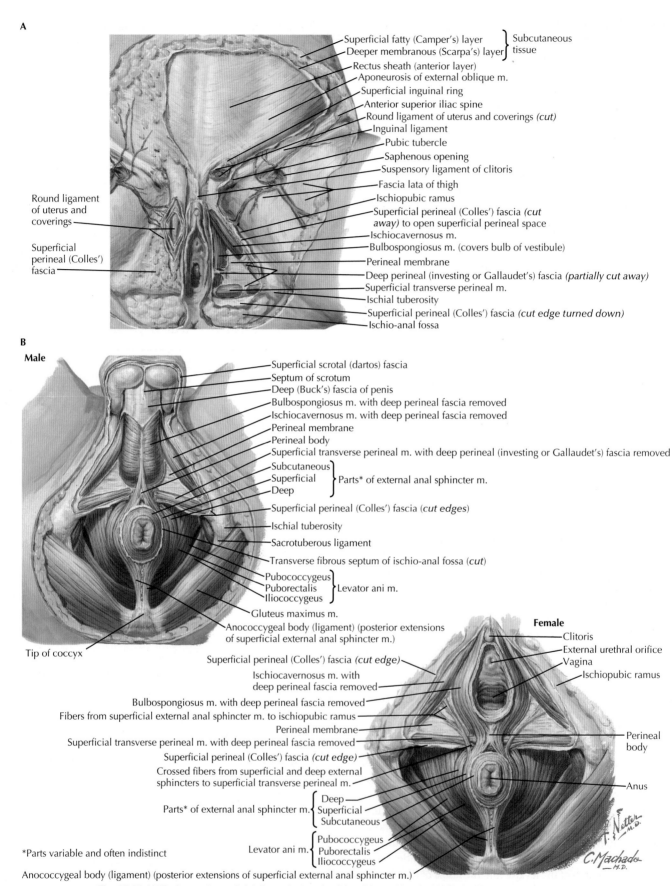

Superficial fatty (Camper's) layer ⎤ Subcutaneous
Deeper membranous (Scarpa's) layer ⎦ tissue
Rectus sheath (anterior layer)
Aponeurosis of external oblique m.
Superficial inguinal ring
Anterior superior iliac spine
Round ligament of uterus and coverings *(cut)*
Inguinal ligament
Pubic tubercle
Saphenous opening
Suspensory ligament of clitoris
Fascia lata of thigh
Ischiopubic ramus
Superficial perineal (Colles') fascia *(cut away)* to open superficial perineal space
Ischiocavernosus m.
Bulbospongiosus m. (covers bulb of vestibule)
Perineal membrane
Deep perineal (investing or Gallaudet's) fascia *(partially cut away)*
Superficial transverse perineal m.
Ischial tuberosity
Superficial perineal (Colles') fascia *(cut edge turned down)*
Ischio-anal fossa

Round ligament of uterus and coverings
Superficial perineal (Colles') fascia

B

Male

Superficial scrotal (dartos) fascia
Septum of scrotum
Deep (Buck's) fascia of penis
Bulbospongiosus m. with deep perineal fascia removed
Ischiocavernosus m. with deep perineal fascia removed
Perineal membrane
Perineal body
Superficial transverse perineal m. with deep perineal (investing or Gallaudet's) fascia removed
Subcutaneous ⎤
Superficial ⎬ Parts* of external anal sphincter m.
Deep   ⎦
Superficial perineal (Colles') fascia *(cut edges)*
Ischial tuberosity
Sacrotuberous ligament
Transverse fibrous septum of ischio-anal fossa *(cut)*
Pubococcygeus ⎤
Puborectalis ⎬ Levator ani m.
Iliococcygeus ⎦
Gluteus maximus m.
Anococcygeal body (ligament) (posterior extensions of superficial external anal sphincter m.)

Tip of coccyx

Female
Clitoris
External urethral orifice
Vagina
Ischiopubic ramus
Perineal body
Anus

Superficial perineal (Colles') fascia *(cut edge)*
Ischiocavernosus m. with deep perineal fascia removed
Bulbospongiosus m. with deep perineal fascia removed
Fibers from superficial external anal sphincter m. to ischiopubic ramus
Perineal membrane
Superficial transverse perineal m. with deep perineal fascia removed
Superficial perineal (Colles') fascia *(cut edge)*
Crossed fibers from superficial and deep external sphincters to superficial transverse perineal m.
Parts* of external anal sphincter m. {
Deep
Superficial
Subcutaneous
Levator ani m. {
Pubococcygeus
Puborectalis
Iliococcygeus

*Parts variable and often indistinct

Anococcygeal body (ligament) (posterior extensions of superficial external anal sphincter m.)

Fig. 12.14 (A) Perineum (superficial dissection) pudendal, pubic, and inguinal regions; (B) anorectal musculature: external sphincter and levator ani.

Muscles of the Superficial Perineal Space—Inferior to Perineal Membrane

Inferior to the perineal membrane is the **superficial perineal space**, which contains erectile tissues of the external genitalia and several muscles that attach to the inferior surface of the perineal membrane. Starting at the perineal body and extending to the ischial tuberosities are the left and right **superficial transverse perineal muscles**. More anteriorly, the **corpus cavernosum** is an erectile body that extends anteriorly along the ischial and inferior pubic ramus on the left and right side. It will contribute to the body of the clitoris or penis. Each corpus cavernosum is covered by the **ischiocavernosus muscle**, but these muscle fibers cease to cover the corpora as they approach the pubic symphysis. Another erectile tissue, the **corpus spongiosum**, is located more medially and is covered by the **bulbospongiosus muscle**. In females this erectile tissue is also known as the bulb of the vestibule. It and its overlying muscle are found just lateral to the labia minora. The corpus spongiosum does not contribute to the body or head of the clitoris. The left and right sides of the bulbospongiosus muscle meet posteriorly at the perineal body and are otherwise separated by the labia minora and vestibule, where the urethral and vaginal openings are located. In males, the corpus spongiosum is sometimes called the bulb of the penis and it surrounds the (spongy) urethra on the midline. The erectile tissue extends along the ventral aspect of the penile shaft before expanding to form the glans of the penis with its urethral opening. The bulbospongiosus muscle does not reach the shaft of the penis and is only present in the perineum. In females and males, the **deep perineal fascia** covers the ischiocavernosus and bulbospongiosus muscles and a variable amount of adipose tissue is found between the deep perineal fascia and the more inferior **superficial perineal (Colles) fascia**, which is continuous with the membranous layer (Scarpa fascia) of the abdomen. Inferior to the superficial perineal fascia is more adipose tissue in the subcutaneous tissue of the perineum, and finally the skin of the perineum (see Fig. 12.14A).

Lateral/Posterior Attachments	• Superficial transverse perineal: inferior aspect of ischial tuberosity
	• Ischiocavernosus: inferior ischial and inferior pubic ramus, covering corpus cavernosum
	• Bulbospongiosus:
	  • Female: perineal body and perineal membrane on each side of the vestibule
	  • Male: perineal body and perineal membrane, covering bulb of penis

Medial/Anterior Attachments	• Superficial transverse perineal: perineal body
	• Ischiocavernosus: attaches to perineal membrane and pubic bones adjacent to corpus cavernosum
	• Bulbospongiosus:
	  • Female: covers vestibular bulbs and greater glands before reaching pubic symphysis.
	  • Male: each side meets at a midline raphe that extends along the corpus spongiosum as far as the pubic symphysis

Functions	• Superficial transverse perineal: stabilize the perineum and perineal body to push superiorly against the pelvic organs.
	• Ischiocavernosus: compression of corpus cavernosum to maintain engorgement of crus of the penis or clitoris.
	• Bulbospongiosus
	  • Female: compression of vestibular gland and bulb to narrow express glandular secretions and narrow vestibular opening.
	  • Male: compression of bulb of the penis to maintain engorgement of penis and expel final drops of semen or urine.

Muscle Testing and Signs of Dysfunction	• Weakness of the perineal muscles can result in perineal pain, sexual dysfunction, or make a patient more prone to prolapse of organs. • There are many factors involved in sexual and urinary dysfunction; however, weakness or atrophy of these muscles may make erection, engorgement, vestibular lubrication, ejaculation, and urination more difficult.
Innervation	• Perineal nerve arising from the pudendal nerve (S2–S4)
Blood Supply	• Perineal artery, deep and dorsal arteries of the penis or clitoris, all branches of internal pudendal artery

Anal Triangle—External Anal Sphincter

The **external anal sphincter** (see Figs. 12.13B, 12.14B, and 12.15) encloses the terminal end of the digestive tract. The nearby internal anal sphincter consists of smooth muscle and will relax involuntarily when the body is preparing to defecate. Thankfully, the external anal sphincter is skeletal muscle under the voluntary control of the inferior rectal (anal) nerve, a branch of the pudendal nerve, and it tends to be contracted at rest and is deliberately relaxed (as is the puborectalis muscle)

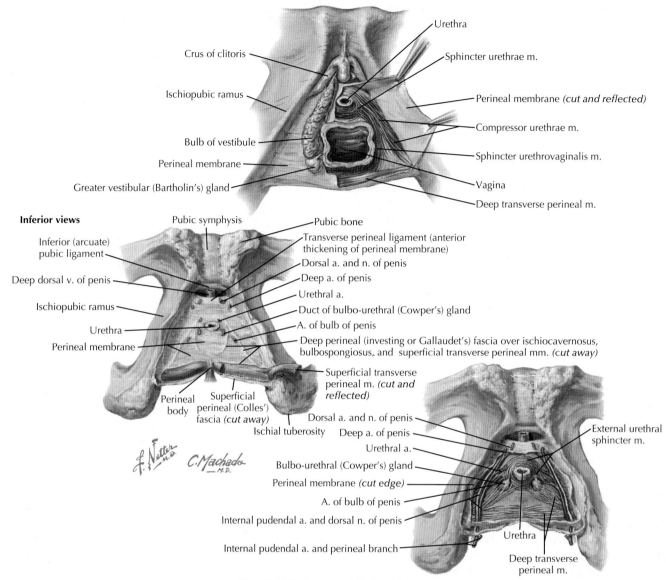

Inferior views

Fig. 12.15 Perineum and Perineal Spaces.

during defecation. The external anal sphincter is described as having **deep, superficial, and subcutaneous parts** but these are not easy to differentiate during dissection. The deep and superficial parts surround the terminal portion of the internal anal sphincter while the subcutaneous part surrounds the anal opening. The posterior aspect of the superficial anal sphincter blends with and contributes to the anococcygeal body while the anterior aspect of the sphincter is anchored to the perineal body (Clinical Correlations 12.15 and 12.16).

CLINICAL CORRELATION 12.15   Kegel Exercises

The muscles of the superficial and deep perineal spaces, pelvic diaphragm, and external anal sphincter are anchored to the connective tissue structures in the area like the perineal body and perineal membrane. Weakness of these muscles can lead to urinary and rectal incontinence and pelvic prolapse. These muscles can be conditioned by Kegel exercises, wherein the muscles of the urogenital, anal, and pelvic areas are clenched and held. Over time these muscles become stronger and better able to support the pelvic organs.

Posterior Attachments	• Anococcygeal body connects to coccyx • Skin of the anal opening
Anterior Attachments	• Surrounds anal opening to reach the perineal body
Functions	• Stabilizes the perineum and perineal body to push superiorly against the pelvic organs. • Contraction at rest keeps the anal opening closed and prevents defecation. Willful relaxation is (hopefully) needed to relax the sphincter in order to allow defecation to occur.
Muscle Testing and Signs of Dysfunction	• If the skin of the anus is stimulated by a light pinprick, a reflexive contraction of the external anal sphincter will occur. This can be done to assess status of the sacral level of the spinal cord or the pudendal nerve (S2–S4). • Dysfunction of the external anal sphincter, particularly spastic paralysis caused by loss of innervation, can result in rectal incontinence since the anal opening is no longer tightly closed by skeletal muscle. Thereafter, defecation may occur any time the internal (smooth muscle) anal sphincter relaxes.
Innervation	• Inferior rectal (anal) nerve, arising from the pudendal nerve (S2–S4)
Blood Supply	• Inferior and middle rectal arteries, both of which arise from the internal iliac artery

CLINICAL CORRELATION 12.16
Episiotomy

Occasionally the head of an infant will have difficulty passing through the birth canal or may be lodged in place. While it is no longer as common as it once was, an incision (episiotomy) can be made in the posterior end of the vaginal opening to prevent perineal tearing and a prolonged delivery. In a median episiotomy, the incision is directed posteriorly toward the perineal body but not so far as the anus. These median episiotomies may heal uneventfully but have been associated with urinary or rectal incontinence or prolapse of the pelvic organs when the perineal body is damaged and no longer acts as a stable anchor for the nearby muscles. Alternatively, the incision can be directed posterolaterally, between the bulb of the vestibule and the external anal sphincter but not far enough laterally to encounter the inferior rectal nerve or vessels or other branches of the pudendal nerve and internal pudendal vessels.

INNERVATION OF THE TORSO

The Spinal Nerves to the Torso

By its very nature, the torso receives innervation from every spinal level from C1 to the Coccygeal spinal nerves (Fig. 12.16). The **posterior rami** of these nerves divide into medial and lateral branches as they move more superficially to innervate the vertebral facet joints, intrinsic muscles of the back, and convey sensations from the overlying skin via **posterior cutaneous branches**. The **anterior rami** of each spinal nerve contribute to the plexuses that supply the neck, upper limbs, lower limbs, and pelvis but also to the muscles and skin of the lateral and anterior

body wall by means of **lateral cutaneous branches** and **anterior cutaneous branches**. On the torso these dermatomes are laid out in a relatively uniform set of strips that descend along the body wall before converging on the anus. There are some "landmark" dermatomes on the torso that are worth noting.

- C2: back of the scalp
- C4: upper shoulders
- T4: covers the nipples
- T10: covers the umbilicus
- L1: across the inguinal area
- S3-Co1: forms a "bullseye" pattern of circular dermatomes around the anus

Nerves of the Neck—Spinal Accessory Nerve, Cervical Plexus, and Phrenic Nerve

While most posterior rami innervate discrete strips of muscle or skin close to their exit from an intervertebral foramen, there are some named posterior rami in the cervical region (see Fig. 9.28). The C1 posterior ramus is the **suboccipital nerve** and is a motor nerve to the suboccipital muscles, which were described in Chapter 9. The C2 posterior ramus creates the large, cutaneous **greater occipital nerve**, which passes through the semispinalis capitis, splenius, and trapezius muscles and then turns superiorly to distribute itself across the majority of the posterior scalp. The C3 posterior ramus also has a cutaneous branch, the **third occipital nerve**, which pierces the muscles of the superior back and conveys sensation from a discrete patch of scalp near the posterior midline. A more lateral lesser occipital nerve comes from anterior rami and will be described with the rest of the cervical plexus.

The spinal accessory nucleus (see Fig. 4.3) is found in the upper cervical spinal cord, between C1 and C5(6). Rootlets from this motor nucleus exit the cord alongside the anterior and posterior roots. However, instead of exiting through the interventricular foramen, these rootlets converge on each other to form the **spinal root of the accessory nerve**, ascend in the spinal canal, and pass superiorly through the foramen magnum. The nerve then turns inferiorly and exits the skull via the jugular foramen alongside the internal jugular vein, cranial nerve IX (glossopharyngeal), and cranial nerve X (vagus). Axons from the nucleus ambiguus bundle together to create the **cranial root of the accessory nerve**, which joins the spinal root of the accessory nerve as it leaves the jugular foramen. However, these axons then leave the accessory nerve to join the vagus nerve. So in the end, only the spinal root of the accessory nerve contributes to the main body of the nerve and its muscular branches. It then descends along the medial aspect of the sternocleidomastoid muscle, innervating it along the way. Roughly midway along the length of the sternocleidomastoid muscle, the spinal accessory nerve travels posteriorly to reach the anterior surface of the trapezius muscle, which it also innervates. In this area it is joined by sensory branches from the cervical plexus that convey sensation from these muscles. Sensory neurons have been found along the rootlets of the spinal accessory nerve, sometimes forming visible ganglia. These may convey proprioceptive information from the sternocleidomastoid and trapezius muscles (Boehm and Kondrashov, 2016).

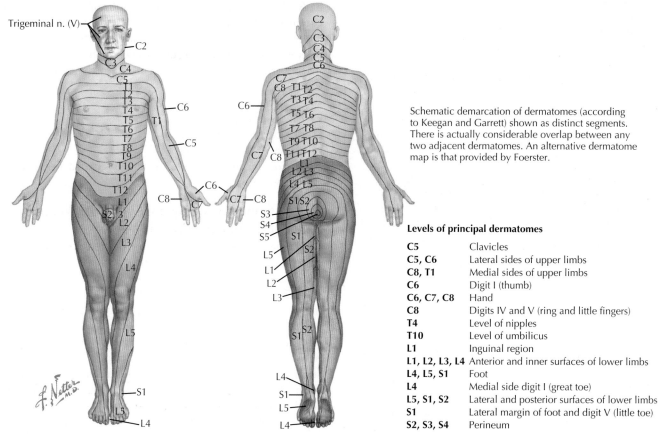

Schematic demarcation of dermatomes (according to Keegan and Garrett) shown as distinct segments. There is actually considerable overlap between any two adjacent dermatomes. An alternative dermatome map is that provided by Foerster.

Levels of principal dermatomes

C5	Clavicles
C5, C6	Lateral sides of upper limbs
C8, T1	Medial sides of upper limbs
C6	Digit I (thumb)
C6, C7, C8	Hand
C8	Digits IV and V (ring and little fingers)
T4	Level of nipples
T10	Level of umbilicus
L1	Inguinal region
L1, L2, L3, L4	Anterior and inner surfaces of lower limbs
L4, L5, S1	Foot
L4	Medial side digit I (great toe)
L5, S1, S2	Lateral and posterior surfaces of lower limbs
S1	Lateral margin of foot and digit V (little toe)
S2, S3, S4	Perineum

Fig. 12.16 Adult Dermatomes: Dermal Sensation.

The **cervical plexus** (Fig. 12.17) arises from the anterior rami of C1–C4 spinal nerves and has motor and cutaneous branches that distribute themselves throughout the cervical region. The **ansa cervicalis** is a loop of motor nerves that lies within the connective tissue on the surface of the carotid sheath. It must be identified and protected during procedures in this area. The anterior rami of C1 and C2 join to create the **superior root of the ansa cervicalis**, while the **inferior root of the ansa cervicalis** consists of axons coming from the anterior rami of C2 and C3. The superior root of the ansa travels along the surface of the hypoglossal nerve as it crosses the carotid sheath. It gives off a **thyrohyoid branch (C1)** that separates from the hypoglossal nerve to reach the geniohyoid and thyrohyoid muscles. More proximally, the superior root leaves the hypoglossal nerve, descends along the carotid sheath and meets the nerves of the inferior root, which creates the distinctive looped shape of the ansa cervicalis. Along its course, the ansa cervicalis gives off motor branches to the superior belly of the omohyoid, sternothyroid, sternohyoid, and inferior belly of the omohyoid muscles.

The cervical plexus also generates cutaneous branches that leave the plexus and travel across the medial and posterior sides of the sternocleidomastoid muscle before they scatter widely to the nearby skin. Because so many cutaneous nerves are clustered in such a small space, the posterior border of the middle of the sternocleidomastoid is referred to as the **nerve point of the neck**. The **lesser occipital nerve (C2)** ascends along the lateral

side of the superior third of the sternocleidomastoid muscle to reach the superolateral neck and posterolateral scalp just posterior to the auricle of the ear. The **great auricular nerve (C2–C3)** conveys cutaneous sensations from the area around the auricle itself. Its posterior branch covers the mastoid process and posterior auricle of the ear (but not the superior portion) and sends a branch through the lobule (inferior part) of the ear to reach the anterior auricle. The anterior branch of the great auricular nerve conveys sensations from a strip of skin along the angle and ramus of the mandible and across the inferior half of the parotid gland. The **transverse cervical nerve (C2–C3)** travels anterior to the sternocleidomastoid and posterior to the platysma muscle and external jugular vein before it divides into superior and inferior branches that convey sensation form the skin of the anterolateral neck. Lastly, the medial, intermediate, and lateral **supraclavicular nerves (C3–C4)** leave the nerve point and descend, fanning out across the inferior neck, superior thorax, and shoulder.

The **phrenic nerve (C3–C5)** (Fig. 12.18, see also Fig. 12.17) arises from branches of the cervical plexus, largely C3 and C4, along with a contribution from C5 to innervate the muscles of the diaphragm. Because of the distance between the cervical region and the diaphragm, this nerve has a long course that exposes it to danger in several locations. Branches of the C3–C5 anterior rami fuse on the anterior surface of the anterior scalene muscle before they pass between the subclavian vein (anteriorly) and artery (posteriorly) and enter the superior

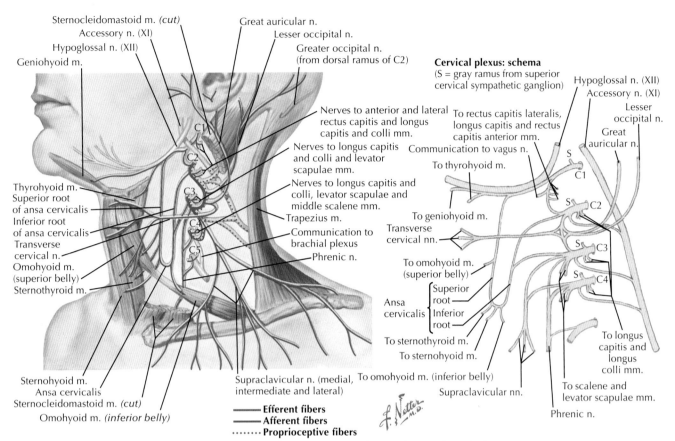

Fig. 12.17 Nerve Supply of the Neck: Cervical Plexus of the Neck.

thoracic aperture. The C5 contribution sometimes does not join the rest of the phrenic nerve on the anterior scalene muscle and descends separately as an **accessory phrenic nerve**, fusing with the C3–C4 branches in the thorax. In the thorax, the left and right phrenic nerves descend deep to the mediastinal pleura and lateral to the parietal pericardium. The phrenic nerve conveys sensation from both of those layers, which becomes important when there is inflammation of the pericardium or medial pleural surfaces. Branches of the phrenic nerve then spread out across the superior surface of the diaphragm and also to the inferior surface via **phrenicoabdominal branches** that pierce the central tendon of the diaphragm. These branches innervate the muscles of the diaphragm and convey sensation from its central area. Sensations from more peripheral areas of the diaphragm are conveyed by nearby intercostal nerves (Clinical Correlations 12.17 and 12.18).

Nerves of the Thorax and Abdomen

The **intercostal nerves** (Fig. 12.19, see also, Fig. 12.8A) are the anterior rami of T1–T11. They travel along the inferior border of their respective ribs (T6 nerve running inferior to the 6th rib) alongside the corresponding intercostal artery and vein. A few exceptions exist: the T1 and T2 intercostal nerves tend to run along the medial aspect of their ribs, rather than on their inferior edge, and the T12 anterior ramus is called the **subcostal nerve** since it has no rib inferior to it. Shortly after entering the intercostal space, these nerves typically give off a small **collateral branch** that parallels its parent nerve but travels in

the inferior part of the space, just superior to the neighboring ribs (e.g., the collateral branch of the T4 intercostal nerve can be found just superior to the 5th rib). These nerves project laterally and then anteriorly, sending muscular branches to all the intercostal muscles, as well as the subcostal and transversus thoracis muscles. The intercostal nerves and vessels run along the deep surface of the internal intercostal muscles and are covered medially by the innermost intercostal muscles in the area of the ribcage where that muscle is present. On the lateral aspect of the thorax, near the midaxillary line each intercostal nerve gives off a **lateral cutaneous branch** that pierces the overlying muscles and subdivides into an anterior and posterior branch that will convey sensation from the skin of the lateral thorax. The T2 lateral cutaneous nerve is special because it also innervates the skin of the axilla and a small region of the medial arm. This branch is called the **intercostobrachial nerve** and may also involve the lateral cutaneous nerve of T3. Near the sternum, the T1–T6 intercostal nerves terminate as **anterior cutaneous branch** that convey sensations from the skin of anterior thoracic wall (Clinical Correlations 12.19–12.21).

In the lower half of the thoracic wall, the thoracic anterior rami do not parallel the ribs and costal cartilages, which arch superiorly to reach the inferior sternum and costal arch (excluding floating ribs 11 and 12), but instead continue anteriorly along the body wall. In the process, the T7–T11 intercostal nerves and the T12 subcostal nerve pass medial to their corresponding rib and enter the abdominal wall, continuing as **thoracoabdominal nerves** (see Fig. 12.19). They are joined

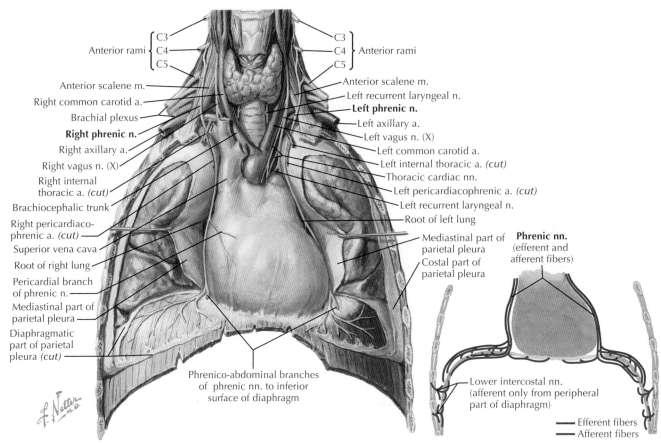

Anterior rami { C3 C4 C5 }
C3 C4 C5 } Anterior rami

Anterior scalene m.
Right common carotid a.
Brachial plexus
Right phrenic n.
Right axillary a.
Right vagus n. (X)
Right internal thoracic a. (cut)
Brachiocephalic trunk
Right pericardiacophrenic a. (cut)
Superior vena cava
Root of right lung
Pericardial branch of phrenic n.
Mediastinal part of parietal pleura
Diaphragmatic part of parietal pleura (cut)

Anterior scalene m.
Left recurrent laryngeal n.
Left phrenic n.
Left axillary a.
Left vagus n. (X)
Left common carotid a.
Left internal thoracic a. (cut)
Thoracic cardiac nn.
Left pericardiacophrenic a. (cut)
Left recurrent laryngeal n.
Root of left lung
Mediastinal part of parietal pleura
Costal part of parietal pleura

Phrenic nn.
(efferent and afferent fibers)

Phrenico-abdominal branches of phrenic nn. to inferior surface of diaphragm

Lower intercostal nn. (afferent only from peripheral part of diaphragm)

—— Efferent fibers
—— Afferent fibers

Fig. 12.18 Phrenic Nerve.

by the anterior ramus of L1, which splits into the **iliohypogastric nerve** and **ilioinguinal nerve**. The thoraco-abdominal, iliohypogastric, and ilioinguinal nerves innervate the external abdominal oblique, internal abdominal oblique, transversus abdominis, rectus abdominis, and pyramidalis muscles, traveling between the internal abdominal oblique and transversus abdominis muscles, and conveying sensations from the abdominal wall by giving off a **lateral cutaneous branch** and an **anterior cutaneous branch** to the overlying skin. The anterior cutaneous branch of the ilioinguinal nerve travels across the surface of the superficial inguinal ring before reaching the skin of the anterior genitalia, labia majora, or scrotum. The **genitofemoral nerve (L1–L2)** travels inferiorly along the anterior surface of the psoas major muscle before piercing the abdominal wall. The **femoral branch of the genitofemoral nerve (L2)** conveys sensation from a small area of the anteromedial thigh; the **genital branch of the genitofemoral nerve (L1)** conveys sensation from the anterior genitalia but also innervates a small portion of the internal abdominal oblique muscle that gives rise to the cremaster muscle, which forms part of the spermatic cord and elevates the testicles when it contracts (Clinical Correlation 12.22).

Nerves of the Pelvis

Most muscles of the pelvis and perineum are innervated by the **pudendal nerve (S2–S4)** (Fig. 12.20), which arises from the anterior division of the sacral plexus (described in Chapter 11)

CLINICAL CORRELATION 12.17 Cervical Plexus Nerve Block

In preparation for procedures of the lateral and anterior neck, the cutaneous nerves of the cervical plexus can be blocked by injecting anesthetic around the nerve point of the neck, which will likely block the lesser occipital, great auricular, transverse cervical, and supraclavicular nerves. Because of its close proximity, the phrenic nerve is often affected by this block, temporarily paralyzing half of the diaphragm.

CLINICAL CORRELATION 12.18 Phrenic Nerve Damage

The phrenic nerve is vulnerable to being damaged anywhere along its extended pathway from C3 to C5 to the diaphragm. As mentioned earlier, it can be affected by a nerve block of the cervical plexus, injured by trauma to the inferior neck, compressed by tumors of the mediastinum, and compromised by demyelinating diseases. In any case, the result is flaccid paralysis of the affected half of the diaphragm, causing it to dome upward into the pleura space/thorax and compromising the ability to breathe.

near the sciatic nerve. It exits the pelvis through the greater sciatic foramen but then passes between the sacrospinous and sacrotuberous ligaments to re-enter the pelvis through the lesser sciatic foramen and travels anteriorly in the ischioanal fossa alongside branches of the internal pudendal vessels. In the ischioanal fossa it gives off its first branch, the **inferior rectal**

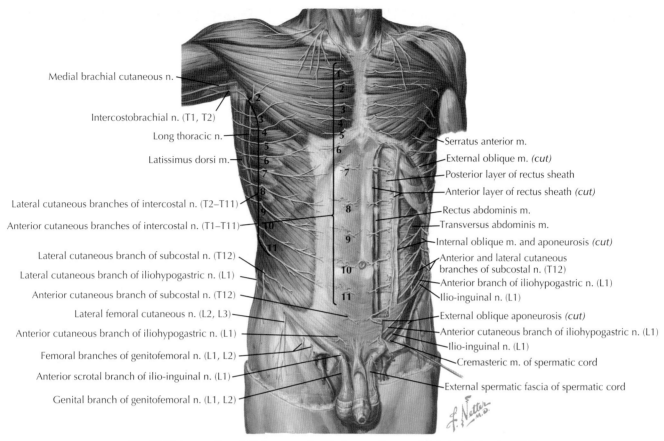

Medial brachial cutaneous n.

Intercostobrachial n. (T1, T2)

Long thoracic n.

Latissimus dorsi m.

Lateral cutaneous branches of intercostal n. (T2–T11)

Anterior cutaneous branches of intercostal n. (T1–T11)

Lateral cutaneous branch of subcostal n. (T12)

Lateral cutaneous branch of iliohypogastric n. (L1)

Anterior cutaneous branch of subcostal n. (T12)

Lateral femoral cutaneous n. (L2, L3)

Anterior cutaneous branch of iliohypogastric n. (L1)

Femoral branches of genitofemoral n. (L1, L2)

Anterior scrotal branch of ilio-inguinal n. (L1)

Genital branch of genitofemoral n. (L1, L2)

Serratus anterior m.

External oblique m. *(cut)*

Posterior layer of rectus sheath

Anterior layer of rectus sheath *(cut)*

Rectus abdominis m.

Transversus abdominis m.

Internal oblique m. and aponeurosis *(cut)*

Anterior and lateral cutaneous branches of subcostal n. (T12)

Anterior branch of iliohypogastric n. (L1)

Ilio-inguinal n. (L1)

External oblique aponeurosis *(cut)*

Anterior cutaneous branch of iliohypogastric n. (L1)

Ilio-inguinal n. (L1)

Cremasteric m. of spermatic cord

External spermatic fascia of spermatic cord

Fig. 12.19 Innervation of Abdomen and of Perineum: Nerves of Anterior Abdominal Wall.

(anal) nerve, which passes medial to the external anal sphincter and skin of the anal opening. The pudendal nerve continues anteriorly within the **pudendal (Alcock) canal**, which is a thickened region of the obturator internus fascia inferior to the arch of the levator ani muscle. As it approaches the urogenital triangle, the pudendal nerve gives off its terminal branches, the dorsal nerve of the clitoris/penis and the perineal nerve.

The **dorsal nerve of the clitoris/penis** travels superior to the perineal membrane in the deep perineal space while the perineal nerve travels inferior to the perineal membrane in the superficial perineal space. The dorsal nerve of the clitoris/penis passes through the deep transverse perineal muscle, innervating some parts of it, particularly the sphincter urethrae muscle. Thereafter it travels along the dorsal aspect of the penis or clitoris and conveys sensation from the skin on the organ, including the glans. The **perineal nerve** branches medially off of the pudendal nerve and divides into deep and superficial branches. The **deep (muscular) branch of the perineal nerve** innervates the bulbospongiosus, ischiocavernosus, superficial transverse perineal, and parts of the deep transverse perineal muscles. The **superficial branch of the perineal nerve** is cutaneous and terminates as the **posterior labial/scrotal nerve** that covers a significant portion of the posterior perineum.

The anterior rami of the S4 and S5 join the small coccygeal nerves to create the **coccygeal plexus**. Branches related to these rami and this plexus will innervate the coccygeus and levator ani muscles. However, some branches of the pudendal nerve

(which contains contributions from S4) may also innervate portions of the levator ani and coccygeus muscles that arise from S3 to S4 anterior rami and travel directly to the muscles which they innervate. A small **anococcygeal nerve** leaves the coccygeal plexus and conveys sensation from the skin around the posterior anus and coccyx (Clinical Correlation 12.23).

Autonomic Innervation of the Torso (Fig. 12.21, See Also Figs. 10.24 and 11.29)

Just like the back and limbs, the sympathetic nervous system innervates sweat glands in the skin, arrector pili muscles of the hair follicles, and smooth muscle sphincters that regulate blood flow to skeletal muscles and skin of the torso. **Preganglionic sympathetic axons** from the **intermediolateral (IML) cell columns** that are present from the T1–L2 levels of the spinal cord project their axons through the anterior spinal roots, spinal nerve, and anterior rami. These axons exit the anterior ramus as **white rami communicans** to reach the **paravertebral ganglia** associated with each spinal level within the **sympathetic chain**. Since they come from the IML cell column, white rami communicans are only present from T1 to L2. These axons distribute themselves along the entire length of the sympathetic chain and the cervical, thoracic, lumbar, and sacral ganglia within it. There is roughly one ganglion per vertebral level, but considerable variation exists and fused, multiple, or absent ganglia may be noted. The single **ganglion impar** connects the left and right sympathetic chains just anterior to the apex of the sacrum.

CLINICAL CORRELATION 12.19   **Intercostal Nerve Block**

To treat thoracic trauma or prior to thoracic surgery, the intercostal nerves of the affected levels can be anesthetized. A needle with the anesthetic agent is passed along the lower edge of the rib, through the skin and into the intercostal muscles. This can be done with or without ultrasound guidance but if the needle is advanced too far, it can pierce the pleura and underlying lung. Loss of sensation anterior to the block indicates that it has been successful.

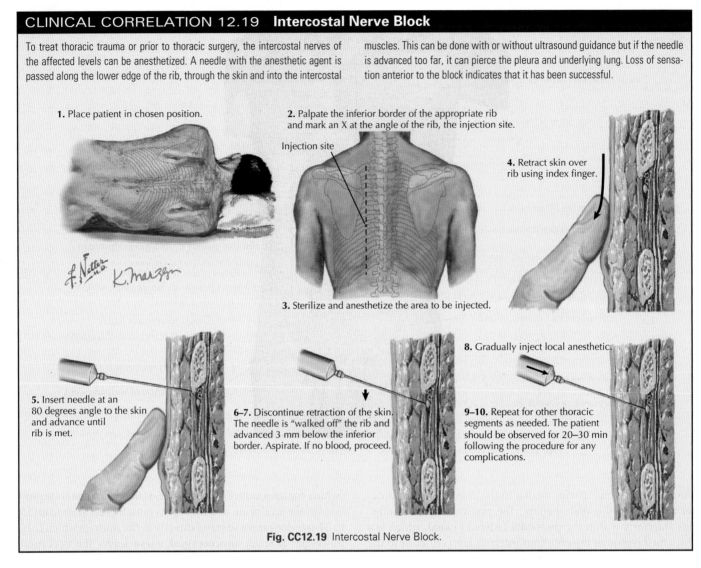

1. Place patient in chosen position.

2. Palpate the inferior border of the appropriate rib and mark an X at the angle of the rib, the injection site.

Injection site

4. Retract skin over rib using index finger.

3. Sterilize and anesthetize the area to be injected.

5. Insert needle at an 80 degrees angle to the skin and advance until rib is met.

6–7. Discontinue retraction of the skin. The needle is "walked off" the rib and advanced 3 mm below the inferior border. Aspirate. If no blood, proceed.

8. Gradually inject local anesthetic.

9–10. Repeat for other thoracic segments as needed. The patient should be observed for 20–30 min following the procedure for any complications.

Fig. CC12.19 Intercostal Nerve Block.

Several splanchnic nerves leave the sympathetic chain to innervate the thoracic, abdominal, and pelvic organs but that is outside the scope of this volume.

To reach the skin and muscles of the neck, preganglionic sympathetic axons in the upper thoracic IML ascend within the sympathetic chain to reach the **inferior cervical**, **stellate** (fused inferior cervical and first thoracic), **middle cervical**, and **superior cervical ganglion** that are located near the superior end of the sympathetic chain and synapse with postganglionic sympathetic nerve cells within them. **Postganglionic sympathetic axons** leave the chain via **gray rami communicans** and join nearby cervical spinal nerves. Thereafter the postganglionic sympathetic axons travel as part of the cervical plexus, phrenic nerve, and brachial plexus (described in the Upper Limb chapter). In addition to sending gray rami communicans to the upper cervical spinal nerves, the superior cervical ganglion also extends postganglionic sympathetic axons onto the outer surface of the nearby external and internal carotid arteries, which convey these axons to targets in the head. There is typically a loop formed by two interganglionic branches between the middle cervical and inferior cervical (or stellate if present) ganglia that wraps around the

anterior and posterior sides of the subclavian artery, the **ansa subclavia**.

The sweat glands, arrector pili muscles, and precapillary sphincters of the skin and skeletal muscles of the thorax, abdomen, and pelvis receive postganglionic sympathetic axons from the **thoracic ganglia**, **lumbar ganglia**, and **sacral ganglia** as well as the ganglion impar. These postganglionic sympathetic axons leave each ganglion as gray rami communicans and join the spinal nerves from T1 to S5. These axons travel as part of the intercostal, subcostal, thoraco-abdominal nerves, lumbar plexus, sacral plexus, and coccygeal plexus to reach their targets in the thorax, abdomen, pelvis, and lower limbs.

THE BLOOD SUPPLY OF THE TORSO

Arteries of the Neck and Thorax

After leaving the left ventricle of the heart, arterial blood is propelled up the **ascending aorta**, the **arch of the aorta**, and then down the **thoracic (descending) aorta**. The ascending aorta supplies blood to the heart itself via coronary arteries and the arch of the aorta has three large arteries that leave it: the

CLINICAL CORRELATION 12.20 Thoracocentesis and Chest Tubes

Unlike an intercostal nerve block, the intent of thoracocentesis is to pass a needle through the tissues of the intercostal space and into the pleural space to sample fluids within it. When drainage is necessary, a chest tube can be placed to remove blood (hemothorax), lymphatic fluid (chylothorax), or air (hemothorax) in the pleural space. The patient is seated so that any fluid will fall to the lower part of the pleural space. A needle or trocar is then inserted into the intercostal space with the patient exhaling to raise the lower edge of the lung. To avoid the intercostal nerve and vessels in the superior part of the intercostal space, as well as the collateral branches along the inferior part of the space, the needle is inserted into the middle of the intercostal space, closer to the inferior rib than the superior rib.

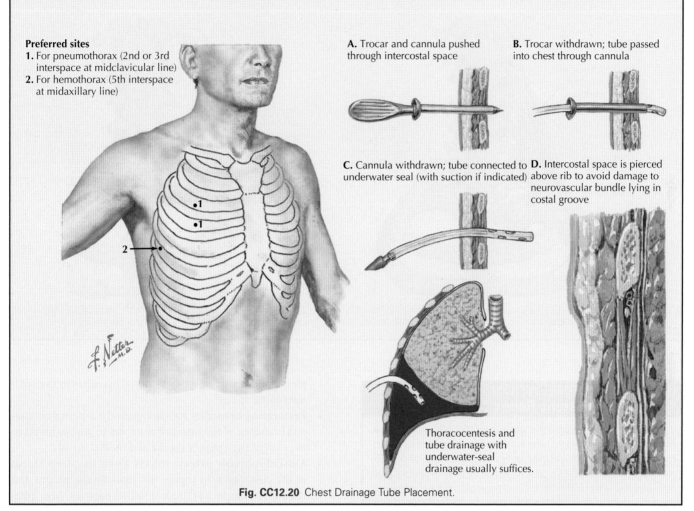

Preferred sites
1. For pneumothorax (2nd or 3rd interspace at midclavicular line)
2. For hemothorax (5th interspace at midaxillary line)

A. Trocar and cannula pushed through intercostal space

B. Trocar withdrawn; tube passed into chest through cannula

C. Cannula withdrawn; tube connected to underwater seal (with suction if indicated)

D. Intercostal space is pierced above rib to avoid damage to neurovascular bundle lying in costal groove

Thoracocentesis and tube drainage with underwater-seal drainage usually suffices.

Fig. CC12.20 Chest Drainage Tube Placement.

brachiocephalic trunk, which subdivides into the **right subclavian artery** and **right common carotid artery**, the **left common carotid artery**, and **left subclavian artery**. The subclavian artery has been discussed in Chapter 10 but will be revisited here with reference to vessels that supply the neck and upper torso. Other branches will be discussed as they pertain to the musculoskeletal system.

Each **common carotid artery** (Fig. 12.22) ascends in the carotid sheath and divides at the **carotid bifurcation** into internal and external carotid arteries, often at the level of the hyoid bone/C3–C4 vertebra (Clinical Correlation 12.24).

- **Internal carotid artery**: ascends without branching and enters the skull via the carotid canal. Inside the skull it gives off branches to the eye, orbit, nasal cavity, and central nervous system.
- **External carotid artery**: gives off many branches to the neck, face, and scalp

- **Superior thyroid artery**: supplies blood to thyroid gland, larynx, infrahyoid, and sternocleidomastoid muscles
- Ascending pharyngeal artery: ascends medially and supplies blood to the pharyngeal muscles and the prevertebral muscles
- Lingual artery provides blood to the tongue and suprahyoid muscles
- Facial artery: provides blood to the muscles and structures of the face, forehead, palate, and salivary glands
- Occipital artery ascends posteriorly to supply blood to the muscles of the superior neck, posterior scalp, and a portion of the auricle of the ear.
- Posterior auricular artery travels posterior to the auricle of the ear. Supplies the auricle, facial nerve, scalp, and parotid gland.
- Superficial temporal artery: provides blood to the parotid gland, part of the auricle, lateral scalp, and facial structures

CLINICAL CORRELATION 12.21 **Cervical Ribs and Thoracic Outlet Syndrome**

Approximately 1% of people have an extra, cervical rib superior to the first thoracic rib. Instead of a costal cartilage, such ribs frequently have a fibrous band that connects it to the superior surface of the 1st rib. On their own, cervical ribs are not problematic although they may create some confusion during radiographic examination; however, the nerves and vessels traveling out of the superior thoracic aperture may become compressed as they arch over this additional rib. When this causes signs related to the T1 dermatome, such as pins-and-needles pain along the medial arm, forearm, and hand, it is often referred to as thoracic outlet syndrome.

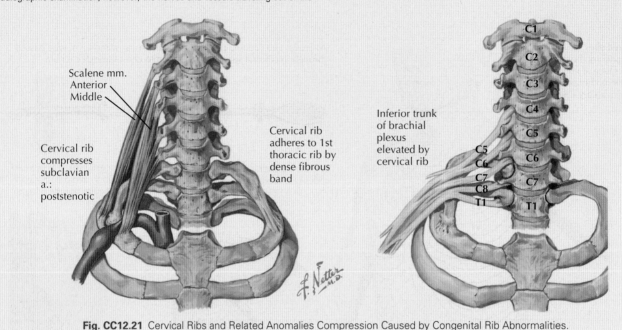

Fig. CC12.21 Cervical Ribs and Related Anomalies Compression Caused by Congenital Rib Abnormalities.

CLINICAL CORRELATION 12.22 **Cremasteric Reflex**

Because the cremaster muscle of the spermatic cord is innervated by the genital branch of the genitofemoral nerve (L1), it can be made to contract involuntarily when the upper thigh is touched gently since that region is innervated by the ilioinguinal nerve (also L1), causing the testicle on the same side to ascend. This rarely used reflex can be used to assess the integrity of the L1 spinal cord.

- Maxillary artery: provides blood to the mandible, maxilla, muscles of mastication, cheek, and nasal cavity

The left and right **subclavian arteries** (Fig. 12.23, see also Fig. 12.8B) leave the superior thoracic aperture and extend toward the upper limbs. The arteries that leave the subclavian artery vary considerably in their branching patterns but typically there are several that perfuse musculoskeletal structures of the torso.

- **Internal thoracic artery:** descends posterior to costal cartilages. It supplies blood to the manubrium, sternal body, xiphoid process, transversus thoracis muscles (which cover the posterior aspect of the vessels), and medial aspect of the pectoralis major muscles.
  - **Anterior intercostal arteries:** travel laterally from the internal thoracic artery in the upper six intercostal spaces to anastomose with posterior intercostal arteries. They supply the intercostal muscles, nearby fascia, and parietal pleura and divide into two terminal branches in the sixth intercostal space.
  - **Perforating branches:** run alongside the anterior cutaneous branches of the intercostal nerves to supply blood to the skin of the anterior thorax and medial breast.
  - **Musculophrenic artery:** travels along the deep aspect of the costal arch to supply the anterior diaphragm and the superior aspect of the abdominal muscles. Also gives rise to anterior intercostal arteries for intercostal spaces 7 to 9.
  - **Superior epigastric artery:** continues inferiorly from the internal thoracic artery into the rectus sheath. It supplies blood to the rectus abdominis muscle and anastomoses with the inferior epigastric artery.
  - **Pericardiacophrenic artery:** a small vessel that leaves the internal thoracic artery and travels alongside the phrenic artery in the mediastinum. It supplies the pericardium and part of the central diaphragm.
- **Vertebral artery:** the 1st segment leaves the superior aspect of the subclavian artery and ascends between the scalene and longus colli muscles to reach the transverse foramen of C6, giving off muscular branches along the way. The 2nd segment passes through the transverse foramina from C6 to C1. In this span it provides radicular and larger segmental medullary arteries to the cervical spinal cord. Once it passes through the transverse foramen of C1, the 3rd segment of the vertebral artery courses posteromedially along the vertebral

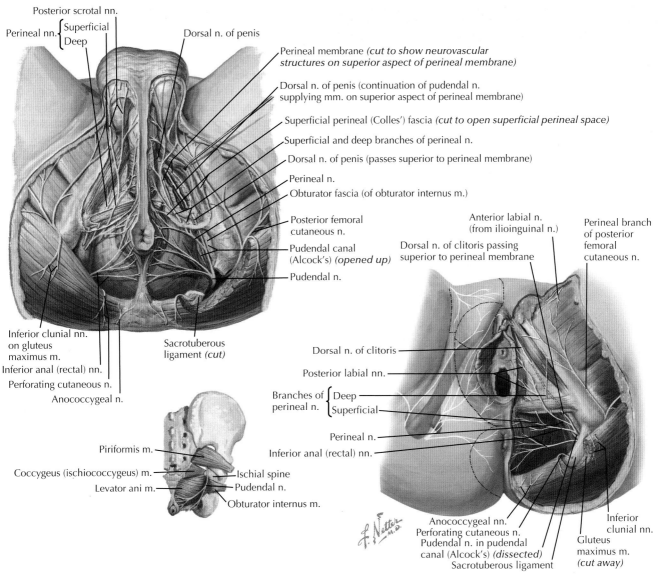

Fig. 12.20 Innervation of the Abdomen, Perineum, and External Genitalia.

groove of the superior atlas. In this region it supplies the muscles via suboccipital arteries (of Salmon) before the 4th segment passes through the atlanto-occipital membrane and dura mater to reach the brainstem.

- **Thyrocervical trunk**: this trunk splits into several arteries, which sometimes branch separately from the subclavian artery.
  - **Inferior thyroid artery**: a large vessel that ascends medially to supply the thyroid gland, parathyroid glands, parts of the inferior pharynx, superior esophagus, larynx, and trachea, as well as the infrahyoid muscles.
  - **Ascending cervical artery**: small vessel that ascends along the scalene and pre-vertebral muscles, which it supplies. It also gives off radicular branches to the spinal cord.
  - **Suprascapular artery**: described in detail in Chapter 10. Passes superior to the brachial plexus to reach the superior border of the scapula and supply blood to the supraspinatus and infraspinatus muscles.

- **Transverse cervical artery** (also called the **cervicodorsal trunk**) gives rise to several branches related to the torso and upper limb.
  - **Superficial cervical artery** (also called superficial branch of transverse cervical artery): runs posteriorly across the lateral cervical region to join the spinal accessory nerve on the anterior aspect of the trapezius. It splits into ascending and descending branches.
  - **Dorsal scapular artery** (also called deep branch of transverse cervical artery): passes posteriorly between the roots of the brachial plexus to reach the levator scapulae, rhomboid minor, and rhomboid major muscles.
- **Costocervical trunk**: branches off of the subclavian artery posterior to the anterior scalene muscle.
  - **Supreme thoracic artery**: branches inferiorly and enters the superior thoracic aperture. It runs along the medial aspects of ribs 1 and 2 and creates the first and second posterior intercostal arteries. These will anastomose with the corresponding anterior intercostal

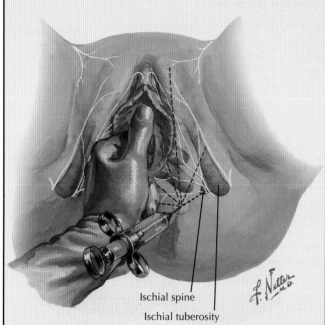

Ischial spine

Ischial tuberosity

Fig. CC12.23 Block Anesthesia of Pudendal and Other Nerves of Perineal Area.

the thorax alongside the long thoracic nerve to supply the serratus anterior muscle, pectoralis major, nearby intercostal muscles, and the lateral breast.

The **thoracic (descending) aorta** (Fig. 12.24, see also Fig. 12.8) is located just to the left of the midline in the superior and posterior mediastinum. As it descends it gives off branches to the esophagus, bronchi, pericardium, and other nearby structures. More pertinent to the musculoskeletal system are the paired **posterior intercostal arteries** (3 to 11) and **subcostal artery** (12) that branch laterally off of the aorta in the thorax and have their own branches.

- **Dorsal branch**: leaves each intercostal or subcostal artery and travels alongside the nearby posterior rami to supply blood to the intrinsic muscles of the back and overlying skin, splitting into a medial and lateral cutaneous branch along the way.
  - **Spinal branches**: enter intervertebral foramina to supply spinal structures
  - **Anterior and posterior radicular arteries**: supply anterior and posterior spinal roots
  - **Segmental medullary arteries**: not present at every level, they branch from the dorsal branches and supply blood into the longitudinal arteries of the spinal cord itself (discussed in Chapter 9) (Clinical Correlation 12.25).
- The intercostal arteries continue anteriorly in the superior part of the intercostal spaces (3 to 11), running just superior to the intercostal nerve and inferior to the intercostal vein. The intercostal arteries anastomose with the anterior intercostal arteries that are derived from the internal thoracic and musculophrenic arteries on the anterior side of the thoracic cage.
  - **Collateral branch**: leaves each intercostal artery just after it enters its intercostal space and travels alongside the collateral branch of the intercostal nerve.
  - **Lateral cutaneous branches**: run alongside the lateral cutaneous branch of the nerve at the same level and supply blood to the muscles and skin of the lateral thorax, as well as some of the breast.

Arteries of the Diaphragm and Abdomen (Fig. 12.25, See Also Figs. 12.9 and 12.23B)

At the T12 vertebral level, the aorta passes through the aortic hiatus of the diaphragm and becomes the abdominal aorta. The abdominal aorta supplies the diaphragm, abdominal organs, kidneys, ureters, adrenal/suprarenal glands, gonads, and the abdominal body wall. The abdominal aorta ends as it bifurcates into the left and right common iliac arteries that travel into the pelvis along with the small median sacral artery. I will list the vessels related to the lower thoracic and abdominal aorta, but the focus will remain on those relevant to the musculoskeletal system. Note that several important vessels of the anterior abdominal wall arise from the internal thoracic artery.

- **Superior phrenic artery**: final branches of the thoracic aorta, these paired arteries supply blood to the posterolateral aspect of the superior diaphragm and anastomose medially with the pericardiacophrenic artery and laterally with the musculophrenic artery.

arteries from the internal thoracic artery. The 2nd posterior intercostal artery also has **dorsal branches** that supply blood to the intrinsic back muscles and spinal branches to the spinal nerves.

- **Deep cervical artery**: a small vessel that ascends and courses posteriorly to supply the posterior intrinsic back muscles. It is essentially the dorsal branch corresponding to the 1st posterior intercostal artery.

Once the subclavian artery crosses the lateral border of the first rib, the vessel changes names to become the **axillary artery** (see Fig. 10.25) to denote its location in the axilla. It is described in detail in Chapter 10. While there are many branches from this vessel, only two arteries are explicitly related to structures of the torso.

- **Superior thoracic artery**: branches from the first section of the axillary artery and supplies blood to the external aspect of intercostal spaces 1 to 2, serratus anterior, subclavius, and pectoralis major muscles. This vessel is easily confused with the supreme thoracic artery from the costocervical trunk.
- **Lateral thoracic artery**: branches from the second section of the axillary artery and descends along the lateral wall of

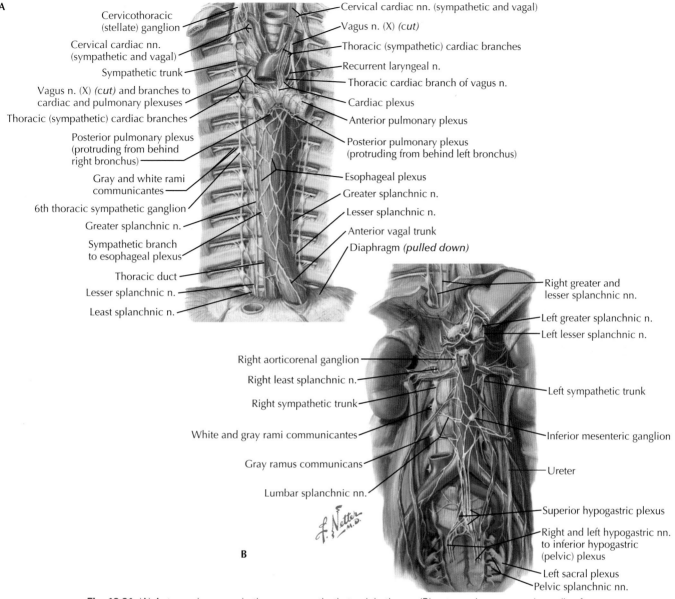

A

Cervicothoracic (stellate) ganglion

Cervical cardiac nn. (sympathetic and vagal)

Sympathetic trunk

Vagus n. (X) (cut) and branches to cardiac and pulmonary plexuses

Thoracic (sympathetic) cardiac branches

Posterior pulmonary plexus (protruding from behind right bronchus)

Gray and white rami communicantes

6th thoracic sympathetic ganglion

Greater splanchnic n.

Sympathetic branch to esophageal plexus

Thoracic duct

Lesser splanchnic n.

Least splanchnic n.

Cervical cardiac nn. (sympathetic and vagal)

Vagus n. (X) (cut)

Thoracic (sympathetic) cardiac branches

Recurrent laryngeal n.

Thoracic cardiac branch of vagus n.

Cardiac plexus

Anterior pulmonary plexus

Posterior pulmonary plexus (protruding from behind left bronchus)

Esophageal plexus

Greater splanchnic n.

Lesser splanchnic n.

Anterior vagal trunk

Diaphragm (pulled down)

Right greater and lesser splanchnic nn.

Left greater splanchnic n.

Left lesser splanchnic n.

Right aorticorenal ganglion

Right least splanchnic n.

Right sympathetic trunk

White and gray rami communicantes

Gray ramus communicans

Lumbar splanchnic nn.

Left sympathetic trunk

Inferior mesenteric ganglion

Ureter

Superior hypogastric plexus

Right and left hypogastric nn. to inferior hypogastric (pelvic) plexus

Left sacral plexus

Pelvic splanchnic nn.

B

Fig. 12.21 (A) Autonomic nerves in thorax: sympathetic trunk in thorax; (B) autonomic nerves and ganglia of abdomen: sympathetic nerves in the abdomen.

- **Inferior phrenic artery**: first branches (usually) of the abdominal aorta, these paired arteries supply blood to the inferior diaphragm and anastomose with branches of the lumbar arteries on the posterior and lateral body wall. They also give rise to small superior suprarenal arteries to the adrenal/suprarenal glands.
- Celiac trunk: supplies blood to all foregut organs: distal esophagus, stomach, proximal duodenum, liver, gall bladder, spleen, and some of the pancreas.
- Superior mesenteric artery: supplies blood to all midgut organs: some of pancreas, distal duodenum, jejunum, ilium, cecum, appendix, ascending colon, and transverse colon.
- Middle suprarenal arteries: supply inner portion of suprarenal/adrenal gland
- Renal arteries: supplies blood to the kidneys, proximal ureter, and part of the suprarenal/adrenal gland via inferior suprarenal arteries.

- Gonadal (testicular or ovarian) arteries: leave the aorta just inferior to the renal arteries and descend along the psoas major and iliacus muscles to reach the ovaries in the pelvis or through the inguinal canal to reach the testes in the scrotum.
- Inferior mesenteric artery: supplies blood to the hindgut organs: descending colon, sigmoid colon, and the superior portion of rectum.
- **Lumbar arteries 1 to 4**: very similar to intercostal and subcostal arteries but found within the abdomen. These supply blood to the muscles and skin of the back and abdominal wall. They also have dorsal branches that also have spinal branches with radicular and segmental medullary arteries leaving them to supply the spinal cord.
- **Median sacral artery**: a tiny final branch of the abdominal aorta, leaving just superior to the bifurcation, which descends along the anterior midline of the sacrum. A

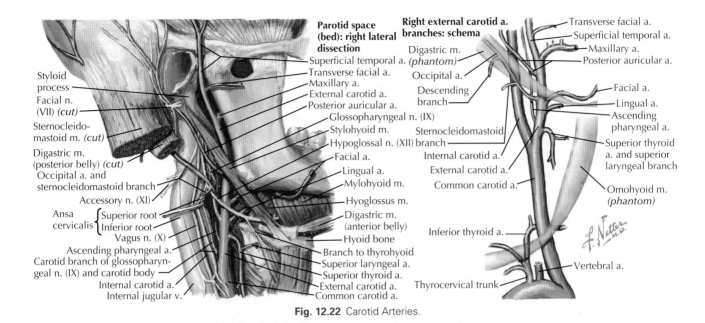

Fig. 12.22 Carotid Arteries.

small **5th lumbar artery** leaves this vessel on both sides. More inferiorly, the median sacral artery anastomoses with branches of the lateral sacral arteries and may supply some blood to the rectum.

After the aortic bifurcation, the common iliac arteries travel medial to the psoas major (with the ureter crossing anteriorly) and split to become the internal and external iliac arteries. These vessels have already been partly described in Chapter 11. In this chapter I will be focusing on those branches that supply the musculoskeletal structures of the pelvis itself.

Arteries of the Pelvis (See Figs. 11.30 and 12.25)

The **internal iliac artery** descends into the lesser pelvis where it splits into many arteries to the muscles of the lower limb, pelvic organs, and the muscles of the pelvis.

- Umbilical artery: leaves the internal iliac artery and travels anteriorly through the lesser pelvis and then along the posterior aspect of the anterior abdominal wall to the umbilicus. During the fetal period this artery carried blood from the fetus to the placenta via the umbilical cord.
  - Patent part: branches from this region of the umbilical artery deliver blood to the superior aspect of the urinary bladder, distal ureter, and ductus deferens.
  - Occluded part: since the umbilical cord is no longer in use after birth, the part of the umbilical artery on the

posterior side of the anterior abdominal wall becomes fibrous and no longer carries blood. Along with its covering of peritoneum, it forms the medial umbilical ligament.

- Obturator artery: described in detail in Chapter 11.
- **Iliolumbar artery**: leaves the posterior aspect of the internal iliac artery and ascends lateral to the lumbar vertebrae. The **lumbar branch** ascends and supplies the psoas major, as well as sending branches to the lower lumbar intervertebral foramina. The **iliac branch** travels parallel to the iliac crest to supply the iliacus muscle and anastomose with the deep circumflex iliac artery. While the median sacral artery technically gives off the 5th lumbar arteries, the iliac branch of the iliolumbar artery acts as a de facto 5th lumbar artery due to its size and course.
- **Lateral sacral artery**: leaves the posterior side of the internal iliac artery and descends along the anterior sacrum, giving off spinal branches that enter the anterior sacral foramina. Near the apex of the sacrum it anastomoses with its counterpart from the other side and the median sacral artery.
- Superior gluteal artery: described in detail in Chapter 11.
- Inferior gluteal artery: described in detail in Chapter 11.
- Inferior vesical artery: supplies the lower urinary bladder and prostate.
- Uterine artery: supplies the body of the uterus and sends off a more inferior vaginal artery. The ureter passes between the two vessels on the way to the posterior wall of the urinary bladder.
- Middle rectal artery: supplies the rectum superior to the levator ani muscle.
- **Internal pudendal artery** (Fig. 12.26): supplies the muscles and skin of the perineum with branches to the anal and urogenital triangles. Like the pudendal nerve, this artery exits the greater sciatic foramen, passes between the sacrospinous and sacrotuberous ligaments, and re-enters the pelvis through the lesser sciatic foramen to reach the ischioanal fossa. It also

A

Internal jugular v.

Common carotid a.

Ascending cervical a.

Phrenic n.

Anterior scalene m.

Transverse cervical a.

Suprascapular a.

Dorsal scapular a.

Costocervical trunk

Thyrocervical trunk

Subclavian a. and v.

Right anterior dissection

Thyroid gland *(reflected)*

Middle cervical sympathetic ganglion

Vagus n. (X)

Inferior thyroid a.

Vertebral a.

Common carotid a.

Recurrent laryngeal n.

Brachiocephalic trunk

Internal jugular v. *(cut)*

Right lateral schematic view

Vertebral a.

Deep cervical a. (ascending to anastomose with descending branch of occipital a.)

Superficial cervical a.

Costocervical trunk

Supreme intercostal a.

1st posterior intercostal a.

2nd posterior intercostal a.

Scapula

External carotid a.

Internal carotid a.

Ascending cervical a.

Inferior thyroid a.

Transverse cervical a.

Common carotid a.

Thyrocervical trunk

Suprascapular a.

Subclavian a.

Internal thoracic a.

B

Axillary a.

Lateral thoracic a.

Anterior intercostal aa.

Intercostal mm. { External / Internal / Innermost

Anastomoses with lower intercostal, subcostal, and lumbar aa.

External oblique m.

Internal oblique m.

Transversus abdominis m.

Ascending branch of deep circumflex iliac a.

Superficial circumflex iliac a.

Superficial epigastric a. *(cut)*

Femoral a.

Cremasteric and testicular aa. and a. to ductus deferens in spermatic cord

Subclavian a.

Internal thoracic aa.

Pericardiacophrenic a. with phrenic n.

Branch to falciform ligament of liver

Musculophrenic aa.

Superior epigastric aa.

Diaphragm

Transversus abdominis m. and aponeurosis

Rectus abdominis mm.

Internal oblique m.

External oblique m.

Posterior layer of rectus sheath

Arcuate line

Inferior epigastric a.

Superficial epigastric a.

Femoral a.

Superficial external pudendal a.

Deep external pudendal a.

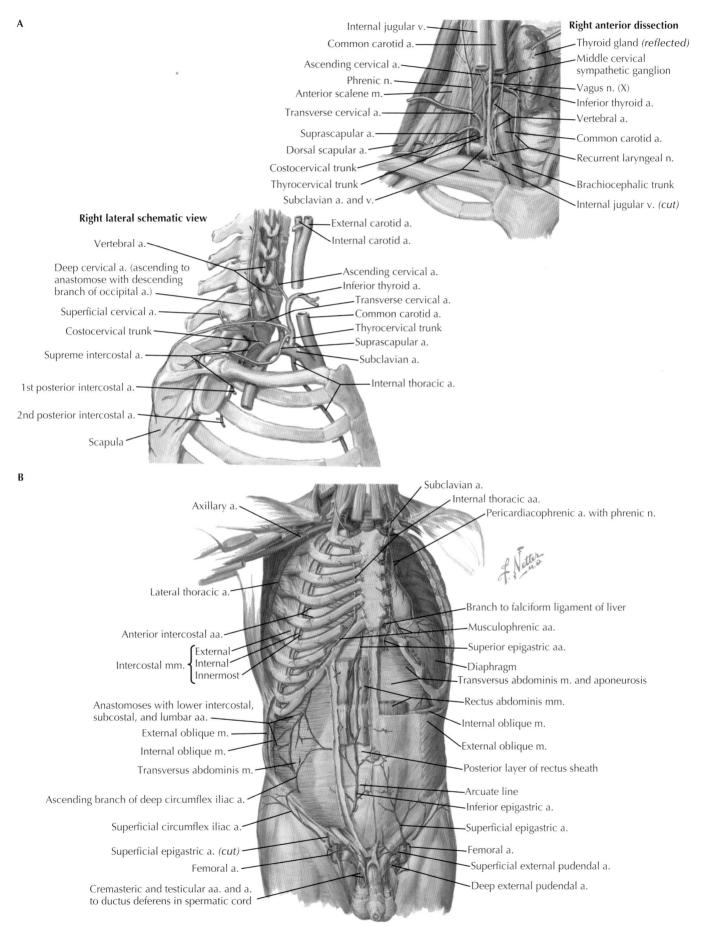

Fig. 12.23 (A) Subclavian artery; (B) arteries of anterior abdominal wall: blood supply of the abdomen.

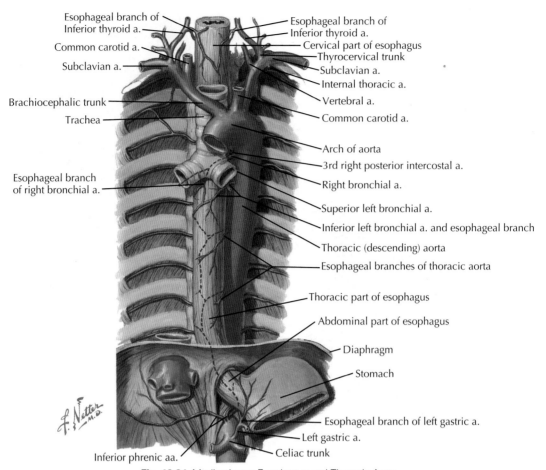

Esophageal branch of Inferior thyroid a.
Common carotid a.
Subclavian a.
Brachiocephalic trunk
Trachea
Esophageal branch of right bronchial a.

Esophageal branch of Inferior thyroid a.
Cervical part of esophagus
Thyrocervical trunk
Subclavian a.
Internal thoracic a.
Vertebral a.
Common carotid a.
Arch of aorta
3rd right posterior intercostal a.
Right bronchial a.
Superior left bronchial a.
Inferior left bronchial a. and esophageal branch
Thoracic (descending) aorta
Esophageal branches of thoracic aorta
Thoracic part of esophagus
Abdominal part of esophagus
Diaphragm
Stomach
Esophageal branch of left gastric a.
Left gastric a.
Celiac trunk
Inferior phrenic aa.

Fig. 12.24 Mediastinum: Esophagus and Thoracic Aorta.

CLINICAL CORRELATION 12.25 The Great Anterior Segmental Medullary Artery

While not every intercostal, subcostal, or lumbar artery gives rise to a segmental medullary artery, they are very important in maintaining adequate blood supply to the spinal cord. Segmental medullary arteries are prominent in the cervical and lumbar levels of the spinal cord; however, the **great anterior segmental medullary artery** (of Adamkiewicz) supplies a significant amount of blood to the lower part of the spinal cord (see Fig. 9.18). It is typically found on the left side branching from one of the inferior intercostal, subcostal, or upper lumbar arteries. Disruption or compression of this artery during thoracic or abdominal procedures can cause ischemia of the spinal cord and permanent neurologic deficits.

travels within the **pudendal canal** formed by the fascia of the obturator internus muscle to reach the urogenital triangle. After giving off the perineal artery, the internal pudendal artery continues into the deep perineal space. Other branches of the internal pudendal artery parallel the nerve branches from the pudendal nerve and share their names.

- **Inferior rectal/anal artery**: exits the pudendal canal posteriorly and crosses the ischioanal fossa medially to supply blood to part of the levator ani, external anal sphincter, and overlying skin.

- **Perineal artery**: leaves the internal pudendal artery and courses medially, inferior to the perineal membrane, and supplies blood to the muscles, glands, and erectile tissues within the superficial perineal space.
  - **Posterior labial/scrotal branches**: supply blood to the skin and tissues of the posterior labia majora or scrotum as well as the ischiocavernosus muscle.
  - **Artery of bulb of vestibule/bulb of penis**: supplies blood to the bulbospongiosus muscle and the deeper corpus spongiosum, the erectile tissue at the core of the bulb of the vestibule or penis.
- **Urethral artery**: medial branch that supplies the external urethral sphincter, which is part of the deep transverse perineal muscle.
- Deep artery of clitoris/penis: a terminal branch that pierces the ischiocavernosus muscle and runs within the core of the corpus cavernosum of the clitoris or penis. It supplies blood to these tissues and is important in the process of engorgement.
- Dorsal artery of clitoris/penis: a terminal branch that passes through the perineal membrane to travel on the dorsal aspect of the clitoris or penis.

The **external iliac artery** (see Figs. 11.30 and 12.25) travels along the superior edge of the arcuate line of the pelvis, giving

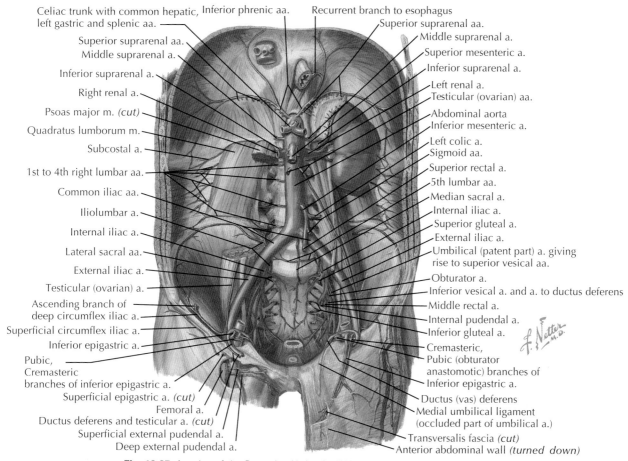

Celiac trunk with common hepatic, left gastric and splenic aa.
Inferior phrenic aa.
Recurrent branch to esophagus
Superior suprarenal aa.
Middle suprarenal a.
Superior suprarenal aa.
Middle suprarenal a.
Superior mesenteric a.
Inferior suprarenal a.
Inferior suprarenal a.
Right renal a.
Left renal a.
Testicular (ovarian) aa.
Psoas major m. (cut)
Abdominal aorta
Quadratus lumborum m.
Inferior mesenteric a.
Left colic a.
Subcostal a.
Sigmoid aa.
1st to 4th right lumbar aa.
Superior rectal a.
5th lumbar aa.
Common iliac aa.
Median sacral a.
Iliolumbar a.
Internal iliac a.
Superior gluteal a.
Internal iliac a.
External iliac a.
Lateral sacral aa.
Umbilical (patent part) a. giving rise to superior vesical aa.
External iliac a.
Obturator a.
Testicular (ovarian) a.
Inferior vesical a. and a. to ductus deferens
Ascending branch of deep circumflex iliac a.
Middle rectal a.
Internal pudendal a.
Superficial circumflex iliac a.
Inferior gluteal a.
Inferior epigastric a.
Cremasteric,
Pubic,
Cremasteric
Pubic (obturator anastomotic) branches of
branches of inferior epigastric a.
Inferior epigastric a.
Superficial epigastric a. (cut)
Ductus (vas) deferens
Femoral a.
Medial umbilical ligament (occluded part of umbilical a.)
Ductus deferens and testicular a. (cut)
Superficial external pudendal a.
Transversalis fascia (cut)
Deep external pudendal a.
Anterior abdominal wall (turned down)

Fig. 12.25 Arteries of the Posterior Abdominal Wall: Blood Supply of the Abdomen.

off two major branches immediately before becoming the femoral artery.

- **Deep circumflex iliac**: leaves the lateral aspect of the external iliac artery and runs parallel to the iliac crest, supplying the iliacus muscle and anastomosing with the iliac branch of the iliolumbar artery. The ascending branch pierces the transversus abdominis muscle to supply it and the abdominal obliques. It forms anastomoses with the superficial circumflex iliac, and musculophrenic arteries on the anterior abdominal wall.
- **Inferior epigastric**: leaves the external iliac artery more medially and ascends the anterior abdominal wall on the posterior side of the rectus abdominis muscle, anastomosing with the superior epigastric artery. When covered by peritoneum, it is called the lateral umbilical ligament on the posterior side of the anterior abdominal wall. Proximally this vessel gives off pubic and obturator branches, with the obturator branch sometimes enlarging to become an accessory obturator artery. It also sends a branch laterally toward the deep inguinal ring to supply an artery to either the cremaster muscle (male) or the round ligament of the uterus (female).

The **femoral artery** (see Figs. 11.31, 12.23B, and 12.25) is primarily involved in supplying blood to the lower limb but there are a few proximal branches to the torso. The rest of the femoral artery is described in detail in Chapter 11.

- **Superficial epigastric artery**: exits the femoral artery and ascends superiorly across the inguinal ligament to supply blood to the skin and superficial fascia of the inferior anterior abdomen up to the level of the umbilicus. It anastomoses with branches from the inferior epigastric artery.
- Superficial circumflex iliac artery leaves the femoral artery and travels laterally across the inguinal ligament to supply the skin and superficial fascia of the lateral abdomen up to the level of the umbilicus. It anastomoses with small branches of the inferior epigastric artery.
- External pudendal artery leaves the medial aspect of the femoral artery and supplies blood to the spermatic cord or round ligament of the uterus as well as the skin and superficial fascia of the superior, anterior external genitalia, scrotum or labia majora.

Veins of the Neck and Thorax (Fig. 12.27)

As with other areas of the body, nearly all arteries are accompanied by veins of the same name that drain blood from the regions that are supplied by the artery. Small veins drain to larger and larger veins until they reach either the **superior vena cava (SVC)** (head, neck, upper limb, torso) or the **inferior vena cava (IVC)** (abdomen, pelvis, lower limb). Both of the vena cavae drain blood to the right atrium of the heart.

Venous blood from the head and neck is drained primarily by a system of jugular veins. The **internal jugular vein** receives

A

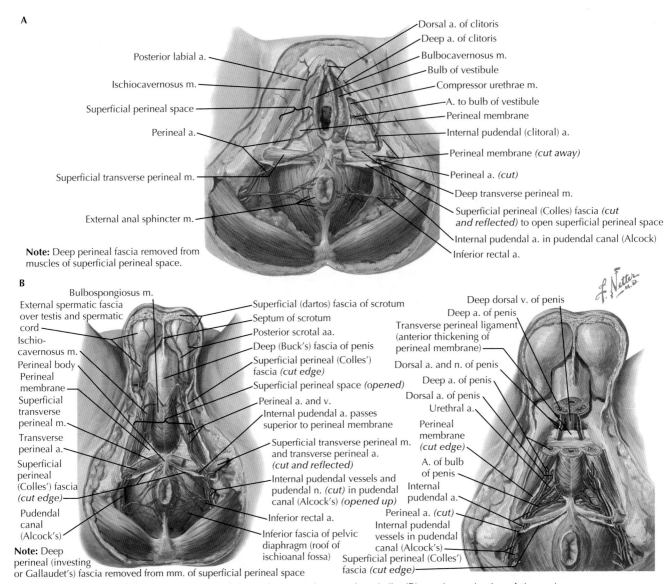

Posterior labial a.

Ischiocavernosus m.

Superficial perineal space

Perineal a.

Superficial transverse perineal m.

External anal sphincter m.

Dorsal a. of clitoris

Deep a. of clitoris

Bulbocavernosus m.

Bulb of vestibule

Compressor urethrae m.

A. to bulb of vestibule

Perineal membrane

Internal pudendal (clitoral) a.

Perineal membrane (cut away)

Perineal a. (cut)

Deep transverse perineal m.

Superficial perineal (Colles) fascia (cut and reflected) to open superficial perineal space

Internal pudendal a. in pudendal canal (Alcock)

Inferior rectal a.

Note: Deep perineal fascia removed from muscles of superficial perineal space.

B

Bulbospongiosus m.

External spermatic fascia over testis and spermatic cord

Ischio-cavernosus m.

Perineal body

Perineal membrane

Superficial transverse perineal m.

Transverse perineal a.

Superficial perineal (Colles') fascia (cut edge)

Pudendal canal (Alcock's)

Superficial (dartos) fascia of scrotum

Septum of scrotum

Posterior scrotal aa.

Deep (Buck's) fascia of penis

Superficial perineal (Colles') fascia (cut edge)

Superficial perineal space (opened)

Perineal a. and v.

Internal pudendal a. passes superior to perineal membrane

Superficial transverse perineal m. and transverse perineal a. (cut and reflected)

Internal pudendal vessels and pudendal n. (cut) in pudendal canal (Alcock's) (opened up)

Inferior rectal a.

Inferior fascia of pelvic diaphragm (roof of ischioanal fossa)

Deep dorsal v. of penis

Deep a. of penis

Transverse perineal ligament (anterior thickening of perineal membrane)

Dorsal a. and n. of penis

Deep a. of penis

Dorsal a. of penis

Urethral a.

Perineal membrane (cut edge)

A. of bulb of penis

Internal pudendal a.

Perineal a. (cut)

Internal pudendal vessels in pudendal canal (Alcock's)

Superficial perineal (Colles') fascia (cut edge)

Note: Deep perineal (investing or Gallaudet's) fascia removed from mm. of superficial perineal space

Fig. 12.26 (A) Blood supply of the perineum and external genitalia; (B) arteries and veins of the perineum: male blood supply of the perineum.

a tremendous amount of blood from the brain as it passes through the jugular foramen of the temporal bone. It then descends deep to the sternocleidomastoid muscle, receiving blood from maxillary, retromandibular, occipital, facial, lingual, superior thyroid, and middle thyroid veins. There is substantial variation and interconnection between these veins, so their exact drainage pattern varies accordingly. The posterior auricular and retromandibular veins drain to the **external jugular vein**, which passes inferiorly on the lateral surface of the sternocleidomastoid muscle. An **anterior jugular vein** may also be present on the anterior surface of the neck, superficial to the suprahyoid and infrahyoid muscles. The external and anterior jugular veins drain to the **subclavian vein**, sometimes forming a common trunk. On each side of the neck, the subclavian veins (carrying blood from the upper limbs) join the internal jugular veins to form the left and right **brachiocephalic veins**. The left brachiocephalic vein crosses anterior to the large arteries leaving the arch of the aorta and descends on the right side of the

superior mediastinum of the thorax. The left brachiocephalic vein receives blood from intercostal spaces 1 to 3 (and perhaps 4) via a single **left superior intercostal vein**. The shorter right brachiocephalic vein directly receives the **1st posterior intercostal vein**. Before they fuse to create the **SVC**, each brachiocephalic vein receives blood from the **vertebral**, inferior thyroid, pericardiacophrenic, and **internal thoracic veins**. The internal thoracic veins drain a wide area and receive blood from the **anterior intercostal**, **superior epigastric,** and **musculophrenic veins**, which drain the anterior intercostal spaces, anterior diaphragm, and anterolateral abdominal wall.

The **posterior intercostal veins** collect blood from the intercostal spaces and thoracic vertebrae, as well as the muscles and skin of the posterolateral thorax and back. Posterior intercostal veins 2 to 11 and the subcostal vein on the right thorax drain into the **azygos vein**, a large, vertical vein that ascends to the right of the thoracic vertebral bodies. A single **right superior intercostal vein** often drains intercostal spaces 2 to 4 into the

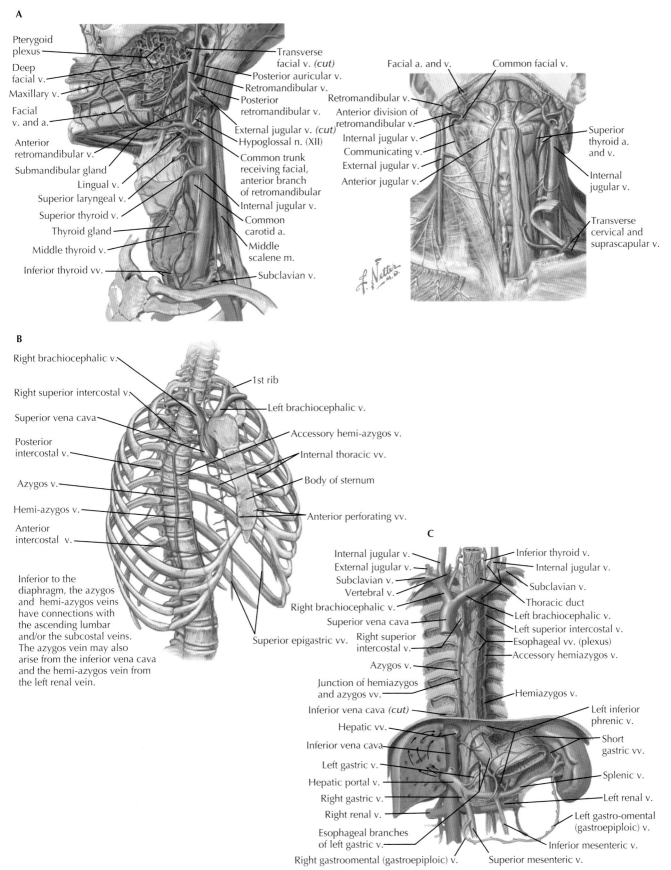

Fig. 12.27 (A) External and internal jugular veins; (B) veins of the internal thoracic wall; (C) mediastinum: azygos system of veins.

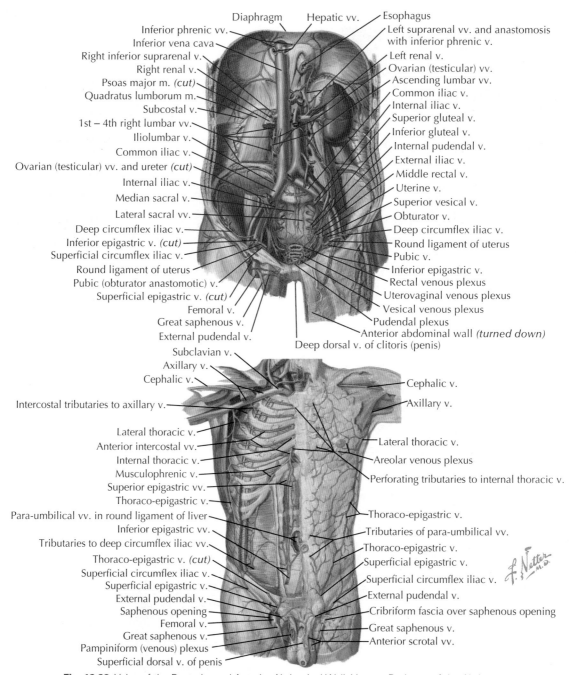

Diaphragm — Hepatic vv. — Esophagus
Inferior phrenic vv. — Left suprarenal vv. and anastomosis with inferior phrenic v.
Inferior vena cava —
Right inferior suprarenal v. — Left renal v.
Right renal v. — Ovarian (testicular) vv.
Psoas major m. (cut) — Ascending lumbar vv.
Quadratus lumborum m. — Common iliac v.
Subcostal v. — Internal iliac v.
1st – 4th right lumbar vv. — Superior gluteal v.
Iliolumbar v. — Inferior gluteal v.
Common iliac v. — Internal pudendal v.
Ovarian (testicular) vv. and ureter (cut) — External iliac v.
Internal iliac v. — Middle rectal v.
Median sacral v. — Uterine v.
Lateral sacral vv. — Superior vesical v.
Deep circumflex iliac v. — Obturator v.
Inferior epigastric v. (cut) — Deep circumflex iliac v.
Superficial circumflex iliac v. — Round ligament of uterus
Round ligament of uterus — Pubic v.
Pubic (obturator anastomotic) v. — Inferior epigastric v.
Superficial epigastric v. (cut) — Rectal venous plexus
Femoral v. — Uterovaginal venous plexus
Great saphenous v. — Vesical venous plexus
External pudendal v. — Pudendal plexus
Subclavian v. — Anterior abdominal wall (turned down)
Axillary v. — Deep dorsal v. of clitoris (penis)
Cephalic v. — Cephalic v.
Intercostal tributaries to axillary v. — Axillary v.
Lateral thoracic v. — Lateral thoracic v.
Anterior intercostal vv. — Areolar venous plexus
Internal thoracic v. — Perforating tributaries to internal thoracic v.
Musculophrenic v. —
Superior epigastric vv. —
Thoraco-epigastric v. — Thoraco-epigastric v.
Para-umbilical vv. in round ligament of liver — Tributaries of para-umbilical vv.
Inferior epigastric vv. — Thoraco-epigastric v.
Tributaries to deep circumflex iliac vv. — Superficial epigastric v.
Thoraco-epigastric v. (cut) — Superficial circumflex iliac v.
Superficial circumflex iliac v. — External pudendal v.
Superficial epigastric v. — Cribriform fascia over saphenous opening
External pudendal v. — Great saphenous v.
Saphenous opening — Anterior scrotal vv.
Femoral v. —
Great saphenous v. —
Pampiniform (venous) plexus —
Superficial dorsal v. of penis —

Fig. 12.28 Veins of the Posterior and Anterior Abdominal Wall: Venous Drainage of the Abdomen.

azygos vein as the **arch of the azygos vein** crosses superior to the right primary bronchus and pulmonary artery to reach the SVC immediately before it enters the right atrium. On the left side, the **hemi-azygos vein** receives venous blood from the left subcostal and posterior intercostal veins 9 to 11 while the **accessory hemi-azygos vein** receives blood from posterior intercostal veins 5 to 8. These veins drain into the azygos vein by crossing the anterior surface of the vertebral column in the vicinity of T9. The azygos system also receives blood from the mediastinum, bronchi, and pericardium. There is significant variation in this set of veins; the accessory hemi-azygos vein may drain to the azygos vein or into the left brachiocephalic vein via the left superior intercostal vein. Sometimes a single

azygos vein is present near the anterior midline of the vertebrae and receives the right and left posterior intercostal veins directly, taking the place of the hemi-azygos and/or accessory hemi-azygos veins.

Veins of the Abdomen and Pelvis (Fig. 12.28, See Also Fig. 12.26A)

The **femoral vein** returns the majority of the blood from the lower limb. Before entering the pelvis, it receives several veins related to the torso. The **superficial epigastric vein** drains the skin and superficial fascia of the inferior abdomen; the **superficial circumflex iliac vein** receives blood from the skin and superficial fascia of the inguinal region and inferior, lateral abdomen; and the **external pudendal vein** drains the anterior aspect of the external genitalia. All these superficial veins pass through the saphenous opening to join the femoral vein. Once the femoral vein passes inferior to the inguinal ligament it is called the **external iliac vein**. The **inferior epigastric** and **deep circumflex iliac veins** drain blood from the inferior rectus sheath and inferior abdomen into the external iliac vein on the posterior side of the anterior abdominal wall.

The **superficial dorsal vein of the clitoris/penis** drains into the external pudendal vein while the **deep dorsal vein of the clitoris/penis** passes inferior to the pubic symphysis and joins veins inside the pelvis near the inferior urinary bladder. **Deep veins of the clitoris/penis, posterior labial/scrotal veins, veins from the bulb of the vestibule/penis,** and **inferior rectal (anal) veins** all drain into the **internal pudendal vein**. The internal pudendal vein runs posteriorly through the pudendal canal and drains into the **internal iliac vein**. Within the lesser pelvis, the internal iliac vein receives venous blood from veins around the rectum, urinary bladder, and internal genitalia. In addition, the **superior and inferior gluteal veins** drain the gluteal region and parts of the lower limb. The **lateral sacral** and **obturator veins** also drain into the internal iliac vein. The internal and external iliac veins fuse to create the common iliac vein. Each common iliac vein receives blood from the **L5 lumbar vein, iliolumbar vein,** and (on the left side) the **median sacral vein** before the right and left common iliac veins join to become the **IVC** at the L5 level.

The IVC runs just to the right of the midline as it ascends within the abdomen. It receives several veins from gastrointestinal, reproductive, and urinary organs. The large right and left renal veins join the IVC near the L1 vertebral level. The right ovarian/testicular vein joins the IVC several centimeters inferior to the right renal vein while the right suprarenal vein joins it several centimeters superior to the right renal vein. The left ovarian/testicular vein and left suprarenal veins drain into the left renal vein, which then joins the IVC. The three hepatic veins empty into the anterior aspect of the IVC shortly before it passes through the diaphragm. These hepatic veins carry venous blood originating from all the foregut, midgut, and hindgut organs to the IVC (see Fig. 12.27C). The **lumbar veins** for levels L1–L4 on both sides drain segmentally to the IVC and also interconnect with each other by means of the **ascending lumbar vein** on each side, which connect to the azygos (right) and hemi-azygos (left) veins as they pass posterior to the diaphragm. Lateral to the hepatic veins, just inferior to the diaphragm are the **inferior phrenic veins**, which drain blood from the inferior aspect of the diaphragm.

Branches of the SVC and IVC are connected in two major places. The ascending lumbar vein (drains to IVC) and subcostal vein (drains to SVC) run along the posterior body wall near the lower thoracic and upper lumbar vertebral bodies. More superficially (see Fig. 12.28), the left and right **thoracoepigastric veins** are present in the superficial fascia of the lateral abdomen. Inferiorly, this vein drains into the femoral vein (IVC) at the saphenous opening; however, it continues superiorly as the **lateral thoracic vein**, which drains into the axillary vein (SVC). These pathways can allow venous blood to bypass

a blockage in either of the vena cavae to reach the right atrium. **Peri-umbilical veins** in the superficial fascia also connect with the thoracoepigastric and lateral thoracic veins. This becomes important when blood flow through the liver and portal vein is compromised, portal hypertension occurs, and venous blood backs up into the peri-umbilical veins and then is shunted to the thoracoepigastric and lateral thoracic veins, expanding them tremendously.

LYMPHATIC DRAINAGE OF THE TORSO (SEE FIGS. 10.28 AND 11.36; FIG. 12.29)

For this text, we are deliberately skimming over the lymphatic drainage of the thoracic, abdominal, and pelvic organs and focusing on the musculoskeletal structures of the torso. As we discussed in Chapter 11, the lymphatic fluid from the lower limbs and pelvis finds its way primarily to the **common iliac lymph nodes** before ascending along the vertebral column, encountering **parietal lymph nodes** along the posterior body wall and large vessels. These include the **left lumbar** (pre-aortic, lateral aortic, and post-aortic) **lymph nodes** near the aorta, the **right lumbar** (pre-caval, lateral caval, post-caval) **lymph nodes**, as well as the **intermediate lumbar lymph nodes** between the two large vessels. **Lumbar trunks** then convey the fluid to the **cisterna chyli** and **thoracic duct**, situated posterior to the aorta and IVC near the level of the renal vessels. Note that the lymphatic fluid from the hindgut, midgut, and foregut (often called **chyle**) joins the chain of lymph nodes on the surface of the aorta (via inferior mesenteric, superior mesenteric, and celiac lymph nodes, respectively) so that the cisterna chyli receives lymphatic fluid from both lower limbs, the pelvis, and all abdominopelvic organs. **Inferior diaphragmatic lymph nodes** near the origin of the inferior phrenic arteries also pass lymph into the cisterna chyli, with other nodes possibly intervening. Lymphatic fluid in the cisterna chyli travels superiorly within the **thoracic duct** on the anterior surface of the vertebral bodies between the esophagus and aorta. The elongated duct is the largest lymph vessel in the body and can often be distinguished by its beaded appearance, caused by the valves within its lumen that prevent retrograde flow of lymph. While it still appears small, between 2 and 4 L of fluid passes through it each day. It must be identified and protected during any surgical procedures in its vicinity. The **arch of the thoracic duct** passes posterior to the left brachiocephalic vein, left internal jugular vein to reach and empty into the angle formed by the left subclavian and internal jugular veins.

The thorax also has parietal lymph nodes that drain the body wall, notably the **superior phrenic lymph nodes** and **intercostal lymph nodes** that are seen near the necks of each rib. Lymph from these nodes drains anteriorly toward the thoracic duct, possibly encountering **prevertebral lymph nodes** along the way. More anteriorly, lymph can pass through a chain of **para-esophageal lymph nodes, paratracheal lymph nodes** (carrying lymph from the lungs), as well as lateral pericardial and anterior pericardial lymph nodes. **Parasternal lymph nodes** are found along the anterior intercostal spaces near the sternum. They receive lymph from the anterior body wall and medial breast, making them a common site where metastatic breast cancer cells may lodge.

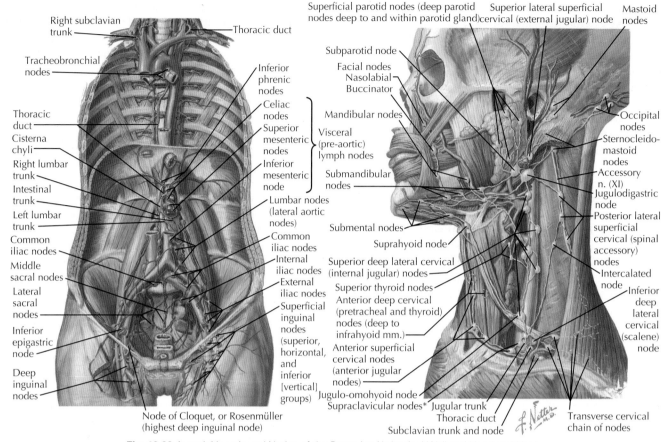

Fig. 12.29 Lymph Vessels and Nodes of the Posterior Abdominal Wall and Head and Neck.

The parasternal lymph nodes and **brachiocephalic lymph nodes** drain into the left or right **bronchomediastinal trunk**, which then drains into the left or right subclavian vein or else into the right lymphatic duct or the thoracic duct on the left.

As we discussed in Chapter 10, lymphatic fluid from the upper limbs is directed toward the axillary lymph nodes. The **lateral (humeral) axillary lymph nodes**, **anterior (pectoral) axillary lymph nodes**, and **posterior (subscapular) lymph nodes** pass their fluid to **central axillary lymph nodes** and **apical axillary lymph nodes**. There are **interpectoral lymph nodes** in between the pectoralis major and minor that drain lymph from the overlying areas into the anterior axillary lymph nodes. Thereafter the fluid will travel to the **supraclavicular lymph nodes** and then reach the **subclavian trunk** that will drain into the **right or left subclavian vein**. On the left side, lymph from the subclavian trunk may join the thoracic duct before reaching the subclavian vein. The parasternal lymph nodes of the anterior thorax have already been noted. Lymphatic drainage from the anterior abdominal wall is roughly divided at the level of the umbilicus. Inferior to the umbilicus, lymph drains into superficial inguinal lymph nodes and thereafter toward the deep inguinal, external iliac, and common iliac lymph nodes. Superior to the umbilicus, lymph drains laterally toward the axillary lymph nodes or medially toward the inferior phrenic and parasternal nodes near the xiphoid process.

In the head, lymph nodes clustered around the base of the skull and jaw send lymphatic fluid inferiorly to other nodes near the jugular veins. Laterally, there are **superficial jugular nodes** located around the sternocleidomastoid muscle and external jugular vein. Between the sternocleidomastoid and trapezius muscles are some **accessory lymph nodes** that run parallel to the spinal accessory nerve. Lymph continues draining to the **deep cervical lymph nodes**. There are also **deep lymph nodes of the anterior neck**, such as the infrahyoid, prelaryngeal, pretracheal, thyroid, and paratracheal lymph nodes. These nodes can drain to the inferior cervical lymph nodes, **jugular lymph trunks**, or directly into the nearby subclavian or internal jugular veins.

NEUROVASCULAR BUNDLES OF THE TORSO

There are several locations in the torso where large vessels run alongside nerves. Injuries in these areas will damage the vessels and the nerves together, causing hemorrhage (pulsatile bleeding from the artery and seeping bleeding from the vein) and de-innervation injuries involving sensory and/or motor losses.

Neck

- **Carotid arteries, internal jugular, vagus nerve, ansa cervicalis, sympathetic chain** (see Figs. 12.4, 12.6, 12.22, 12.23A, and 12.27A): one of the largest bundles in the body with disastrous consequences if it is traumatized. Only the internal jugular vein, vagus nerve, and carotid arteries are bundled in the carotid sheath but the proximity of the ansa cervicalis on the anterior aspect of the sheath and the sympathetic chain posteriorly make them an important consideration. Trauma restricted to the anterior sheath might damage the ansa cervicalis and result in tilt of the hyoid bone and difficulty swallowing due to paralysis of the suprahyoid and/or infrahyoid muscles. If the carotid sheath is entered, damage to the internal jugular vein (most anterior) would cause massive nonpulsatile hemorrhage. Injury to the carotid arteries (most posterior) would cause pulsatile hemorrhage and blood spray. Damage of the vagus nerve (between the vein and artery) would result in loss of some parasympathetic input to the thoracic and abdominal organs, causing tachycardia (persistently fast heartbeat), persistently widened airways, and lack of GI gland secretion and peristalsis. This may become a consideration during rehabilitation if the patient survives. Posterior to the carotid sheath and anterior to the cervical vertebrae is the sympathetic chain. Damage to this structure would result in sympathetic loss to the head and neck and possibly thoracic organs. This will manifest (if the patient survives) with Horner syndrome (see Clinical Correlation 8.1).

- **Lesser occipital nerve and occipital vessels** (see Figs. 12.17 and 12.22): this bundle leaves the lateral neck and travels posteriorly to reach the superolateral neck and posterior scalp. Trauma in this area could affect the bundle, causing a loss of sensation superior to the injury and bleeding.
- **Great auricular nerve and posterior auricular vessels** (see Figs. 12.17 and 12.22): this bundle leaves the lateral neck and travels posterior to the auricle of the ear to perfuse and innervate the area over the mastoid process and posterolateral scalp. Trauma in this area could affect the bundle, causing a loss of sensation superior to the injury as well as bleeding.
- **Spinal accessory nerve and superficial cervical vessels** (see Fig. 9.17): the spinal accessory nerve exits the jugular foramen of the temporal bone and descends between the sternocleidomastoid and trapezius muscles (which it innervates) before continuing inferiorly on the anterior surface of the trapezius. The superficial cervical (superficial branch of transverse cervical) artery joins it on the trapezius and descends along with it. Damage to this bundle would result in weakness of the lower part of the trapezius muscle and hemorrhage.

Thorax

- **Phrenic nerve and pericardiacophrenic artery** (see Fig. 12.18): the phrenic nerve has a very long course from the cervical region to the diaphragm, making it prone to injury in the lower cervical and upper thoracic regions. In the mediastinum, the phrenic nerve falls alongside the pericardiacophrenic vessels and runs in the lateral aspect of the pericardium. This bundle is unlikely to be damaged in this region but could be affected by enlarged lymph nodes.
- **Intercostal and subcostal nerves and vessels** (see Fig. 12.8 and CC12.19): these nerves and vessels run parallel to each other immediately medial and inferior to the corresponding rib, protected by the costal groove. These bundles can be damaged by external trauma or rib fractures. This can result in paralysis of the intercostal, subcostal, and transversus thoracis muscles at the same level. It will also affect a portion of the abdominal obliques, transversus abdominis, and rectus abdominis muscles. While this will not obliterate movement of the ribcage or abdomen, it will compromise inhalation, exhalation, and torso rotation somewhat. Sensation along the associated dermatome will also be noted if the lateral and anterior cutaneous branches are affected.

Pelvis

- Several of these bundles (e.g., superior gluteal, inferior gluteal, and obturator nerves and vessels) were discussed in Chapter 11.
- **Pudendal nerve and internal pudendal vessels** (see Figs. 12.20 and 12.26): run together starting in the greater sciatic foramen, passing between the sacrotuberous and sacrospinous ligaments, and reentering the pelvis through the lesser sciatic foramen. In the ischioanal fossa the bundle travels within the pudendal canal, formed by the fascia of the obturator internus muscle. The bundle gives off the inferior rectal (anal) nerve and vessels in the posterior ischioanal fossa. Damage to this bundle can be caused by perianal trauma and would result in hemorrhage and possible anal incontinence due to de-innervation of the external anal sphincter. The remaining nerve and vessel branches parallel each other through the ischioanal fossa. Damage to these branches can cause loss of sensation along the posterior labia majora or scrotum as well as the clitoris or penis. Urinary incontinence can result from paralysis of the external urethral sphincter and sexual dysfunction can be caused by problems with the erectile tissues and muscles of the external genitalia.

REFERENCE

Boehm KE, Kondrashov P. Distribution of neuron cell bodies in the intraspinal portion of the spinal accessory nerve in humans. *Anat Rec.* 2016;299:98–102.

Etymology of Selected Terms From Their Latin, Greek, and Arabic Sources

- Greek = Gr
- Latin = La
- Arabic = Ar

A

Ab (La): away from
Ad (La): toward
Al Batan (Ar): abdomen
An (Gr): without
Ante (La): before
Aqua (La): water
Arth (Gr): joint

B

(al) Bazali (Ar): draining
Bi (La): two, doubled
Blast (Gr): bud
Brachi (Gr): arm
Brevi (La): short

C

Capit (La): head
Carania (Ar): cornea
Cardi (Gr): heart
Cartilag (La): gristle
Caud (La): tail
Cephal (Gr): head
Cervi (La): neck
Chondro (Gr): cartilage
Chori (Gr): membrane
Circ (La): ring
Circum (La): around
Cocc (Gr): berry
Condyl (Gr): knob
Contra (La): against
Cost (La): rib

D

Dactyl (Gr): finger or toe
De (La): from, out of
Delt (Gr): triangle

Derm (Gr): skin

Derm (Gr): skin
Di (Gr): two, double
Du (La): two, double
Dur (La): hard
Dys (Gr): difficult, bad

E

E (La): outward
Ecto (Gr): outer
Ef (La): away from
En (Gr): into
Encephal (Gr): brain
Endo (Gr): inner
Epi (Gr): over
Epithel (Gr): covered
Erythro (Gr): red
Ex (La): out from
Extra (La): more, additional

F

Fasci (La): bundle, band
Femo (La): thigh
Fenestra (La): window
Fibra (La): fiber, thin hair
Foramen (La): opening
Fractura (La): break

G

Ganglion (Gr): knot, swelling
Gastero (Gr): stomach
Glia (Gr): glue
Gloss (Gr): tongue

H

Hemato (Gr): blood
Histo (Gr): tissue
Homo (Gr): similar
Homo (La): man
Hydra (Gr): water
Hyper (Gr): over, above
Hypo (Gr): under

I

Ilio (La): intestine
Immuno (La): secure

K

Kafili (Ar): sponsoring
Kara (Ar): head, skull
Karotides (Gr): neck arteries
Kypho (Gr): bent

L

Labi (La): lip
Lamina (La): sheet
Lat (La): broad
Lateral (La): side
Lemma (Gr): peel, shell
Leuko (Gr): white
Lingua (La): tongue

M

Macro (Gr): large, long
Male (La): evil
Mandibul (La): jaw
Mast (Gr): breast
Mater (La): mother
Medi (La): middle
Medulla (La): marrow
Melano (Gr): black
Micro (Gr): small
Mini (La): smallest
Mono (Gr): one
Morph (Gr): form
Mort (La): death
Muta (La): change
Myo (Gr): muscle

N

Nari (La): nostril
Naso (La): nose
Necros (Gr): death
Neo (Gr): new
Nuch'a (Ar): related to spine

O

Olfact (La): smell
Oo (Gr): egg

Opercul (La): cover
Optikos (Gr): vision
Oro (La): mouth
Ortho (Gr): straight
Os (La): bone
Ossic (La): small bone
Osteon (Gr): bone
Oto (Gr): ear
Ov (La): egg

P

Palp (La): touch
Papilla (La): nipple
Peri (Gr): around
Phleb (Gr): vein
Pili (La): hair
Pleur (Gr): side of body
Pneumo (Gr): lungs
Poly (Gr): many
Pons (La): bridge
Post (La): behind
Ptery (Gr): wing

Q

Quadra (La): four

R

Radius (La): rod, spoke
Retro (La): behind
Rhino (Gr): nose

S

Safin (Ar): conspicuous
Sclerosis (Gr): hardness
Sub (La): under
Supra (La): above
Synapsis (Gr): junction

T

Tacti (La): touch
Tardi (La): late, slow
Tri (La): three

V

Viscera (La): organs

Medical Eponyms Related to the Musculoskeletal System

Anatomists endeavor to use descriptive terminology when identifying structures of the body so that the name conveys some useful information about the structure itself. Despite this, many anatomical eponyms (structures named after their discoverer or as an homage to a person or group) are still used in clinical settings. I have included the most common eponyms in the main body of the text for convenience, but also wanted to provide a more comprehensive list so that the reader can quickly relate an obscure eponym to a structural term.

A

Abernethy's fascia = iliac fascia

Achilles tendon = calcaneal tendon

Adamkiewicz, artery of = great anterior segmental medullary artery

Adam's apple = laryngeal prominence

Alcock's canal = pudendal canal

Arnold's nerves = there seem to be several, one of which is the greater occipital nerve

Arnold, tract of = frontopontine fibers

B

Bell's nerve = long thoracic nerve

Bertin's ligament = iliofemoral ligament (also Bigelow's ligament)

Betz cell = giant pyramidal neuron

Bigelow's ligament = iliofemoral ligament (also Bertin's ligament)

Bochdalek's triangle = lumbocostal triangle

Bogros, space of = retroinguinal space

Bourgery's ligament = oblique popliteal ligament (also Winslow, ligament of)

Boxer's muscle = serratus anterior muscle

Brodie's bursa = semimembranosus bursa

Burdach's nucleus = cuneate nucleus

Burdach's tract = cuneate fasciculus

Burn's ligament = falciform margin of saphenous opening (also Hey's ligament)

C

Camper's fascia = subcutaneous (intermediate) investing abdominal fascia

Casserio's muscle = brachialis muscle

Casserio's nerve = medial cutaneous nerve of the arm (also Wrisberg, nerve of)

Chassaignac's space = retromammary space between subcutaneous tissue and pectoralis major muscle

Chassaignac's tubercle = carotid tubercle of C6 vertebra

Chopart's joint = transverse tarsal joint

Chopart's ligament = bifurcate ligament

Cloquet's node = intermediate deep inguinal lymph node(s)

Colles' ligament = reflected ligament (part of inguinal ligament)

Cooper's fascia = cremaster fascia of spermatic cord

Cooper's ligament = pectineal ligament (part of inguinal ligament)

D

Douglas, line of = arcuate line

F

Fallopian ligament = inguinal ligament (also Poupart's and Vesalius' ligament)

Flechsig's tract = posterior/dorsal spinocerebellar tract

Flood's ligaments = glenohumeral ligaments

Forel, decussation of = ventral tegmental decussation

G

Gallaudet's fascia of the abdomen = superficial layer of investing abdominal fascia

Gallaudet's fascia of the perineum = perineal fascia

Gasserian ganglion = trigeminal ganglion

Gerdy's ligament = suspensory ligament of axilla

Gerdy's tubercle = anterolateral tubercle of tibia

Gimbernat's ligament = lacunar ligament (part of inguinal ligament)

Golgi tendon organ = tendon organ

Goll's nucleus = gracile nucleus

Goll's tract = gracile fasciculus

Gower's tract = anterior/ventral spinocerebellar tract

Grynfeltt, triangle of = superior lumbar triangle (also Lesshaft, triangle of)

Gutrie's muscle = external urethral sphincter and deep transverse perineal muscle

Guyon's canal = ulnar canal

H

Haller's arches = medial and lateral arcuate ligaments

Haversian canal = osteal or central canal of dense bone

Haversian folds = synovial folds of synovial membrane
Henle's ligament = conjoint tendon
Hesselbach's fascia = cribriform fascia of saphenous opening
Hesselbach's triangle = inguinal triangle
Hey's ligament = falciform margin of saphenous opening (also Burn's ligament)
Hortega cells = microglial cells
Humphrey, ligament of = anterior meniscofemoral ligament
Hunter's canal = adductor canal
Hyrtl's muscle = iliopsoas muscle

L

Langer lines = tension/cleavage lines of skin
Lecomte's pronator of ulna = articularis cubiti muscle
Lesshaft, triangle of = superior lumbar triangle (also Grynfeltt, triangle of)
Lisfranc's joint = tarsometatarsal joints
Lisfranc's ligament = cuneometatarsal interosseous ligaments
Lisfranc's tubercle = scalene tubercle of the 1st rib
Lissauer's tract = posterolateral tract
Lister's tubercle = dorsal tubercle of distal radius
Louis, angle of = sternal angle (also angle of Ludwig)
Ludwig, angle of = sternal angle
Luschka, foramen of = lateral aperture of roof of 4th ventricle
Luschka, joints of = uncovertebral joints
Luys, nucleus of = subthalamic nucleus

M

Magendie, foramen of = median aperture of roof of 4th ventricle
Maissiat, bandelette of = iliotibial tract
Mauchart's ligaments = alar ligaments of the dens
Meissner corpuscle = sensory epithelial cell
Merkel cell = tactile epithelial cell
Meynert's decussation = dorsal tegmental decussation
Mohrenheim's fossa = infraclavicular fossa
Monakow's tract = rubrospinal tract
Monro, foramen of = interventricular foramen
Morgagni, triangle of = sternocostal triangle

N

Node of Ranvier = myelin sheath gap

P

Pacchioni bodies = arachnoid granulations
Pacinian corpuscles = lamellar corpuscles
Parona, space of = deep part of anterior compartment of forearm
Pecquet, cistern of = cisterna chyli
Petit, triangle of = (inferior) lumbar triangle
Pirogov's angle = angle formed by conjunction of internal jugular and subclavian veins
Pirogov's aponeurosis = bicipital aponeurosis

Poupart's ligament = inguinal ligament (also fallopian and Vesalius' ligament)

R

Reil, island of = insular lobe
Retzius, cave of = retropubic space
Riolan, muscle of = cremaster muscle
Robert, ligament of = posterior meniscofemoral ligament (also Wrisberg, ligament of)
Rolando, sulcus of = central sulcus
Rosenmüller's node = proximal deep inguinal node(s)
Roser-Nealton line = from lateral view, a line between anterior superior iliac spine and ischial tuberosity.
Rouget cell = pericyte
Russel, uncinated bundle of = uncinate fasciculus of cerebellum

S

Scarpa's fascia = membranous layer of abdominal subcutaneous tissue
Scarpa's nerve = nasopalatine nerve
Scarpa's triangle = femoral triangle
Schmidt-Lanterman incisure = myelin incisure
Schmorl's nodes = herniation of nucleus pulposis into spongy part of vertebral bodies
Sharpey fibers = perforating collagen fiber bundle
Sibson's fascia = suprapleural membrane
Soemmering's substance = substantia nigra
Spiegel's line = linea semilunaris
Stieda's process = posterior process of talus
Sylvian aqueduct = cerebral aqueduct
Sylvian artery = middle cerebral artery
Sylvian fissure/sulcus = lateral sulcus

T

Thiele's muscle = superficial transverse perineal muscle
Türck, column of = anterior corticospinal tract

V

Vesalius' ligament = inguinal ligament (also fallopian and Poupart's ligament)
Vieussens' annulus = ansa subclavia
Virchow's node = firm and enlarged supraclavicular lymph node, specifically on the left side
Volkmann's canal = transverse canal of dense bone
Volkmann's triangle = posterolateral corner of the distal tibia

W

Waldeyer's fascia = inferior fascia of pelvic diaphragm
Weitbrecht, foramen of = weak area between superior and middle glenohumeral ligaments

Wernekink's decussation = decussation of the superior cerebellar peduncles

Willis, circle of = cerebral arterial circle

Willis' nerve = spinal accessory nerve, cranial nerve XI

Winslow, ligament of = oblique popliteal ligament (also Bourgery's ligament)

Wormian bone = sutural bone

Wrisberg, ligament of = posterior meniscofemoral ligament (also Robert, ligament of)

Wrisberg, nerve of = medial cutaneous nerve of arm (also Casserio's nerve)

INDEX

Note: Page numbers followed by *f* indicate figures and *t* indicate tables.